Helicobacter Pylori: A Worldwide Perspective 2014

Editor

Buzás György Miklós

Budapest

Hungary

CONTENTS

FOREWORD

I am honoured to be able to contribute to this new and exciting eBook about Helicobacter in the 21st century, coming as it does from Budapest, an area central too much of the thinking about gastrointestinal and infectious diseases over the past 150 years. The eBook has excellent credentials for describing new knowledge in these areas.

The editor, BUZÁS GYÖRGY MIKLÓS, has attracted well known and active global researchers to update us on basic sciences, clinico-pathological correlations, newest treatments and diagnostic methods. All these facts are cleverly wrapped in a comprehensive, country-specific description of the epidemiology of the ubiquitous and fascinating bug, Helicobacter.

In summary, I am delighted to see such an authoritative, expertly produced and well referenced eBook which will be a milestone in Helicobacter science. By starting here, newcomers will immediately achieve an understanding of the field, thereby being well grounded towards making their own discoveries.

Barry Marshall, AC Nobel Laureate
FRACP FAA FRS
Clinical Professor of Microbiology and Medicine
University of Western Australia
Australia

PREFACE

The discovery of *H. pylori* almost 30 years ago triggered a paradigm shift in the medical community's thinking about the pathogenesis and treatment of peptic ulcers, chronic gastritis, functional dyspepsia and other conditions. In the past 3 decades, it has generated an overwhelming amount of literature, including over 30,000 articles in peer-reviewed journals, dozens of books written in English - but also in many other languages - dedicated to the bacterium, congresses/congress sessions on all continents and many national, international and continental consensus statements. The major benefit of diagnosing and eradicating *H. pylori* was a change in the natural course of peptic ulcer disease, preventing its complications – a feat not achieved with any other treatment -, and improving the quality of life of the patients; regimens directed against the infections also proved to be cost-efficient in many parts of the world. The contributions of *H. pylori*-related basic research to the progress of bacteriology, therapeutics, genetics and many other fields all deserve a mention.

Knowledge about *H. pylori* has been widely distributed in hundreds of medical journals published worldwide. Several eBooks have already been published but unfortunately, due to the long editorial times, most become outdated shortly after their release. This is why after being invited by Bentham Publishers I was very keen to propose and compile the content of an eBook which will offer all the advantages of rapid and worldwide distribution. The preliminary content and structure of the eBook was peer-reviewed and approved by the publisher.

The initial goal of this eBook is to give a broad perspective of *Helicobacter pylori* research in all major continents/geographic areas. To achieve this, more than 100 personalised letters were sent to potential contributors from 35 states, asking them to contribute with a review chapter. The subject for each author was chosen after careful review of their specific research field. Many international experts answered promptly and positively, while others proposed as co-authors their collaborators or PhD recipients: thus the list of contributors contains well-known experts and specialists along with "rising stars". Unfortunately there were experts who declined the opportunity to write a chapter, but I fully understand their position. To my greatest surprise, I was unable to obtain contributions from the world most populous countries, even after repeated invitations. All in all, however, 20 chapters were finally submitted covering most, if not all fields of *H. pylori* research, ranging from microbiology, biochemistry and epidemiology to clinical aspects, meta-analysis of therapeutic results, *etc.* Particular emphasis was laid on presenting the local features of each country/continent, although this resulted in some overlaps.

In spite of a relatively tight deadline and many other appointments/duties, all of the contributors forwarded their chapters in due course. I greatly appreciate their effort and am very grateful to all the authors for what they achieved. I sincerely hope that we will succeed in compiling an eBook unique in both, structure and content.

Finally, my thanks goes to the staff of Bentham Science who published the eBook. We all hope the readers will enjoy it.

Görgy Miklós Buzás
Budapest
Hungary

List of Contributors

Baršić, Neven

Department of Gastroenterology and Hepatology, Sestre milosrdnice University Hospital Center, Vinogradska 29, 10 000 Zagreb, Croatia

Bessède, Emile

INSERM-U853 Laboratoire de Bacteriologie – C.H.U. Pellegrin, Place Amelie Raba-Leon, 33076 Bordeaux – Cedex, France

Bodánszky, Hedvig

Semmelweis University 1st Department of Pediatrics, 1083 Budapest Bókay J. utca 53. Hungary

Buzás, György Miklós

Ferencváros Health Centre Non-Profit Ltd., Department of Gastroenterology, 1095 Budapest, Mester utca 45. Hungary

Ciobanu, Lidia

University of Medicine and Pharmacy Iuliu Haţieganu 3rd Medical Clinic, 400162 Cluj-Napoca Str.Croitorilor 19-21. Romania

Coelho, Luiz Gonzaga Vaz

Rua dos Otoni 705/601, 30150-270 Belo Horizonte MG, Brazil

Colquhoun, Amy

University of Alberta Division of Gastroenterology, 7-142 Katz, University of Alberta, Edmonton AB, Canada T6G 2E1

Cseh, Áron

First Department of Pediatrics Semmelweis University, 1083 Budapest Bokay János utca 53. Hungary

Czimmer, József

First Department of Medicine Medical and Health Centre University of Pécs, 7624 Pécs Ifjúság út 13. Hungary

Dumitraşcu, Dan Liviu

University of Medicine and Pharmacy Iuliu Haţieganu Cluj-Napoca 2nd Medical Department, 400006 Cluj-Napoca Str.Clinicilor 2-4. Romania

Duvnjak, Marko

Department of Gastroenterology and Hepatology Sestre milosrdnmice University Hospital Center, Vinogradska 29 10 000 Zagreb, Croatia

Fagan-Garcia, Katherine

University of Alberta Division of Gastroenterology, 7-142 Katz University of Alberta, Edmonton AB, Canada T6G 2E1

Francesco, Vicenzo de

University of Foggia Department of Medical Sciences Section of Gastroenterology, Foggia 71100, Viale L. Pinto, Italy

Fiorilli, Giulia

University of Siena Department of Medical and Surgical Sciences and Neurosciences, Policlinicop S.Maria alle Scotte Via le Bracci 8 53100 Siena, Italy

Figura, Natale

University of Siena Department of Medical and Surgical Sciences and Neurosciences, Policlinicop S. Maria alle Scotte v.le Bracci 8 53100 Siena, Italy

Gisbert, Javier P.

Playa de Mojácar 29. Urb. Bonanza. 28669 Boadilla del Monte, Madrid, Spain

Goodman, Karen J.

University of Alberta Division of Gastroenterology, 7-142 Katz, University of Alberta, Edmonton AB, Canada T6G 2E1

Graham, David Y.

Michael E.DeBakey Veterans Affair Center, RM 3AQ-320 (111D), 2002 Holcombe Boulevard Houston TX 77030, USA

Hagymási, Krisztina

Semmelweis University 2nd Medical Clinic, 1088 Budapest, Szentkirályi utca 46. Hungary

Hastings, Emily, V.

University of Alberta Division of Gastroenterology, 7-142 Katz, University of Alberta, Edmonton AB Canada T6G 2E1

Herszényi , László

Semmelweis University 2nd Medical Clinic, 1088 Budapest Szentkirályi utca 46. Hungary

Hibi, Toshifumi

Keio University School of Medicine Department of Internal Medicine, Division of Gastroenterology and Hepatology, 35 Shinanomachi, Shinjuku-ku 160-8582 Tokyo, Japan

Kusters, Johannes G.

Department of Medical Microbiology, University Medical Center, Utrecht, Heidelberglaan 100, 3584 CX Utrecht, The Netherlands

Langone, Francesco

University of Siena Department of Medical and Surgical Sciences and Neurosciences, Policlinicop S.Maria alle Scotte, Via le Bracci 8, 53100 Siena, Italy

Lee, Sun-Young

Department of Internal Medicine Konkuk University School of Medicine, 120-1 Neungdong-ro, Gwangjin-gu, Seoul 143-729. Korea

Lehours, Lehours

INSERM-U853, Laboratoire de Bacteriologie – C.H.U. Pellegrin, Place Amelie Raba-Leon, 33076 Bordeaux – Cedex France

Lerotić, Ivan

Department of Gastroenterology and Hepatology, Sestre milosrdnice University Hospital Center, Vinogradska 29. 10 000 Zagreb, Croatia

Mégraud, Francis

INSERM-U853, Laboratoire de Bacteriologie – C.H.U. Pellegrin, Place Amelie Raba-Leon 33076 Bordeaux – Cedex France

Moretti, Elena

University of Siena Department of Medical and Surgical Sciences and Neurosciences Policlinico S.Maria alle Scotte, v.le Bracci 8. 53100 Siena, Italy

Mózsik, Gyula

University of Pécs Medical and Health Center First Department of Medicine, 7624 Pécs Ifjúság u. 13. Hungary

Nishizawa, Toshihiro

National Tokyo Medical Center Department of Gastroenterology and Hepatology, 2-5-1 Higashigaoka, Meguro-ku, 152-8902 Tokyo, Japan

Niv, Yaron

Department of Gastroenterology Rabin Medical Center, 39 Jabotinski Street, 49100 Petach Tikva, Israel

Rokkas, Theodore

Henry Durant Hsopital, 192b Alexandras Ave, 11521 Athens, Greece

Shiotani, Akkiro

Division of Gastroenterology Department of Internal Medicine Kawasaki Medic al School, 577 Matsushima Kurashiki City, Okayama Prefecture 701-0192. Japan

Shmuely, Haim

Department of Gastroenterology Rabin Medical Center, 39 Jabotinski Street, 49100 Petach Tikva, Israel

Sierra, Mónica S.

University of Alberta Division of Gastroenterology, 7-142 Katz, University of Alberta, Edmonton AB. Canada T6G 2E1

Suzuki, Hidekazu

Keio University School of Medicine Department of Internal Medicine Division of Gastroenterology and Hepatology Toyko, Japan

Szabó, Imre László

First Department of Medicine Medical and Health Centre University of Pécs, 7642 Pécs Ifjúság út 13. Hungary

Talebi, Amin Bezmin Abadi

Department of Medical Microbiology University Medical Center Utrecht, Heidelberglaan 100. 3584 CX Utrecht, The Netherlands

Taulescu, Marian

University of Agricultural Sciences and Veterinary Medicine Pathology Department, 3-5 Calea Mănăştur 400372 Cluj-Napoca, Romania

Tomašić, Vedran

Department of Gastroenterology and Hepatology, Sestre milosrdnice University Hospital Center, Vinogradska 29. 10 000 Zagreb, Croatia

Tulassay, Zsolt

Semmelweis University 2nd Medical Clinica, 1088 Budapest, Szentkirályi utca 46. Hungary

Vaglio, Leonardo

Department of Biomedical Sciences Applied Biology Section University of Siena, v.le Bracci 8. 53100Siena Italy

Veres, Gábor

University Semmelweis 1st Department of Pediatrics, 1083 Budapest Bókay J. utca 53, Hungary

Yamaoka, Yoshio

Department of Environmental abnd Preventive Medicine, Oita University, Faculty of Medicine, Yufu-City, Oita, Japan

Send Orders for Reprints to reprints@benthamscience.net
Helicobacter Pylori: A Worldwide Perspective 2014, **2014, 3-10**

CHAPTER 1

Main Bacteriologic Features of *Helicobacter pylori*

Amin Talebi Bezmin Abadi and Johannes G. Kusters*

Department of Medical Microbiology, University Medical Center Utrecht, Utrecht, The Netherlands

Abstract: *H. pylori* is an S-shaped microaerophilic, gram-negative bacterium which colonizes the epithelial stomach surface of half the world's population. The colonisation of *H. pylori* in human stomachs results in chronic gastritis and sometimes ulcers or gastric cancer. Infection mostly occurs during childhood and unless treated lasts for life. Treatment of *H. pylori* is relatively complicated and requires antibiotics to which the bacterium is sensitive. Thus a microbiological culture determining antibiotic resistance is a prerequisite for rational antibiotic treatment. Unfortunately, routine clinical practice is often done without such a culture, and hence, the treatment is frequently empirical, not based on antibiotic resistance data. In this chapter we will elaborate on how to isolate and culture this fastidious bacterium.

Keywords: *Helicobacter pylori*, morphology, genome, ulcers, chronic gastritis, plasmids, gene regulation, strain diversity.

INTRODUCTION

Helicobacter pylori is a gram-negative bacterium that colonises the gastric mucosa of more than half of the world's population [1]. The prevalence of infection is higher in developing countries and is influenced by socioeconomic conditions and ethnic backgrounds. The bacterium measures approximately 1μm in width and 2 to 4μm in length and is highly motile with its 2 to 6 uni-polar, 3 μm long-sheathed flagella. The human stomach seems to be the principal reservoir of infection and person-to-person contact is thought to be the main route of transmission. The bacterium resides in the mucous layer of the human stomach and duodenum, and unless treated persists there for decades. This colonisation initially results in a mild inflammation but can eventually lead to chronic active gastritis, peptic ulcer disease, gastric cell carcinoma and MALT lymphomas [2]. While *Helicobacter*- like species were already described two centuries ago [3], the

***Address correspondence to Johannes G. Kusters:** Department of Medical Microbiology, University Medical Center Utrecht, The Netherlands; Tel: +31 88 7553687; Fax: + 31 88 75 55426; E-mail: h.kusters@umcutrecht.nl first description of a successful culture dates back to thirty years ago when Marshall and Warren isolated this bacterium [4]. As they believed the organism represented a slow-growing *Campylobacter*-like organism (CLO) they named it *Campylobacter pyloridis* before changing it shortly thereafter to *Campylobacter pylori* [5, 6]. Subsequently related CLOs from the stomachs of various animals were subsequently identified and it became clear that this bacterium might resemble *Campylobacter* in many aspects, but it also differed in important features such as morphology, fatty acid content, and 16S rRNA sequence. Consequently, *Campylobacter pylori* together with the other CLOs were transferred to the new genus *Helicobacter*, order *Campylobacterales* of the ε subdivision of the *Proteobacteria* [6]. To date, the genus *Helicobacter* consists of more than 20 recognised species, with many species awaiting formal recognition [6]. Members of the genus Helicobacter are all microaerophilic organisms and in most cases are catalase and oxidase positive. Many but not all species, are also urease positive. *Helicobacter pylori* belongs to the subgroup of gastric *Helicobacter* species which have adapted to the low pH of the stomach. *H. pylori* can produce large amounts of the enzyme urease, on which the bacterium depends on for its survival in the highly acidic gastric lumen [7]. The spiral morphology and its flagella render the bacterium highly motile thus allowing it to penetrate the viscous mucus layer of the stomach where the pH is less acidic, facilitating the growth of *H. pylori*.

Isolation and Culture of *H. pylori*

Histology and microbiological culture are the gold standard for the detection of *H. pylori* infections. Microbiological culture has the advantage over histology that it allows for the determination of antimicrobial resistance, but both techniques require the availability of a gastric bioptic sample obtained by endoscopy. In routine clinical practice, the diagnosis is often based on non-invasive diagnostic tests such as the faecal antigen and urea breath tests. Serology is also used for routine clinical diagnosis, but due to its lower specificity and sensitivity it is more appropriate in large epidemiological studies. Both culture and histology can suffer from sampling errors as the colonisation of *H. pylori* is patchy, and strains can display a preferential antrum or corpus location. Hence it is advisable to test a minimum of two biopsy samples, one from the corpus, and one from the antrum.

When one attempts to culture *H. pylori* it is important to realise that this is a fastidious microorganism requiring a microaerobic environment and complex media for its growth. Optimal growth is obtained at 2-5% O_2, 5-10% CO_2, and high humidity. Growth occurs at 34-40°C, with an optimum of 37°C. While it may sound strange for a bacterium whose natural habitat is the acidic gastric mucosa, *H. pylori* is in fact a neutralophile and can only survive short exposures to pH<4.0. Survival at an acidic pH is enhanced by the presence of urea in the medium [1, 7]. Growth occurs at a neutral pH, and in the absence of urea bacterial growth is only observed at the relatively narrow pH range of 5.5 to 8.0 [8]. For optimal growth culture-media need to be supplemented with blood or serum (or more defined substances) as a source of nutrients and protection against the toxic effects of long-chain fatty acids [9]. *H. pylori* has an extremely narrow host and organ targeting range and seems highly adapted to this niche as infection is usually lifelong.

Many genome sequences of *H. pylori* lack several of the common biosynthetic pathways of enteric bacteria [10, 11]. As a consequence, reasonable growth can only be obtained on rich media supplemented with lysed blood or serum. Synthetic media that support the growth have been described but as these require the addition of several amino acids they are not very practical to use [12, 13]. For routine isolation and culture of *H. pylori,* most labs use Columbia or Brucella agar plates supplemented with horse or sheep blood. To isolate the primary colonies, these plates can be supplemented with selective antibiotic mixtures (vancomycin, trimethoprim, cefsoludin, amphotericin B and/or polymyxin B) to suppress the growth of fungi and other microbes present in the gastric biopsy sample [14, 15]. Isolation rates of *H. pylori* from gastric biopsy samples are highly variable and range from 30-95%, depending on the technical expertise of the microbiology laboratory [1]. In addition bacterial or fungal overgrowth or inappropriate transport conditions may also result in failure to isolate the organism. Upon the initial inoculation the freshly inoculated plates should be ideally kept in a humid micro-aerobic atmosphere for at least three days before being inspected for the first time. Plates need to be incubated for a long time as it can sometimes take up to two weeks before colonies appear. *H. pylori* typically grows in very small, translucent, smooth colonies [1]. Meanwhile, to facilitate the detection of

H. pylori colonies, the plates can be supplemented with triphenyltetrazolium chloride. This makes *H. pylori* appear as dark red pinpoint colonies with a golden shine [16, 17]. *H. pylori* is urease, catalase, and oxidase positive, and these characteristics are often used in the initial identification. With subsequent subcultures of the primary isolates, most *H. pylori* strains tend to adapt rapidly to the lab-specific growth conditions and as a consequence good growth can generally be achieved following 2 to 4 days of incubation. Although usually spiral-shaped, the bacterium can appear as a rod or coccoid shaped, especially after prolonged *in vitro* culture or antibiotic treatment [18].While it is mostly believed that these coccoids represent dead bacteria that cannot be cultured *in vitro* [18], some have suggested that coccoid forms represent a viable, non-culturable state [19]. Once an *H. pylori* culture reaches the stationary phase, the growth rate not only declines but the bacteria in the culture also undergo a rapid morphological transformation into the coccoid form [18]. Thus a prolonged culture does not lead to an increase in viable bacteria, but rather leads to a transition into an uncultivable coccoid state. Hence when one wants to prepare frozen stocks of *H. pylori,* it is crucial to freeze them while still in the mid-logarithmic growth phase with more than 90% spiral-shaped cells. *H. pylori* can be stored in the long term at −80°C in brain heart infusion or Brucella broth supplemented with either 15 to 20% glycerol or 10% dimethyl sulfoxide.

Genome, Plasmids, Gene Regulation and Strain Diversity

To date there are approximately 250 whole genome sequences for *H. pylori* present in the public databases. The average size is approximately 1.6 Mbp, with a G+C content of ~40%. The genome encodes ~1,500 genes, including two copies of the 16S, 23S, and 5S rRNA genes [10, 11]. In addition, many strains carry one or more plasmids, but in contrast to most other bacteria these plasmids do not seem to carry any antibiotic resistance genes or virulence genes [20]. There are also some reports on *H. pylori*-infecting bacteriophages, but there is a lack of detailed characterisation [21-23]. Understanding of the virulence and metabolism of *H. pylori* has also been greatly facilitated by the availability of genomic sequences of *H. pylori* [10, 11, 24]. Many of the biochemical deficiencies of *H. pylori* that were described in the pre-genome era were indeed confirmed by the lack of the corresponding genes in the sequenced genomes [11, 24]. However, many of these analyses are based on *in silico* predictions and often lack convincing experimental validation; for a more in-depth discussion of the pathogenicity and virulence of *H. pylori,* we would like to refer to the specialized chapters on this subject. While many bacterial pathogens have a clonal distribution, *H. pylori* is genetically very heterogeneous. This results in every *H. pylori*-positive subject having his/her own personal strain [25]. Often there is even clear difference between the strains of children that were infected by the *H. pylori* strain transferred from one of their parents. This rapid genetic evolution may represent an adaptation mechanism of *H. pylori* to the different gastric conditions and host-mediated immune responses [26]. In *H. pylori,* genetic heterogeneity is thought to occur *via* both rearrangements and deletions of existing sequences as well as *via* the introduction of novel sequences [27, 28]. These novel sequences can often be recognised by their aberrant G+C content and seldom seem to carry genes that are putatively involved in virulence. A good example of this is the cag PAI, but other plasticity regions have been identified and were suggested to carry potential virulence factors [29-32]. In addition to these major insertion and deletion events, functional genetic diversity is observed at the nucleotide level. Most notably, mutations appear in homopolymeric nucleotide tracts where the insertion/deletion of a single nucleotide results in transcriptional and translational phase variations and mutation [27, 28]. As this phase variation seems to occur often in homopolymeric G or C tracts *via* reversible slipped-strand mispairing generating single base pair deletions/insertions which cause a shift in translation of the affected gene, this mechanism results in phase variation *via* a single mutation. This can result in major phenotypic changes that are fully reversible as they are generated by single base pair insertion/deletion. Several important *H. pylori* virulence genes, such as the *sabA*, *sabB*, *hopZ*, and *oipA* outer membrane protein-encoding genes, display such phenotypic variation, as do lipopolysaccharide (LPS) biosynthetic enzymes [33, 34]. This makes phase variation a very simple and basic form of gene regulation, ensuring that part of the bacterial population is prepared for sudden unexpected environmental changes. In addition, *H. pylori* reacts to other changes in environmental conditions in a more classical way by increasing the transcription of genes which encode factors that counteract the effect of these environmental changes. In other bacteria, this classical gene regulation is often controlled by two-component regulatory systems but genome analysis revealed an apparent lack of these two-component regulatory systems in *H. pylori* [35]. Also other transcriptional regulator systems are relatively scarce in *H. pylori* as it seems to contain only three sigma factors (σ80, σ28, and σ54), two metalloregulatory proteins, two heat shock regulators and a few other regulatory proteins [35]. Initially this was considered a consequence of the fact that *H. pylori* is only found in human gastric mucosa, a niche that was considered to offer relatively stable conditions. Transcriptional profiling studies indicate that approximately half of the *H. pylori* genomes are expressed under *in vitro* conditions and that the expression of ~10% of the *in vitro* transcribed genes displays changes when environmental conditions are altered. The finding that *H. pylori* regulates gene expression in response to environmental stresses suggests that the gastric mucosa may not be the relatively stable environment previously assumed.

ACKNOWLEDGEMENT

Declared None.

CONFLICT OF INTEREST

The author(s) confirm that this chapter content has no conflict of interest.

REFERENCES

[1] Kusters JG, van Vliet AH, Kuipers EJ. Pathogenesis of *Helicobacter pylori* infection. Clin Microbiol Rev 2006;19:449-90.

[2] Go MF. Natural history and epidemiology of *Helicobacter pylori* infection. Aliment Pharmacol Ther 2002;16:3-15.

[3] Bizzozero G. Ueber die schlauchförmigen Drüsen des Magendarmkanals und die Beziehungen ihres Epithels zu dem Oberflächenepithel der Schleimhaut. Dritte mitteilung. Archiv Mikroskopische Anat 1893; 43:82-152.

[4] Marshall BJ, Royce H, Annear DI, Goodwin CS, Pearman JW, Warren JR, Armstrong JA. Original isolation of Campylobacter pyloridis from human gastric mucosa. Microbios letters 1984; 25: 83-88.

[5] Romaniuk PJ, Zoltowska B, Trust TJ, Lane DJ, Olsen GJ, Pace NR,Stahl DA. Campylobacter pylori, the spiral bacterium associated with human gastritis, is not a true Campylobacter sp. J Bacteriol 1987; 169: 2137-41.

[6] Dewhirst FE, Fox JG, On SL. Recommended minimal standards for describing new species of the genus Helicobacter. Int J Syst Evol Microbiol 2000; 50: 2231-7.

[7] Fox JG. The non-*H. pylori* helicobacters: their expanding role in gastrointestinal and systemic diseases. Gut 2002; 50: 273-83.

[8] Scott DR, Marcus EA, Weeks DL, Sachs G. Mechanisms of acid resistance due to the urease system of *Helicobacter pylori*. Gastroenterology 2002; 123: 187-95.

[9] Stingl K, Altendorf K, Bakker EP. Acid survival of *Helicobacter pylori*: how does urease activity trigger cytoplasmic pH homeostasis? Trends Microbiol 2002; 10: 70-4.

[10] Taneera J, A. P. Moran, S. O. Hynes, H. O. Nilsson, W. Al-Soud, and T. Wadstrom. Influence of activated charcoal, porcine gastric mucin and beta-cyclodextrin on the morphology and growth of intestinal and gastric Helicobacter spp. Microbiology 2002; 148: 677-84.

[11] Alm RA, Ling LS, Moir DT, King BL, Brown ED, Doig PC, *et al.* Genomic-sequence comparison of two unrelated isolates of the human gastric pathogen *Helicobacter pylori.* Nature 1999; 397: 176-80.

[12] Berg DE, Hoffman PS, Appelmelk BJ, Kusters JG. The *Helicobacter pylori* genome sequence: genetic factors for long life in the gastric mucosa. Trends Microbiol 1997;5:468-74.

[13] Nedenskov P. Nutritional requirements for growth of *Helicobacter pylori.* Appl Environ Microbiol 1994; 60:3450-3.

[14] Reynolds DJ, C. W. Penn. Characteristics of *Helicobacter pylori* growth in a defined medium and determination of its amino acid requirements. Microbiology 1994; 140:2649-56.

[15] Dent JC, McNulty CAM, Uff JC, Wilkinson SP, Gear MWL. Spiral organisms in the gastric antrum. Lancet 1987;ii:96.

[16] Skirrow MB. Campylobacter enteritis: a "new" disease. Br Med J 1977;2:9-11.

[17] Queiroz DM, Mendes EN, RochaG. Indicator medium for isolation of Campylobacter pylori. J Clin Microbiol 1987; 25:2378–2379.

[18] Kusters JG, Gerrits MM, Van Strijp JA, Vandenbroucke-Grauls CM. Coccoid forms of *Helicobacter pylori* are the morphologic manifestation of cell death. Infect Immun 1997;65:3672-9.

[19] Azevedo NF, Almeida C, Cerqueira L, Dias S, *et al.* Coccoid Form of *Helicobacter pylori* as a Morphological Manifestation of Cell Adaptation to the Environment.Appl Environ Microbiol 2007; 73:3423–3427.

[20] Hofreuter D, Haas R. Characterization of Two Cryptic *Helicobacter pylori* Plasmids: a Putative Source for Horizontal Gene Transfer and Gene Shuffling. J Bacteriol 2002; 184:2755-66.

[21] Schmid EN, von Recklinghausen G, Ansorg R. Bacteriophages in Helicobacter (Campylobacter) pylori. J Med Microbiol 1990; 32:101-4.

[22] Lehours P V, F, Bjursell, M, Melefors O, Advani, R, Glavas, S, Gueguenîat, J, Gontier J, Lacomme, S, Alves Matos, A, Menard, A, Mégraud, F, Engstrand, L, Andersson, A. Genome Sequencing Reveals a Phage in *Helicobacter pylori.* mBio 2011;2.

[23] Luo CH, Chiou PY, Yang CY, Lin NT Genome, integration, and transduction of a novel temperate phage of *Helicobacter pylori.* J Virol 2012; 86: 8781-92.

[24] Doig P, de Jonge BL, Alm RA, Brown ED, Uria-Nickelsen M, Noonan B, Mills SD, Tummino P, Carmel G, Guild BC, Moir DT, Vovis GF, Trust TJ *Helicobacter pylori* physiology predicted from genomic comparison of two strains. Microbiol Mol Biol Rev 1999;63:675-707.

[25] Kansau I, Raymond J, Bingen E, Courcoux P, Kalach N, Bergeret M, Braimi N, Dupont C, Labigne A. Genotyping of *Helicobacter pylori* isolates by sequencing of PCR products and comparison with the RAPD technique. Res Microbiol 1996;147:661-9.

[26] Kuipers EJ, Israel DA, Kusters JG, Gerrits MM, Weel J, van Der Ende A, van Der Hulst RW, Wirth HP, Höök-Nikanne J, Thompson SA, Blaser MJ. Quasispecies development of *Helicobacter pylori* observed in paired isolates obtained years apart from the same host. J Infect Dis 2000; 181:273-82.

[27] Achtman M, Suerbaum S. Sequence variation in *Helicobacter pylori.* Trends Microbiol 2000; 8: 57-58.

[28] Falush D, Kraft C, Taylor NS, Correa P, Fox JG, Achtman M, Suerbaum S. Recombination and mutation during long-term gastric colonization by *Helicobacter pylori*: estimates of clock rates, recombination size, and minimal age. Proc Natl Acad Sci USA 2001; 98: 15056-15061.

[29] McGee DJ, Mobley HL. Mechanisms of *Helicobacter pylori* infection: bacterial factors. Curr Top Microbiol Immunol 1999;241:155-80.

[30] de Jonge R, Kusters JG, Timmer MS, Gimmel V, Appelmelk BJ, Bereswill S, *et al.* The role of *Helicobacter pylori* virulence factors in interleukin production by monocytic cells. FEMS Microbiol Lett 2001;196:235-8.

[31] Talebi Bezmin Abadi A, Taghvaei T, Wolfram L, Kusters JG. Infection with *Helicobacter pylori* strains lacking dupA is associated with an increased risk of gastric ulcer and gastric cancer development. J Med Microbiol 2012;61:23-30.

[32] Nguyen LT UT, Tsukamoto Y, Kuroda A, Okimoto T, Kodama M, Murakami K, Fujioka T, Moriyama M. *Helicobacter pylori* dupA gene is not associated with clinical outcomes in the Japanese population. Clin Microbiol Infect 2010;16:1264-9.

[33] de Vries N, Duinsbergen D, Kuipers EJ, Pot RG, Wiesenekker P, Penn CW, van Vliet AH, Vandenbroucke-Grauls CM, Kusters JG. Transcriptional phase variation of a type III restriction-modification system in *Helicobacter pylori.*J Bacteriol 2002; 184: 6615-6623.

[34] Appelmelk BJ, Shiberu B, Trinks C, Tapsi N, Zheng PY, Verboom T, Maaskant J, Hokke CH, Schiphorst WE, Blanchard D, Simoons-Smit IM, van den Eijnden DH, Vandenbroucke-Grauls CM. Phase variation in *Helicobacter pylori* lipopolysaccharide.Infect Immun 1998; 66:70-76.

[35] de Vries N, van Vliet AHM, Kusters JG. Chapter 29; Gene Regulation. In *Helicobacter pylori*: Physiology and Genetics. Washington (DC): ASM Press; 2001.

CHAPTER 2

Virulence Factors of *Helicobacter pylori*

Yoshio Yamaoka[1, 2,*] and David Y. Graham[2]

[1]Department of Environmental and Preventive Medicine, Oita University Faculty of Medicine, 1-1 Idaigaoka, Hasama-machi, Yufu-City, Oita 879-5593, Japan and [2]Department of Medicine-Gastroenterology, Baylor College of Medicine and Michael E. Debakey Veterans Affairs Medical Center, 2002 Holcombe Blvd. Houston, Texas 77030, USA

Abstract: *Helicobacter pylori* is a Gram-negative bacterium living in the stomach of its human host. The infection causes chronic gastric mucosal inflammation and is etiologically related to gastritis-associated diseases, gastric cancer and peptic ulcer disease. As with other chronic infectious diseases associated with a long latent period (*e.g.*, syphilis and tuberculosis), clinical manifestations develop in only a minority of infected individuals. The outcome for any of these diseases is dependent on the interplay between host, environmental, and bacterial factors. The variable virulence of *H. pylori* in relation to the presence or absence of a specific virulence factor reflects the differences in risk of a clinical outcome. The best-studied virulence factors are the vacuolating cytotoxin A (VacA) and cytotoxin-associated gene A product (CagA). This chapter will discuss the clinical relevance of typing *H. pylori* virulence factors CagA and VacA. Approximately 1,600 genes make up the *H. pylori* genome suggesting that there may be other unidentified virulence factors, many likely to be discovered using whole-genome sequencing.

Keywords: *Helicobacter pylori,* gastric cancer, peptic ulcer, virulence factors, vacuolating cytotoxin (VacA), cytotoxin-associated gene A product (CagA), next-generation sequencers.

INTRODUCTION

Helicobacter pylori is a spiral, microaerophilic, Gram-negative bacterium and a significant human pathogen. Infection causes gastric inflammation, which

[*]**Address correspondence to Yoshio Yamaoka:** Department of Environmental and Preventive Medicine, Oita University Faculty of Medicine, Yufu-City, Oita, Japan; Tel: +81-97-586-5740; Fax: +81-97-586-5749; E-mail: yyamaoka@oita-u.ac.jp

increases the risk of duodenal ulcer disease, gastric ulcer disease, gastric adenocarcinoma, and mucosa-associated lymphoid tissue (MALT) primary B-cell lymphoma. Gastric cancer remains the fourth most common cancer and second leading cause of cancer-related deaths worldwide (http://globocan.iarc.fr/). The prevalence of *H. pylori* has been decreasing in developed countries, coincident with improved sanitation and standards of living, but still affects at least 50% of the world's population especially in developing countries. *H. pylori* is thus known as a 'submerging' rather than an 'emerging' pathogen. While the infection, typically acquired in childhood is life-long, most infected individuals do not exhibit recognizable symptoms although they may suffer unrecognized manifestations of the infection such as iron deficiency anemia. Approximately 20% to 30% of infected individuals develop clinically recognized diseases. In countries with a high prevalence of *H. pylori* infections such as Africa and South Asia, the primary clinical illness is duodenal ulcer disease, which is often unrecognized unless specifically diagnosed. In the absence of medical care, the lack of disease recognition has been erroneously thought to represent the absence of disease and called the African and Asian enigmas [1] (Table **1**).

The pattern of gastritis can predict the outcome of an *H. pylori* infection. In tropical and semitropical Africa and South Asia, most patients with non-atrophic gastritis produce robust acid secretions, and if a disease develops, it will likely be peptic ulcer. In contrast, the clinical manifestation of gastric ulcer and gastric cancer is tightly associated with atrophic gastritis which is reflected in the high incidence of gastric cancer in Japan, Korea and the northern and mountainous areas of China. The pathogenesis of the different clinical outcomes is multi-factorial with environmental factors (especially diet) often playing a dominant role, *e.g.*, atrophic gastritis is common in East Asia where diets are seasonal and food preservation relies on salt. However, host factors especially those governing the severity of the immune response also affect the outcome of the infection in the individual patient. In addition, virulence factors of *H. pylori* also play a role in clinical outcomes. In this chapter, we describe the best studied virulence factors vacuolating cytotoxin (VacA) and cytotoxin-associated gene A product (CagA), and discuss their roles as clinically relevant *H. pylori* virulence factors.

Table 1: Incidence of gastric cancer in 2008

Geographic Region		Total		Male		Female	
		Total Numbers	**ASR**	**Total Numbers**	**ASR**	**Total Numbers**	**ASR**
World total		989598	**14.1**	640556	**19.8**	349042	**9.1**
Asia		727500	**18.6**	484244	**25.9**	243256	**11.7**
	East Asia	601314	**30.0**	408208	**42.4**	193106	**18.3**
	West Asia	14879	**9.4**	9248	**12.6**	5631	**6.7**
	Southeast Asia	43281	**8.6**	24926	**10.9**	18355	**6.7**
	South-Central Asia	68037	**5.3**	41871	**6.7**	26166	**3.9**
Latin America and Caribbean		65360	**11.7**	39401	**15.7**	25959	**8.4**
	South America	47244	**12.4**	29312	**17.3**	17932	**8.4**
	Central America	14144	**10.9**	7671	**12.7**	6473	**9.3**
	Caribbean	3972	**8.5**	2418	**11.2**	1554	**6.1**
Europe		146939	**10.3**	87548	**14.7**	59391	**7.0**
	Central-East Europe	73940	**14.7**	43292	**22.2**	30648	**9.7**
	South Europe	32873	**10.1**	19953	**14.0**	12920	**6.8**
	West Europe	27457	**6.5**	16530	**9.0**	10927	**4.4**
	North Europe	12669	**6.2**	7773	**8.6**	4896	**4.2**
Oceania		2728	**5.5**	1746	**7.5**	982	**3.7**
North America		24401	**4.2**	15051	**5.8**	9350	**2.8**
Africa		22659	**4.0**	12557	**4.7**	10102	**3.3**

ASR: age-standardized incidence rates per 100,000 population.

Data were obtained from GLOBOCAN databases, which provide access to the most recent estimates (2008) for the incidence of and mortality from 27 major cancers worldwide and are organized by the International Agency for Research on Cancer (IARC) (http://globocan.iarc.fr/).

In addition to the ASR for geographic regions, 20 countries with ASRs that are equal to or more than 17.0 for the total (male and female) with total number of gastric cancers more than 100 are listed.

vacA (Vacuolating Cytotoxin)

The *vacA* gene encoding a vacuolating cytotoxin is present in most *H. pylori* strains. Until recently, the biological role of *vacA* in disease pathogenesis was unclear and most observations based on *in vitro* experiments did not demonstrate its clinical relevance. VacA was identified because it induced vacuolation in some cell lines *in vitro*. Detailed study of this *in vitro* activity showed multiple cellular activities, such as membrane-channel formation, cytochrome *c* release from mitochondria leading to apoptosis, and binding to cell-membrane receptors, resulting in the initiation of a proinflammatory response [2-4]. VacA also can specifically inhibit T-cell activation and proliferation, although it is not clear whether these results, seen *in vitro*, are observed *in vivo* [5-7]. More recent evidence suggests that the primary role of VacA is related to autophagy, assisting in the production of the vacuole in which intracellular *H. pylori* can survive [8]. This is probably the most important role of VacA *in vivo*, and possibly its only important role in clinical disease.

The structure of the *vacA* gene varies with differences at the signal (s) regions (s1 and s2) and middle (m) regions (m1 and m2). These differences contribute to variations in the *in vitro* vacuolating activity of different *H. pylori* strains [9] (Fig. **1**) with s1/m1 strains being the most cytotoxic. Although s2/m2 strains have no *in vitro* cytotoxic activity, and s1/m2 strains have reduced activity, their effects on autophagy remain unstudied [9]. Risk of peptic ulcer or gastric cancer correlates best with the severity of inflammation produced by the infecting strain, and few studies have attempted to control for other variables known to be associated with inflammation. Studies from Western countries have suggested that patients infected with *vacA* s1 or m1 strains are at increased risk for developing peptic ulcers and/or gastric cancer compared to those infected with s2 or m2 strains [9-11]. It is possible that the overall inflammatory response is reduced because s2 or m2 strains are less able to enter and survive within epithelial cells, and may explain these epidemiological data. In East Asia, most *H. pylori* strains possess the *vacA* s1 genotype, and the s region genotypes are independent of clinical outcomes; however, the biological basis for these observations reported from Western countries remains unknown [12,13].

The m1 genotype is common in Northeast Asian countries, such as Japan and South Korea, and the m2 genotype is predominant in Southeast Asia (*e.g.*, Taiwan and Vietnam) [13,14]. Because the incidence of gastric cancer is higher in northern regions than in southern regions of East Asia, it is possible that the m region plays a role in these regional differences. The north-south difference is also evident in Vietnam with the m1 genotype and gastric cancer more prevalent in Hanoi than Ho Chi Minh City [15]. Okinawa consists of several small islands in southwestern Japan. Although the prevalence of *H. pylori* in Okinawa is not different from other parts of Japan, the incidence of gastric cancer in Okinawa (6.3 deaths/100,000 population) is the lowest in Japan (mean mortality rate of Japan, 11.8 deaths/100,000 population in 2009) (http://www.ncc.go.jp/). It is important to note that Okinawa is a tropical region with a markedly different diet and salt intake from mainland Japan, and was originally populated by non-Japanese (*i.e.*, most of the *H. pylori* strains possess the *vacA* s1/m1 genotype in mainland Japan [13] compared to less than 70% of the strains in Okinawa [16]). Of the 337 strains evaluated from Okinawa we found that the *vacA* s1/m2 genotype was uncommon in this with only *H. pylori* gastritis (17.3%), and even less common in gastric ulcer (7.9%) (P = 0.04); *vacA* s2/m2 was higher in gastritis (22.4%) than in gastric ulcer (11.9%), duodenal ulcer (10.5%), and gastric cancer (4.2%) (P = 0.04, P = 0.01, and P = 0.04, respectively). We did not compare the genotype with extent, severity, pattern of gastritis, or inhabitants' country of origin. However, even in East Asia in areas where non-s1/m1 strains are common, *vacA* m genotypes roughly correlated with risk of different *H pylori*-related diseases.

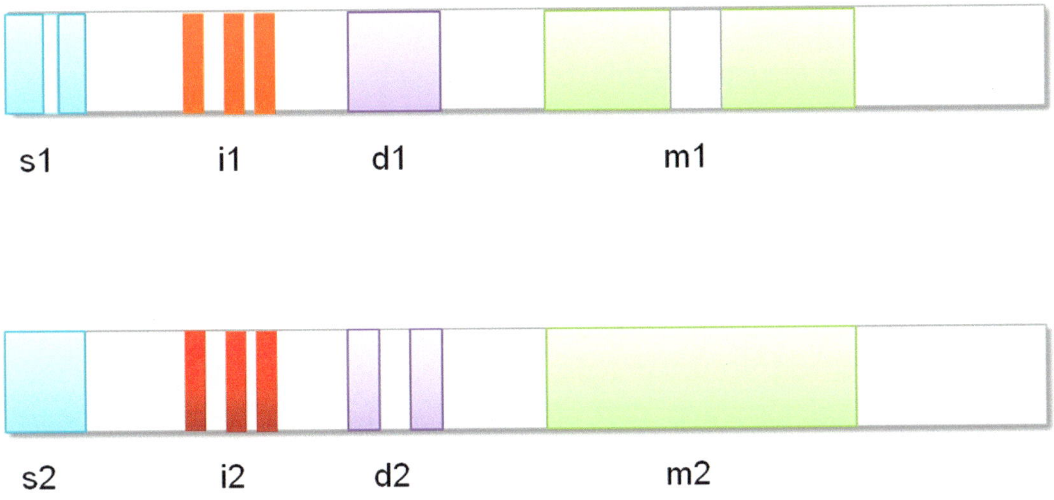

Figure 1: Structural polymorphism in the *vacA* gene. The *vacA* s1 genotype has a 27-bp deletion as compared to the s2 genotype. The *vacA* i region can be classified into 2 types (i1 and i2, shaded in orange and red, respectively) according to the amino acid sequences denoted as clusters A, B, and C (from left to right). The *vacA* d2 genotype has a 69- to 81-bp deletion as compared to the d1 genotype. The *vacA* m1 genotype has a 73-bp deletion as compared to the m2 genotype. As shown in this figure, typical types of clinical isolates are either *vacA* s1/i1/d1/m1 or s2/i2/d2/m2 types.

The *vacA* s1 and m1 genotypes are subdivided into 3 types: s1a, s1b, and s1c [9]; m1a, m1b, and m1c, respectively [17]. The *vacA* s1c and m1b genotypes are common in East Asia, whereas the s1a and m1c genotypes are common in South Asia [13,17]. The *vacA* m1c is the predominant genotype in Central Asia (Calcuttans and ethnic Kazakhs) [13] and the m1a genotype common in Africans and ethnic Europeans [13]. Both the s1a and s1b genotypes are common in ethnic Europeans, whereas s1b genotypes are especially common in the Iberian Peninsula and Latin America [18]. The s1b genotype is predominant in Africa [18]. However, it currently remains unclear whether subtypes of the s1 and m1 genotypes correlate with clinical outcomes or to differences in the extent, severity, or distribution of gastritis.

A third region of *vacA*, known as the intermediate (i) region, has been identified between the s region and the m region [19] (Fig. **1**). All s1/m1 strains are classified as i1 genotype, and all s2/m2 strains as i2 genotype. Although s1/m1 strains can be classified as either i1 or i2 genotype, it has been suggested that i1 strains are possibly more pathogenic. In another study, an intermediate variant (i3) was identified in Turkish strains (25.7%) [20]. Originally, it was reported that, in Iran, the *vacA* i genotype was more useful in identifying risk of gastric cancer than typing the s or m regions. A subsequent study suggested that the *vacA* i genotype is related to peptic ulcers in Iraq and Italy [21,22]. Another study showed that the polymorphisms at amino acid position 196 of *vacA*, which is located in the i region, are associated with severe outcomes in South Korea [23]. However, in East and Southeast Asia, no associations are found between the i region and clinical outcomes [24]. Finally, a study from Portugal examined patients with progression to more severe histological diagnoses after a mean of 12.8 year follow-up and reported that *vacA* i genotyping did not improve the prediction of progression in relation to other *vacA loci*, s and m regions [25]. A fourth disease-related region identified between the i region and the m region has been described as the deletion or d region [26] (Fig. **1**). The d region is divided into a d1 genotype (no deletion) and d2 genotype with a 69- to 81-bp deletion. In Western strains, the d1 genotype was associated with mucosal atrophy. Almost all East Asian strains are classified as s1/i1/d1, d genotypes thus, d genotyping is less useful as a marker for clinical outcomes. Overall, genotyping of the *vacA* i and d regions has provided interesting but not clinically useful data and no information on the involvement of these genotypes in pathogenesis.

CagA (Cytotoxin-Associated Gene A Product)

cagA, which encodes a highly immunogenic protein (CagA) is located at one end of the *cag* pathogenicity island (PAI). The approximately 40-kbp region of the PAI is believed to have been incorporated into the *H. pylori* genome by horizontal transfer from an unknown source [27]. The *cag* PAI encodes a type-IV secretion system (T4SS) (*i.e.*, molecular syringe), which injects CagA and possibly other proteins into host cells. One of the proteins, CagL is a protein that covers the pilus and acts as a specialized adhesin to connect the T4SS to the target cell [28]. CagL binds to and activates host cell $\alpha_5\beta_1$ integrins for delivery of CagA across the host cell membrane. The injected CagA then interacts with various target molecules in host cells including the cytoplasmic Src homology-2 domain of Src homology-2 phosphatase (SHP-2), which is known to have oncogenic activity [29]. Studies of Mongolian gerbils showed that gastric cancer develops in animals infected with wild-type *H. pylori* but not in gerbils infected with isogenic *cagA* mutants [30,31]. However, it is difficult to produce gastric cancer by *H. pylori* infection of Mongolian gerbils. An interesting study showed that gastric cancer and other malignant neoplasms occur in some transgenic mice with an artificially introduced CagA protein [32]. These results provide evidence that CagA may act as a bacterial oncoprotein when integrated into the host genome; however, whether this is relevant to clinical infection in which it is injected only into gastric cells is unknown.

Almost all *H. pylori* isolates from East Asia are *cagA*-positive, whereas 20% to 40% of isolates from Western countries do not possess *cagA* (*i.e.*, *cagA*-negative) [13]. In Western countries, infection with *cagA*-positive strains is associated with a greater inflammatory response and an increased risk of peptic ulcer and/or gastric cancer compared to infection with *cagA*-negative strains [33,34]. Almost all *cagA*-positive strains are also *vacA* s1 (either m1 or m2), whereas almost all *cagA*-negative strains are classified as *vacA* s2/m2 strains [9]. Both *cagA*-positive and *cagA*-negative infections are associated with the development of peptic ulcer and gastric cancer but the risk is typically lower and likely correlates with the lower inflammatory response to the infection.

CagA-positive strains have been subdivided into East Asian and Western types according to the sequence located in the 3′ region of *cagA* [35,36]. This repeat-region was initially classified into 2 types (*i.e.*, first repeat and second repeat). The sequence of the second-repeat region differs between East Asian and Western strains [13,35-37]. Each region contains the tyrosine phosphorylation site motif: Glu-Pro-Ile-Tyr-Ala (EPIYA). The first-repeat regions have been renamed EPIYA-A and EPIYA-B segments and the second-repeat region in Western and East Asian strains as EPIYA-C and EPIYA-D segments, respectively [29] (Fig. **2**). Each CagA sequence is assigned a sequence type based on the EPIYA segments in the sequence (*i.e.*, ABC, ABCC, ABCCC *etc.* for Wester-type CagA and ABD *etc.* for East Asian-type CagA) (Fig. **2**).

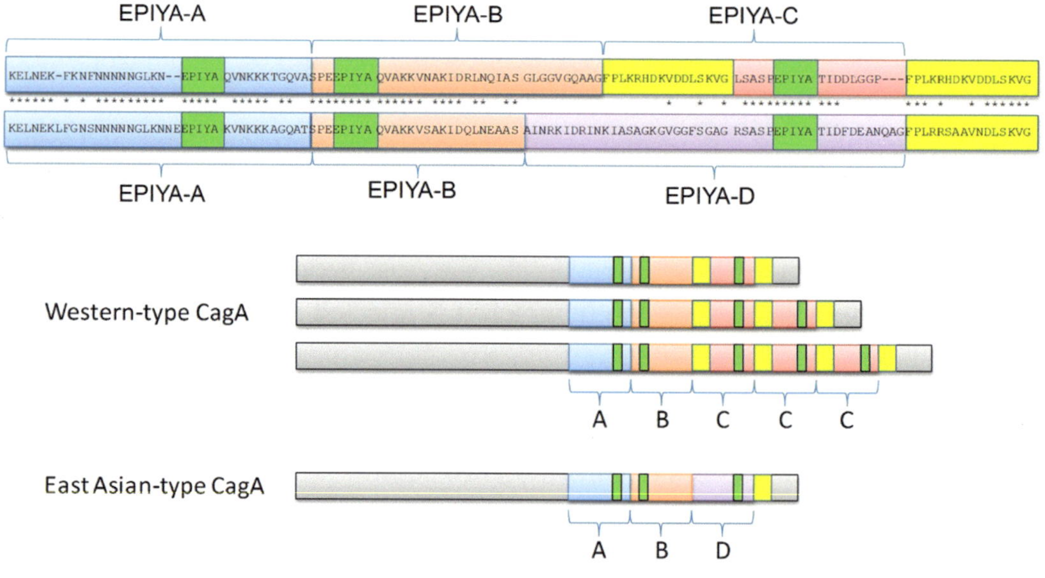

Figure 2: Structural polymorphism in CagA. Western-type CagA contain the EPIYA-A, EPIYA-B, and EPIYA-C segments; whereas East Asian-type CagA contain the EPIYA-A, EPIYA-B and EPIYA-D segments, but do not possess the EPIYA-C segment. EPIYA-motif in each segment represent the tyrosine phosphorylation sites of CagA. The sequence flanking the tyrosine phosphorylation site of the EPIYA-D segment (EPIYATIDF), but not the EPIYA-C segment (EPIYATIDD), matches perfectly the consensus high-affinity binding sequence for the SH2 domains of SHP2.

In vitro experiments have shown that CagA with a EPIYA-D segment has a higher binding ability for SHP-2 than CagA with a EPIYA-C segment [29]. Epidemiological studies from Thailand and South Korea also showed that individuals infected with East Asian-type *cagA* strains are at increased risk of peptic ulcer or gastric cancer compared with those infected with Western-type *cagA* strains [23,38]. Similarly, the difference in incidences of gastric cancer between Okinawa and mainland Japan also correlate with the difference in prevalence of Western-type *cagA* strains in Okinawa compared with other areas of Japan [16]. In our study from Okinawa, the East Asian-type *cagA* genotype was significantly more prevalent in strains derived from gastric ulcers (83.2%) and gastric cancer (87.5%) than those with only gastritis (60.2%) ($P < 0.001$ and $P = 0.01$, respectively) and those derived from duodenal ulcer (64.0%) ($P = 0.001$ and 0.02, respectively). In contrast, there was no significant difference between the prevalence of East Asian-type *cagA* in duodenal ulcers (64.0%). These data suggest that the pattern of gastritis in individuals with East Asian-type CagA had more rapid progression of gastric damage and more extensive and severe atrophic gastritis overall. It remains unclear whether the increased risk of cancer was related to the the Japanese had migrated to Okinawa from an area with a high incidence of gastric cancer as they would be more likely to retain that risk after migration. In contrast their children and grandchildren would be likely to have lower and steadily falling risks similar to the surrounding population. In mainland Japan, the incidence of gastric cancer fell approximately 60% between 1965 and 1995 despite no change in *H. pylori* infection or infecting strain. Such a rapid change is most consistent with changes in the environment especially diet. Importantly, the highest incidence of gastric cancer is found in the mountains of Costa Rica, an area in which East Asian-type *H. pylori* strains are absent. Overall, careful epidemiologic studies comparing place of birth, diet, and histology over time will be required to determine whether the East Asian-type *cagA* is specifically related to the development of gastric cancer.

A number of second-repeat regions have been reported to be associated with gastric cancer both in East Asian and Western countries [35,36]. For example, the incidence of gastric cancer is higher in Colombia than in the US (age-standardized incidence rates per 100,000 population = 4.1), and 57% of Colombian isolates have 2 EPIYA-C segments compared with only 4% of the isolates from the U.S.

[14]. Subsequent studies have confirmed the association of gastric cancer with strains with multiple EPIYA-C segments compared with those infected with a single segment [35,36,39,40]. Recent *in vitro* data have shown that C-terminal Src tyrosine kinase (Csk), which is an important molecule involved in intracellular signaling systems, prefers to bind EPIYA-A and EPIYA-B motifs [41]. We recently reported that c-Src can only phosphorylate EPIYA- C and D motifs, while c-Abl phosphorylates EPIYA-A, -B, -C and -D motifs [42]. These data suggest that EPIYA-A, -B, -C and -D motifs all play some role. We previously showed that the number of repeats could be easily changed in the stomach [36,37]. The incidence of gastric cancer fell rapidly in most countries over the same 50 years described in the Japan study above. It is possible that the *H. pylori* with *cagA* containing multiple repeats also decreased. This concept is supported by studies in children where despite the high prevalence of multiple repeats in the infected elderly this pattern is not found in children [43]. Importantly, strains with an increased number of repeats has been shown to be sensitive to acid [36], suggesting that the number of repeats is a *post hoc* event occurring in response to the development of atrophic gastritis and not the cause. The overall correlation of any *cagA* genotype with an outcome is potentially a surrogate marker for a biologically important event or events; however, such an event is currently unknown.

Detection of Genomic Changes

The rapid advances in sequencing technology have provided new rapid methods to identify novel putative virulence factors [44-46]. McClain *et al.* compared the genome sequences of an isolate obtained from a patient with gastric cancer (strain 98-10) with an isolate from a patient with gastric ulcer (strain B128) to search for strain-specific genes of strain 98-10 associated with gastric cancer using a next-generation sequencer [47]. Kawai *et al.* used this approach to study the evolution of East Asian strains using 20 whole genomes of Japanese, Korean, Amerindian, European, and West African strains [45]. A phylogenetic analysis revealed greater divergence between the East Asian strains and the Western strains in genes related to virulence factors, especially those related to outer membrane proteins and lipopolysaccharide synthesis enzymes. Genomic changes during infection also have been studied. The whole-genome sequence of strain HPAG1 was determined with the whole-genome shotgun method, and the data obtained were used to design a custom microarray [48]. Genotyping of isolates that were obtained from patients with chronic atrophic gastritis revealed that genes are gained and lost during the progression of the disease. Whole-genome transcriptional profiling also identified genes associated with the adaptation of *H. pylori* to chronic atrophic gastritis. A chronological comparison of the whole genome was performed on 5 sets of *H. pylori* strains from Colombia with isolation intervals of 3 to 16 years using the next-generation sequencing technology to identify genomic changes occurring in the same stomach [49]. Data obtained from the massively parallel sequencing technology should provide valuable candidates for novel virulence factors.

CONCLUSIONS

Of the approximately 1,600 genes contained in the *H. pylori* genome, it is likely that only a fraction of potential virulence genes have been identified. Comparative genomic techniques and the sequential sampling of the stomach during the course of the infection may provide an opportunity to correlate changes in bacteria with environmental factors, such as diet (*e.g.*, salt intake), which are critical determinants of outcome. Future studies should examine putative virulence factors as groups or as part of a virulence complex rather than individually. This approach is likely to provide a more complete understanding of the underlying mechanism of *H. pylori*-induced gastric inflammation that leads to severe gastroduodenal diseases by combining bacterial virulence factors with other factors, such as the environment and host.

ACKNOWLEDGMENTS

His report is based on work supported in part by grants from the National Institutes of Health (DK62813), grants-in-aid for Scientific Research from the Ministry of Education, Culture, Sports, Science, and Technology (MEXT) of Japan (22390085 and 22659087), Special Coordination Funds for Promoting Science and Technology from MEXT of Japan, and a Research Fund at the Discretion of the President, Oita University. Dr. Graham is supported in part by the Office of Research and Development Medical Research Service Department of Veterans Affairs, Public

Health Service grants DK067366 and DK56338 which funds the Texas Medical Center Digestive Diseases Center. The contents are solely the responsibility of the authors and do not necessarily represent the official views of the VA or NIH.

CONFLICT OF INTEREST

The author(s) confirm that this chapter content has no conflict of interest.

REFERENCES

[1] Graham DY, Lu H, Yamaoka Y. African, Asian or Indian enigma, the East Asian *Helicobacter pylori*: facts or medical myths. J Dig Dis 2009;10:77-84.

[2] Atherton JC. The pathogenesis of *Helicobacter pylori*-induced gastro-duodenal diseases. Annu Rev Pathol Mech Dis 2006;1:63-96.

[3] Cover TL, Blanke SR. *Helicobacter pylori* VacA, a paradigm for toxin multifunctionality. Nat Rev Microbiol 2005;3:320-32.

[4] Kusters JG, van Vliet AH, Kuipers EJ. Pathogenesis of *Helicobacter pylori* infection. Clin Microbiol Rev 2006;19:449-90.

[5] Boncristiano M, Paccani SR, Barone S, *et al.* The *Helicobacter pylori* vacuolating toxin inhibits T cell activation by two independent mechanisms. J Exp Med 2003;198:1887-97.

[6] Gebert B, Fischer W, Weiss E, Hoffmann R, Haas R. *Helicobacter pylori* vacuolating cytotoxin inhibits T lymphocyte activation. Science 2003;301:1099-102.

[7] Sundrud MS, Torres VJ, Unutmaz D, Cover TL. Inhibition of primary human T cell proliferation by *Helicobacter pylori* vacuolating toxin (VacA) is independent of VacA effects on IL-2 secretion. Proc Natl Acad Sci U S A 2004;101:7727-32.

[8] Raju D, Hussey S, Ang M, *et al.* Vacuolating cytotoxin and variants in Atg16L1 that disrupt autophagy promote *Helicobacter pylori* infection in humans. Gastroenterology 2012;142:1160-71.

[9] Atherton JC, Cao P, Peek RM, Jr., *et al.* Mosaicism in vacuolating cytotoxin alleles of *Helicobacter pylori.* Association of specific *vacA* types with cytotoxin production and peptic ulceration. J Biol Chem 1995;270:17771-7.

[10] Sugimoto M, Zali MR, Yamaoka Y. The association of *vacA* genotypes and *Helicobacter pylori*-related gastroduodenal diseases in the Middle East. Eur J Clin Microbiol Infect Dis 2009;28:1227-36.

[11] Sugimoto M, Yamaoka Y. The association of *vacA* genotype and *Helicobacter pylori*-related disease in Latin American and African populations. Clin Microbiol Infect 2009;15:835-42.

[12] Yamaoka Y, Kodama T, Gutierrez O, *et al.* Relationship between *Helicobacter pylori iceA, cagA*, and *vacA* status and clinical outcome: studies in four different countries. J Clin Microbiol 1999;37:2274-9.

[13] Yamaoka Y, Orito E, Mizokami M, *et al. Helicobacter pylori* in North and South America before Columbus. FEBS Lett 2002;517:180-4.

[14] Yamaoka Y. Mechanisms of disease: *Helicobacter pylori* virulence factors. Nat Rev Gastroenterol Hepatol 2010;7:629-41.

[15] Uchida T, Nguyen LT, Takayama A, *et al.* Analysis of virulence factors of *Helicobacter pylori* isolated from a Vietnamese population. BMC Microbiol 2009;9:175.
[16] Matsunari O, Shiota S, Suzuki R, *et al.* Association between *Helicobacter pylori* virulence factors and gastroduodenal diseases in Okinawa, Japan. J Clin Microbiol 2012;50:876-83.
[17] Mukhopadhyay AK, Kersulyte D, Jeong JY, *et al.* Distinctiveness of genotypes of *Helicobacter pylori* in Calcutta, India. J Bacteriol 2000;182:3219-27.
[18] Sugimoto M, Yamaoka Y. The association of *vacA* genotype and *Helicobacter pylori*-related disease in Latin American and African populations. Clin Microbiol Infect 2009;15:835-42.
[19] Rhead JL, Letley DP, Mohammadi M, *et al.* A new *Helicobacter pylori* vacuolating cytotoxin determinant, the intermediate region, is associated with gastric cancer. Gastroenterology 2007;133:926-36.
[20] Chung C, Olivares A, Torres E, *et al.* Diversity of VacA intermediate region among *Helicobacter pylori* strains from several regions of the world. J Clin Microbiol 2010;48:690-6.
[21] Hussein NR, Mohammadi M, Talebkhan Y, *et al.* Differences in virulence markers between *Helicobacter pylori* strains from Iraq and those from Iran: potential importance of regional differences in *H. pylori*-associated disease. J Clin Microbiol 2008;46:1774-9.
[22] Basso D, Zambon CF, Letley DP, *et al.* Clinical relevance of *Helicobacter pylori cagA* and *vacA* gene polymorphisms. Gastroenterology 2008;135:91-9.
[23] Jones KR, Jang S, Chang JY, *et al.* Polymorphisms in the intermediate region of VacA impact *Helicobacter pylori*-induced disease development. J Clin Microbiol 2011;49:101-10.
[24] Ogiwara H, Graham DY, Yamaoka Y. *vacA* i-region subtyping. Gastroenterology 2008;134:1267.
[25] Ferreira RM, Figueiredo C, Bonet C, *et al.* *Helicobacter pylori vacA* intermediate region genotyping and progression of gastric preneoplastic lesions. Am J Gastroenterol 2012;107:145-6.
[26] Ogiwara H, Sugimoto M, Ohno T, *et al.* Role of deletion located between the intermediate and middle regions of the *Helicobacter pylori vacA* gene in cases of gastroduodenal diseases. J Clin Microbiol 2009;47:3493-500.
[27] Censini S, Lange C, Xiang Z, *et al.* *cag*, a pathogenicity island of *Helicobacter pylori,* encodes type I-specific and disease-associated virulence factors. Proc Natl Acad Sci U S A 1996;93:14648-53.
[28] Kwok T, Zabler D, Urman S, *et al.* *Helicobacter* exploits integrin for type IV secretion and kinase activation. Nature 2007;449:862-6.
[29] Hatakeyama M. Oncogenic mechanisms of the *Helicobacter pylori* CagA protein. Nat Rev Cancer 2004;4:688-94.
[30] Franco AT, Israel DA, Washington MK, *et al.* Activation of beta-catenin by carcinogenic *Helicobacter pylori*. Proc Natl Acad Sci U S A 2005;102:10646-51.
[31] Franco AT, Johnston E, Krishna U, *et al.* Regulation of gastric carcinogenesis by *Helicobacter pylori* virulence factors. Cancer Res 2008;68:379-87.
[32] Ohnishi N, Yuasa H, Tanaka S, *et al.* Transgenic expression of *Helicobacter pylori* CagA induces gastrointestinal and hematopoietic neoplasms in mouse. Proc Natl Acad Sci U S A 2008;105:1003-8.
[33] van Doorn LJ, Figueiredo C, Sanna R, *et al.* Clinical relevance of the *cagA, vacA,* and *iceA* status of *Helicobacter pylori*. Gastroenterology 1998;115:58-66.
[34] Yamaoka Y, Kikuchi S, El-Zimaity HM, *et al.* Importance of *Helicobacter pylori oipA* in clinical presentation, gastric inflammation, and mucosal interleukin 8 production. Gastroenterology 2002;123:414-24.

[35] Yamaoka Y, Kodama T, Kashima K, Graham DY, Sepulveda AR. Variants of the 3' region of the *cagA* gene in *Helicobacter pylori* isolates from patients with different *H. pylori*-associated diseases. J Clin Microbiol 1998;36:2258-63.

[36] Yamaoka Y, El-Zimaity HM, Gutierrez O, *et al.* Relationship between the *cagA* 3' repeat region of *Helicobacter pylori,* gastric histology, and susceptibility to low pH. Gastroenterology 1999;117:342-9.

[37] Yamaoka Y, Osato MS, Sepulveda AR, *et al.* Molecular epidemiology of *Helicobacter pylori*: separation of *H. pylori* from East Asian and non-Asian countries. Epidemiol Infect 2000;124:91-6.

[38] Vilaichone RK, Mahachai V, Tumwasorn S, *et al.* Molecular epidemiology and outcome of *Helicobacter pylori* infection in Thailand: a cultural cross roads. *Helicobacter* 2004;9:453-9.

[39] Argent RH, Kidd M, Owen RJ, *et al.* Determinants and consequences of different levels of CagA phosphorylation for clinical isolates of *Helicobacter pylori*. Gastroenterology 2004;127:514-23.

[40] Azuma T, Yamakawa A, Yamazaki S, *et al.* Correlation between variation of the 3' region of the *cagA* gene in *Helicobacter pylori* and disease outcome in Japan. J Infect Dis 2002;186:1621-30.

[41] Selbach M, Paul FE, Brandt S, *et al.* Host cell interactome of tyrosine-phosphorylated bacterial proteins. Cell Host Microbe 2009;5:397-403.

[42] Mueller D, Tegtmeyer N, Brandt S, *et al.* c-Src and c-Abl kinases control hierarchic phosphorylation and function of the CagA effector protein in Western and East Asian *Helicobacter pylori* strains. J Clin Invest 2012.

[43] Yamaoka Y, Reddy R, Graham DY. *Helicobacter pylori* virulence factor genotypes in children in the United States: clues about genotype and outcome relationships. J Clin Microbiol 2010;48:2550-1.

[44] Fischer W, Windhager L, Rohrer S, *et al.* Strain-specific genes of *Helicobacter pylori*: genome evolution driven by a novel type IV secretion system and genomic island transfer. Nucleic Acids Res 2010.

[45] Kawai M, Furuta Y, Yahara K, *et al.* Evolution in an oncogenic bacterial species with extreme genome plasticity: *Helicobacter pylori* East Asian genomes. BMC Microbiol 2011;11:104.

[46] McClain MS, Shaffer CL, Israel DA, Peek RM, Jr., Cover TL. Genome sequence analysis of *Helicobacter pylori* strains associated with gastric ulceration and gastric cancer. BMC Genomics 2009;10:3.

[47] McNamara D. *Helicobacter pylori* infection and the pathogenesis of gastric cancer: a paradigm for host-bacterial interactions. 2008.

[48] Oh JD, Kling-Backhed H, Giannakis M, *et al.* The complete genome sequence of a chronic atrophic gastritis *Helicobacter pylori* strain: evolution during disease progression. Proc Natl Acad Sci U S A 2006;103:9999-10004.

[49] Kennemann L, Didelot X, Aebischer T, *et al.* *Helicobacter pylori* genome evolution during human infection. Proc Natl Acad Sci U S A 2011;108:5033-8.

Send Orders for Reprints to reprints@benthamscience.net
Helicobacter Pylori: A Worldwide Perspective 2014, **2014, 25-79**

CHAPTER 3

Epidemiology, Transmission and Public Health Implications of *Helicobacter pylori* Infection in Western Countries

Mónica S. Sierra*, Emily V. Hastings, Katharine Fagan-Garcia, Amy Colquhoun, and Karen J. Goodman

University of Alberta Division of Gastroenterology, Edmonton, Canada

Abstract: Across western countries, the observed prevalence of *H. pylori* infection ranges from 4% to 95% in adults and 4% to 82% in children, with estimates varying by country and subpopulation within countries. Reported incidence ranges from 0 to 7.3% per year in adults, with higher rates observed among travelers to high prevalence areas. Reported incidence ranges from 0 to 1.7% per month in children under 2 years old and 0.11% to 16% per year in 2- to 18-year olds. Reported elimination rates in children range from 0.37% to 35% per year. Evidence points to direct person-to-person contact as the predominant mode of transmission. Factors linked to increased prevalence in adults include residential crowding, institutionalization, and having hepatitis A virus. In children, *H. pylori* infection is associated with age, indicators of poor socioeconomic status such as residential crowding and parents' education level, and migration from high prevalence areas. Factors associated with elimination of *H. pylori* in childhood are age, sex, ethnicity, and antibiotic use. Recurrence of *H. pylori* infection after successful treatment is not frequently observed in western countries. Studies investigating the relationship between intrafamilial clustering of *H. pylori* infection and *H. pylori* recurrence have had inconsistent results. Development of cost-effective prevention strategies requires more evidence pertaining to transmission pathways and risk factors, as well as more effective treatments, particularly for high prevalence subpopulations.

Keywords: *H. pylori* infection, western countries, prevalence, incidence, elimination, recurrence, transmission.

NATURAL HISTORY OF *H. PYLORI* INFECTION

At onset, *Helicobacter pylori* infection has non-specific dyspeptic symptoms and generally goes undetected, thus few acute cases have been observed [1-3]. Evidence suggests that acute infection sometimes resolves spontaneously without

*__Address correspondence to Mónica S. Sierra:__ University of Alberta Division of Gastroenterology, Edmonton, Canada; E-mail:MonicaSierra@med.ualberta.ca

the development of detectable antibodies [2,4]. In other cases the infection persists indefinitely, generating specific anti-*H. pylori* IgG, generally detectable while the infection is present [2,4]; antibody titers often, but not always, reduce to undetectable levels following elimination of the infection [2,4]. Because of obstacles to studying the course of acute cases, it is not known what proportion of acute *H. pylori* infections become chronic [1,2,4]. Chronic *H. pylori* infection is nearly always accompanied by chronic gastritis [1,2,4] and occasionally leads to duodenal ulcers, gastric ulcers, and, more rarely, gastric carcinoma [1-4]. Chronic gastritis and peptic ulcer disease are more common in older and low-income populations [4]. Chronic *H. pylori*-associated gastritis is generally asymptomatic, particularly in children; symptomatic diseases associated with long-term infection generally occur in adults [1,2,4].

Initially, epidemiologic studies of *H. pylori* infection focused on adults; this focus changed with growing evidence that most infections are acquired in childhood [3]. Epidemiologic evidence shows that the prevalence of *H. pylori* infection is much higher in developing countries than in the developed world, with estimates in the range of 22 to 95% and 1 to 58%, respectively [3,5,6]. The prevalence of *H. pylori* infection varies by geographic location, ethnicity, socioeconomic status, and age [1,3]. In developing countries, most people become infected during childhood; in developed countries, a smaller percentage of children become infected and the prevalence of infection increases with age [3,7]. The aim of this chapter is to provide a summary of the evidence pertaining to the epidemiology, transmission, and public health implications of *H. pylori* infection in countries in the western part of the world, specifically: Western Europe, North America, and Oceania.

EPIDEMIOLOGY OF *H. PYLORI* INFECTION IN WESTERN COUNTRIES

Occurrence

Measures of occurrence of *H. pylori* infection reported in the literature include estimates of prevalence, incidence rates and elimination rates. The prevalence is the proportion of persons in a defined population who have *H. pylori* infection at a point in time. Incidence and elimination measures have as their numerator the number of *H. pylori* infection events (infections acquired or eliminated) in a defined population during a specific period of time. Incidence and elimination rates have as their denominator the person-time at risk of an infection event. Given that new *H. pylori* infections are not generally detected at onset, acquisition of *H. pylori* infection is inferred if tests that classify the infection status of an individual change from negative to positive from one exam to the next. Similarly, the elimination (loss or clearance) of *H. pylori* infection is inferred when the infection status of an individual changes from positive to negative from one exam to the next. Longitudinal studies of *H. pylori* infection are limited to testing for *H. pylori* at designated intervals and classifying subjects as having or not having a prevalent infection at each follow-up exam; therefore, the time of infection events can only be known to occur at some point during the interval between observations. To estimate the denominator for incidence or elimination rates, investigators must make assumptions about the average time of infection events within intervals.

A systematic review of the *H. pylori* literature was conducted to identify high quality reviews published in Ovid-Medline between 2000 and 2012. To identify published reviews, *Helicobacter pylori* (both as a medical subject heading and free text term) was combined using the set operator "OR" with the terms: *helicobacter* infections, isolation and purification, diagnosis, pathology, therapy, and transmission. These key terms were linked with the "AND" operator to the following terms either in the abstract, title, or as free text: prevalence or incidence, acquisition or persistence, elimination. The search was limited to review articles published in English. High quality reviews were defined as reports published in an epidemiology journal or reviews that met the following criteria: (a) listed one of the following key words: systematic review, meta-analysis, critical review, comprehensive review (in the title, abstract, or text); or (b) explicitly listed the criteria that were used to include or exclude study reports.

The selected review papers were scrutinized for reports of prevalence, incidence, or elimination of *H. pylori* infection in a non-infirm population from an identified geographic location in a western country (Western Europe, North America, including Greenland, and Oceania). Original sources were consulted when detailed information regarding sample size, detection method, population characteristics, or confidence intervals were not available in the review paper; in those instances the original source is also cited. The restriction to non-infirm populations excluded studies of patients being evaluated for symptoms; it included studies of people in non-clinical settings or clinical settings with non-infirm people, such as vaccination trials or prenatal care.

A second literature review was conducted to identify cohort studies of *H. pylori* infection in non-infirm populations of children from an identified geographic location in a western country (Western Europe, North America, including Greenland, and Oceania). To identify published reports, *Helicobacter pylori* (both as a medical subject heading and free text term) was combined using the set operator "OR" with the term *helicobacter* infections. These key terms were linked with the "AND" operator to the following terms either in the abstract, title, or as free text: incidence, acquisition or persistence, elimination or clearance. The search was limited to "all child (0 to 18 years)" and articles published in English. Articles were included in the review if the following information was included in the abstract or text: (a) incidence, (b) elimination or clearance, or (c) event counts and person-time at risk or person-time of follow-up.

Estimates of prevalence, incidence rates and elimination rates are presented in tables showing the study location, population and *H. pylori* detection method. In addition, factors examined in association with these estimates are summarized in tables showing the study location and classifying associations as positive, inverse or null. Reported associations are further subdivided by their statistical precision (precise *vs.* imprecise), with associations for which precision was not reported included in the imprecise category.

Prevalence

Prevalence in Adults

Across varied populations of adults in western countries, the reported prevalence of *H. pylori* infection ranges from 10% to 95% (Tables **1, 2**). Low prevalence has been observed in general populations within the United States and Denmark [1], and among pregnant women seeking antenatal care in a study by Blecker and Vandenplas (1993) in Brussels, Belgium (as cited in [2]). Conversely, high prevalence has been observed in a Canadian Aboriginal population in a study by

Bernstein *et al.* (1999) (as cited in [8]), in a Finnish study by Aromaa *et al.* (1996) (as cited in [9]), as well as in studies of institutionalized persons in the Netherlands and Australia, by Bohmer (1997) and Lambert (1995), respectively (as cited in [1,9]).

Table 1: Prevalence of *H. pylori* infection in adults in Western Countries.

Study Location, Year, and Author	**Study Population**		**Detection Method**	**Age Range (Years)**	**Sample Size**	**Prevalence (%)**
Western Europe						
Belgium[2] 1993 Blecker	Asymptomatic pregnant women seeking antenatal care in Brussels		Serology	20-29 30-40	213 276	12 23
Belgium[5, [10]] 2008 De Schryver	Workers Cases: caretakers of institutionalized children with intellectual disability at 2 institutions Controls: administrative workers (volunteers for a check-up for cardiovascular risk factors)		Serology	20-50 Mean 36 (SD= 8.0) Mean 39 (SD= 7.9)	587 390	41 29
Denmark[4] 1996 Andersen	General population		Serology	30-60	3,589	26
Denmark[4] 1993	General population, EUROGAST Study group[13]		Serology	25-34 55-64	157	15 30
England[2, [11]] 1994 Webb	Male factory employees in Stoke on Trent	Non-manual occupation Manual occupation	Serology	18-65 18-65	65 406	22 22[9] 40 40[9]
England and Wales[3]	Male participants in two cohort studies[11] between		Serology	35-64	116	47

Table 1: contd...

1991 Forman	1975-1982					
England[3] 1997 Wald	Professional men attending the British United Provident Association medical center in London during 1975-1982		Serology	35-64	1,296	46
Finland[3] 1996 Aromaa	Participants randomly selected from the 1966-1972 Mobile Clinic Unit of the Social Insurance Institution screening examinations across Finland		Serology	32-85	146	83
France[2, 14, [12]] 1989 Megraud	Random sample of adults attending a health checkup center		Serology	20-29 30-39 40-49 50-59 ≥60	105 299 285 324 45	25 26 30 35 30
Germany[6] Weyerman n 2009	Parents of children enrolled in a birth cohort study, Ulm	Mothers German Turkish Other Fathers German Turkish Other	UBT SAT	Mean 31.8 Mean 34.2	613 551 17 45 662 605 11 46	17 13 77 44 18 16 64 35
Italy[2] 1994 Palli	Random sample of residents of four geographic areas in Italy: Forli, Imola, Florence, Genoa & Cagliari		Serology	35-49 50-64	234 335	36 47
Italy[5] 2008 Zagari	Residents of two northern villages who participated in earlier population-based survey		UBT and biopsy[10]	≥ 32 Mean 59	1,033	58

Table 1: contd...

Ireland[6, [13]] 2006 Rowland	Parents of children enrolled in a cohort study	Mothers Fathers	UBT	Not reported	286 136	45 51
Norway[3] 1999 Hansen	Participants from two studies[12] during 1974-1978		Serology	34-68	983	63
Norway[7] 2009 Breckan	Representative sample of healthy adults		SAT	18-85	1,414	33
Spain[4] 1998 Senra-Varela	General population		Serology	Adults	332	43
Sweden[3] 1997 Siman	Volunteers at the health screening intervention program of the Prevention Section of the Department of Medicine at the University Hospital of Malmo		Serology	38-70	224	49
United Kingdom[4] 1995 Harris	Institutionalized persons Healthy controls		Serology	18-106 18-80+	424 267	87 41
United Kingdom[4] 1994 Webb	Male volunteers		Serology	18-64	471	37
United Kingdom[7] 2009 Jackson	Healthy adults (randomly selected)		Serology	18-70	2,437	26
Wales[2] 1992 Mendall	Consecutive patients attending a health screening clinic in Gwynedd and North West Clwyd	Non-manual occupation Manual occupation	Serology	21-30 41-50 51-60 21-30 41-50 51-60	137 131 65 138 108 43	33 34 52 46 46 58

Table 1: contd...

Wales[4] 1998 Strachan	General population in South Wales		Serology	45-59	1,796	70
North America						
Canada[1] 1990 Drumm	Parents of upper endoscopy patients at the Hospital for Sick Children, Toronto Ontario		Serology	Mean 47	67	49
Canada[1] 1994 Veldhuyzen van Zanten	Participants in a study of *Coxiella burnetii* infection, randomly selected from the provincial medical insurance registry, Nova Scotia		Serology	18-72 20-29 30-39 40-49 50-59 60-69 70-79	316 28 68 79 51 72 16	38 21 28 39 41 47 50
Canada[1] 1997 Pérez-Pérez	Stored serum samples selected from healthy persons	Canada	Serology	>20 23-65	469 265	35 46
Canada[1] 1998 Hodgins	Cord blood samples, consecutive births in Southern Quebec		Serology	Materna l age range	99	10
Canada[1] 1998 Hodgins	Cord blood samples, consecutive Inuit births in Nunavik, northern Quebec		Serology	Materna l age range	100	27
Canada[1] 1999 Bernstein	Residents of a Wasagamack Cree community, northern Manitoba		Serology	Adult ages	306	95
Greenland[1] 2003 Milman	Population survey participants		Serology	22-76	71	47
United States[2, [14]] 1991 Graham	Residents of Houston, Texas recruited through newspapers and flyers	European-American African-American	Serology and UBT	20-29 40-49 50-69 20-29 40-49 50-69	39 38 65 38 34 54	12 38 50 42 75 90

Table 1: contd...

United States[3] 1991 Parsonnet	Participants in a multiphasic health checkup		Serology	44-90	111	60
United States[3] 1991 Nomura	Japanese American men born between 1900 and 1919, who participated in the Honolulu Heart Program, Hawaii		Serology	56-85	109	76
United States[4] 1992 Malaty	Healthy volunteers in Texas	Hispanic Black White	Serology	20-75	89 89 89	65 66 26
United States[4] 1995 Replogle	Outpatients in California		Serology	20-39	556	27
United States[4] 1993	General population in Minnesota, EUROGAST Study Group[13]		Serology	25-34 55-64	198	15 34
United States[1, [15]] 2006 Zhu	Rural village residents, Norton Sound, Alaska		Serology	18-75+ 18-24 25-34 35-44 45-54 55-64 65-74 75+	610	80 72 82 85 77 87 78 63
Oceania						
Australia[8, [16]] 1993 Cullen	Randomly selected participants in the Busselton Population Study with an oversampling of males		Serology	41.3-65	141	35
Australia[4] 1998 Lin	General population		Serology	20-80	273	38

Table 1: contd...

Australia[4, 17] 1998 Lin	Random selection of dental staff matched by age and sex to randomly selected practicing gastroenterologists and gastroenterology nurses Dental students matched by age and sex to a random sample of the urban population (using the phonebook)	Dentist Gastroenterologist Dental nurses Gastroenterology nurses Dental students, 5th year Dental students, 1st year Urban population	Serology	Mean 42 Mean 32 Mean 24 Mean 19	92 187 40 108 33 30 14	23 33 18 30 18 16 18
Australia[4] 1995 Lambert	Institutionalized patients (mentally and physically disabled) Population controls, sex and age matched		Serology	19-47	122	75 23
New Zealand[4] 1996 Fraser	Workers	All European Maori Pacific Islander	Serology	40-64	579 190 195 194	56 36 57 73

UBT, urea breath test; SAT, stool antigen test
[1] As cited in reference [8]
[2] As cited in reference [2]
[3] As cited in reference [9]
[4] As cited in reference [1]
[5] As cited in reference [18]
[6] As cited in reference [19]
[7] As cited in reference [20]
[8] As cited in reference [4]
[9] Adjusted for age
[10] *H. pylori*-positive status defined by positive result on at least two of the following: urea breath test, histology, rapid urease test
[11] Participants of the British United Provident Association study and the Caerphilly Collaborative Study
[12] Participants of the Norwegian JANUS cohort study (blood donors in Oslo from 1973-1985 for the Study of Cardiovascular Disease) and participants from the Norwegian Counties Study
[13] From the EUROGAST Study Group. Includes participants from Algeria, Belgium, Denmark, Germany, Greece, Iceland, Italy, Japan, Poland, Portugal Slovenia, United Kingdom, United States
[14] Prevalence estimated from Fig. **1** pg. 1871

Estimates of *H. pylori* prevalence vary by country and by subpopulation within countries (Tables **1**, **2**). For instance, in Canada, Hodgins *et al.* (1998) reported a prevalence of 10% among women of maternal age in southern Quebec, while Bernstein *et al.* (1999) reported a prevalence of 95% in the Wasagamack Cree community in Northern Manitoba (as cited in [8]). In Australia, Cullen *et al.* (1993) and Lin *et al.* (1998) reported prevalences of 35% and 38%, respectively, in the general population (as cited in [4] and [1], respectively), while Lambert *et al.* (1995) reported a prevalence of 75% among institutionalized mentally and physically disabled patients (as cited in [1]).

The prevalence of *H. pylori* infection appears to increase with age (Table **2**); however, this increase is believed to reflect a cohort effect rather than an increased risk in older age groups. Reported *H. pylori* prevalence is higher among ethnic groups that have relatively low socioeconomic status on average (Tables **1-3**). In the United States, the prevalence has been shown to be considerably higher among African or Hispanic Americans compared to non-Hispanic whites. Differences based on ethnicity have also been found in other geographic regions: for example, in a New Zealand study, Fraser *et al.* (1996) reported 1.4- and 1.8-fold increases in *H. pylori* prevalence among Maori and Pacific Islander workers, respectively, compared to European workers (as cited in [1]). Factors linked to increased *H. pylori* prevalence in several studies were residential crowding, institutionalization, and infection with hepatitis A virus (Table **3**). Studies that compare *H. pylori* prevalence across occupations have reported inconsistent results. Many of the studies that investigated potential predictors of *H. pylori* prevalence report results that are too imprecise to draw conclusions, and this may explain much of the inconsistency across studies.

Table 2: Prevalence of *H. pylori* infection in combined populations of adults and children in Western Countries.

Study Location, Year, and Author	**Study Population**		**Detection Method**	**Age Range (Years)**	**Sample Size**	**Prevalence (%)**
Western Europe						
Ireland[4] 1997 Murray	General population		Serology	12-64	4,724	50

Table 2: contd...

Netherlands[4, [21]] 1997 Bohmer	Residents of institutes for the mentally disabled		Serology	11-89	338	83
Sweden[6, [22]] 2005 Kivi	Parents and siblings of 10- to 14-year-old children enrolled in a *H. pylori* study	*H. pylori+* index child: Mother Father Siblings *H. pylori-* index child: Mother Father Siblings	Serology	 ND ND 0-23 ND ND 0-23	 50 35 99 98 70 125	 94 91 66 36 41 11
North America						
Canada[1] 1999 McKeown	Residents of Inuit communities: Chesterfield Inlet and Repulse Bay, Nunavut		Serology	All ages	256	51
Greenland[1] 2005 Koch	Participants in a population-based cohort study during 1996-1998		Serology	15-87	685	58
United States[4] 1991 Graham	Healthy volunteers in Texas	Blacks Whites	Serology	15-80	246 239	70 34
United States[4] 1994 Smoak	Army recruits		Serology	17-26	938	26
United States[4] 1995 Hyams	Navy and Marine Corps personnel		Serology	17-50	1,000	25
Canada[1] 1990 Drumm	Random sample from the Hospital for Sick Children, Toronto, Ontario		Serology	Mean 16	37	14

Table 2: contd...

Oceania						
Australia[1,4,] [23] 1993 Mitchell	Family members of index children infected with *H. pylori*	 Grandparents Parents Siblings	Serology	1-49 ND 22-49 1-21	69 1 41 27	77 100 80 70
Australia[5] 2008 Moujaber	Age-stratified random sampling from 8000 banked diagnostic laboratory samples		Serology	1-59	2,413	15
New Zealand[2] [24] 1986 Morris	Blood donors		Serology	15-20 21-30 31-40 41-50 51-60 61-70	175 165 93 35 12 3	32 33 45 54 33 0
		All Maori Cook Island Samoan Tongan		15-70	462 192 85 129 56	37 21 39 44 70

ND, no data provided in report

[1] As cited in reference [8]

[2] As cited in reference [2]

[3] As cited in reference [9]

[4] As cited in reference [1]

[5] As cited in reference [18]

[6] As cited in reference [19]

Table 3: Predictors of *H. pylori* Prevalence in Adults in Western Countries.

Factor	**Positive Association**	**Inverse Association**	**Null Association**			
	Precise	**Imprecise**	**Precise**	**Imprecise**	**Precise**	**Imprecise**
Race/Ethnicity						
Non-Caucasian *vs.* Caucasian						
Black or Hispanic *vs.* White						

Factor	Positive Association	Inverse Association	Null Association			
	Precise	Imprecise	Precise	Imprecise	Precise	Imprecise
African American or Hispanic *vs.* White	United States 2,4, [25-27]	United States[4]				
Cook Island or Samoan *vs.* Tongan		New				
Zealand[4] [24]						
Chinese *vs.* Chinese-Australian			Australia[2,7]			
Japanese *vs.* Chinese-Australian						Australia[2,7]
Occupation						
Endoscopy & non-endoscopy physicians *vs.* controls[8]	Germany[4,] [28]					
Endoscopy & non-endoscopy nurses *vs.*						
controls[8]	Germany[4,] [28]	Germany[4,] [28]				
Endoscopy & medical staff *vs.* controls[8]	Germany[4,] [28]					
Gastroenterologists *vs.* blood donors	Australia[2]					
Gastroenterology nurses *vs.* blood donors			Australia[2]			
General practitioners *vs.* blood donors		Australia[2]				
Gastroenterologists & endoscopy staff *vs.* controls[8]	Germany[2,] [29]					
Physicians *vs.* nurses, endoscopy- *vs.* non-endoscopy physicians, endoscopy- *vs.* non-endoscopy staff						Germany[4,] [28]
Endoscopy- *vs.* non-endoscopy nurses	Germany[4,] [28]					

Factor	**Positive Association**	**Inverse Association**	**Null Association**			
	Precise	**Imprecise**	**Precise**	**Imprecise**	**Precise**	**Imprecise**
Dental assistants *vs.* dentists	United States [2]					
Dentists *vs.* gastroenterologists				Australia[4], [17]		
Dental nurses *vs.* gastroenterology nurses						Australia[4], [17]
Dental students *vs.* random sample of urban population		Australia[4], [17]				
Dental hygienists & students *vs.* dentists		United States [2]				
≤3 years of work in the gastroenterology or endoscopy unit *vs.* >3 years				Germany[4], [30]		
≥5 years of work in institutes for the mentally disabled						
vs. <5 years	The Netherlands [21]					
Nurses *vs.* staff with little direct contact with patients	The Netherlands[4], [21]					
Years in a job with public contact	Australia [31]					
Submarine crews *vs.* air force crews	Germany[2], [32]					
***H. pylori*-Positive Spouse**						
Yes *vs.* no	Germany[4], [33]					United States[2], [34]
Length of cohabitation with an infected partner						
(≤15 years *vs.* >15)	Germany[4], [33]					
Duration of cohabitation with an infected partner						United States[2], [34]
Partner born outside the United States						United States[2], [34]

Factor	Positive Association	Inverse Association	Null Association			
	Precise	**Imprecise**	**Precise**	**Imprecise**	**Precise**	**Imprecise**
Crowding						
More than one person/room in childhood home	England[2]					
Australia [31]						
Share a bed during childhood *vs.* not	England[2]					
Domestic crowding during childhood	England[2]					
Institutionalized schizophrenic patients *vs.* blood donors	Belgium[4]					
≥15 years living in institution for mentally disabled *vs.* <15 years	Netherlands[4], [21]					
Hospitalization length						United States[2], [26]
Hygiene Practices						
Use of chopsticks to eat from communal dishes *vs.* not	Australia[4], [35]					
Drinking Water Source						
Non-municipal water supply *vs.* municipal water supply		Germany[6]				
Hot water in household during childhood	England[2]					
Hepatitis A Virus Infection						
Seropositive *vs.* seronegative	Germany[3]					
Italy[3]						
United Kingdom[3]						
United States[3], [36]	Italy[3]					
Dental Plaque						
High score *vs.* low score	Australia[4]					

Factor	Positive Association	Inverse Association	Null Association			
	Precise	**Imprecise**	**Precise**	**Imprecise**	**Precise**	**Imprecise**
<1 dentist visit per year *vs.* >1	Australia[4]					
Contact with Animals						
Poultry workers *vs.* no job-related contact with animals						France[2]
Livestock slaughterers *vs.* no job-related contact with animals				France[2]		
Direct Contact with Feces						
Regularly *vs.* never	Belgium[5]					
Sometimes *vs.* never		Belgium[5]				
Alcohol Consumption						
Yes *vs.* no				New Zealand[4], [37]		Australia[4], [31]
United States[4, 9], [38]						
High *vs.* low intake			Germany[4], [39-41]	Germany[4], [41]		
United States[4], [25]						
Moderate *vs.* low intake			United States[4], [25]	Germany[4], [39-41]		
Smoking						
Current or ex-smoker *vs.* never smoker	United States[4, 9], [38]	Australia[4], [42]				
United States[4], [25]						
Germany[4], [39]				Australia[4], [31]		
United States[4, 9], [38]						
San Marino[4], [43]						
New Zealand[4], [37]						
Female: current *vs.* never smoker	Australia[4], [42]					
Male: current *vs.* never smoker						Australia[4], [42]
Black ethnicity: current smoker *vs.* not current						

Factor	Positive Association	Inverse Association	Null Association			
	Precise	**Imprecise**	**Precise**	**Imprecise**	**Precise**	**Imprecise**
White ethnicity: current smoker *vs.* not current	United States[4], [25]					
Smoking intensity						
Age at smoking initiation						Australia[4], [42]
Sexual Orientation						
Regular homosexual contact *vs.* never			United States [2], [27]			
HIV Infection						
Seropositive *vs.* seronegative		United States [2], [27]				

[1] As cited in reference [3].
[2] As cited in reference [2].
[3] As cited in reference [44].
[4] As cited in reference [1].
[5] As cited in reference [18].
[6] As cited in reference [45].
[7] Control groups included: random sample of children (aged 5-17 years) without acute abdominal symptoms, healthy medical students, blood donors, and a random sample of 58 patients without acute peptic ulcer or acute gastritis. Controls were matched by age and sex.
[8] Controls were individuals who did not work in the field of medicine.
[9] From the EUROGAST Study Group. Includes participants from Algeria, Belgium, Denmark, Germany, Greece, Iceland, Italy, Japan, Poland, Portugal, Slovenia, United Kingdom, United States.

b. Prevalence in Children

Prevalence of *H. pylori* in groups of children in western countries ranged from 4% to 82% (Table **4**). Low *H. pylori* prevalence has been observed among French, Finnish, German and urban Canadian children (as cited in [2,3]). High prevalence has been reported for African refugee children living in Australia (Cherian [2008], as cited in [18]), Canadian children from the rural Wasagamack Cree community in Northern Manitoba (Sinha *et al.* (2002), as cited in [8]), and Turkish children living in Germany (Rothenbacher (1998, 1999), as cited in [3]).

Age, indicators of poor socioeconomic status such as residential crowding and parents' education level, and migration from high prevalence areas are major determinants of *H. pylori* prevalence (Tables **4** and **5**), although as with the adult literature many of the studies have insufficient statistical power, which may explain some of the inconsistencies across studies. In general, prevalence increases with age except within some narrow age ranges in children. In a national survey of 6- to19-year-old children in the United States by Staat *et al.* (1996), the prevalence of the *H. pylori* infection was 17% in 6-9 year olds, 26% in 10-14 year olds, and 29% in 15-19 year olds (as cited in [3]). In the Wasagamack Cree community in Northern Manitoba, Canada, Sinha *et al.* (2002) reported that the prevalence by age group was 20% in 0-1 year olds and 70% in 7-9 year olds (as cited in [8]). In Sweden, Granstrom *et al.* (1997) found that the prevalence was 5% in 1.5 year olds, 10% in 2 year olds, 8% in 4 year olds, and 3% in 11 year olds (as cited in [3]). Other risk factors linked with an increased prevalence of *H. pylori* infection include sources of drinking water, the presence of *H. pylori* infection in siblings or parents, as well as poor nutritional status. Antibiotic use and the presence of pets in the household have been linked to a decreased prevalence of *H. pylori* infection in children.

Overall, high prevalence of *H. pylori* infection in adults in particular populations corresponds to high prevalence of this infection in children from the same populations. These findings suggest that the prevalence of *H. pylori* infection remains high in certain geographical regions and subpopulations of the western world, particularly among low-income groups and immigrants from high prevalence areas [3,6,46].

Table 4: Prevalence of *H. pylori* Infection in Children in Western Countries.

Study Location, Year, and Author	**Study Population**		**Detection Method**	**Age Range (Years)**	**Sample Size**	**Prevalence (%)**
Western Europe						
Belgium[2] 1993 Blecker	Minor elective surgery patients of high socioeconomic status, Brussels	Belgian African	Serology	0-17 0-17	472 40	4 18
Finland[3] 1995 Ashorn	Participants in a multicenter cohort study of atherosclerosis precursors		Serology	3-18	461	10
Finland[3] 1996 Ashorn	Infants delivered at university hospital in Tampere		Serology	2	195	6
France[5, [3]] 1994 Vincent	Institutionalized children (neurologically impaired)		Serology, culture, histology[8]	3.5-19	117	38

Table 4: contd...

Germany[3] 1998, 1999 Rothenbacher	School fitness exam attendees in Ulm	1996 study German Turkish 1997 study German Turkish	UBT	5-8	945 685 105 1,143 874 118	13 6 45 11 5 44
Germany[47] 2004 Krumbiegel	Children from 2 rural counties in Leipzig	Landkreis Leipziger Land Muldentalkreis	UBT	2nd graders	1,884 1,119 765	6 6 7
Greece[3] 1990 Pateraki	Attendees at multiple vaccination clinics		Serology	1-10	188	39
England[3] 1996 O'Donohoe	School children in London		Serology	5-13	640	17
Italy[3] 1997 Perri	School children in S. Giovanni Rotondo		UBT	4-18	304	28
Italy[3] 1999 Dominici	Small town residents in Campogalliano		Serology	12-16	186	30
Ireland[3] 1997 Murray	National surveys, Northern Ireland		Serology	12-19	661	24
Portugal [48] 2011 Oleastro	Random selection of vaccination program attendees at health care centers in Lisbon		SAT	0-15 0-5 6-10 11-15	844 403 276 165	32 20 (16-24) 37 (31-43) 52 (44-59)
Scotland[3] 1994 Patel	School children in Edinburgh		Salivary IgG	11	554	11
Sweden[3] 1997 Granstrom	Vaccine trial participants, Stockholm		Serology	1.5 2 4 11	239 237 185 201	5 10 8 3
Switzerland[3] 1999 Boltshauser	Preschool children in St. Gallen	Children of immigrant parents	UBT	5-7	432 359 73	7 4 19

Table 4: contd...

North America						
Canada[1] 1999 McKeown	Residents of Inuit communities, Repulse Bay, Nunavut		Serology	0-15	28	32
Canada[1] 2002 Sinha	Residents of Wasagamack Cree community, northern Manitoba		SAT	0-12 0-1 7-9	163 22 23	56 20 70
United States[2], [49] 1991 Fiedorek	Minor surgery outpatients, Arkansas Children's Hospital	Euro-American African-American	Serology	3-10 3-10	141 36	24 42
United States[3], [50] 1991 Malaty	Volunteers recruited through newspapers and flyers in Houston, Texas	 Black White	UBT	1-18	69 30 39	22 37 8
United States[3] 1996 Staat	National Health and Nutrition Examination Survey III (weighted to represent United States demographics)		Serology	6-19 6-9 10-14 15-19	2,581 869 902 810	25 17 26 29
United States[3] 1999 Redlinger	Hispanic residents of El Paso, Texas		Serology	4-7	365	21
United States[3] 1999 Malaty	Participants in a community-based cohort study, Bogalusa, Louisiana	Black White	Serology	7-9	62 150	40 11
Oceania						
Australia[4] 2008 Cherian	African refugees attending health assessments		SAT	<16	193	82
New Zealand[3] 1996 Fraser	School children in South Auckland		Serology	11-12	299	32[6]
New Zealand[3] 1998 Fawcett	Participants in a birth cohort, Dunedin		Serology	11	561	7

UBT, urea breath test; SAT, stool antigen test.

[1] As cited in reference [8].

[2] As cited in reference [2].

[3] As cited in reference [9].
[4] As cited in reference [18].
[5] As cited in reference [3].
[6] Estimated using data from report.
[8] *H. pylori*-positive status defined by positive serology and culture, or positive serology and at least two positive of: histology; urease test; inflammatory reaction of the mucosa.

Table 5: Predictors of *H. pylori* Prevalence in Children in Western Countries.

Factor	Positive association		Inverse association		Null association	
	Precise	Imprecise	Precise	Imprecise	Precise	Imprecise
Child's Sex						
Boys *vs.* girls		Portugal [48]		Germany[1]		United States [1,2, [46]]
Girls *vs.* Boys		England[2]		US[1, [51]]		Wales[2]
Child's age						
Younger *vs.* older age			Portugal [48] US[1, [46]]			
Age per 1 year increase	United States [1, [51]]	United States [1, [6]] United States - Mexico[6, [7]]			Wales[2]	
Race/Ethnicity						
Non-Hispanic Black Mexican-American *vs.* Non-Hispanic White	United States [1, [6]]					
Black *vs.* White		United States[2]				
Maori or Pacific Islander *vs.* European	New Zealand[1]					
Antibiotic Use						
No *vs.* yes			Germany[1]			
Nutritional Status						
Diminished growth (height centiles)		Italy[1, [52]]				
Diminished growth (<25th	Italy[1, [52]]					

Factor	Positive association		Inverse association		Null association	
	Precise	Imprecise	Precise	Imprecise	Precise	Imprecise
centile), at ages 8.5-14 years						
Migration from / Residence in High Prevalence Region						
Non-Caucasian (African or Mediterranean background) *vs.* Caucasian	Belgium[1, [53]]	Belgium[1, [53]]				
Immigrant father	Australia[1]					
Immigrant mother		Australia[1]				
Other ethnicity living in Germany or German living elsewhere during infancy *vs.* German living in Germany during infancy	Germany[1,3, [54]]					
Age child moved to a lower prevalence area	Germany[1]					
Mexico *vs.* United States residence		United States - Mexico [7]				
Born in United States *vs.* Canada			United States[1]			
Mexican Americans born outside the United States or Canada *vs.* born in the United States or Canada	United States [1, [6]]					
Lived in Mexico >6 months *vs.* did not live in Mexico >6 months		United States [1, [46]]				
Area of Residence						
Suburban *vs.* urban residence				United States [2]		
Rural *vs.* urban	United States	United		United		United States

Factor	Positive association		Inverse association		Null association	
	Precise	Imprecise	Precise	Imprecise	Precise	Imprecise
residence	1, [46]	States [2]		States [1]		1
Living and born in Gwynedd *vs.* not		Wales[2]				
Living in but not born in Gwynedd *vs.* not						Wales[2]
Crowding / Family Composition / Personal Contact						
Number of siblings	England[2] Germany[1]	England[2] Germany[1]				
Birth order						Germany[1]
Childhood household density				Wales[2]		Wales[2]
Persons per room in home	England[2] Scotland[1] United States [1, [6]]	England[2]		England[2]		
Household crowding, high *vs.* low	United States [1, [46]]	United States [1, [55]]				United States [1, [55]]
Household crowding, medium *vs.* low		United States [1, [46]]				
Number of children living in home	England[2]	England[2] Portugal [48]				
Square meter per person living in home		Germany[1]				
Sharing a bed	Wales[2] England[2]					
Sharing a bed with a positive sibling	Ireland[3]					
Sharing a bedroom						England[2]
Daycare, nursery or kindergarten attendance	Portugal [48]		United States [1]			
Years of residence in an institution		France[1, [56]]				

Factor	Positive association		Inverse association		Null association	
	Precise	Imprecise	Precise	Imprecise	Precise	Imprecise
Living in an institution since birth	France[1, [56]]					
***H. pylori* Status of Parents**						
1 seropositive parent *vs.* none	Italy[1] United States [1, [50]]	United States [1, [51]]				
2 seropositive parents *vs.* none	United States [1, [51]]	Italy[1]				
***H. pylori* Status of Mother**						
Positive *vs.* negative	Germany[1, 3, [57]] Ireland[3] United States-Mexico[6, [7]]					
***H. pylori* Status of Father**						
Positive *vs.* negative	Ireland[3]	Germany[1, 3, [57]]				
***H. pylori* Status of Siblings**						
1+ positive sibs *vs.* all negative or no sibs		Germany[3]				
Family History of Ulcer						
Mother's history: positive *vs.* negative	Germany[1, [58]]					
Father's history: positive *vs.* negative		Germany[1, [58]				
Parents' Smoking						
Father smokes *vs.* does not smoke	United States [1, [59]]					
Mother smokes *vs.* does not smoke			United States [1, [59]]			
Socioeconomic Indicators						
Low *vs.* high income	United States [2]	United States [2]				
Below *vs.* above poverty line		United States [1, [6]]				

Factor	**Positive association**		**Inverse association**		**Null association**	
	Precise	**Imprecise**	**Precise**	**Imprecise**	**Precise**	**Imprecise**
Lower *vs.* higher social stratification		England[2] Scotland[1]		England[2] Scotland[1]		
Occupation-based social class: Manual *vs.* non-manual Middle *vs.* upper Lower *vs.* upper	Wales[2]	Australia[1] Australia[1]				
Father's occupation, manual *vs.* non-manual	England[2]					
Blue collar workers and farmers *vs.* white collar workers	Italy[1], [51]					
Low education of parents or parent	United States[1], [6,46] Spain[1]			Portugal [48]		
High *vs.* low education of the mother or father				Germany[1]		
Rents *vs.* owns house			Scotland[1]			
Household has *vs.* does not have refrigerator						England[2]
Number of indoor bathrooms				United States - Mexico[6], [7]		
Household has *vs.* does not have indoor toilet		England[2] United States [1], [46]				
Water Source						
City *vs.* well water						United States[2]
Drinking water from other *vs.* public source	Germany[4], [47]					United States [1],[46]
Piped water in home *vs.* no piped		United States [1],[46]				

Factor	Positive association		Inverse association		Null association	
	Precise	Imprecise	Precise	Imprecise	Precise	Imprecise
water						
Household Pets						
Pet ownership: any *vs.* none		Germany[1, [60]]	United States [1, 2, [6,49]]	Portugal [48]		England[2]
Pet ownership, cat or rabbit		Germany[1, [60]]				
Pet ownership, Guinea pig or bird				Germany[1, [60]]		
Contact with dogs outside house				Germany[1, [60]]		
Contact with cats or rabbits outside house		Germany[1, [60]]				

[1] As cited in reference [3].
[2] As cited in reference [2].
[3] As cited in reference [19].
[4] As cited in reference [45].
[5] As cited in reference [1].
[6] Includes data for the United States and the Mexico border.
[7] As cited in reference.

Incidence

Incidence Rates

In adults, the reported incidence of *H. pylori* infection ranges from 0 per year to 7.3% per year (Table **6**). However, the annual incidence rate reported from most studies was between 0 and 1.0%. Higher incidence rates were observed among travelers to high prevalence areas. For instance, in a cohort study by Taylor *et al.* (1997), the incidence rate was 7.3% per year in army personnel who served in the Persian Gulf from August 1990 to April 1991 (as cited in [61]) (Table **6**). The estimated incidence of *H. pylori* infection in children living in western countries is higher than in adults, particularly in early childhood. Among children aged 2 to 18 years, the incidence rate ranged from 0.11% to 16% per year (Table **7**). Particularly high incidence rates were observed in children in Portugal (12% per year) [48] and in children residing in a Canadian First Nations community (16% per year) [62]. In children under 2 years of age, the reported incidence rate ranged from 0 to 1.7% per month. The highest incidence in this age group was observed among children residing along the United States–Mexico border (1.7% per month; 95% Confidence Interval (CI): 1.4, 2.0) [63] (Table **8**).

Varied rates of *H. pylori* acquisition have been observed in children living in the United States. In the Bogalusa Heart Study conducted in Louisiana, Malaty *et al.* (1999) reported an incidence rate of 22% per year for children aged 7 to 21 years [64]; however, in a subsequent analysis, Malaty *et al.* (2002) reported a rate of 1.4% per year among children aged 1 to 21 years [65]. In a study conducted in California, Perry *et al.* (2006) reported a rate of 6.8% per year for children 2 to 17 years old [66] (Table **7**). The variation in rates within the same country may be attributable in part to the different age ranges of study subjects and random variation from small sample sizes.

Factors Associated with the Incidence of *H. pylori* Infection

Numerous risk factors for acquisition of *H. pylori* infection were investigated in cohort studies examining *H. pylori* incidence; however, few risk factors were examined in more than one study (Table **9**). The factors that were examined most frequently in association with *H. pylori* infection were age, sex, socioeconomic indicators (particularly mother's education), and antibiotic use. Other common factors analyzed were family income, breastfeeding practices, mother's or parents' age, presence of infected siblings, drinking water source, number of siblings, and place of residence.

Age-specific *H. pylori* incidence rates were estimated in 10 cohort studies. The highest age-specific incidence rates were reported in the birth cohort living along the United States-Mexico border, where incidence rates were 1.1% per month (CI: 0.77, 1.6) in 0-0.5 year olds, 2.1% per month (CI: 1.6, 2.8) in 0.5-1 year olds, 1.6% per month (CI: 1.1, 2.4) in 1-1.5 year olds, and 2.1% per month (CI: 1.4, 3.1) in 1.5-2 year olds [63]. In a cohort of 195 Finnish children, the incidence rate was 0.13% per month among 1 year olds and 0.31% per month among 2 year olds [67] (Tables **7**, **8**, and **9**). *H. pylori* incidence rates appear to decrease with age. In a United States study, observed incidence rates decreased steadily over age (2.1% per year in the 4-5 year age group, 1.5% per year in the 7-9 year age group, 1% per year in the 13-15 year age group, and 0.3 % per year in the 21-23 year age group) [65]. In Ireland, the highest observed incidence rate was for children between 2 and 3 years of age (5.1% per year) [13]. A steady decrease in the incidence rate was observed for the subsequent three age groups studied, plateauing thereafter around zero (4.2% per year in the 3-4 year age group, 2.1% per year in the 4-5 year age group, 0 in the 5-6 year age group, 0.68% per year in the 6-7 year age group, and 0year in the 7-8 year age group). In these studies, the incidence of *H. pylori* infection appears to peak at 2-3 years of age and decline thereafter.

Sex is another factor examined in association with acquisition of *H. pylori* infection in childhood. Studies investigating this relationship have reported conflicting results. In a study conducted in New Zealand, the rate of *H. pylori* acquisition was 3 times higher in boys than in girls [68]. However, no clear difference was observed between boys and girls in the studies conducted in the United States [65] or along the United States–Mexico border [63] (Table **9**).

Studies assessing the relationship between household crowding (large number of people per room, sharing of beds, high housing density) and *H. pylori* infection have also reported conflicting results. Household crowding was positively associated with the incidence of *H. pylori* infection in a study conducted in Ireland [13]; however, it was inversely associated with the incidence of *H. pylori* in a birth cohort study conducted along the United States–Mexico border [69] (Table **9**).

Having an *H. pylori*-positive mother or an *H. pylori*-positive sibling has been found to be positively associated with the incidence of *H. pylori* infection. In studies conducted in Ireland [13] and Italy [70], children who had *H. pylori*-seropositive mothers were more likely to acquire *H. pylori* infection than those with *H. pylori*-seronegative mothers (rate ratios ranged from 1.21 to 3.34; Table **9**). Evidence from two studies showed that children born to *H. pylori*-positive mothers tested seropositive for *H. pylori* infection in early infancy, and children born to seronegative mothers tested seronegative [67,71]; however, in these studies, all children that tested seropositive at birth tested seronegative between 3-7 months of age, suggesting that seropositivity at birth was due to maternally acquired antibodies. A study conducted in Belgium showed that children born to seropositive mothers did not readily acquire *H. pylori* infection during the first year of life; among 67 of these children tested by urea breath test around 15 months of age, only 1 tested positive [71]. Children with *H. pylori*-seropositive siblings were more likely to acquire *H. pylori* infection than those with *H. pylori*-seronegative siblings in an Irish study [13]. Similarly, in the birth cohort study conducted along the United States–Mexico border, children with an older sibling who was persistently positive for *H. pylori* were more likely to acquire *H. pylori* than those who did not have a sibling with a persistent infection, particularly if the difference in age between the siblings was 3 years or less [72] (Table **9**).

The effect of socioeconomic indicators such as income, social stratum, socioeconomic status, mother's years of education, urban or rural residence, and drinking water source on the acquisition of *H. pylori* infection was evaluated in numerous studies (Table **9**). Risk factors linked with an increased incidence rate of *H. pylori* infection in more than 1 study included low socioeconomic status and limited education of the mother. The relationship between drinking water source and the incidence of *H. pylori* infection was inconsistent across studies (Table **9**).

In summary, acquisition of *H. pylori* infection in western countries is infrequent and appears to occur most often in young children. However, the highest incidence rates have been reported in settings where poverty and crowding are common. Most of the studies observed differences between infected and uninfected children corresponding to age and indicators of low socioeconomic status. Findings for other risk factors were inconsistent, possibly due to differing definitions of variables and insufficient study sizes.

Elimination

Elimination rates

Reports from 4 cohort studies mentioned apparent eliminations of *H. pylori* infection in adults (Table **7**), but just 1 estimated an elimination rate. Veldhuyzen van Zanten (1993) reported an elimination rate of 1.6% per year (CI: 0.62, 8.5) among residents of Nova Scotia aged 18-72 years [73]. Ten studies estimated the elimination rate of *H. pylori* infection in children (Table **8**). Reported elimination rates in children from western countries ranged from 0.37% to 35% per year, with the highest elimination rate observed among German children (35% per year, CI: 20, 54) [74]. In the study conducted along the United States–Mexico border, the estimated risk of *H. pylori* elimination from one follow-up visit to the next was 68% (CI: 61, 74) [75]. As with incidence rates, the wide range of reported elimination rates is likely due, in part, to differences in age ranges, cohort sizes, and follow-up schedules.

Factors Associated with the Elimination of *H. pylori* Infection

Factors associated with elimination of *H. pylori* infection are age, antibiotic use, sex, and ethnicity. These factors were investigated in 3 of the 10 cohort studies that examined elimination rates (Table **10**). Age was identified as a risk factor for elimination in the study conducted along the United States–Mexico border [63], as well as in a study conducted in Italy [70]; these studies suggested that elimination of *H. pylori* infection may occur most frequently during early childhood (Tables **7** and **8**). Three studies investigated the effect of antibiotic use on the elimination of *H. pylori* infection with inconsistent results. Each of these studies, however, observed spontaneous elimination of *H. pylori* that did not appear related to antibiotic use. For example, Perri *et al.* (1998) examined 48 *H. pylori*-positive Italian children aged 4.5-18.5 years every 6 months for 2 years to observe whether *H. pylori* infection was eliminated spontaneously [76]. After 2 years of follow-up, 8 children had negative results by urea breath test; 2 of these children had received antibiotics for other infections during the study period. However, the proportion of children who became *H. pylori*-negative was the same in children who took antibiotics during follow-up (2 of 12) and those who did not (6 of 36) [76]. Given the wide CI on the risk ratio for this comparison (RR: 1.0, CI: 0.23, 4.3), this study has insufficient data to draw conclusions about the effect of antibiotics taken for other illnesses on the *H. pylori* elimination rate. Rothenbacher *et al.* (2002) reported that German children who took antibiotics were more likely to eliminate *H. pylori* infection than children who did not take antibiotics [74]. Further investigation of *H. pylori* elimination by antibiotic type indicated that elimination of the infection was weakly associated with the use of penicillins or macrolides; the infection was eliminated in one of three children aged 1 and 2 years old who took cephalosporin or sulphonamide, while the infection was not eliminated in any of the 4 year old children who reported cephalosporin or sulphonamide use. Three eliminations were identified among children who did not take antibiotics during follow-up (one of six children aged 1 and 2 years, and two of four children aged 4 years) [74]. Similarly, spontaneous clearances of *H. pylori* infection were observed among children along the United States-Mexico border who were not exposed to antibiotics; however, the frequency of clearance was even higher among those who used antibiotics [75]. Of 197 children who tested positive by urea breath test and who provided data regarding antibiotic usage, 66% of those who did not take antibiotics tested negative for *H. pylori* at a later follow-up exam, 72% of those who took 1 or more systemic antibiotic courses of any type tested negative later, and 79% of those who took 1 or more *H. pylori*-effective antibiotic courses tested negative later. Furthermore, incidental exposure to antibiotics appeared to reduce the duration of the infection [75] (Table **9**).

No consistent pattern of association appears for sex and elimination of *H. pylori* infection (Table **9**). Boys appeared to be less likely to eliminate *H. pylori* infection than girls in a New Zealand study [68], with an estimated elimination rate ratio of 0.43 (no confidence interval reported). However, no clear association between sex and the elimination rate was observed in a study conducted in the United States [65] (Table **9**). Racial/ethnic differences in the *H. pylori* elimination rate were reported for a biracial cohort of children followed from 7-9 years of age to adulthood in the United States [64,65]. In the 2002 published report from this study, black children had 0.47 times the rate of elimination compared to white children (no confidence interval reported). It is unclear, however, whether these differences are confounded by socioenvironmental factors.

In summary, evidence suggests that spontaneous elimination of *H. pylori* infection occurs frequently in childhood, with little data on the occurrence of spontaneous elimination of this infection in adults. Evidence regarding factors associated with elimination of *H. pylori* infection is scant.

Table 6: Cohort studies of *H. pylori* infection in adults in Western Countries.

Location and Reference	**Study Population**	**Detection Method**	**Follow-Up Interval**	**No. of Exams**	**Study Duration(Years)**	**Sample Size**	**Age Range (Years)**	**IR %/Year (95% CI)**	**Eliminations (n) / *H. pylori*+ at Baseline (n)**
Western Europe									
Finland[1, [77]] 1996	Participants in gastritis studies	Serology (IgG, IgA)	1974, 1976-91	>2	Mean 15	181	Mean 53 (SD 12)	0.4 (0.23,	ND

Location and Reference	Study Population	Detection Method	Follow-Up Interval	No. of Exams	Study Duration(Years)	Sample Size	Age Range (Years)	IR %/Year (95% CI)	Eliminations (n) / *H. pylori*+ at Baseline (n)
Sipponen	with normal, non-infected gastric mucosa	and histology						0.80)	
Finland[1, [78]] 1997 Kosunen	Randomly selected residents of Vammala	Serology (IgG, IgA)	1973-94	2	Mean 21	126	15-74	0.3 (0.2, 0.6)	8 (98)
Switzerland [79] 2008 Tschopp	Sewage workers Municipal workers[2] Sewage workers Municipal workers[2]	Serology IgA IgG	Yearly	5		778	16-68	0.11 0.10 0.15 0.18	ND
North America									
Canada[1, [73]] 1994 Veldhuyzen van	Random sample, provincial medical	Serology	Before 1972	2-3	Mean 1.4	316	18-72	1.0 (0.31, 4.3)	3 (120)[3]
Zanten	insurance registry in Nova Scotia								
United States[1, [80]] 1992 Parsonnet	Epidemiologists	Serology	1969, 1987-88	2	Mean 8.5	287	26-35	0.5 (0.3, 0.9)	6 (63)
Oceania									
Australia[1, [16]] 1993 Cullen	Randomly selected participants of the Busselton Population Study (community based) with an oversampling of males for the purposes of a sleep study	Serology	1969 1978 1990	3	Mean 21	86	20-65	0.33 (0.08, 0.59)	4 (8)
Studies Focusing on Foreign Travel									
United States[1, [81]] 1997 Taylor	Army personnel in Persian Gulf service from August 1990 to April 1991	Serology	1990, 1991	3	Mean 0.5	111	19-35	7.3 (3.1, 13.5)	ND
Sweden[1] 1995 Lindkvist	Young Swedes traveling to developing countries	Serology	ND	2	Mean 0.7	103	12-31	0.0 (0.0, 5.1)	ND
United States[1, [82]] 1999 Becker	North American missionaries serving in developing countries	Serology	1967, 1984	2	Mean 7.4	259	Mean 39	1.9 (1.4, 2.7)	ND
United States[1, [36]] 1995	United States military personnel deployed to South America, West	Serology	1989, 1991	2-3	Mean 0.5	601	Mean 22	1.9 (0.60, 4.4)	ND

Location and Reference	Study Population	Detection Method	Follow-Up Interval	No. of Exams	Study Duration(Years)	Sample Size	Age Range (Years)	IR %/Year (95% CI)	Eliminations (n) / *H. pylori*+ at Baseline (n)
Hyams	Africa, Mediterranean								

IR, incidence rate; CI, confidence interval; IgA, immunoglobulin A antibodies; IgG, immunoglobulin G antibodies; ND, no data available in report.

[1] As cited in reference [61].

[2] Municipal workers include garbage collectors, gardeners, workers maintaining waterways, public transport workers and forestry workers.

[3] Estimated annual elimination rate: 1.6% (CI: 0.62, 8.5).

Table 7: Cohort studies of *H. pylori* infection in children 2 years of age and younger in Western Countries.

Location and Reference	Study Population	Detection Method	Follow-up Interval	No. of Exams	Study Duration(Years)	Sample Size	Age Range (Years)	IR %/Month (95% CI)	ER %/Month (95% CI)
Western Europe									
Belgium[71] 1994 Blecker	Prenatal clinic patients	Serology and UBT	12-15 months	2	1.25	67	0-1.25	0.13[4]	ND
Finland[67] 1996 Ashorn	Subjects in university hospital study of childhood diarrhea	Serology[1]	Ages 1,7, 12,18,24 months	4	2	195	0-2 Sub-intervals: 0-1 1-2	0.47[7] 0.13 (0.03, 0.37)[7] 0.31 (0.12, 0.61)[7]	ND
Germany[83] 2006 Weyermann	Newborns, mothers, and partners recruited in hospital	SAT	Ages 1,2, 3 years	3	3	841	1-2 2-3	0.09 (0.04, 0.17)[4] 0.12 (0.01, 0.02)[4]	ND
Italy[70] 2009 Baldassarre	Prenatal patients recruited at a teaching hospital	SAT	Ages 1, 6, 12, 18 months	4	1.5	180	0-1.5 Sub-intervals: 0-0.08 0.08-0.5 0.5-1 0.08-1.5	3.0 (1.1, 6.7)[4] 0.0 (0, 0.002)[4]	[3] 11.4 (1.4, 41)[4] 16.7 (3.4, 49)[4]
Sweden[84] 1997 Granström	Vaccine trial subjects	Serology[1]	Ages 6, 8, 10 months; 1, 1.5, 2	6	11		Sub-intervals: 0.83-1.5 1.5-2	0.53[7] 1.1[7]	[6]
North America									
United States and Mexico[63] 2005 Goodman	Children born to women recruited at maternal-child	UBT	Ages 6, 12, 18, 24 months	4	2	468	0-2 Sub-intervals: 0–0.5 0.5-1	1.7 (1.4, 2.0) 1.1 (0.77, 1.6) 2.1 (1.6, 2.8)	ND

	clinics in El Paso and Ciudad Juarez						1-1.5 1.5-2	1.6 (1.1, 2.4) 2.1 (1.4, 3.1)	
Updated in Broussard 2009[75]			Every 6 months, ages 6-84 months	13	7	218	0-7	ND	68 (61, 74)[2]
United States[66] 2006 Perry	Hispanic immigrant families in California	SAT	3 months	1	1	175	<2	1.7 (0.98, 2.8)[7]	ND

IR, incidence rate; ER, elimination rate, CI, confidence interval; UBT, urea breath test; SAT, stool antigen test; ND, no data presented in the report.
[1] Used stored samples from studies conducted for other purposes.
[2] Risk.
[3] All *H. pylori*-positive children spontaneously cleared the infection by 0.5 years of age.
[4] Incidence rate calculation based on the number of events and person-time follow-up presented in text.
[5] Reported no evidence of spontaneous clearance.
[6] Most children infected at younger ages had lost their infection by 11 years of age.
[7] Reported annual rate; rate divided by 12 to obtain monthly rate.

Table 8: Cohort studies of *H. pylori* infection in children aged 2 to 18 years in Western Countries.

Location and Reference	Study Population	Detection Method	Follow-up Interval	No. of Exams	Study Duration (Years)	Sample Size	Age Range, (Years)	IR %/Year (95% CI)	ER %Year (95% CI)
Western Europe									
Finland[85] 1995 Ashorn	Participants in a multicenter atherosclerosis study	Serology[a]	3 years	4	9	74	3-12	0.30	6.3
France[86] 1999 Ganga-Zandzou	Asymptomatic children	Endoscopy	Yearly	2	2	18	Mean 7.4 years (SD±4.4 years)	ND	3.8
Germany[74] 2002 Rothenbacher	Asymptomatic children	SAT	Yearly	2	1.3	180	1-4	7 (3, 14)	35 (20, 54)
Germany[83] 2006 Weyermann	Newborns, mothers, and partners	SAT	Ages 1, 2, 3 years	3	3	890	0-3 3	0.60	ND
Ireland[13] 2006 Rowland	Healthy children recruited by family doctors	UBT	Yearly	5	4	262 181 256 256 230	1.9-4 Sub-intervals: 2-3 3-4	5.1 (1.6, 11.8) 4.2 (1.9, 8.0) 2.1	[b]

Location and Reference	Study Population	Detection Method	Follow-up Interval	No. of Exams	Study Duration (Years)	Sample Size	Age Range, (Years)	IR %/Year (95% CI)	ER %Year (95% CI)
						200 85	4-5 5-6 6-7 7-8	(0.67, 4.8) 0.0 (0.0, 1.6) 0.68 (0.02, 3.8) 0.0 (0.0, 8.02)	
Italy[76] 1998 Perri	School children, *H. pylori*-positive	UBT	6 months	5	2	48	4.5-18.5	ND	10.6 (5.1, 19.4)[d]
Portugal[48] 2011 Oleastro	Vaccination program attendees	SAT	6 months	5	3	296	0-15 By age groups: 0-5 6-10 10-15 16-19	12 (8.7, 14.7) 11.5 (7.4, 16) 13 (8.0, 19) 10.5 (4.3, 19) 0.0 (0.0, 60)	ND
Sweden[84] 1997 Granström	Vaccine trial participants	Serology[a]	Ages 2,4, 11 years	6	11	294	0.5-11 Sub-intervals: 2-4 4-11	2.4 0.0	[c]
Sweden[87] 2002 Granquist	Children with α-1-antitrypsin deficiency detected at birth	Serology[a]	Ages 4,8, 12,16,18 years	5	14	168	4-18	0.12[d]	0.96[d]
North America									
Canada[62] 2004	Residents of rural First	SAT	Yearly	2	1	50	1-13	16	ND
Sinha	Nations (aboriginal community)								
United States[66] 2006	Hispanic immigrant families in	SAT Serology	3 months	1	1	304	<2-18+ 2-17	6.8 (4.6-9.8)	ND 3.1

Location and Reference	**Study Population**	**Detection Method**	**Follow-up Interval**	**No. of Exams**	**Study Duration (Years)**	**Sample Size**	**Age Range, (Years)**	**IR %/Year (95% CI)**	**ER %Year (95% CI)**
Perry	California						≥18	5.3 (2.4-9.6) 3.0 (0.9-6.5) 3.7	
United States[64] 1999 Malaty	Bogalusa Heart Study participants, Louisiana	Serology[a]	12 years	2	12	212	7-21	22	1.8
Updated in Malaty 2002[65]	Bogalusa Heart Study participants, Louisiana (different from 1999 subjects)		ND	8	20	226	1-21 Sub-intervals: 4-5 7-9 13-15 21-23	1.4 2.1 1.5 1.0 0.30	ND
Oceania									
New Zealand[68] 1998 Fawcett	Dunedin health study participants	Serology[a]	10 years	2	10	465	11-21	0.11	0.37
Update of Fawcett 2005[88]			Ages 11, 21, 26 years	3	16	452	11-26 Sub-intervals: 11-21 11-26	0.53 0.11 0.44	0.11 0.35 0.04

IR, incidence rate; ER, elimination rate, CI, confidence interval.
[a] Used stored samples from studies conducted for other purposes.
[b] Reported no evidence of spontaneous clearance.
[c] Most children infected at younger ages had lost their infection by 11 years of age.
[d] Incidence or elimination rate calculation based on the number of events and person-time follow-up presented in text.

Recurrence

Gisbert (2005) reviewed the evidence regarding the recurrence of *H. pylori* infection [89]. Evidence indicates that the *H. pylori* recurrence rate after eradication is relatively low in western countries (estimated mean annual reinfection rate, 4.6% per year, CI: 4.2, 5.0). Recurrence of *H. pylori* infection can result from either recrudescence of an infection temporarily suppressed by antibiotic therapy, or reinfection after successful eradication of *H. pylori*. Gisbert points out that recrudescence may be responsible for most recurrences for two reasons: 1) recurrences decrease with time and decline sharply after the first year, and 2) genetically identical microorganisms have been identified before and after eradication therapy. Furthermore, using antibiotic therapy known to have lower efficacy increases the frequency of *H. pylori* recurrence. Gisbert suggests that selecting a lower cut-off value for the urea breath test may provide better diagnostic accuracy for monitoring *H. pylori* clearance given evidence that patients deemed cured who later suffer a recurrence have higher post-treatment breath test values within the negative range on average.

Factors Associated with the Recurrence of *H. pylori* Infection

Intrafamilial clustering of *H. pylori* infection has been investigated for its potential role in recurrence; however, findings have been inconclusive. In a treatment trial conducted in the United Kingdom by Farrell *et al.* (2004), fifty families each with an *H. pylori*-infected pediatric index child (mean age 9.5 years) were randomized into an 'index case treatment' group (only the index case was treated) or a 'family unit treatment' group (all infected family members were treated) (as cited in [89]). Families were followed for a mean of 62 months and tested with the urea breath test. In the 'index case treatment' group the reinfection rate was 2.4% per year and in the 'family unit treatment' group the reinfection rate was 0.7% per year (p-value=0.31) [90]. While the p-value on this comparison is relatively high, it should be noted that only 3 children in the 'index case treatment' group were reinfected with *H. pylori.* In a study conducted in Spain by Gisbert (2002), 120 patients were followed for one year to investigate the role of the partner's infection status on reinfection after *H. pylori* clearance (as cited in [89]). By the end of follow-up, 8 reinfections occurred (recurrence rate, 6.8% per year). Of the 8 reinfected subjects, 7 spouses were *H. pylori*-positive (87%), and of the 112 non-reinfected subjects 85 spouses were *H. pylori*-positive (76%) (odds ratio (OR)=2.9, CI: 0.29, 29; adjusted by age, breath test value, and anti-*H. pylori* therapy). Further molecular analysis of *H. pylori* strains in 3 subjects and their spouses revealed that the strains were different in all cases [91]. In conclusion, there is very little data on predictors of *H. pylori* recurrence in western countries.

H. pylori Transmission Pathways in Western Countries

Despite extensive research employing diverse disciplinary approaches to investigate how *H. pylori* spreads, the major modes of transmission have not been clearly identified. While much evidence suggests that spread commonly occurs through contact with digestive tract secretions from infected human hosts, the relative importance of fecal-oral, oral-oral or gastric-oral (through regurgitation) pathways remains uncertain. Further, it remains unclear whether water or other environmental reservoirs play a major role in the endemicity of the infection [1,3].

Evidence of Direct Person-to-Person Transmission

Several studies have attempted to investigate intrafamilial transmission of *H. pylori* as the major source of infection; however, inconsistent findings have been reported across studies (Tables **3**, **5**, and **9**).

Moderate to strong associations between maternal prevalence of *H. pylori* infection and child's prevalence of *H. pylori* infection have been observed in studies conducted in Germany and Ireland (as cited in [19]), as well as along the United States–Mexico border [7]. From a study conducted in Ulm, Germany, Weyermann (2009) reported a strong association of maternal *H. pylori* status at the time of the child's birth with the child's *H. pylori* status at age 3 years [19]. Children with an *H. pylori*-positive mother had 13 times the odds of *H. pylori* positivity than those with an *H. pylori*-negative mother (OR=13.0, CI: 3.0, 55.2; adjusted for *H. pylori* status of spouse and of siblings, nationality of parents, and single-child status). It is worth noting, however, that while the *H. pylori* prevalence among German 3 year olds born to *H. pylori*-negative mothers was just 0.9%, it was still quite low, at 10.9%, among those born to *H. pylori*-positive mothers. Blecker *et al.* (1994) followed from birth infants born to *H. pylori*-positive women recruited at an antenatal care clinic in Belgium [71]. At birth, 35 of the newborns had positive anti-*H. pylori* IgG and were tested for anti-*H. pylori* IgM and IgG levels every 3 months for 1 year. By 12 months IgG levels were negative in all 35 of these newborns and all tested negative throughout the year for IgM, a marker of active *H. pylori* infection. From the same study population of *H. pylori* infected mothers, 67 children were tested with the urea breath test at the ages of 12 and 15 months: only one had a positive breath test. These results suggest that *H. pylori* was not transmitted readily to the infants by their infected mothers. Similar results were reported by Ashorn *et al.* (1996) for a birth cohort study of Finnish children followed until 2 years of age [67]; maternal antibodies for *H. pylori* were found in 21 children as measured by serum IgG antibodies, although these antibodies disappeared in 20 children before the age of 7 months and no new acquisitions of *H. pylori* were identified in these children.

Positive associations of inconsistent magnitude between the paternal prevalence of *H. pylori* infection and the child's prevalence have been reported from studies conducted in Australia, Italy, Germany, Ireland, and the United States (as cited in [3,19]). Some studies have investigated family history of peptic ulcer as a proxy for *H. pylori* infection in childhood. In a study by Brenner *et al.* (1998), maternal history of ulcer was associated with an increased prevalence of *H. pylori* infection in German children; however, paternal history of ulcer was minimally associated with the prevalence of *H. pylori* infection in children (as cited in [3]).

Epidemiologic evidence provided by studies conducted in Australia, Germany (as cited in [1,3,19]), and along the United States-Mexico border [72], shows a positive association between having an *H. pylori*-positive sibling and acquiring *H. pylori* infection. In the United States-Mexico birth cohort study, having an older sibling with persistent *H. pylori* infection was strongly associated with the incidence of *H. pylori* infection in younger siblings (hazard ratio=2.8, CI: 1.6, 4.9); the association was even stronger when the age between siblings was 3 years or less (hazard ratio=3.7, CI: 1.5, 8.7) [72]. Similar patterns of sibling transmission were observed when results were stratified by country of residence [72].

Several studies carried out in England, Germany, Ireland, Scotland, United States, Wales (as cited in [2,3]), Portugal [48], and along the United States–Mexico border [69], investigated the effect of variables associated with household crowding and/or family composition (birth order, number of siblings, number of children currently living in the household, number of children <18 years in the household, crowding index, number of people per room, square meter per person in home, and sharing a bedroom or bed) on the frequency of *H. pylori* infection (Tables **3** and **5**). In several studies, the prevalence of *H. pylori* infection increased as the number of siblings increased (Tables **3** and **5**). Bed-sharing was also a predictor of *H. pylori* prevalence in children; sharing a bed with an *H. pylori*-infected sibling was strongly associated with *H. pylori* prevalence in a study by Farell *et al.* (2005) in Ireland, (as cited in [19]). Other indicators of household crowding have inconsistent associations with *H. pylori* prevalence or incidence across studies.

Evidence of direct person-to-person transmission of *H. pylori* has been generated by studies that examine exposure to crowded settings such as institutions for the disabled, daycare centers, and submarines. In studies by Oleastro *et al.* (2011) in Portugal [48] and by Vincent *et al.* (1994) in France (as cited in [3]), residence in an institution and nursery school or kindergarten attendance was related to an increased prevalence of *H. pylori* in childhood. Conversely, in a study by Staat *et al.* (1996), daycare attendance was inversely related with the prevalence of *H. pylori* in children from the United States (as cited in [3]).

Fecal-Oral Route

Bin Saeed (2010) conducted a systematic review to evaluate evidence of the relationship between hepatitis A virus (HAV) and *H. pylori* infection [44]. Known to be spread primarily though fecal-oral transmission, HAV has been used as a proxy for ingestion of fecal matter contaminated with pathogens; thus positive associations between positivity for HAV and *H. pylori* infection are viewed as evidence of a shared transmission pathway (Table **3**). Moderate to strong associations between positivity for HAV and *H. pylori* were observed in studies of adult populations by Rudi *et al.* (1997) in Germany; Luzza *et al.* (1997), Pretolani *et al.* (1997), and Stroffolini *et al.* (1998) in Italy; *et al.* Hyams (1995) in the United States; and Webb *et al.* (1996) in the United Kingdom (ORs ranging between 1.9 and 5.7) (as cited in [44]). The strong associations between HAV and *H. pylori* observed in the 3 studies conducted in Italy became weaker after adjustment for potential confounders. Bin Saeed concluded that the reported associations between positivity for HAV and *H. pylori* are typically overestimated as the associations become weak after controlling for confounding factors (age and socioeconomic related factors).

Studies from the United States (as cited in [3]), the United States-Mexico border [7,69], Switzerland [79], and England (as cited in [2]) have investigated several factors as proxies for fecal-oral transmission of *H. pylori* infection with inconsistent results (Tables **3**, **5**, **6** and **9**). The birth cohort study of children living along the United States-Mexico border examined various indicators of fecal-oral transmission [69]. Minimal associations with the incidence of *H. pylori* infection were observed for the mother's hand washing habits after changing diapers, the type of sanitary facility (flush toilet, latrine), or having a sewer connection to the house. Likewise, a cohort study among workers in Switzerland did not find a difference in the incidence of *H. pylori* infection when comparing sewage workers to municipal workers (incidence rates were 0.11% per year and 0.10% per year, respectively) [79].

Oral-Oral Route

Dental plaque has been implicated as a possible source of *H. pylori* infection; however, attempts to identify the bacterium in the mouth through bacterial culturing techniques have yielded inconclusive results [1]. In a study by Peach *et al.* (1997), the prevalence of *H. pylori* infection among adults in Australia was associated with high plaque score (OR=1.7, CI: 1.1, 2.7) and with visiting the dentist less than once a year (OR=4.4, CI: 0.8, 23.0) (as cited in [1]). An exposure investigated as a potential vehicle for oral-oral transmission is chopstick use, associated with the practice of family members eating from the same bowl. In a study by Chow *et al.* (1995), the prevalence of *H. pylori* among Chinese immigrants in Melbourne, Australia was associated with the use of chopsticks independently of age and socioeconomic status (crude OR=2.0 (p-value <0.047) for males and OR=2.5 (p-value <0.001) for females; adjusted OR=1.7 (p-value 0.014) for females and OR=1.4 (p-value 0.031) for males and females) [35]; however, chopstick use among immigrants may be related to other factors associated with acculturation.

Gastro-Oral Route

Evidence of gastro-oral transmission of *H. pylori* comes from a study of gastroenteritis and *H. pylori* infection in Hispanic immigrant families in the United States [66]. Exposure to an *H. pylori*-infected household member with gastroenteritis was strongly associated with the acquisition of a new *H. pylori* infection when compared to exposure to an *H. pylori*-infected household member without gastroenteritis (OR=4.8, CI: 1.4, 17; adjusted for age, sleeping density, and proportion of household contacts completing both visits). When an *H. pylori*-infected household member had gastroenteritis accompanied by vomiting and/or diarrhea, the risk of acquiring a new *H. pylori* infection was 6 times higher than the risk when exposed to an *H. pylori*-infected household member with gastroenteritis but with no vomiting or diarrhea (OR=6.3, CI: 1.6, 24; adjusted for age, sleeping density, proportion of household completing both visits, and a random household effect). The positive association for exposure to a household member suffering from vomiting with or without diarrhea was considerably stronger than the positive association observed for exposure to a household member suffering from diarrhea alone. These results suggest that *H. pylori* is spread most readily when the infected host suffers from gastroenteritis, particularly if it is accompanied by vomiting.

Evidence of Waterborne Transmission

The role of water in *H. pylori* transmission has been explored in a few epidemiologic studies (Tables **3** and **5**). In a study by Herbarth *et al.* (2001), German children who used a non-municipal water source had almost 3 times the odds of *H. pylori* infection compared to children who used municipal water supplies as their source of drinking water (OR=2.8, CI: 1.0, 8.2) (as cited in [45]). In the United States-Mexico birth cohort study, children who consumed bottled water had a lower incidence of *H. pylori* compared to those who used municipal water (incidence rate ratio=0.71, CI: 0.50, 1.0) [69]. However, further details of this study reported by Travis *et al.* (2007) showed imprecise weak or null associations between the incidence of *H. pylori* infection and drinking water quality (municipal purified, municipal not purified, and bottled/vending machine), child's bathing water source, and bathing or swimming in a river or pool and [69].

Evidence of Zoonotic Transmission

Humans appear to be the principal reservoir for *H. pylori* infection. Although *H. pylori* has been isolated from nonhuman primates and domestic cats (as cited in [1]), evidence to support zoonotic transmission as a major mode of spread is lacking. Associations between contact with animals (pets or farm animals) and the prevalence or incidence of *H. pylori* infection in childhood has been investigated in studies conducted in Portugal [48], along the United States–Mexico border [69]; and in the United States, England, and Germany (as cited in [2,3]). Minimal to null associations were observed in the majority of studies that investigated such relationships (Tables **3** and **5**). The studies conducted in the United States by Fiedorek *et al.* (1991) (as cited in [2]) and Staat *et al.* (1996) (as cited in [3]), revealed that *H. pylori* prevalence was lower in children whose family had a pet in the house than in those without pets. However, these findings might be explained by higher socioeconomic status associated with pet ownership.

Evidence of Iatrogenic Transmission

Historical studies have revealed a few instances in which transmission of *H. pylori* appears to have occurred in patient care and clinical research settings through gastroscopes and gastric pH electrodes (as cited in [2]). Given that endoscopic examinations are routinely conducted for the diagnosis and treatment of gastrointestinal diseases, the potential for iatrogenic transmission of *H. pylori* through contaminated gastroscopes has been investigated. A few studies have shown that the potential for transmission of *H. pylori* during gastroscopy depends on the protocols followed for disinfecting gastroscopes. Cronmiller *et al.* (1999) found in a study conducted in Rochester, New York (as cited in [1]) that manual pre-cleaning alone did not completely remove *H. pylori* from endoscopes, although it reduced the absolute number of bacteria [92]. They reported that *H. pylori* transmission can be prevented by manual cleaning followed by ≥20 minutes of immersion in glutaraldehyde and ethanol drying or by the automated STERIS system [92]. A study conducted by Fantry *et al.* (1995) in Baltimore, (as cited in [1]), revealed that endoscopes were contaminated with *H. pylori* after 61% of procedures performed on *H. pylori*-infected patients. They reported that all endoscopes were negative for *H. pylori* after both manual and automated disinfection [93]. Nurnberg *et al.* (2003) [94] studied 400 German patients undergoing upper gastrointestinal endoscopy to determine whether conventional cleaning and disinfection techniques avoid the risk of endoscopic *H. pylori* transmission. They found that 42% (54/128) of the endoscopes used on *H. pylori*–positive patients were contaminated before cleaning and disinfection. After manual cleaning and disinfection, 1 of 54 endoscopes was contaminated with *H. pylori,* indicating that the cleaning and disinfection procedures employed may be insufficient to eliminate *H. pylori* from endoscopes. However, the patient who was examined with the contaminated endoscope tested *H. pylori*-seronegative 5 months after the endoscopic examination [94]. In summary, it appears that current guidelines for disinfecting gastroscopes minimize iatrogenic spread of *H. pylori*, although it may occur in rare instances.

PUBLIC HEALTH IMPLICATIONS

Epidemiologic studies published in western countries show consistently that *H. pylori* infection occurs most frequently in low-income communities with overcrowding and poor sanitation. Incidence rates of *H. pylori* infection in western countries are relatively low on average, with the highest rates occurring in early childhood, particularly in subgroups of children in which poverty and crowding are common. Evidence regarding the frequency of spontaneous elimination of *H. pylori* infection is scant, although findings from 3 cohort studies suggest that spontaneous elimination of *H. pylori* infection frequently occurs in childhood; all 3 of these studies observed elimination of *H. pylori* infection in children who did not take antibiotics for other illnesses.

Given that the development of cost-effective measures aimed at reducing health risks from *H. pylori* infection requires accurate information on the occurrence of this infection by person, place, and time, as well as identification of determinants of acquisition and persistence, limitations of the available evidence should be noted. Most of the evidence comes from cross-sectional studies, which have the limitation of temporal ambiguity and thus cannot differentiate factors that influence the acquisition of *H. pylori* infection from those that determine its persistence. Several of the longitudinal studies included in this review were limited by infrequent follow-up visits; this is an important limitation because longer intervals increase the probability of missing changes in *H. pylori* infection status, with correspondingly increased underestimation of infection events. Some of the studies that used methods to control for confounding used suboptimal methods for ascertaining important confounders, such as antibiotic intake, which may have resulted in inadequate control of confounding. Furthermore, epidemiologic research on *H. pylori* infection in human populations relies on methods for detection of the bacterium with variable accuracy across geographic locations and age groups [4]. A common limitation across the studies reviewed here is insufficient use of bias analysis methods for optimal interpretation of study results [95].

Research aimed at developing effective vaccines against *H. pylori* has encountered formidable obstacles; few candidates for human trials have emerged and prospects for success remain unclear [96]. The literature includes very little investigation of other interventions aimed at preventing *H. pylori* infection, perhaps due to persisting uncertainty regarding modes of transmission and risk factors for acquisition. Without evidence from such research, there is no basis for implementing primary prevention measures. For example, there is no clear evidence that treatment of infected family members reduces recurrence in individuals treated for *H. pylori* infection, thus it is difficult to justify screening and treating asymptomatic family members to protect treated individuals.

The small body of public health research pertaining to *H. pylori* infection has focused on infection control measures to reduce the risk of adverse health consequences of the infection. These measures rely on screening people to identify those who are infected and offering therapy to eliminate the infection. One obstacle to this approach is the need for more effective treatments against *H. pylori*, particularly for high-prevalence subpopulations, given that these groups often have relatively high treatment failure rates [97]. Even given suboptimal treatment regimens, however, a growing body of evidence shows that most *H. pylori* screening and treatment strategies considered are cost-effective for prevention of *H. pylori*-associated disease outcomes in most populations studied. The evidence is less compelling, however, for comparing the cost-effectiveness of alternative public health strategies, such as targeting population subgroups or using alternate detection methods and schedules for screening.

From a review of the health economics of *H. pylori* infection, Moayyedi (2007) [98] concluded that existing cost-effectiveness studies provide compelling evidence that a test and treat strategy for *H. pylori* is cost-effective compared to endoscopic investigation and acid-suppressive maintenance therapy for the management of peptic ulcer disease and dyspepsia, although the cost-effectiveness of this approach to the management of dyspepsia is reduced in the United States due to the higher cost of treatment. In contrast, Moayyedi concluded that there is insufficient information to justify population screening and treatment strategies for *H. pylori*-associated disease prevention in western countries.

Recent evidence comes from a community-based intervention in Odense, Denmark that randomized around 20,000 40- to-64-year-old residents to *H. pylori* screening and treatment or no intervention [18]. After 5 years, investigators estimated the effect of the program on rates of *H. pylori*-associated diseases, health care costs, and health related quality of life. The clearest benefit of the program was a 33% reduction in the incidence of peptic ulcers. The cost of dyspepsia related health care was lower in the screened group, but the savings were exceeded by the program costs. While the intervention was not cost saving, it might be considered cost-effective for prevention of peptic ulcer disease, given that the total expenditure could be considered reasonable for the number of peptic ulcer cases prevented.

Despite the sizable body of literature published on the epidemiology of *H. pylori* infection in western countries, several questions remain regarding how *H. pylori* spreads and which factors determine acquisition, elimination, and recurrence of the infection. These gaps in knowledge limit the development of effective interventions that may prevent the spread of *H. pylori* infection in vulnerable western populations.

ACKNOWLEDGEMENT

While contributing to this chapter, Mónica S. Sierra was supported by the Canadian Institutes of Health Research (FRN 115031), Emily V. Hastings was supported by a graduate studentship from The Nasivvik Centre for Inuit Health and Changing Environments, Katharine Fagan-Garcia was supported by the ArcticNet Network of Centres of Excellence, Amy Colquhoun was supported by a Vanier Canada Graduate Scholarship funded by the Canadian Institutes of Health Research, and Karen J. Goodman was supported by a Health Senior Scholar award from Alberta Innovates Health Solutions.

CONFLICT OF INTEREST

The authors do not have any financial conflict of interest to disclose.

REFERENCES

[1] Brown L: *Helicobacter pylori*: epidemiology and routes of transmission. Epidemiol Rev 2000; 22: 283-97.

[2] Goodman KJ, Correa P: The transmission of *Helicobacter pylori*. A critical review of the evidence. Int J Epidemiol 1995; 24: 875-87.

[3] Torres J, Pérez-Pérez G, Goodman K, Atherton J, Gold B, Harris P *et al.*: A comprehensive review of the natural history of *Helicobacter pylori* infection in children. Arch Med Res 2000; 31: 431-69.

[4] Goodman KJ, Cockburn M: The role of epidemiology in understanding the health effects of *Helicobacter pylori*. Epidemiology 2001; 12: 266-71.

[5] Frenck JRW, Clemens J: *Helicobacter* in the developing world. Microbes and Infection 2003; 5: 705-13.

[6] Staat MA, Kruszon-Moran D, McQuillan G, Kaslow R: A population-based serologic survey of *Helicobacter pylori* infection in children and adolescents in the United States. J Infect Dis 1996; 174: 1120-23.

[7] O'Rourke K, Goodman KJ, Grazioplene M, Redlinger T, Day R: Determinants of Geographic Variation in *Helicobacter pylori* Infection among Children on the US-Mexico Border. Am J Epidemiol 2003; 158: 816-24.

[8] Goodman KJ, Jacobson K, Veldhuyzen van Zanten S: *Helicobacter pylori* infection in Canadian and related Arctic Aboriginal populations. Can J Gastroenterol 2008; 22: 289-95.

[9] *Helicobacter* and Cancer Collaborative Group: Gastric cancer and *Helicobacter pylori*: a combined analysis of 12 case control studies nested within prospective cohorts. Gut 2001; 49: 347-53.

[10] De SA, Cornelis K, Van WM, Moens G, Devlies G, Derthoo D *et al.*: The occupational risk of *Helicobacter pylori* infection among workers in institutions for people with intellectual disability. Occupational and Environmental Medicine 2008; 65: 587-91.

[11] Webb PM, Knight T, Greaves S, Wilson A, Newell DG, Elder J *et al.*: Relation between infection with *Helicobacter pylori* and living conditions in childhood: evidence for person to person transmission in early life. BMJ (Clinical Research Ed) 1994; 308: 750-53.

[12] Megraud F, Brassens-Rabbe MP, Denis F, Belbouri A, Hoa DQ: Seroepidemiology of Campylobacter *pylori* infection in various populations. J Clin Microbiol 1989; 27: 1870-73.

[13] Rowland M, Daly L, Vaughan M, Higgins A, Bourke B, Drumm B: Age-specific incidence of *Helicobacter pylori*. Gastroenterology 2006; 130: 65-72.

[14] Graham DY, Malaty HM, Evans DG, Evans DJ, Klein PD, Adam E: Epidemiology of *Helicobacter pylori* in an asymptomatic population in the United States. Gastroenterol 1991; 100: 1495-1501.

[15] Zhu J, Davidson M, Leinonen M, Saikku P, Gaydos CA, Canos DA *et al.*: Prevalence and persistence of antibodies to herpes viruses, Chlamydia pneumoniae and *Helicobacter pylori* in Alaskan Eskimos: the GOCADAN Study. Clin Microbiol Infect 2006;, 12: 118-22.

[16] Cullen DJE, Collins BJ, Christiansen KJ, Epis J, Warren JR, Surveyor I *et al.*: When is *Helicobacter pylori* infection acquired? Gut 1993; 34: 1681-82.

[17] Lin SK, Lambert JR, Schembri MA, Nicholson L, Johnson IH: The prevalence of *Helicobacter pylori* in practising dental staff and dental students. Austr Dental J 1998; 43: 35-9.

[18] Azevedo NF, Huntington J, Goodman KJ: The epidemiology of *Helicobacter pylori* and public health implications. *Helicobacter* 2009; 14: 1-7.

[19] Weyermann M, Rothenbacher D, Brenner H: Acquisition of *Helicobacter pylori* infection in early childhood: independent contributions of infected mothers, fathers, and siblings. Am J Gastroenterol 2009; 104: 182-89.

[20] Ford AC, Axon AT: Epidemiology of *Helicobacter pylori* infection and public health implications. *Helicobacter* 2010; 15: 1-6.

[21] Bohmer CJ, Klinkenberg-Knol EC, Kuipers EJ, Niezen-de Boer MC, Schreuder H, Schuckink-Kool F *et al.*: The prevalence of *Helicobacter pylori* infection among inhabitants and healthy employees of institutes for the intellectually disabled. Am J Gastroenterol 1997; 92: 1000-04.

[22] Kivi M, Johansson AL, Reilly M, Tindberg Y: *Helicobacter pylori* status in family members as risk factors for infection in children. Epidemiol Infect 2005; 133: 645-52.

[23] Mitchell HM, Bohane T, Hawkes RA, Lee A: *Helicobacter pylori* infection within families. International Journal of Medical Microbiology 1993; 280: 128-36.

[24] Morris A, Nicholson G, Lloyd G, Haines D, Rogers A, Taylor D: Seroepidemiology of *Campylobacter pyloridis*. NZ Med J 1986; 99: 657-59.

[25] Fontham ETH, Ruiz B, Perez A, Hunter F, Correa P: Determinants of *Helicobacter pylori* infection and chronic gastritis. Am J Gastroenterol 1995; 90: 1094-104.

[26] Thoene J, Burken M, Hopkins RJ, Russell RG, Morris JG: Seropositivity to Helicobacter-*pylori*: Lack of association with length of hospitalization. Journal of Clinical Microbiology 1991; 29: 1392-96.

[27] Polish LB, Douglas JM, Jr., Davidson AJ, Perez-Perez GI, Blaser MJ: Characterization of risk factors for *Helicobacter pylori* infection among men attending a sexually transmitted disease clinic: lack of evidence for sexual transmission. J Clin Microbiol 1991;, 29: 2139-43.

[28] Braden B, Duan LP, Caspary WF, Lembcke B: Endoscopy is not a risk factor for *Helicobacter pylori* infection--but medical practice is. Gastrointest Endoscopy 1997; 46: 305-310.

[29] Reiff A, Jacobs E, Kist M: Seroepidemiological study of the immune response to *Campylobacter pylori* in potential risk groups. European Journal of Clinical Microbiology and Infectious Diseases: Official Publication of The European Society of Clinical Microbiology 1989; 8: 592-96.

[30] Rudi J, Toppe H, Marx N, Zuna I, Theilmann L, Stremmel W *et al.*: Risk of infection with *Helicobacter pylori* and hepatitis A virus in different groups of hospital workers. Am J Gastroenterol 1997; 92: 258-62.

[31] Peach HG, Pearce DC, Farish SJ: *Helicobacter pylori* infection in an Australian regional city: prevalence and risk factors. Med J Austr 1997,;167: 310-13.

[32] Hammermeister I, Janus G, Schamarowski F, Rudolf M, Jacobs E, Kist M: Elevated risk of *Helicobacter pylori* infection in submarine crews. European Journal of Clinical Microbiology and Infectious Diseases: Official Publication of The European Society of Clinical Microbiology 1992; 11: 9-14.

[33] Brenner H, Rothenbacher D, Bode G, Dieudonne P, Adler G: Active infection with *Helicobacter pylori* in healthy couples. Epidemiology and Infection 1998; 122: 91-5.

[34] Perez-Perez GI, Witkin SS, Decker MD, Blaser MJ: Seroprevalence of *Helicobacter pylori* infection in couples. J Clin Microbiol 1991; 29: 642-44.

[35] Chow TK, Lambert JR, Wahlqvist ML, Hsu-Hage BH: *Helicobacter pylori* in Melbourne Chinese immigrants: evidence for oral-oral transmission *via* chopsticks. J Gastroenterol Hepatology 1995; 10: 562-69.

[36] Hyams KC, Taylor DN, Gray GC, Knowles JB, Hawkins R, Malone JD: The risk of *Helicobacter pylori* infection among U.S. military personnel deployed outside the United States. Am J Trop Med Hyg 1995; 52: 109-12.

[37] Fraser AG, Scragg R, Metcalf P, McCullough S, Yeates NJ: Prevalence of *Helicobacter pylori* infection in different ethnic groups in New Zealand children and adults. Austr N Z J Med 1996; 26: 646-51.

[38] Epidemiology of, and risk factors for, *Helicobacter pylori* infection among 3194 asymptomatic subjects in 17 populations. The EUROGAST Study Group. Gut 1993; 34: 1672-76.

[39] Brenner H, Rothenbacher D, Bode G+, Adler G: Relation of Smoking and Alcohol and Coffee Consumption to Active *Helicobacter pylori* Infection: Cross Sectional Study. Brit Med J 1997; 315: 1489-92.

[40] Brenner H, Berg G, Lappus N, Kliebsch U, Bode G, Boeing H: Alcohol Consumption and *Helicobacter pylori* Infection: Results from the German National Health and Nutrition Survey. Epidemiology 1999; 214-18.

[41] Brenner H, Rothenbacher D, Bode G, Adler G: Inverse graded relation between alcohol consumption and active infection with *Helicobacter pylori*. Am J Epidemiol 1999; 149: 571-76.

[42] Lin SK, Lambert JR, Nicholson L, Lukito W, Wahlqvist M: Prevalence of *Helicobacter pylori* in a representative Anglo-Celtic population of urban Melbourne. J Gastroenterol Hepatol 1998; 13: 505-10.

[43] Gasbarrini G, Pretolani S, Bonvicini F, Gatto MR, Tonelli E, M+¬graud F *et al.*: A population based study of *Helicobacter pylori* infection in a European country: the San Marino Study. Relations with gastrointestinal diseases. Gut 1995; 36: 838-44.

[44] BinSaeed AA: Is there a link between seropositivity to *Helicobacter pylori* and hepatitis A virus? A systematic review. [Review] [34 refs]. Int J Infects Dis 2010; 14: e567-e571.

[45] Bellack NR, Koehoorn MW, MacNab YC, Morshed MG: A conceptual model of water's role as a reservoir in *Helicobacter pylori* transmission: a review of the evidence. Epidemiology and Infection 2006; 134: 439-49.

[46] Redlinger T, O'Rourke K, Goodman K: Age distribution of *Helicobacter pylori* seroprevalence among young children in a United States/Mexico border community: evidence for transitory infection. Am J Epidemiol 1999; 150: 225-30.

[47] Krumbiegel P, Lehmann I, Alfreider A, Fritz GJ, Boeckler D, Rolle-Kampczyk U *et al.*: *Helicobacter pylori* determination in non-municipal drinking water and epidemiological findings. Isotopes in Environmental and Health Studies 2004; 40: 75-81.

[48] Oleastro M, Pelerito A, Nogueira P, Benoliel J, Santos A, Cabral J *et al.*: Prevalence and incidence of *Helicobacter pylori* Infection in a healthy pediatric population in the Lisbon area. *Helicobacter* 2011; 16: 363-72.

[49] Fiedorek SC, Malaty HM, Evans DL, Pumphrey CL, Casteel HB, Evans DJ *et al.*: Factors influencing the epidemiology of *Helicobacter pylori* infection in children. Pediatrics 1991; 88: 578-82.

[50] Malaty HM, Graham DY, Klein PD, Evans DG, Adam E, Evans DJ: Transmission of *Helicobacter pylori* infection. Studies in families of healthy individuals. Scand J Gastroenterol 1991; 26: 927-32.

[51] Dominici P, Belentani S, Di Biase AR, Saccoccio G, Le Rose A, Masutti F *et al.*: Familial clustering of *Helicobacter pylori* infection: population based study. Brit Med J 1999; 319: 537-41.

[52] Perri F, Pastore M, Leandro G, Clemente R, Ghoos Y, Peeters M *et al.*: *Helicobacter pylori* infection and growth delay in older children. Arch Dis Childhood 1997; 77: 46-9.

[53] Blecker U, Hauser B, Lanciers S, Peeters S, Suys B, Vandenplas Y: The prevalence of *Helicobacter pylori*-positive serology in asympatomatic children. J Pediatr Gastroenterol Nutr 1993; 16: 252-56.

[54] Rothenbacher D, Bode G, Berg G, Gommel R, Gonser T, Adler G *et al.*: Prevalence and determinants of *Helicobacter pylori* infection in preschool children: a population-based study from Germany. Int J Epidemiol 1998; 27: 135-41.

[55] Elitsur Y, Short JP, Neace C: Prevalence of *Helicobacter pylori* Infection in Children from Urban and Rural West Virginia. Digestive Diseases and Sciences 1998; 43: 773-78.

[56] Vincent P, Gottrand F, Pernes P, Husson MO, Lecomte-Houcke M, Turck D *et al.*: High prevalence of *Helicobacter pylori* infection in cohabitating children. Epidemiology of a cluster, with special emphasis on molecular typing. Gut 1994; 35: 313-16.

[57] Rothenbacher D, Bode G, Berg G, Knayer U, Gosner T, Adler G *et al.*: *Helicobacter pylori* among preschool children and their parents: evidence of parent-child transmission. J Infect Dis 1999; 179: 398-402.

[58] Brenner H, Rothenbacher D, Bode G, Adler G: Parental History of gastric or duodenal ulcer and prevalence of *Helicobacter pylori* infection in preschool children: population based study. Brit Med J; 1998, 316: 665.

[59] Brenner H, Rothenbacher D, Bode G, Gommel R, Berg G, Adler G: Parental smoking and infection with *Helicobacter pylori* among preschool children in Southern Germany. Epidemiology 1998; 9: 545-49.

[60] Bode G, Rothenbacher D, Brenner H, Adler G: Pets are not a risk factor for *Helicobacter pylori* infection in young children: results of a population-based study in Southern Germany. Pediatr Infect Dis J 1998; 17: 909-12.

[61] Everhart JE: Recent developments in the epidemiology of *Helicobacter pylori.* Gastroenterol Clin N Am 2000; 29: 559-78.

[62] Sinha SK, Martin B, Gold BD, Song Q, Sargent M, Bernstein CN: The incidence of *Helicobacter pylori* acquisition in children of a Canadian First Nations Community and the potential for parent-to-child transmission. *Helicobacter* 2004; 9: 59-68.

[63] Goodman KJ, O'Rourke K, Day RS, Wang C, Nurgalieva Z, Phillips CV *et al.*: Dynamics of *Helicobacter pylori* infection in a US-Mexico cohort during the first two years of life. Int J Epidemiology 2005; 34: 1348-55.

[64] Malaty HM, Graham D, Wattigney W, Srinivasan S, Osato M, Berenson G: Natural history of *Helicobacter pylori* infection in childhood: 12-year follow-up cohort study in a biracial community. Clinical infectious diseases: an official publication of the Infectious Dis Soc Am 1999; 28: 279-82.

[65] Malaty HM, El-Kasabany A, Graham D, Miller C, Reddy S, Srinivasan S *et al.*: Age at acquisition of *Helicobacter pylori* infection: a follow-up study from infancy to adulthood. Lancet 2002, 2: 9310.

[66] Perry S, de la Luz SM, Yang S, Haggerty TD, Hurst P, Perez-Perez G *et al.*: Gastroenteritis and transmission of *Helicobacter pylori* infection in households. Emerg Infect Dis 2006; 12: 1701-08.

[67] Ashorn M, Miettinen A, Ruuska T, Laippala P, Maki M: Seroepidemiological study of *Helicobacter pylori* infection in infancy. Arch Dis Childhood Fetal & Neonatal Edition 1996; 74: F141-F142.

[68] Fawcett JP, Shaw JP, Brooke M, Walker A, Barbezat GO: Seroprevalence of *Helicobacter pylori* in a longitudinal study of New Zealanders at ages 11 and 21. Austr N Z J Med 1998; 28: 585-89.

[69] Travis PB, Goodman KJ, O'Rourke KM, Groves FD, Sinha D, Nicholas JS *et al.*: The association of drinking water quality and sewage disposal with *Helicobacter pylori* incidence in infants: the potential role of water-borne transmission. Journal of Water and Health 2010; 8: 192-203.

[70] Baldassarre ME, Monno R, Laforgia N, Fumarola L, Fanelli M, Sgobba C *et al.*: The source of *Helicobacter pylori* infection in the neonatal period. J Perinat Med 2009; 37: 288-92.

[71] Blecker U, Lanciers S, Keppens E, Vandenplas Y: Evolution of *Helicobacter pylori* positivity in infants born from positive mothers. J Ped Gastroenterol Nutr 1994; 19: 87-90.

[72] Cervantes DT, Fischbach LA, Goodman KJ, Phillips CV, Chen S, Broussard CS: Exposure to *Helicobacter pylori*-positive siblings and persistence of *Helicobacter pylori* infection in early childhood. J Ped Gastroenterol and Nutr 2010; 50: 481-85.

[73] Veldhuyzen van Zanten SJO, Pollak PT, Best LM, Bezanson GS, Marrie T: Increasing prevalence of *Helicobacter pylori* infection with age: continuous risk of infection in adults rather than cohort effect. J Infect Dis 1994; 169: 434-37.

[74] Rothenbacher D, Bode G, Brenner H: Dynamics of *Helicobacter pylori* infection in early childhood in a high-risk group living in Germany: loss of infection higher than acquisition. Aliment Pharmacol Ther 2002; 16: 1663-68.

[75] Broussard CS, Goodman KJ, Phillips CV, Smith MA, Fischbach LA, Day RS *et al.*: Antibiotics taken for other illnesses and spontaneous clearance of *Helicobacter pylori* infection in children. Pharmacoepidemiol Drug Safety 2009; 18: 722-29.

[76] Perri F, Pastore M, Clemente R, Festa V, Quitadamo M, Niro G *et al.*: *Helicobacter pylori* infection may undergo spontaneous eradication in children: a 2-year follow-up study. J Ped Gastroenterol Nutr 1998; 27: 181-83.

[77] Sipponen P, Kosunen TU, Samloff IM, Heinonen OP, Siurala M: Rate of *Helicobacter pylori* Acquisition among Finnish Adults A 15-Year Follow-up. Scandinavian Journal of Gastroenterol 1996; 31: 229-32.

[78] Kosunen TU, Aromaa A, Knekt P, Salomaa A, Rautelin H, Lohi P *et al.*: *Helicobacter pylori* antibodies in 1973 and 1994 in the adult population of Vammala, Finland. Epidemiol Infect 1997; 119: 29-34.

[79] Tschopp A, Joller H, Jeggli S, Widmeier S, Steffen R, Hilfiker S *et al.*: Hepatitis E, *Helicobacter pylori* and peptic ulcers in workers exposed to sewage: a prospective cohort study. Occupational and Environmental Medicine 2009; 66: 45-50.

[80] Parsonnet J, Blaser MJ, Pérez-Pérez GI, Hargrett-Bean N, Tauxe RV: Symptoms and risk factors of *Helicobacter pylori* infection in a cohort of epidemiologists. Gastroenterol 1992; 102: 41-6.

[81] Taylor DN, Sanchez JL, Smoak BL, DeFraites R: *Helicobacter pylori* Infection in Desert Storm Troops. Clin Infect Dis 1997; 25: 979-82.

[82] Becker SI, Smalligan RD, Frame JD, Kleanthous H, Tibbitts TJ, Monath TP *et al.*: Risk of *Helicobacter pylori* infection among long-term residents in developing countries. Am J Trop Med Hyg 1999; 60: 267-70.

[83] Weyermann M, Adler G, Brenner H, Rothenbacher D: The mother as source of *Helicobacter pylori* infection. Epidemiology 2006; 17: 332-34.

[84] Granstrom M, Tindberg Y, Blennow M: Seroepidemiology of *Helicobacter pylori* infection in a cohort of children monitored from 6 months to 11 years of age. J Clin Microbiol 1997; 35: 468-70.

[85] Ashorn M, Mäki M, Hällström M, Uhari M, Akerblom H, Viikari J *et al.*: *Helicobacter pylori* infection in Finnish children and adolescents. A serologic cross-sectional and follow-up study. Scand J Gastroenterol 1995; 30: 876-79.

[86] Ganga-Zandzou PS, Michaud L, Vincent P, Husson MO, Wizla-Derambure N, Delassalle EM *et al.*: Natural outcome of *Helicobacter pylori* infection in asymptomatic children: a two-year follow-up study. Pediatrics 1999; 104: 216-21.

[87] Granquist A, Bredberg A, Sveger T, Axelsson I: A longitudinal cohort study on the prevalence of *Helicobacter pylori* antibodies in Swedish children and adolescents. Acta Paediatrica 2002; 91: 636-40.

[88] Fawcett JP, Barbezat GO, Poulton R, Milne BJ, Xia HH, Talley NJ: *Helicobacter pylori* serology in a birth cohort of New Zealanders from age 11 to 26. World Journal of Gastroenterology 2005; 11: 3273-76.

[89] Gisbert JP: The Recurrence of *Helicobacter pylori* Infection: Incidence and Variables Influencing It. A Critical Review. Am J Gastroenterol 2005; 100: 2083-99.

[90] Farrell S, Milliken I, Doherty GM, Murphy JL, Wootton SA, McCallion WA: Total Family Unit *Helicobacter pylori* Eradication and Pediatric Re-Infection Rates. *Helicobacter* 2004; 9: 285-88.

[91] Gisbert JP, Arata IG, Boixeda D, Barba M, Cantón R, Plaza AG *et al.*: Role of partner's infection in reinfection after *Helicobacter pylori* eradication. Eur J Gastroenterol Hepatol 2002; 14: 865-71.

[92] Cronmiller JR, Nelson DK, Jackson DK, Kim CH: Efficacy of conventional endoscopic disinfection and sterilization methods against *Helicobacter pylori* contamination. *Helicobacter* 1999; 4: 198-203.

[93] Fantry GT, Zheng QX, James SP: Conventional cleaning and disinfection techniques eliminate the risk of endoscopic transmission of *Helicobacter pylori*. Am J Gastroenterol 1995; 90: 227-32.

[94] Nurnberg M, Schulz HJ, Ruden H, Vogt K: Do conventional cleaning and disinfection techniques avoid the risk of endoscopic *Helicobacter pylori* transmission? Endoscopy 2003; 35: 295-99.

[95] Rothman KJ, Greenland S, Lash TL: Bias Analysis. In Modern Epidemiology. Third edition Philadelphia: Lippincott-Raven; 2008, pp 345-380.

[96] Czinn SJ, Blanchard T: Vaccinating against *Helicobacter pylori* infection. Nature Rev Gastroenterol Hepatol 2011; 8: 133-140.

[97] Graham DY, Fischbach LA: *Helicobacter pylori* treatment in the era of increasing antibiotic resistance. Gut 2010; 59: 1143-53.

[98] Moayyedi P: The health economics of *Helicobacter pylori* infection. Best pract Res Clin Gastroenterol 2007; 21: 347-61.

CHAPTER 4

Helicobacter pylori in Japan: Epidemiology, Diagnosis and Treatment

Hidekazu Suzuki[1,*], Toshihiro Nishizawa[2] and Toshifumi Hibi[1]

[1]Division of Gastroenterology and Hepatology, Department of Internal Medicine, Keio University School of Medicine, Tokyo, Japan and [2]Division of Gastroenterology, National Hospital Organization Tokyo Medical Center

Abstract: *Helicobacter pylori* (*H. pylori*) infection is the main cause of gastritis, gastroduodenal ulcer and gastric cancer. Evidence for the prevention of metachronous gastric cancer has been established in Japan. The committee of the Japanese Society for Helicobacter Research has revised the guidelines for diagnosis and treatment of *H. pylori* infection in 2009. *H. pylori* eradication therapy achieved a grade A recommendation, being useful for the treatment of gastric or duodenal ulcer, for the treatment and prevention of *H. pylori*-associated diseases such as gastric cancer, and for inhibiting the spread of *H. pylori* infection. According to Japanese guidelines, first-line therapy for treating *H. pylori* infection consists of proton pump inhibitor (PPI) with amoxicillin and clarithromycin given for 7 days. Even with the recommended regimens, eradication failure is still seen in more than 20% of the patients. The recommended second-line therapy is PPI with amoxicillin and metronidazole for 7 days. In case of second-line treatment failure, a PPI + amoxicillin + fluoroquinolone or high-dose PPI/amoxicillin therapy is recommended in Japan.

Keywords: *Helicobacter pylori*, eradication, Japan

INTRODUCTION

Helicobacter pylori (*H. pylori*) infection is one of the most prevalent infectious diseases worldwide with an estimation of 40-50% of the world population. *H. pylori* has been identified as a group 1 carcinogen by the World Health Organization and is associated with the development of gastric cancer [1]. In experimental studies, *H. pylori* eradication has been shown to have a prophylactic effect on gastric cancer [2-5]. In human beings, the beneficial effect of *H. pylori* eradication on the reduction in gastric cancer incidence has been also reported [6].

*Address correspondence to Hidekazu Suzuki: Division of Gastroenterology and Hepatology, Department of Internal Medicine, Keio University School of Medicine, Tokyo, Japan; Tel: +81 3 5363 3914, Fax: +81 3 5363 3967; E-mail: hsuzuki@akeio.jp

Before the modern discovery of intra-gastric bacteria by Warren and Marshall, several reports dealt with spiral gastric bacteria as long ago as 1890 [7]. The modern discovery of *H. pylori* might have been delayed because in 1954, Palmer denied the existence of microorganisms in the human stomach, claiming that spiral bacteria were seen only post-mortem because microorganisms could not survive in the acidic gastric environment [8]. However, microorganisms had been described in the gastric mucosa since the 1890s. For example, in Japan, Kasai and Kobayashi of the Kitasato Institute reported propagation of a spirochete-like organism, probably *Helicobacter felis*, from the stomach of dogs and cats, but not from laboratory animals [9]. They showed that when rabbits infected with these spirochetes were also inoculated with the *virus fixe* (attenuated rabies virus), marked hemorrhagic lesions occurred in the gastric mucosa. They also demonstrated that spirochetes inoculated into the gastric mucosa of the mouse could be eradicated by arsamino (a modern equivalent of arsaminol is thought to be bismuth, a close relative of arsenic). Seventy years then elapsed before scientists again attempted to treat gastric diseases associated with "spirochetes," that is, *Helicobacter* infection.

Epidemiology

It is known that approximately half the population of Japan is infected with *H. pylori.*

Now, the prevalence of *H. pylori* infection is 4.0-6.7% in children, because the hygienic environment was improved.

Konno *et al.* investigated transmission by DNA fingerprinting analysis of cultured *H. pylori* from pediatric patients and their family members. Forty-two index patients with a mean age of 11.7 years (range, 4-19) were diagnosed as having *H. pylori* gastritis with or without duodenal/gastric ulcer disease. A total of 66 family members for whom the results of the *H. pylori* stool antigen test and/or serum *H. pylori* IgG test were positive underwent endoscopic examination and biopsy or aspiration of gastric juice for *H. pylori* culture. The extraction of *H. pylori* genomic DNA and PCR-based RAPD analysis were performed. Thirty-two (76%) of the 42 patients showed DNA fingerprint patterns identical to those of at least one of the respective family members. The patterns of 29 (69%) of the analyses of the *H. pylori* infected patients were identical to those of their mothers. The patterns for 7 patients were identical to those of their fathers, and those for 6 of the latter patients were also identical to those of their mothers. The rate of fingerprint patterns identical to those of the index patients was significantly higher in those of mothers compared with those of fathers ($P < 0.01$). Mother-to-child transmission is the predominant route of *H. pylori* infection in Japan [10].

Bacterial Resistance

In patients with clarithromycin-resistant *H. pylori*, it has been reported that the eradication rate achieved with clarithromycin-based regimens shows a marked decrease. Clarithromycin resistance has also been reported to develop after unsuccessful eradication therapy, suggesting that inadequate therapy increases the risk of bacterial resistance [11]. When patients are treated with clarithromycin in the pediatric, respiratory, and otorhinolaryngology fields, clarithromycin resistance is possibly being created. A 5-year nationwide survey of bacterial resistance was conducted by the Japanese Society for Helicobacter Research from 2002 to September 2007 to determine the status of bacterial resistance in Japan and investigate guidelines for future eradication therapy [12]. At the 2008 meeting of the Japanese Society for Helicobacter Research, it was reported that the mean national clarithromycin resistance rates from 2002 to 2006 were 18.9%, 21.2%, 27.7%, 29.0%, and 27.2%. The mean nationwide clarithromycin resistance rate determined by the Japanese Society of Chemotherapy was 7.0% (21 / 302) in 2000, so there has been an increase of resistance by approximately 20% over several years. From the above results, it appears that the incidence of clarithromycin-resistant *H. pylori* is increasing rapidly, so a decrease of the eradication rate achieved by the therapy currently available under the national health insurance scheme is a concern.

H. pylori has been considered to seldom become resistant to amoxicillin. Nishizawa *et al.* reported that a high resistance rate to amoxicillin was observed in *H. pylori* after two or three unsuccessful eradication [13]. The resistance rates to amoxicillin in the group of no history of eradication treatment, one treatment failure, two treatment failures, and three treatment failures were 13.6%, 26.5%, 49.5% and 72.7%, respectively. The high level resistance rates to amoxicillin in the group of no history of eradication treatment, one treatment failure, two treatment failures, and three treatment failures were 0%, 0.9%, 6.1% and 18.2%, respectively. (Isolates were considered high level resistant and resistant to amoxicillin if the minimal inhibitory concentration (MIC) was 0.5 μg/ml and 0.06 μg/ml, respectively.) The bacterial DNA was amplified by PCR, and the *PBP1* genes were sequenced. High level resistant strains to amoxicillin had 1-3 substitutions, and low level resistant strains (MIC 0.06-0.25 μg/ml) had 0-2 substitutions. The accumulation of *PBP1* mutations could result in a gradual increase in amoxicillin resistance.

The prevalence of *H. pylori* resistance to metronidazole (MET) has been reported to range between 5% and 12% in Japan [14,15]. Recently, we examined the initial *in vitro* mechanism of resistance acquisition of *H. pylori* to MET [16]. In that study, after 10 MET-susceptible strains were cultured on plates containing sub-inhibitory concentrations of MET, the MIC of MET for 90% of strains increased to levels of the MET-resistant strains. Especially, in the MET-resistance-induced strains, the expression of the TolC efflux pump (hefA) was significantly increased under MET exposure, suggesting that overexpression of hefA may be the initial step in the acquisition of MET resistance in *H. pylori*. On the other hand, MET is a prodrug that is converted to its active form when its nitro group is reduced and superoxide radicals, which are directly toxic to the bug, are generated. Then, another major mechanism for MET resistance would be explained by the mutation of *rdxA* [17], a coding gene of nitroreductase of *H. pylori*. We also reported the third mechanism of MET resistance by the mutation of the transcriptional regulator, ferric uptake regulator (Fur), of *H. pylori*, a direct suppressor of the iron-cofactored superoxide dismutase SodB, which is essential for protection against superoxide attack. We demonstrated that in some MET-resistant strains, SodB activity was induced in a dose-dependent manner on exposure to MET and that, under MET exposure, the generation of superoxide radicals in MET-resistant strains was significantly reduced as compared with that in the MET -susceptible strains [18]. These MET-resistant strains carried the amino acids mutation of Fur (C78Y, P114S; mutant-type Fur) [18]. The binding affinity of the mutant-type Fur to an operator sequence on the sodB promoter (Fur-Box) was significantly reduced [18].

Primary resistance of *H. pylori* to fluoroquinolones has been reported 15% in Japan. Nishizawa *et al.* reported a high resistance rate (47.9%) to gatifloxacin (8-methoxy fluoroquinolone) after eradication failure in Japan [19]. Resistance to fluoroquinolones is easily acquired, and the resistance rate is relatively high in countries with a high consumption rate of these drugs.

The prevalence of the resistance to tetracycline and rifampins has fortunately remained low in Japan [15]. Suzuki *et al.* investigated the minimal inhibitory concentration of rifabutin and also the point mutations of the *rpoB* gene in 48 strains of *H. pylori* isolated from patients of a general hospital and 46 strains isolated from patients at a specialized hospital for chronic respiratory diseases [20]. Although all the strains isolated from the patients at the general hospital were susceptible to rifabutin, eight of the 46 strains (17.4%) isolated from the patients at the specialized hospital for chronic respiratory diseases showed resistance to rifabutin; six of these eight strains also showed point mutations of the *rpoB* gene. In particular, the MICs were high for the strains isolated from patients with a past history of treatment with rifampicin.

Diagnosis

When attempting to detect *H. pylori* infection before and after eradication therapy, the following tests are used. (1. Tests requiring endoscopic biopsy: (i) rapid urease test (ii) histology (iii) culture, 2. Tests not requiring endoscopic biopsy: (i) urea breath test (ii) measurement of *H. pylori* antibody (iii) measurement of *H. pylori* antigen in feces) Employing two tests are covered by the national health insurance scheme in Japan.

ABC Method

According to the ABC method, it is recommended that the risk for gastric cancer be stratified into four groups according to the anti-*H. pylori* IgG antibody titer before eradication of *H. pylori* and the serum pepsinogen (PG) levels, as follows: group A [*H. pylori* (-)PG(-)], group B [*H. pylori* (+)PG(-)], group C [*H. pylori* (+)PG(+)], and group D [*H. pylori* (-)PG(+)] [21] (Table **1**). For the PG method, the cutoff points for identifying the risk of gastric cancer should be 70 μg/l for pepsinogen I and 3 for the PG I/II ratio.

Table 1: ABC method by *H. pylori* IgG and serum pepsinogen levels.

Group	**A**	**B**	**C**	**D**
H. pylori IgG	−	+	+	−
Pepsinogen method	−	−	+	+
Endoscopic feature	Normal	Chronic gastritis	Chronic Atrophic gastritis	Intestinal metaplasia
Gastric cancer risk	None	Low	Middle - High	High
Recommended endoscopic examination interval	−	3 years	1-2 years	1 year

Cohort studies in 4,655 normal male individuals who could be followed up for 8 years show that gastric cancer developed only in individuals infected with *H. pylori* and did not develop in normal individuals testing negative for *H. pylori*. With the progression of *H. pylori*-induced gastritis, the risk of gastric cancer increased in a stepwise fashion from chronic gastritis [*H. pylori*(+)PG(-), group B] (HR: 7.13, 95%CI: 0.95-53.33) to atrophic gastritis [*H. pylori*(+)PG(-), group C] (HR:14.85, 95%CI: 1.96-107.7) and finally to severe atrophic gastritis with intestinal metaplasia [*H. pylori*(-)PG(+), group D] (HR: 61.85, 95%CI: 5.6-682.64) [22]. The ABC method was introduced in 2007 at some institutions and cities in Japan.

The interval for screening by the ABC method need not be yearly, and an interval of 5 years or so is recommended. It is recommended that endoscopic examination be performed at least once every 3 years for group B, at least once every 1-2 years for group C, and annually for group D, and that group A be excluded from the examination.

Guideline for the Management of *H. pylori* Infection in Japan: 2009 Revised Edition

It has been reported that *H. pylori* eradication from the residual gastric mucosa after endoscopic treatment of early gastric cancer, such as endoscopic mucosal resection (EMR), has an inhibitory effect on the occurrence of metachronous gastric cancer [23]. As this report was not based on a randomized controlled study, a multicenter randomized clinical trial was subsequently conducted in

Japan Gastro Study Group that demonstrated an inhibitory effect of eradication therapy on metachronous gastric cancer [6]. The committee of the Japanese Society for Helicobacter Research has revised the guidelines for diagnosis and treatment of *H. pylori* infection [24]. *H. pylori* eradication therapy achieved a grade A recommendation, being useful for the treatment of gastric or duodenal ulcer, for the treatment and prevention of *H. pylori*-associated diseases such as gastric cancer, and for inhibiting the spread of *H. pylori* infection.

When the gastric mucosa is infected with *H. pylori*, gastritis occurs. *H. pylori* infection often persists throughout life, and can lead to various upper gastrointestinal (GI) tract diseases, such as atrophic gastritis, gastro-duodenal ulcer, gastric adenocarcinoma, gastric MALT lymphoma, and hyperplastic gastric polyps. In addition, *H. pylori* infection influences gastric function, including gastric acid secretion [25] and motility [26], and alters the intra-gastric environment. An association between *H. pylori* infection and some diseases occurring outside the GI tract, such as idiopathic thrombocytopenic purpura (ITP) and iron-deficiency anemia, has also been indicated. Although not all infected people have the above-mentioned diseases, they form a high-risk population for such complications. Successful eradication improves histologic gastritis and may prevent various diseases associated with *H. pylori*, and may lead to reduction of medical costs in the future. As failure of eradication due to drug resistance may occur or treatment may have to be discontinued due to adverse reactions, providing a careful explanation about this therapy to patients and obtain their informed consent are required before starting *H. pylori* eradication therapy.

First-Line Therapy

One week of triple therapy using a proton pump inhibitor (PPI) combined with amoxicillin (750mg, b.i.d) and clarithromycin (400mg or 200mg, b.i.d) is recommended as the treatment of first choice for eradicating *H. pylori* in Japan [27]. The success rate of the triple therapy has recently fallen to 80% or below because of increasing incidence of clarithromycin resistance.

Second-Line Therapy

One week of triple therapy using a (PPI) combined with amoxicillin (750mg, b.i.d) and metronidazole (250mg, b.i.d) is recommended as the treatment of second choice in Japan.

The Tokyo *H. pylori* Study Group examined the eradication rate in response to the second-line regimen consisting of (PPI), amoxicillin, and metronidazole by conducting a multicenter study in the Tokyo metropolitan area [28]. Intention-to-treat (ITT) and per-protocol (PP) analyses revealed an eradication rate of 87.6 and 90.6%, respectively.

Murakami *et al.* reported that the eradication rates following second-line treatment of *H. pylori* infection with the PPI+ amoxicillin + metronidazole regimen was 97 % for infections with metronidazole-sensitive strains and 82 % for infections with metronidazole-resistant strains. Therefore, it would be difficult to predict the effect of metronidazole-containing second-line treatment regimens by only determining the MIC of metronidazole. Nishizawa *et al.* previously reported that a eradication resistance index was defined as: [Pre-treatment urea breath test result (‰)] x [amoxicillin MIC (μg/ml)] x [metronidazole MIC (μg/ml)] [29]. When a cutoff value of 3 was used, the eradication resistance index predicted the response to therapy with a specificity of 81.8 %, sensitivity of 93.8 %, and accuracy of 92.5 %.

Third-Line Therapy (Not Covered by the National Health Insurance Scheme)

Currently, a standard third-line therapy still remains to be established, and European guidelines recommend culture before the selection of a third-line treatment based on the microbial sensitivity to the antibiotics. *H. pylori* isolates after two eradication failures are often resistant to both metronidazole and clarithromycin. Therefore, these two drugs are not recommended for inclusion in third-line regimens.

If second-line eradication therapy fails, a PPI + amoxicillin + fluoroquinolone or high-dose PPI/amoxicillin therapy are recommended in Japan [24].

Fluoroquinolones exert their antimicrobial activity by inhibiting the enzyme DNA gyrase. This enzyme, in addition to relaxing super-coiled DNA, introduces negative super-coils into the DNA causing the bacterial chromosome to be maintained in a negatively super-coiled state [30]. In addition, the enzyme is involved in DNA replication, recombination and transcription [19]. Several studies have shown that the "quinolone resistance-determining region" of the *gyrA* gene plays a critical role in the resistance of *H. pylori* to fluoroquinolone [31].

Recently novel fluoroquinolones were developed, and superior *in vitro* activity of gatifloxacin over that of levofloxacin against *H. pylori* was reported. Furthermore, garenoxacin (des-fluoro(6) quinolone) and sitafloxacin show activities four-fold or greater than those of gatifloxacin [32]. Nishizawa *et al.* investigated the efficacy of gatifloxacin-based triple therapy (gatifloxacin 400 mg o.d., amoxicillin 500mg q.d.s. and rabeprazole 10 mg q.d.s.) as a third-line treatment for *H. pylori* eradication, administered after assessment of the susceptibility of the organisms to gatifloxacin and the presence of *gyrA* mutations [33]. Successful eradication of *H. pylori* was achieved in 63.6%, as assessed by both ITT and PT analysis. The eradication rate was 100% in the patients infected with gatifloxacin-susceptible bacteria and/or bacteria without *gyrA* mutations, but only 33.3% in those infected with gatifloxacin-resistant bacteria or bacteria with *gyrA* mutations.

The increase in gastric pH induced by antisecretory drugs is crucial in order to allow antibiotics exerting the best activity against *H. pylori*. By increasing intra-gastric pH, antisecretory drugs allow the microorganism to reach the growth phase and become more sensitive to antibiotics such as amoxicillin. Moreover, PPIs exert an antibacterial action against *H. pylori*. *H. pylori* has been considered to seldom become resistant to amoxicillin, so high-dose dual therapy might be a promising option as an alternative treatment regimen. Furuta *et al.* reported an excellent eradication rate of 87.8% (43/49) with dual therapy using rabeprazole (10 mg, q.i.d.) and amoxicillin (500 mg q.i.d.) for 2 weeks as the third rescue regimen for eradication of *H. pylori* [34].

Future Perspective

Recommended first-line therapies are effective and well tolerated, but the wide use over the year has led to failure of those regimens in more than 20%. Failure is mainly due to increasing antibiotic resistance, in particular against clarithromycin. The challenge for the future is the development of improved therapies. In countries such as Japan where dreaded diseases such as gastric cancer seem to stem from *H. pylori*, the twenty-first century may be the time to totally eradicate this troublesome organism from the entire population.

ACKNOWLEDGEMENTS

This work was supported by a Grant-in-Aid for Scientific Research B (22300169 to H.S.), Grant-in-Aid for challenging Exploratory Research (24659103, to H.S.), from the Japan Society for the Promotion of Science, a Research Fund of Mitsukoshi Health and Welfare Foundation (to H.S.), a grant from the Smoking Research Foundation (to H.S.) and the Keijo Gijuku Academic Development Fund (to H.S).

CONFLICT OF INTEREST

None declared

REFERENCES

[1] Suzuki, H., Nishizawa, T., and Hibi, T. *Helicobacter pylori* eradication therapy. Future Microbiol 2010; 5: 639-648.

[2] Nishizawa, T., Suzuki, H., Masaoka, T., Minegishi, Y., Iwasahi, E., and Hibi, T. *Helicobacter pylori* eradication restored sonic hedgehog expression in the stomach. Hepatogastroenterology 2007; 54:697-700.

[3] Nishizawa, T., Suzuki, H., Nakagawa, I., Minegishi, Y., Masaoka, T., Iwasaki, E., and Hibi, T. Early *Helicobacter pylori* eradication restores sonic hedgehog expression in the gastric mucosa of Mongolian gerbils. Digestion 2009; 79:99-108.

[4] Nishizawa, T., Suzuki, H., Nakagawa, I., Minegishi, Y., Masaoka, T., Iwasaki, E., and Hibi, T. Rebamipide-promoted restoration of gastric mucosal sonic hedgehog expression after early *Helicobacter pylori* eradication. Digestion 2009; 79:259-262.

[5] Suzuki, H., Iwasaki, E., and Hibi, T. *Helicobacter pylori* and gastric cancer. Gastric Cancer 2009;12:79-87.

[6] Fukase, K., Kato, M., Kikuchi, S., Inoue, K., Uemura, N., Okamoto, S., Terao, S., Amagai, K., Hayashi, S., and Asaka, M. Effect of eradication of *Helicobacter pylori* on incidence of metachronous gastric carcinoma after endoscopic resection of early gastric cancer: an open-label, randomised controlled trial. Lancet 2008;372:392-397.

[7] Marshall, B.J., and Warren, J.R. Unidentified curved bacilli in the stomach of patients with gastritis and peptic ulceration. Lancet 1984; 1:1311-1315.

[8] Palmer, E.D. Investigation of the gastric mucosa spirochetes of the human. Gastroenterology 1954; 27:218-220.

[9] Kasai, K., and Kobayashi, R. The stomach spiochete occurring in mammals. J Parasitol 1919; 6:1-10.

[10] Konno, M., Yokota, S., Suga, T., Takahashi, M., Sato, K., and Fujii, N. Predominance of mother-to-child transmission of *Helicobacter pylori* infection detected by random amplified polymorphic DNA fingerprinting analysis in Japanese families. Pediatr Infect Dis J 2008; 27:999-1003.

[11] Hirata, K., Suzuki, H., Nishizawa, T., Tsugawa, H., Muraoka, H., Saito, Y., Matsuzaki, J., and Hibi, T. Contribution of efflux pumps to clarithromycin resistance in *Helicobacter pylori*. J Gastroenterol Hepatol 2010; 25 Suppl 1:S75-79.

[12] Kobayashi, I., Murakami, K., Kato, M., Kato, S., Azuma, T., Takahashi, S., Uemura, N., Katsuyama, T., Fukuda, Y., Haruma, K., *et al.* Changing antimicrobial susceptibility epidemiology of *Helicobacter pylori* strains in Japan between 2002 and 2005. J Clin Microbiol 2007; 45:4006-4010.

[13] Nishizawa, T., Suzuki, H., Tsugawa, H., Muraoka, H., Matsuzaki, J., Hirata, K., Ikeda, F., Takahashi, M., and Hibi, T. Enhancement of amoxicillin resistance after unsuccessful *Helicobacter pylori* eradication. Antimicrob Agents Chemother 2011;55:3012-3014.

[14] Tsugawa, H., Suzuki, H., Nakagawa, I., Nishizawa, T., Saito, Y., Suematsu, M., and Hibi, T. Alpha-ketoglutarate oxidoreductase, an essential salvage enzyme of energy metabolism, in coccoid form of *Helicobacter pylori*. Biochem Biophys Res Commun 2008; 376:46-51.

[15] Nishizawa, T., Suzuki, H., and Hibi, T. Quinolone-Based Third-Line Therapy for *Helicobacter pylori* Eradication. J Clin Biochem Nutr 2009; 44:119-124.

[16] Tsugawa, H., Suzuki, H., Muraoka, H., Ikeda, F., Hirata, K., Matsuzaki, J., Saito, Y., and Hibi, T. Enhanced bacterial efflux system is the first step to the development of metronidazole resistance in *Helicobacter pylori*. Biochem Biophys Res Commun 2011; 404:656-660.

[17] Goodwin, A., Kersulyte, D., Sisson, G., Veldhuyzen van Zanten, S.J., Berg, D.E., and Hoffman, P.S. Metronidazole resistance in *Helicobacter pylori* is due to null mutations in a gene (rdxA) that encodes an oxygen-insensitive NADPH nitroreductase. Mol Microbiol 1998;28:383-393.

[18] Tsugawa, H., Suzuki, H., Satoh, K., Hirata, K., Matsuzaki, J., Saito, Y., Suematsu, M., and Hibi, T. Two amino acids mutation of ferric uptake regulator determines *Helicobacter pylori* resistance to metronidazole. Antioxid Redox Signal 2011;14:15-23.

[19] Nishizawa, T., Suzuki, H., Kurabayashi, K., Masaoka, T., Muraoka, H., Mori, M., Iwasaki, E., Kobayashi, I., and Hibi, T. Gatifloxacin resistance and mutations in gyra after unsuccessful *Helicobacter pylori* eradication in Japan. Antimicrob Agents Chemother 2006;50:1538-1540.

[20] Suzuki, S., Suzuki, H., Nishizawa, T., Kaneko, F., Ootani, S., Muraoka, H., Saito, Y., Kobayashi, I., and Hibi, T. Past rifampicin dosing determines rifabutin resistance of *Helicobacter pylori*. Digestion 2009;79:1-4.

[21] Miki, K. Gastric cancer screening by combined assay for serum anti-*Helicobacter pylori* IgG antibody and serum pepsinogen levels - "ABC method". Proc Jpn Acad Ser B Phys Biol Sci 2011;87:405-414.

[22] Ohata, H., Kitauchi, S., Yoshimura, N., Mugitani, K., Iwane, M., Nakamura, H., Yoshikawa, A., Yanaoka, K., Arii, K., Tamai, H., et al. Progression of chronic atrophic gastritis associated with *Helicobacter pylori* infection increases risk of gastric cancer. Int J Cancer 2004;109:138-143.

[23] Uemura, N., Mukai, T., Okamoto, S., Yamaguchi, S., Mashiba, H., Taniyama, K., Sasaki, N., Haruma, K., Sumii, K., and Kajiyama, G. Effect of *Helicobacter pylori* eradication on subsequent development of cancer after endoscopic resection of early gastric cancer. Cancer Epidemiol Biomarkers Prev 1997;6:639-642.

[24] Asaka, M., Kato, M., Takahashi, S., Fukuda, Y., Sugiyama, T., Ota, H., Uemura, N., Murakami, K., Satoh, K., and Sugano, K. Guidelines for the management of *Helicobacter pylori* infection in Japan: 2009 revised edition. Helicobacter 2009;15:1-20.

[25] Suzuki, H., Minegishi, Y., Nomoto, Y., Ota, T., Masaoka, T., van den Brink, G.R., and Hibi, T. 2005. Down-regulation of a morphogen (sonic hedgehog) gradient in the gastric epithelium of *Helicobacter pylori*-infected Mongolian gerbils. J Pathol 2005;206:186-197.

[26] Saito, Y., Suzuki, H., Tsugawa, H., Suzuki, S., Matsuzaki, J., Hirata, K., and Hibi, T. Dysfunctional gastric emptying with down-regulation of muscle-specific microRNAs in *Helicobacter pylori*-infected mice. Gastroenterology 2011;140:189-198.

[27] Suzuki, H., Masaoka, T., Nomura, S., Hoshino, Y., Kurabayashi, K., Minegishi, Y., Suzuki, M., and Ishii, H. Current consensus on the diagnosis and treatment of *H. pylori*-associated gastroduodenal disease. Keio J Med 2003;52:163-173.

[28] Matsuhisa, T., Kawai, T., Masaoka, T., Suzuki, H., Ito, M., Kawamura, Y., Tokunaga, K., Suzuki, M., Mine, T., Takahashi, S., *et al.* Efficacy of metronidazole as second-line drug for the treatment of *Helicobacter pylori* Infection in the Japanese population: a multicenter study in the Tokyo Metropolitan Area. Helicobacter 2006;11:152-158.

[29] Nishizawa, T., Suzuki, H., Masaoka, T., Iwasaki, E., and Hibi, T. A new eradication resistance index as a predictor of metronidazole-containing second-line treatment of *Helicobacter pylori*. Digestion 2007;76:215-220.

[30] Matsuzaki, J., Suzuki, H., Tsugawa, H., Nishizawa, T., and Hibi, T. Homology model of the DNA gyrase enzyme of *Helicobacter pylori*, a target of quinolone-based eradication therapy. J Gastroenterol Hepatol 2010; 25 Suppl 1:S7-10.

[31] Nishizawa, T., Suzuki, H., Umezawa, A., Muraoka, H., Iwasaki, E., Masaoka, T., Kobayashi, I., and Hibi, T. Rapid detection of point mutations conferring resistance to fluoroquinolone in gyrA of *Helicobacter pylori* by allele-specific PCR. J Clin Microbiol 2007;45:303-305.

[32] Suzuki, H., Nishizawa, T., Muraoka, H., and Hibi, T. Sitafloxacin and garenoxacin may overcome the antibiotic resistance of *Helicobacter pylori* with gyrA mutation. Antimicrob Agents Chemother 2009; 53:1720-1721.

[33] Nishizawa, T., Suzuki, H., Nakagawa, I., Iwasaki, E., Masaoka, T., and Hibi, T.. Gatifloxacin-based triple therapy as a third-line regimen for *Helicobacter pylori* eradication. J Gastroenterol Hepatol 2008;23 Suppl 2:S167-170.

[34] Furuta, T., Sugimoto, M., Kodaira, C., Nishino, M., Yamade, M., Uotani, T., Ikuma, M., and Shirai, N. The dual therapy with 4 times daily dosing of rabeprazole and amoxicillin as the 3rd rescue regimen for eradication of *H. pylori*. Hepatogastroenterology 2010; 57:1314-1319.

CHAPTER 5

Helicobacter pylori in South-Eastern Asia

Sun-Young Lee*

Department of Internal Medicine, Konkuk University School of Medicine, Seoul, Korea

Abstract: South-Eastern Asia is a subregion of Asia, consisted of the countries that are geographically South of China, East of India, West of New Guinea and North of Australia. South-Eastern Asian countries such as Korea, Japan, Singapore, Malaysia, Thailand, Vietnam, Indonesia, and the Philippines are known as endemic area of *Helicobacter pylori* infection. Food, lifestyle, and prevalence of *H. pylori* infection, physiological functions, and genetic factors are widely different in these countries. Although the prevalence of *H. pylori* infection has been declining in the Asian countries, *H. pylori* infection is still a health treat in South-Eastern Asia, and thus consensus on eradication has been actively implemented. *H. pylori* eradication is indicated for *H. pylori*-positive patients with the gastritis-associated diseases such as peptic ulcer disease, gastric cancer, or primary gastric B-cell lymphoma (MALToma). In areas with a high prevalence of gastric cancer, eliminating *H. pylori* infection through improvements had an impact in reducing the burden of gastric cancer. The currently recommended first-line therapy for *H. pylori* infection is proton pump inhibitor (PPI), amoxicillin and clarithromycin for 7 days. Classic quadruple therapy is consistent with bismuth, PPI, metronidazole, and tetracycline. Increasing rate of resistance to clarithromycin and metronidazole has led to reduced efficacy of PPI-based triple therapy. Further salvage therapy includes levofloxacin-based triple therapy; and rifabutin-based triple therapy. In this chapter, peculiarities on the aspect of epidemiology, diagnosis, treatment on *H. pylori* infection in South-Eastern Asian countries, excluding those countries which are mentioned in other chapters, will be discussed.

Keywords: Asian enigma, Asia-Pacific guideline, epidemiology, functional dyspepsia, gastric cancer, human migration, Korean guideline, phytoceuticals, probiotics epidemiology.

PREVALENCE OF *HELICOBACTER PYLORI* INFECTION

Prevalence rates vary widely between different geographical regions and ethnic groups. Due to an improvement in of socioeconomic status, hygiene and living

***Address correspondence to Sun-Young Lee:** Department of Internal Medicine Konkuk University School of Medicine, Seoul, South Korea; Tel: + 82 2030-7747; Fax: +82 2030-7748; E-mail: sunyoung@kuh.ac.kr conditions, the prevalence of *H. pylori* has declined rapidly in Asia from developing countries to more industrialized and developed countries. In the Philippines, there was a decreasing trend in the prevalence of gastric ulcer (from 68.13% to 33.48%) and duodenal ulcer (from 76.67% to 36.50%) during 7 year period, and this was associated with a corresponding decrease in *H. pylori* prevalence [1]. In Korea, a follow-up study on the seropositivity of 15,916 subjects with *H. pylori* infection showed that there is a significant decline in 2005 (59.6%) compared with that of 1998 (66.9%) in the prevalence [2]. Seroprevalence of *H. pylori* was significantly higher in subjects aged 50-59 years, males, low income group, and subjects from provinces. Notably, there is a gender-related difference in the prevalence of *H. pylori* infection manifesting as a lower rate of infection in young women and an earlier plateau of infection rate in men [3]. The overall prevalence of *H. pylori* increased with age group across ethnicity and gender in Northern Peninsular Malaysia [4]. Significantly higher numbers of males were infected compared to female, but such trend was only observed among older adult groups. In Vietnam, the prevalence of *H. pylori* infection is high in Vietnam and especially high in a large urban area, such as the city of Hanoi [5]. The risk for infection in the rural area of Hatay was 40% lower than in the urban population of Hanoi. In Thailand, semi-arid plateau, mountain, jungle and fertile plain communities had high incidences of *H. pylori* infection varying from 54.0 to 67.1% while the coastal and peninsular communities had low incidences of 32% [6].

Table 1: Factors known to be associated with *Helicobacter pylori* prevalence in adults

Factors in Childhood
Age (early childhood)
Infected sibling
Geographic area
Household income
Mother's education
Poor living conditions (sanitation)
Source of drinking water
Crowding (number of person per room)
Types of housing

Current knowledge implies that acquisition of *H. pylori* seems to occur predominantly in childhood and a major role of intrafamilial spread is now beyond controversy. Although a seroconversion rate of 2.13% per year suggests that new infections occur continuously even during late adulthood [7], early childhood has been demonstrated as the period of transmission of infection and identified an infected sibling as an important risk factor (Table **1**) [8].

Geographic area, household income, mother's education, poor living conditions, sanitation, drinking water source, age, gender, crowding (number of person per room), and types of housing in childhood are known as significant factors of *H. pylori* infection supporting an oral-fecal route of spread besides an oral-oral route of spread. Interestingly, *H. pylori* was associated with unsanitary practices whereas protection was associated with consumption of tea and locally produced foods, "pegaga" and “budu" in Malaysia [9].

In countries with different races, there is an ethnic difference in prevalence (Table **2**).

Table 2: *Helicobacter pylori* prevalence in countries with different races such as Thailand, Malaysia, or Singapore

Prevalence	Ethnic Differences
Highest	Indian
to	Chinese
Lowest	Malays

In Thailand, *H. pylori* infection was found in 48.2% of dyspeptic patients with high incidence in the age-group 31-60 years (63.7%) [6], and the East-Asian genotype is the most common among Chinese (85%) and Thai-Chinese (55%) when compared to ethnic Thai [10]. The ethnicity of the mother among mixed Thai-Chinese marriages predicted the genotype of the child's *H. pylori*. For example, when the mother was Chinese, 84% had East Asian type *vs.* 29% when the mother was Thai. In Malaysia, *H. pylori* infection prevalence rate is highest in Indians adults, followed Chinese and low in Malays [4]. Prevalence rates among the Malays ranged from 11.9 to 29.2%, while the Chinese ranged from 26.7 to 57.5%, and those of Indians in two studies were 49.4 and 52.3% [11]. The pattern of infection in a multiracial population in Malaysia points to a 'racial cohort' phenomenon. In Singapore, Indians have the highest prevalence of infection followed by Chinese and Malays [12]. The Malays have the lowest prevalence of

H. pylori and peptic ulcer among the three races in Singapore, whereas Indians have a higher prevalence of *H. pylori* antibodies but a lower frequency of peptic ulcer than the Chinese.

Human Migration and *H. pylori*

H. pylori has been shown to follow the routes of human migration by their geographical origin. The genome of *H. pylori* has evolved over the millennia since its migration out of Africa along with its human host, and thus present day isolates of *H. pylori* have molecular markers that reflect population migrations [13]. Currently, the global *H. pylori* population has been divided into six ancestral populations, three from Africa, two from Asia and one from Europe [14].

The human population history in Southeast Asia was shaped by numerous migrations and population expansions, and there are housekeeping gene sequences of the human stomach bacterium *H. pylori* from various countries in Southeast Asia [15]. *H. pylori* accompanied at least three ancient human migrations into Southeast Asia. First is a migration from India introducing hpEurope bacteria into Thailand, Cambodia and Malaysia. Second is a migration of the ancestors of Austro-Asiatic speaking people into Vietnam and Cambodia carrying hspEAsia bacteria. Third is a migration of the ancestors of the Thai people from Southern China into Thailand carrying *H. pylori* of population hpAsia2. Moreover, the *H. pylori* sequences reflect the migrations of Chinese to Thailand and Malaysia within the last 200 years spreading hspEasia strains, and migrations of Indians to Malaysia within the last 200 years distributing both hpAsia2 and hpEurope bacteria. The distribution of the bacterial populations seems to strongly influence the incidence of gastric cancer as countries with predominantly hspEAsia isolates exhibit a high incidence of gastric cancer while the incidence is low in countries with a high proportion of hpAsia2 or hpEurope strains [15].

Phylogenetic studies have shown that *H. pylori* isolates amongst Chinese and Indians are distinctive while Malays have Indian and other strains suggesting a more recent acquisition of the bacterium from Indians [16]. The majority of the Malay and Indian *H. pylori* isolates share the same origin while the Malaysian Chinese *H. pylori* is distinctive. The Malay population, known to have a low infection rate of *H. pylori*, was likely to be initially *H. pylori* free and gained the pathogen only recently from cross infection from other populations.

Asian Enigma

The incidence rate of gastric adenocarcinoma in Asia tends to mirror the seroprevalence rate of *H. pylori* infection, but regional variations exist that do not match the distribution of infection prevalence rates (Table **3**).

Table 3: Variability in gastric cancer rates across Asia (Asian paradox)

Countries with High Incidence Rate of Gastric Cancer	Countries of Low Incidence Rate of Gastric Cancer Despite High Prevalence of *H. pylori* Infection
Korea	Malaysia
Japan	Indonesia
China	Sinagpore
	India
	Bangladesh
	Pakistan
	Thailand

The great variability in gastric cancer rates across Asia, with very high incidences in Japan and Korea, and exceedingly low incidences in ethnic Malays, whether in Malaysia or Indonesia [17]. Malays are populations with high seroprevalence rates of *H. pylori* infection that paradoxically have low incidence rates of gastric adenocarcinoma. In general, *H. pylori* infection is more frequent in less developed Asian countries like India, Bangladesh, Pakistan, and Thailand and is acquired at early age than in more developed Asian countries like Korea, Japan, and China [18]. Seroprevalence of *H. pylori* infection in adult populations of India, Bangladesh, Pakistan and Thailand varies from 55% to 92%. In contrast, seroprevalence of *H. pylori* in Korean, Chinese and Japanese adults is around 50%. However, nnual incidence rate of gastric cancer in Indonesia, Bangladesh, and Thailand is between 1.3-10.6 per 100,000 populations, whereas that in Korea, China, and Japan is 10-100 times higher [19]. Similar enigma has been reported from Africa as compared to the West.

Such diverse clinical outcomes are related to bacterial virulence factors, concomitant environmental factors, host susceptibility and immune response. For example, despite the high prevalence of *H. pylori*, Indians have a relatively low prevalence of peptic ulcer disease and a low incidence of gastric cancer. This paradox with regards to gastric cancer has been termed the "Indian enigma" [20]. Chinese race, *H. pylori* infection, low level of education, smoking, and high intake of salted fish and vegetables were identified as significant independent risk factors for gastric cancer, while high intake of fresh fruits and vegetables was protective for gastric cancer. Bacterial strain differences between races may be putative but this observation may also indicate gastroprotective environmental factors or a lower genetic susceptibility to develop cancer in the Indians.

Gastric Cancer Incidence Based on Genetic Differences

To explain the Asian paradox (incidence of gastric cancer being extremely low despite high prevalence of *H. pylori* infection), genetic difference must be considered. There are studies that help the understanding of the genetic variation between ethnicities, which may influence *H. pylori* susceptibility and the outcome of infection. A study showed the association between polymorphisms related to immune and cancer-related pathways and *H. pylori* infection among the major ethnicities such as Chinese, Malay and Indian, resident in Singapore and Malaysia as well as the association between these polymorphisms and gastric cancer development in ethnic Chinese patients [21]. The prevalence of 16 polymorphisms varied significantly among the ethnicities. In the Chinese subgroup, nominally significant associations were shown between EBBR2+1963G (rs1801200) and *H. pylori* infection, between PTGS2-1195G (rs689466) and an increased risk of gastric cancer on adjusting for *H. pylori* status, and between IL1B-1473C (rs1143623) and a decreased risk of gastric cancer. It has been also hypothesized that strains possessing specific combinations of these motifs may be responsible for gastric cancer development. The prevalence of cagA and the EPIYA motifs with regard to number, class, and patterns in strains from the three major ethnic groups differed between the Malaysian and Singaporean populations in relation to disease development [22]. All 126 isolates possessed cagA, with the majority encoding EPIYA-A (97.6%) and all encoding EPIYA-B. However, while the cagA of 93.0% of Indian functional dyspepsia (FD) isolates encoded EPIYA-C as the third motif, 91.8% of Chinese FD isolates and 81.7% of Chinese gastric cancer isolates encoded

EPIYA-D. Of Malay FD isolates, 61.5% and 38.5% possessed EPIYA-C and EPIYA-D, respectively. Although *H. pylori* strains with distinct cagA-types are circulating within the primary ethnic groups resident in Malaysia and Singapore, these genotypes appear unassociated with the development of gastric cancer in the ethnic Chinese population. The phenomenon of distinct strains circulating within different ethnic groups, in combination with host and certain environmental factors, may help to explain the rates of gastric cancer development in Malaysia.

In Singapore-Chinese population, polymorphisms in NQO1, IL-10 and PTPN11, in combination with *H. pylori* status, could be used to identify individuals who are more likely to develop intestinal metaplasia and therefore gastric cancer [23]. When comparing the effects of *H. pylori* infection on gastropathy between Indonesian and Japanese patients, the percentages of Indonesian and Japanese patients who were *H. pylori*-positive at the antrum or body of the stomach were similar (68% and 59.5%) [24]. Of those who were *H. pylori*-positive, more Japanese patients had high levels of polymorphonuclear cells, mononuclear cells, glandular atrophy, and intestinal metaplasia in both the antrum and body of the stomach than Indonesian patients. In similar, histopathological findings in stomach tissue using an updated Sydney System and the frequencies of interleukin (IL)-1beta polymorphisms are thought to be associated with an increased risk of gastric cancer [25]. When endoscopic-guided biopsies from three regions of the stomach and the -511 T-to-C polymorphism in the IL-1beta gene were examined in 228 Japanese, 116 Chinese, 159 Thai and 83 Vietnamese patients with gastric diseases, *H. pylori* colonization, inflammation and activity were more severe in the Japanese and Thai populations than in the Chinese and Vietnamese populations and these scores were more antrum-predominant in the Thai and Vietnamese populations than in the Japanese and Chinese populations, with the most severe degree of atrophy and intestinal metaplasia occurring in the angulus region of the Japanese population. The IL-1 beta polymorphisms did not differ among the four populations overall, but in cases with severe mucosal atrophy (pepsinogen I/II ratio <3.0), the CC polymorphism was dominant in the Japanese population and the TT+TC polymorphism was dominant in the Chinese population. In Thias, a low serum pepsinogen I/II ratio combined with positivity for *H. pylori* IgG, and a IL-1beta-511 C/C genotype may be independent risk factors for gastric cancer in Thais [26]. The C/C genotype was found more frequently in the gastric cancer group than in the group with a normal gastric mucosa.

A recent study showed the possible contribution of *H. pylori* virulence factors to geographic differences in the incidence of gastric cancer across East and Southeast Asia [27]. In their study, 66 isolates from Cambodian patients that had previously been assigned to two genetic populations based on sequences of seven housekeeping genes, namely hpEurope and hpEastAsia, subpopulation hspEAsia. These strains were characterized with respect to vacA polymorphism and cagA status by PCR, and the CagA C-terminal region was sequenced. We also sequenced the complete cagA gene from 10 hpEurope and 10 hspEAsia strains chosen at random. The cagA gene was present in 92.4% of the 66 isolates and was mainly of Western type, whrereas hpEAsia strains carrying East-Asian CagA and the m1-type vacA allele (15.2%) were less frequent among the 66 Cambodian isolates than reported in East Asian countries, a finding that might partly explain the intermediate incidence of gastric cancer in Cambodia, and by extension, in Southeast Asia (except for Vietnam). The observed high prevalence of s1a alleles (34.4%) and Western CagA (28.1%) among hspEAsia strains indicates frequent introgression of European vacA and cagA alleles into East Asian *H. pylori* strains. Interestingly, the incidence of gastric cancer differs among cities in Vietnam, and it has been suggested that virulence factors associated with *H. pylori* are partly responsible. The vacA m1 genotype was significantly more common in strains isolated in Hanoi, where the incidence of gastric cancer is higher, than in strains from Ho Chi Minh. VacAm1 is not only associated with gastric carcinogenesis, but also with peptic ulcer and might contribute to the difference in the prevalence of peptic ulcer and gastric cancer between Hanoi and Ho Chi Minh [28]. These results explain why the age-standardized incidence rate of gastric cancer in the northern city of Hanoi is higher than that in the southern city of Ho Chi Minh.

With regard to East Asian type CagA gene which is one of the important virulence factors of *H. pylori*, there is extreme sequence heterogeneity on 3' region of cagA gene, demonstrated by the sequence analysis of cagA of *H. pylori* strains isolated from the patients with gastric discasc [29]. The CagA sequences analysis in 21 and 12 *H. pylori* DNA samples obtained from Japanese and Thai individuals, respectively, by the molecular phylogenetic method showed that the sequences were more conserved in the Thai individuals than in the Japanese individuals [30]. Although CagA sequences from almost all Thai individuals were concentrated in one branch, CagA sequences from Japanese individuals were uniformly distributed throughout the consensus tree. These results suggest that the difference in the CagA sequences between asymptomatic healthy Japanese and Thai individuals may be linked to the incidence of gastric cancer in Japan and Thailand. Taken as a whole, the low prevalence of cagA-positive *H. pylori* strain as well as the low prevalence of East-Asian genotype cagA-positive strains may contribute to the low gastric cancer incidence in Thailand. East Asian genotype was the most common among Chinese (85%) and Thai-Chinese (55%) [10]. Gastric cancer was common among ethnic Chinese with East Asian genotype. In similar, *H. pylori*-infected Filipinos can be considered to be at a low risk of developing gastric cancer. A study from the Philippines showed that most (73.7%) of the isolated strains were Western CagA-positive [31].

DIAGNOSIS

Diagnostic tests for *H. pylori* infection are divided into invasive and noninvasive tests (Table **4**). Noninvasive tests include urea breath test and serology (blood, urine, or stool), whereas invasive tests include histology (hematoxylin & eosin stain, Giemsa stain, Warthin-Starry stain, and Gram stain), culture, rapid urease test, and polymerase chain reaction (PCR).

Table 4: Commonly used tests for diagnosis of *H. pylori* infection

Invasive Test	**Noninvasive Test**
Histology	Urea breath test
Hematoxylin & eosin stain	Serology
Giemsa stain	Blood
Warthin-Starry stain	Urine
Gram stain	Stool
Culture	
Rapid urease test	
Polymerase chain reaction	

Helicobacter *pylori* Serology

Noninvasive tests play significant roles in the test-and-treat approach for the management of *H. pylori.* The performance of anti-*H. pylori* enzyme-linked immunosorbent assay (ELISA) can be improved by adjusting new cut-off values. For example, using a cut-off value at a titer of 20 U/ml, the overall *H. pylori* seroprevalence in the healthy blood donors was 57% [32]. In-house serum ELISA test for *H. pylori* antibodies also provides a good sensitivity with acceptable specificity, whereas urine ELISA was unable to produce satisfactory sensitivity or specificity [33]. In similar, immunoblot (Helico Blot 2.1, Genelabs Diagnostics, Singapore) assay with current infection marker (CIM) is known for good performance [34]. Immunochromatography (Assure *H. pylori* Rapid Test, Genelabs Diagnostics, Singapore) with CIM was found to be more specific and accurate than the conventional ELISA (AccuBind ELISA, Monobind, USA), and may be useful for noninvasive diagnosis of *H. pylori* infection. In addition, the rapid blood test kits showed high specificity and positive predictive value (97-100%), while sensitivity and negative predictive value ranged widely (43%-80% and 47%-73%, respectively) [35]. Majority of tests are accurate for the diagnosis of *H. pylori* infection, but the secretory IgA-based techniques in saliva and gastric juice seem to be inappropriate for determining *H. pylori* status due to their low sensitivities [36].

With regard to serology using urine or stool samples, the RAPIRUN test is useful for the diagnosis of *H. pylori* infection in the Vietnamese population, showing high specificity, acceptable sensitivity, noninvasiveness, convenience, and rapidity [37]. Besides, the efficacy of a new polyclonal **e**nzyme immunoassay for the detection of *H. pylori* antigen in stool by determining the optimal cut-off value in the screening population [38]. Sensitivity, specificity, positive and negative predictive values, and accuracy of the stool antigen test were 93.1%, 94.6%, 95.1%, 92.3%, and 93.8%, respectively. The performance of a new stool antigen test was comparable to that of other methods in the diagnosis of *H. pylori* infection for the screening population, even in the presence of atrophic gastritis/intestinal metaplasia.

Stool test is very useful in children, especially in developing countries where noninvasive methods such as urea breath test are often not available. The rapid immunochromatography for *H. pylori* stool antigen (rapid HpSA) test is a recently-developed method for detection of *H. pylori* infection [39]. The rapid HpSA and HpSA ELISA are reliable methods of detection of *H. pylori* infection even in the pediatric population before and after eradication therapy. However, in patients with upper gastrointestinal bleeding, the stool antigen test by using commercially available monoclonal enzyme immunoassay (Amplified IDEIA HpStAR, Dako, Denmark) yielded a low sensitivity and accuracy, and therefore not reliable for the diagnosis of *H. pylori* infection [40].

Rapid Urease Test

The most commonly used rapid urease test remains the Campylobacter-like organism (CLO) test, which generates accurate readings only after 24 hours. Although several types of rapid urease test have been reported, some large endoscopy units use their own homemade unbuffered ultra-rapid urease test.

Positive finding of the CLO test is markedly reduced depending on the degree of atrophic gastritis and intestinal metaplasia in both antrum and body [41]. In similar, the sensitivity of rapid urease test for detecting *H. pylori* is limited in patients presented with bleeding peptic ulcers. Exposure of gastric biopsy specimens to blood for four hours significantly decreased the sensitivity of the biopsy rapid urease test for *H. pylori* detection [42].

Urea Breath Test

The carbon urea breath test is generally considered to be a simple, noninvasive and accurate test for the detection of *H. pylori* infection both before and after treatment. The urea breath test is considered to be the test of choice to confirm the eradication [43]. Besides, follow-up endoscopy is necessary for a gastric ulcer in areas with high incidence of gastric cancer.

Determining the optimal cutoff value of a 13C-urea breath test is important, and it is proposed that *H. pylori* eradication therapy might be beneficial for patients with FD with a delta 13C-urea breath test of >58.2 per thousand [44]. False negative results of 13C urea breath test were common and increased with prolonged use of acid pump antagonist. Just like PPI, revaprazan also had anti-urease activity and most patients reverted to positive results by 2 weeks after the cessation of taking the medication [45].

Histology, Giemsa Stain, PCR, Smear, and Culture

Upper gastrointestinal endoscopically biopsied specimens are usually sent for the diagnosis of *H. pylori* infection. The biopsy is recommended in the body instead of antrum in the subjects with atrophic gastritis and/or intestinal metaplasia for the modified Giemsa staining or Warthin-Starry silver staining [43]. With regard to the site of biopsy for *H. pylori* diagnosis in gastric cancer patients, a study showed that upper body greater curvature was the most sensitive and specific biopsy site to detect *H. pylori* due to less atrophy and less intestinal metaplasia [46]. A study on diagnostic tests with regard to grade of atrophic gastritis and/or intestinal metaplasia showed that any one of biopsy-based test or serology was excellent for identifying current *H. pylori* infection among individuals without atrophic gastritis or intestinal metaplasia and/or young patients (<40 year). However, a combination of at least two tests was necessary in the presence of atrophic gastritis or intestinal metaplasia [47].

Sensitivity and specificity are important for tests used to defect *H. pylori* infection from gastric biopsy specimens, and molecular methods, such as PCR and nested PCR, are sensitive methods for *H. pylori* detection. Nested PCR is a highly sensitive direct method to detect *H. pylori* infection from biopsy specimens [48]. When there is a discrepancy between Giemsa and anti-*H. pylori* antibody stains, PCR can be used to confirm the organism. *Camplylobacter hyointestinalis* is the most common cause of non-*H. pylori*-related Giemsa positive infection, and is associated with lower grades of neutrophil activity and chronic inflammation than East Asian CagA *H. pylori*-related infection [29].

Gastric imprint smears stained with Diff-Quik method is a rapid, cheap, and reliable method for the detection of *H. pylori* and have their best results when complemented with histology. However, imprint smears did not provide added value over histology with regards to inflammation and metaplasia [49].

Culture depends on the factors that influence the successful isolation of *H. pylori* from human gastric biopsies. When each of the gastric biopsies was inoculated onto chocolate blood agar media and incubated for up to 2 weeks, the success rate for culture of *H. pylori* from gastric biopsies increased when two biopsies were taken and inoculated on chocolate blood agar media with and without antibiotics [50]. These results support the histological observation of patchy colonization of *H. pylori* in the stomach.

TREATMENT

In South-Eastern Asian countries with a higher prevalence of *H. pylori* infection, it is not possible to eradicate everyone with *H. pylori* infection due to its low cost-effectiveness. For this reason, current indications for *H. pylori* eradication vary among Asian countries (Table **5**) [51].

Table 5: Current indications for *H. pylori* eradication in Asia [43,51-54]

	Indications for *H. pylori* Eradication
Asia-Pacific guideline	**Recommendation A (randomized controlled trial)** • Peptic ulcer disease • Mucosa-associated lymphoid tissue lymphoma • Patients' wishes • Non-ulcer dyspepsia • NSAIDs users • Communities with high incidence of gastric cancer **Recommendation B (well conducted clinical trial)** • Atrophic gastritis • After gastric cancer resection • First degree relatives of gastric cancer • Before long-term aspirin therapy • Gastroesophageal reflux disease with long-term PPI therapy **Recommendation C (expert opinion)** • Unexplained iron deficiency anemia • Idiopathic thrombocytopenic purpura
Korean guideline	**Definite indications** • Peptic ulcer including scar • Marginal zone B cell lymphoma • After resection of early gastric cancer **Recommended indications** • First relatives of gastric cancer patients • Unexplained iron deficiency anemia • Chronic idiopathic thrombocytopenic purpura

Table 5: contd....

	Possible indications • Atrophic gastritis • Non-ulcer dyspepsia Long-term use of NSAIDs
Japanese guideline	**Evidence level I (systematic review/meta-analysis)** • Gastric/duodenal ulcer • Idiopathic thrombocytopenic purpura • Atrophic gastritis • Functional dyspepsia **Evidence level II (randomized controlled clinical trial)** • After endoscopic treatment of early gastric cancer • Gastric hyperplastic polyp • Reflux esophagitis **Evidence level III (non-randomized controlled clinical studies)** • Gastric mucosa-associated lymphoid tissue lymphoma • Iron deficiency anemia • Chronic urticaria
Chinese guideline	**Necessary** • Peptic ulcer • Early gastric cancer after operation • Gastric mucosa-associated lymphoid tissue lymphoma • Chronic gastritis associated with atrophy and erosions **Supportive** • Chronic gastritis associated with symptoms of functional dyspepsia • Planned long-term use of NSAIDs • Family history of gastric cancer • Iron deficiency anemia of unknown cause • Idiopathic thrombocytopenic purpura • Other *H. pylori*-related gastric diseases such as lymphocytic gastritis, gastric hyperplastic polyps, and Menetrier's disease • Patient wishing *H. pylori* eradication

Indications

Current guidelines are based on the available evidence or on good clinical practice rather than randomised controlled trials [43, 52-54]. Peptic ulcer, mucosa-associated lymphoid tissue (MALT) lymphoma, early gastric cancer, iron deficiency anemia, idiopathic thrombocytopenic purpura, chronic atrophic gastritis, and FD are the common indications. Somc guidclines also include consideration of the patient's wishes, communities with a high incidence of gastric cancer, family history of gastric cancer, long-term use of nonsteroidal anti-inflammatory drugs (NSAIDs)/aspirin or PPI therapy, or gastroesophageal reflux disease. Notably, lymphocytic gastritis and Ménétrier's disease are indications for *H. pylori* eradication in China [53], whereas gastric hyperplastic polyps less than 1 cm in size and chronic urticaria are indications in Japan [54].

1. Gastric Diseases

Acute gastritis related to recent *H. pylori* infection includes nodular gastritis, follicular gastritis, lymphocytic gastritis, hemorrhagic gastritis, granulomatous gastritis, hypertrophic gastritis, Ménétrier's disease, and congestive gastropathy; these conditions are more reversible than chronic gastritis [51,55]. They are therefore assigned as supportive indications for *H. pylori* eradication, since this approach has been shown to be effective in their treatment. Nodular gastritis is related to a new onset of *H. pylori* infection occurs in adult, since some individuals show an immature and aggressive tissue response [56]. It can be improved by *H. pylori* eradication, and disappearance of nodularity on endoscopy is accompanied by a decrease in follicular gastritis score. Besides, *H. pylori*-associated enlarged-fold gastritis can be distinguished from tumorous condition by eradicating *H. pylori* in patients with gastric giant folds [57]. When analyzed by endoscopic ultrasound, subjects who underwent *H. pylori* eradication showed both clinical and morphologic resolution of protein losing enteropathy and hypertrophic gastric folds.

Atrophic gastritis and metaplastic gastritis indicate chronic *H. pylori* infection, whereas nodular gastritis, hemorrhagic gastritis, and hypertrophic gastritis are endoscopic findings of recent *H. pylori* infection [51,55]. Although *H. pylori* eradication therapy clearly improves histologic gastritis, there are conflicting opinions about the reversibility of gastric mucosal atrophy and intestinal metaplasia after eradication therapy. One reason for these controversial results may be that various studies have included not only closed-type and open-type chronic atrophic gastritis, but also complete-type and incomplete-type intestinal metaplasia. It remains an issue of particular interest to determine at which stage *H. pylori* eradication should be performed, and at which point the disease has progressed to the "point of no return" becoming irreversible in a stepwise model of changes in the gastric mucosa after *H. pylori* infection that lead to intestinal-type gastric cancer. The endoscopic diagnosis of open-type chronic atrophic gastritis and metaplastic gastritis was related to higher levels of caudal type homeobox 2 (Cdx2) expression than closed-type chronic atrophic gastritis and nonatrophic/nonmetaplastic cases [58]. This finding suggests that Cdx2 expression is an early change that is correlated with the presence of histological intestinal metaplasia. It occurs before endoscopic metaplastic gastritis, and the risk of development of intestinal-type gastric cancer will continue to remain high during the process of gastric carcinogenesis in open-type chronic atrophic gastritis and metaplastic gastritis, but not in closed-type chronic atrophic gastritis and nonatrophic/nonmetaplastic cases. This strongly indicates that cancer development after eradication depends on the presence of extensive chronic atrophic gastritis before eradication. In summary, *H. pylori* eradication can result in the arrest or reversal of histological and molecular changes in the gastric epithelium that may be surrogate intermediates in the progression towards gastric cancer in closed-type chronic atrophic gastritis, rather than in open-type chronic atrophic gastritis. When considering that metachronous cancer still develops after successful eradication in open-type chronic atrophic gastritis, the identification of the so-called 'point of no return' might be somewhere between closed-type and open-type chronic atrophic gastritis.

The role of *H. pylori* infection in FD remains controversial. In a double blind, randomized, placebo-controlled trial of *H. pylori* eradication for FD in Singapore showed that on intention-to-treat analyses, symptom resolution was observed in 24% of patients on active treatment and 7% on placebo; the difference in proportion of patients with symptom resolution was statistically significant [59]. *H. pylori* eradication rates perprotocol and intention-to-treat were 80.0 and 68.3%, on active treatment and 5.6 and 4.9% on placebo. Among patients with *H. pylori* eradicated on active treatment the symptom resolution rate was 39% (10 of 26), whereas it was 3% (one of 35) among patients in the placebo group who had persistent *H. pylori* infection. In multivariate analysis, posttreatment *H. pylori* status was the only predictor of symptom resolution. The majority of patients, 91.5%, had ulcer-like dyspepsia; heartburn and acid regurgitation were uncommon, and no increase was observed after treatment. In contrast to Western populations, the results suggest that patients with FD in Asia would benefit from treatment for *H. pylori* infection with as much as a 13-fold increased chance of symptom resolution following its eradication.

2. Patient's Wishes Including Family History of Gastric Cancer

There are people in countries with a high prevalence of gastric cancer, who desire *H. pylori* eradication, especially if they have a family history of gastric cancer. A recent Korean study on population attributable fraction of infection-related cancer showed that up to one-quarter of cancer cases and deaths would be preventable through control of infectious agents [60]. In addition, there is growing evidence that *H. pylori* strains of East-Asian type cytotoxin-associated gene A (cagA) are related to gastric cancer. The prevalence of the East Asian CagA-positive strain was shown to be associated with the high mortality rates of gastric cancer in Asia. A Korean study on the association between *H. pylori* and gastric cancer by the virulence factors (CagA and VacA) showed that CagA seropositivity was significantly associated with a higher gastric cancer among *H. pylori*-infected subjects [61]. However, it is not yet indicated to eradicate all East-Asian cagA-positive cases since most of *H. pylori* infections in this region are East Asian type. For instance, in the author's recent study, 94% of *H. pylori*-infections among Korean subjects were of East-Asian cagA type [29].

In subjects with family history of gastric cancer, *H. pylori* detection and prophylactic eradication of the infection should be offered especially when the subject is less than 40 year-old. Siblings of patients who develop gastric cancer before 40 years of age have a higher *H. pylori* infection rate and higher prevalence of intestinal metaplasia at the body, and show a higher multivariate-adjusted odd ratio for gastric cancer [62]. Since gastric cancer in patients younger than 40 year-old is closely associated with *H. pylori* infection rather than genetic causes, eradication may be adopted as a strategy for the prevention or early detection of cancer in young subjects. First-degree relatives of gastric cancer patients might be at an increased risk of developing gastric cancer, as judged by significantly higher prevalence of *H. pylori*, chronic atrophic gastritis, and intestinal metaplasia [63,64]. Compared with healthy controls, first-degree relatives of patients with gastric cancer had a higher prevalence of hypochlorhydria, and of gastric atrophy than patients with non-ulcer dyspepsia matched for *H. pylori* prevalence [65]. Notably, among the relatives of cancer patients, the prevalence of atrophy and hypochlorhydria is increased only in those with *H. pylori* infection. Further, it is, greater in relatives of patients with familial cancer than among relatives of sporadic cancer index patients, and increases with age. Eradication of *H. pylori* resolved the gastric inflammation, hypochlorhydria and atrophy in half of the subjects [65].

3. Extragastric Diseases

Emerging evidences on the effect of *H. pylori* eradication in a diverse range of extragastric diseases suggests that *H. pylori* eradication could be used successfully in those that are unresponsive to conventional therapy. Routine screening and eradication of *H. pylori* have not previously been recommended, and thus a test-and-treat approach should be recommended in certain situations. *H. pylori* eradication can be considered when there is evidence that the extragastric disease is mediated by *H. pylori*-related cytotoxins and/or cytokines and *H. pylori* eradication leads to improvement of the extragastric symptoms. The higher prevalence of *H. pylori* infection in particular diseases cannot be considered as an indication for *H. pylori* eradication, because of confounding factors, including the effect of contamination. *H. pylori* infection should be also sought for and treated in patients with unexplained iron deficiency anemia and idiopathic thrombocytopenic purpura. Diminished halitosis after eradication suggested a causal link between *H. pylori* infection and halitosis [66]. These studies indicate that *H. pylori* eradication may reduce the production of substances responsible for bad breath detected by chromatographic documentation of volatile sulfur compounds.

Other rare extragastric diseases include central nervous system, eye, and hepatobiliary lesions. Parkinson's disease, Alzheimer's disease, and migraine headache can be improved after *H. pylori* eradication. Motor fluctuations of *H. pylori*-infected patients with Parkinson's disease following eradication [67]. When the authors monitored motor fluctuations of the "wearing-off" or "delayed-on" types in 30 *H. pylori* non-infected and 35 *H. pylori*-infected Parkinson's disease patients, L-dopa onset time was longer and on-time duration was shorter in *H. pylori*-infected patients than in non-infected patients. *H. pylori* eradication improved the L-dopa delayed onset time and short on-time duration, thereby demonstrating that *H. pylori* infection could interfere with the absorption of L-dopa and provoke motor fluctuations. Besides, *H. pylori* eradication has been reported to positively influence glaucoma indices, suggesting a possible causal link between *H. pylori* and glaucoma [68]. In addition, *H. pylori* has been reported to promote hepatic fibrosis and increase the risk of tumor growth factor-β1-mediated tumorigenesis, while the organism can be detected in patients with hepatolithiasis, choledocholitihiasis, and cholangiocarcinoma [69,70]. Although these studies suggest a link between *H. pylori* and hepatobiliary diseases, there are no data on significant improvement after eradication. A more reproducible evidence base and some insight into pathogenic mechanisms are needed for certain conditions.

4. Others

To date, it is not well defined whether to treat all *H. pylori*-positive patients taking a PPI and/or antiplatelet agents. Notably, the opinions and clinical practice patterns for the management of anticoagulation and antiplatelet medications differ significantly between Eastern and Western endoscopists [71]. Since there is a tendency among Eastern endoscopists to think that Asians are more prone to bleeding than Caucasians, *H. pylori* eradication might be considered more seriously in East Asians to prevent drug-induced ulcers. *H. pylori* testing should be considered in patients receiving long-term maintenance treatment with PPI, NSAIDs, and aspirin.

Regimen

In Asia, the currently recommended first-line therapy for *H. pylori* infection is PPI-based triple therapy with amoxicillin and clarithromycin for 7 days due to high metronidazole resistance [72]. In the case of treatment failure, one or two weeks of quadruple therapy (PPI+metronidazole+tetracycline+bismuth) is recommended. There is no standard third-line therapy, and some regimens that incorporate levofloxacin, moxifloxacin, and rifabutin can be used. New regimens such as sequenterapytial or concomitant therapy are suggested as alternative treatment for *H. pylori.* Sequential, concomitant therapy, dual therapy, and tailored therapy are being tried these days [73].

1. First-Line Therapy

The current regime using PPI, amoxycillin and clarithromycin is highly tolerable and effective and should continue to be recommended as a first-line therapy for *H. pylori* eradication in our setting. Notably, higher dose amoxicillin regime gives a significantly higher eradication than a lower dose amoxicillin [72]. Side effects of first-line therapy include bitter taste, epigastric pain, diarrhea, nausea or vomiting, loss of appetite, dizziness, or allergic skin rash [74]. Of all, diarrhea is the most common complaint, but shows a significantly low rate of moderate to severe diarrhea with the rifaximin containing regimen [75]. With regard to the types of PPI, high-dose rabeprazole-based triple therapy is more effective than its low-dose equivalent or omeprazole in eradicating *H. pylori* infection [76].

2. Second-Line Therapy

Increasing levels of bacterial antibiotic resistance decrease the eradication efficiency of *H. pylori* eradication. The eradication rate of first-line therapy has decreased from 2001 to 2007 while that of second-line therapy has remained the same in Korea [77]. Quadruple therapy using a PPI, bismuth, metronidazole, and tetracycline is a standard second-line therapy. Besides this regimen, 2-week high dose PPI-amoxicillin dual therapy followed by a PPI-amoxicillin-levofloxacin triple therapy were highly successful in achieving eradication in *H. pylori* treatment failures [78]. In addition, a retrial of quadruple therapy before use of a third-line therapy may be safe and effective for patients who fail to respond to second-line quadruple therapy [79].

With regard to the duration of therapy, two-week bismuth-containing quadruple therapy was more effective than the 1-week treatment, and should be considered for second-line treatment in Korea [80]. The eradication rates were 77.2% with 1-week group and 93.6% with 2-week group, respectively. The adverse events increased as the treatment durations increased from 7 to 14 days (20.0% and 42.5%, respectively).

Regimens that incorporate levofloxacin, moxifloxacin, and rifabutin can be also considered as a second-line therapy. The 10-day moxifloxacin-based triple therapy was found to have a high eradication rate with few side effects and good drug compliance in Korea [81]. Eradication rates by intention-to-treat and per-protocol analyses in the 10 days and 14 days groups were not statistically different. The 10 days group was significantly superior to the 14 days group in terms of side effect rates, and discontinuation rates due to lower side effects and higher compliance.

Supplements for the Treatment

Since the role of *H. pylori* infection is promoting carcinogenesis rather than acting as a direct carcinogen, eradication alone cannot be the right answer for preventing *H. pylori*-associated gastric cancer [82]. Therefore, a non-antimicrobial approach has been suggested to attain microbe-associated cancer prevention through controlling *H. pylori*-related chronic inflammatory processes and mediators responsible for carcinogenesis.

1. Phytoceutical

Phytoceutical, plant products that are active onbiological systems, includes Korean red ginseng, green tea, red wine, flavonoids, broccoli sprouts, garlic, probiotics and flavonoids [82]. It is known to inhibit *H. pylori* colonization, decrease gastric inflammation by inhibiting cytokine and chemokine release, and repress precancerous changes by inhibiting nuclear factor-kappa B DNA binding, inducing profuse levels of apoptosis and inhibiting mutagenesis. It cannot be a standard treatment for *H. pylori* infection, but can be a mighty weapon for either suppressing or modulating the disease-associated footprints of *H. pylori* infection.

In vitro and *in vivo* efficacy of Korean red ginseng of mitigating *H. pylori*-associated gastric atrophy suggest that Korean red ginseng may prevent *H. pylori*-associated gastric cancer in predictable ways [83]. Besides, the pH and concentration-dependent antibacterial activity of crude urushiol extract from the sap of the Korean lacquer tree (Rhus vernicifera Stokes) against 3 strains (NCTC11637, 69, and 219) of *H. pylori* was found by the agar dilution method [84]. Interestingly, the changes were observed within 10 min following incubation with the 1x minimal inhibitory concentrations of urushiol, and thus suggest that urushiol has potential as a rapid therapeutic against *H. pylori* infection by disrupting the bacterial cell membrane.

In Thailand, some plants used in Thai traditional medicine to treat gastrointestinal ailments inhibit the growth of *H. pylori* [85]. Methanol extracts of *Myristica fragrans* (aril) inhibited the growth of all *H. pylori* strains with minimum inhibitory concentration (MIC) of 12.5 micrograms/ml; extracts from *Barringtonia acutangula* (leaf) and *Kaempferia galanga* (rhizome) had an MIC of 25.0 micrograms/ml; *Cassia grandis* (leaf), *Cleome viscosa* (leaf), *Myristica fragrans* (leaf) and *Syzygium aromaticum* (leaf) had MICs of 50.0 micrograms/ml. Extracts with an MIC of 100.0 micrograms/ml included *Pouzolzia pentandra* (leaf), *Cycas siamensis* (leaf), *Litsea elliptica* (leaf) and *Melaleuca quinquenervia* (leaf). These data indicate that these plants may have chemopreventative activities and thus may partly explain the reduced incidence of gastric cancer in Thailand.

2. Probiotics

There are some controversies on the effect of probiotics on *H. pylori* eradication. An *in vitro* study showed that probiotics administration increased expression of suppressor of cytokine signaling (SOCS)-2 and SOCS-3 which were mediated through signal transducers and activation of transcription (STAT)-1/STAT-3 activation and Janus kinase (JAK)2 inactivation [86]. Another study also showed that *H. pylori* eradication was effective in inhibiting the growth and adherence of *cagA*-positive *H. pylori* to gastric epithelial cells [87]. The optimal density of *Lactobacillus acidophilus (L. acidophilus)* that has a maximum inhibitory effect on *H. pylori* in peptic ulcer patients has been reported [88]. Ten microliters of each density of *L. acidophilus* was dropped onto each quadrant of a previously inoculated *H. pylori* plate and then the plate was kept under microaerophilic conditions for 72 hours. As a result, *L. acidophilus* has an inhibitory effect on *H. pylori* isolated from peptic ulcer patients. Approximately an equal density of L. acidophilus on *H. pylori* has the most favorable effect, and could enhance antibiotic therapy for *H. pylori* eradication in humans.

Although there are several clinical studies about probiotics that showed positive results for improving eradication rates by reducing side effects [86-89], there are opposite results on the role of probiotics on *H. pylori* eradication. There was no additional benefit of mucoprotective agents in eradication rates when the following 3 groups were compared: PPI-based 7-day triple therapy, the same triple therapy plus *Saccharomyces boulardii* for 4 weeks, and the same 7-day triple therapy plus *S. boulardii* and mucoprotective agent for 4 weeks [90]. Moreover, addition of yogurt containing probiotics to moxifloxacincontaining second-line treatment neither improved eradication rates nor reduced the adverse event [91].

Sequential Therapy

Since the eradication rates following standard triple therapy for *H. pylori* infection are declining worldwide, sequential therapy such as a 5-day dual therapy (20 mg of rabeprazole and 1 g of amoxicillin, twice daily) followed by a 5-day triple therapy (20 mg of rabeprazole, 500 mg of clarithromycin, and 500 mg of metronidazole, twice daily) has been introduced. The eradication rate was significantly higher in the sequential group (87.9%) compared with the standard triple group (76.0%), whereas the incidence of adverse events was similar [92]. A prospective, randomised, controlled study showed that the 10-day sequential therapy achieved significantly higher eradication rates than the 14-day standard PPI-based triple therapy in Korea [93]. The 10-day sequential treatment for *H. pylori* was well tolerated and provided a high eradication rate [94,95].

The eradication rate of 10 day sequential therapy in genotypic clarithromycin-resistant *H. pylori* group identified by molecular PCR detection in Thai patients [96]. Point mutations at A2143G and A2142G were detected in 11.3% of the patients, and overall eradication rate was 94%. The eradication rate in the group with point mutation was significantly lower than the eradication rate in the group without point mutation. Sequential therapy is highly effective in clarithromycin-sensitive but is less effective in clarithromycin-resistant *H. pylori*.

Eradication in Special Conditions

The optimal therapeutic regimen for *H. pylori* infection has not been established in end-stage renal disease patients receiving hemodialysis. A 7-day triple therapy with low-dose OAC (omeprazole 40 mg daily, amoxicillin 500 mg daily, and clarithromycin 500 mg daily) regimen showed efficacy and safety for eradication of *H. pylori* infection in end-stage renal disease patients receiving hemodialysis [97].

In patients with liver cirrhosis or chronic hepatitis with a peptic ulcer, the PPI-based triple therapy consisted of PPI, 1000 mg of amoxicillin, and 500 mg of clarithromycin achieved high eradication rates for *H. pylori* infection without significant side effects [98]. The eradication rate of *H. pylori* was similar between the liver cirrhosis and chronic hepatitis groups; 82.6% and 88.1%, respectively. In addition, there were no significant differences in eradication rates between the patients with Child-Pugh class A and Child-Pugh class B/C disease. The side effects in each group were generally mild. Only the serum alanine aminotransferase (ALT) levels showed a significant correlation with the success of *H. pylori* eradication in both the liver cirrhosis and chronic hepatitis groups.

Regarding the effect of *H. pylori* eradication therapy on gastric ulcer healing after endoscopic mucosal resection, the ulcer reduction ratio was significantly higher in the subjects with successful *H. pylori* eradication [99]. No differences were observed between the noneradicated groups with regard to drug compliance, adverse drug event rates, or bleeding rates. *H. pylori* eradication therapy should be recommended since it improves the ulcer healing rate after endoscopic mucosal resection.

Antibiotics Resistance

There appears to be an increasing rate of resistance to clarithromycin and metronidazole in parts of Asia, leading to reduced efficacy of PPI-based triple therapy. For example, the distribution of minimal inhibitory concentrations (MIC) for amoxicillin, clarithromycin, metronidazole, tetracycline, azithromycin, and fluoroquinolone (ciprofloxacin, levofloxacin, and moxifloxacin) have shifted to higher concentrations from 1987 to 2003 in *H. pylori* strains isolated from Korean patients [100]. From 2001 to 2007, the eradication rates of first-line therapy (PPI, amoxicillin 1,000 mg, and clarithromycin 500 mg x twice a day) were 81.3%, 83.7%, 80.1%, 80.7%, 82.0%, 75.9%, and 77.5% with a decreasing trend [101]. In addition, the eradication rate of second-line therapy therapy (PPI bid, metronidazole 500 mg tid, tetracycline 500 mg qid, and bismuth 300 mg qid) was 77.3%, 86.2%, 95.6%, 95.9%, 89.6%, 83.2%, and 86.4% from 2001 to 2007 without decreasing trend. Therefore, even with currently most effective treatment regimen, about 10-20% of patients will fail to obtain the eradication of *H. pylori* infection.

Salvage therapies that can be used are as follow. First is the standard triple therapy that has not been previously used. Second is the bismuth-based quadruple therapy. Third is the levofloxacin-based triple therapy. Fourth is the rifabutin-based triple therapy. Fifth is the sequential therapy. After the failure of two or more eradication treatments, bacterial resistance to antibiotics should be evaluated and the regimen of third-line therapy should be selected according to each antimicrobial susceptibility. Multiple eradication failures should be handled on a case-by-case basis by specialists.

1. Metronidazole Resistance

There is a significant rise in the prevalence of metronidazole resistance over [102]. Since there has been a gradual increase in the proportion of Singapore patients with metronidazole resistant strains of *H. pylori*, the efficacy of a nitroimidazole containing regime in eradicating *H. pylori* was evaluated [103]. A high proportion of our patients with metronidazole resistant strains of *H. pylori* failed eradication therapy when a nitroimidazole containing regimen was used. Eradication rate was only 56% (9/16) among those with metronidazole resistant strains, whereas 88% (42/48) among those with metronidazole sensitive strains. Hence, in a population with a high prevalence of metronidazole resistance, the use of non-nitroimidazole-based therapy may be more efficacious.

In Malaysia, there was a high prevalence of resistance to metronidazole 68/90 (75.5%) [104]. No resistance was detected for clarithromycin, levofloxacin, amoxicillin, and nitrofurantoin/furazolidone. Resistance to rifampicin/rifabutin was for breakpoints of 1 and 4 μg/mL of 14.4 and 2.2% respectively in their study.

In Thailand, metronidazole resistant strains and cagA 2a gene of *H. pylori* infection was commonly found in patients with FD [105]. In patients with epigastric pain syndrome, presence of cagA 2a gene was significantly higher in metronidazole resistant than metronidazole sensitive strains. In Thailand, the resistance rates were 30.2% for metronidazole, 9.2% for ciprofloxacin, 5% for clarithromycin, 2.4% for amoxicillin, and 1.7% for erythromycin and tetracycline [106]. Single, double, and more than double antimicrobial resistances were found in 27.7, 6.7 and 2.5%, respectively.

Of South-Eastern Asian countries, Jakarta showed the highest resistance rates for metronidazole [107]. The resistance rates of the isolates were 100% for metronodazole, 27.8% for clarithromycin, 19.4% for amoxicillin, 6.9% for ciprofloxacin, norfloxacin and ofloxacin, 2.8% for sparfloxacin and gatifloxacin, and 1.4% for levofloxacin and moxifloxacin. Fluoroquinolons have the lowest resistance compared to amoxicillin, clarithromycin and metronidazole.

2. Clarithromycin Resistance

The rates of eradication largely depends on the clarithromycin-sensitivity. Resistance to clarithromycin can be determined by using restriction fragment length polymorphism (RFLP) in domain V of 23S rRNA [108]. Analysis of the 23S rRNA gene mutations is based on the generation of restriction sites for two restriction enzymes: BbsI and BsaI, which correspond to the base substitutions characteristic of clarithromycin resistance from A to G at positions 2142 and 2143, respectively. Of 105 Malaysian subjects, only 1 had the BbsI mutation (base substitution at A2142G) and 2 had the BsaI mutation (base substitution at A2143G). Taken as a whole, only 3 of 105 (2.9%) samples harbored clarithromycin resistant strains in Malaysia [108]. Clarithromycin resistance is an uncommon occurrence among Malaysian isolates of *H. pylori* strains and the mutations A2142G and A2143G detected were associated with low-level resistance.

Notably, a high rate of clarithromycin resistant *H. pylori* isolates are reported in Thailand [109]. Primary *H. pylori* resistance to clarithromycin was observed in 16 of 69 patients (23.2%). The eradication rates were 90.6% (48/53) and 56.3% (9/16) in patients with clarithromycin sensitive and clarithromycin resistant *H. pylori* strains, respectively. These results indicate that pretreatment resistance to clarithromycin has a significant impact on treatment failure with clarithromycin-based regimen.

Clarithromycin resistance of *H. pylori* is rapidly increasing these days [110,111]. There was an increasing tendency for the emergence of strains with dual resistance to metronidazole and clarithromycin, although overall resistance to metronidazole did not increase recently [111]. Among clarithromyin-resistant strains that have A2143G mutations are not eradicated by PPI-based triple therapy. Therefore,

A2143G was an important 23S rRNA mutation associated with clarithromycin resistance and affected the *H. pylori* eradication efficacy. When DNA sequences of the 23S rRNA gene in 21 primary clarithromycin-resistant and 64 secondary clarithromycin-resistant strains were determined by PCR amplification and nucleotide sequence analyses, two mutations of the 23S rRNA gene, A2143G and T2182C, were observed in primary clarithromycin-resistant isolates [112]. In secondary isolates, dual mutation of A2143G+T2182C was frequently observed. In addition, A2143G+T2182C+ T2190C, A2143G+T2182C+C2195T, and A2143G+T2182C +A2223G were observed in secondary isolates. These results indicate that secondary isolates show a greater variety of 23S rRNA gene mutation types than primary isolates, and triple mutations of secondary isolates are associated with A2143G+T2182C in *H. pylori* isolated from Korean patients. Both low-dose clarithromycin triple therapy (omeprazole 20 mg, amoxicillin 1000 mg, and clarithromycin 250 mg or omeprazole 20 mg, amoxicillin 1000 mg, and clarithromycin 500 mg) and tinidazole-containing triple therapy (omeprazole 20 mg, tinidazole 500 mg, and clarithromycin 500 mg) are effective and safe regimens for *H. pylori* eradication [113].

3. Fluoroquinolone Resistance

Fluoroquinolone resistance of *H. pylori* is known to be dependent on mutations in the QRDR of gyrA. A study that evaluated on the distribution of gyrA point mutations and to evaluate the impact of the mutations on second-line *H. pylori* eradication therapy showed that fluoroquinolone resistance of *H. pylori* was caused by gyrA Asn-87 and Asp-91 point mutations [114]. The Asn- 87 mutation seems to be an important determinant of failure of fluoroquinolone-containing triple eradication therapy based on eradication results.

The 7-day moxifloxacin-containing triple therapy produced an unacceptably low eradication rate [115]. Increasing the duration of therapy was expected to increase the eradication rate, but the expected increased did not materialize, most likely because of coincident marked increase in the prevalence of resistance to moxifloxacin. Moxifloxacin resistance in 2007-2008 was 28.2%. Side-effect increased with treatment duration (*i.e.*, 9.8, 12.2, and 25.4% at 7, 10, and 14 days, respectively).

4. Mixed Resistance

Antibiotic-susceptible and -resistant *H. pylori* can be present simultaneously in the same host [116]. Of treatment-failure patients, some show mixed infections with both antibiotic-susceptible and -resistant *H. pylori* strains. These results suggest that continuing genomic diversities in the same strain may play an important role in modulating the antibiotic-heteroresistant *H. pylori in vivo.*

Considerable number of patients with treatment failure have *H. pylori* strains resistant to two or more antimicrobial agents (multi-drug resistance, MDR). Notably, in Malaysia, the resistance rates of the antibiotics used in primary treatment of *H. pylori* infections are low, and multi-antibiotic-resistant strains are uncommon [117]. The resistance rates were noted to be 37.4% (metronidazole), 2.1% (clarithromycin), 1% (levofloxacin and ciprofloxacin), and 0% (amoxicillin and tetracycline) with high metronidazole MICs of ≥256 μg/mL among the resistant strains. Resistance to one type of antibiotic was observed in 36.4% of the strains where mono-resistance to metronidazole was the most common. Resistance to ≥2 antibiotics was noted in 3.3% of isolates, and infections with mixed populations of metronidazole-sensitive and -resistant strains were also observed.

PROGNOSIS

Improvement After *H. pylori* Eradication

H. pylori positive patients with the gastritis-associated diseases such as gastric ulcer, duodenal ulcer, gastric cancer, and primary gastric B-cell lymphoma can be improved after *H. pylori* eradication. Majority of patients show improvement of dyspepsia symptoms after eradication treatment [118]. Restored tissue levels of ghrelin and improved status of appetite can be achieved with gastric ulcer healing and *H. pylori* eradication [119]. Gastric ghrelin mRNA expression significantly increase after either ulcer healing or *H. pylori* eradication, whereas gastric TNF-alpha mRNA expression decrease after ulcer treatment and *H. pylori* eradication. In parallel with these changes, the visual analog scales for hunger and prospective food consumptions are significantly increase after ulcer healing and *H. pylori* eradication. With regard to reflux esophagitis, *H. pylori* eradication increase the prevalence of erosive esophagitis to the level of *H. pylori*-negative individuals [120].

In areas with a high prevalence of gastric cancer, eliminating *H. pylori* infection have the greatest impact in reducing the burden of gastric cancer. A long-term follow-up (9.4 years), large-size (n=1790) Korean study showed that atrophy can be improved after *H. pylori* eradication, but not intestinal metaplasia [121]. Although the compartment theory has not been well investigated in gastric carcinogenesis in relation to incomplete-type and complete-type intestinal metaplasia, a study showed that *H. pylori* eradication prior to development of incomplete-type intestinal metaplasia improves corpus gastritis and may prevent gastric cancer [122]. When sonic hedgehog and Cdx2 expression in corpus gastritis was compared after *H. pylori* eradication between 70 subjects at high risk for gastric cancer and 30 controls, residual inflammation at the corpus lesser curve was more frequently detected in the cancer group than in the controls. In addition, sonic hedgehog and Cdx2 expression were more frequently noticed in the mucosa with incomplete-type intestinal metaplasia rather than in those without incomplete-type intestinal metaplasia. These findings suggest that cellular phenotype of gastric intestinal metaplasia may be an important factor in the reduction of cancer incidence after *H. pylori* eradication, and that incomplete-type intestinal metaplasia is a more progressive form toward gastric carcinogenesis than complete-type intestinal metaplasia. Therefore, to prevent gastric cancer, *H. pylori* eradication is best performed before the development of intestinal metaplasia.

Reinfection

In Asia, high reinfection rates in the community makes *H. pylori* cure a temporary event, and this also has resulted in there being fewer indications for *H. pylori* eradication in Asian countries than in Western guidelines. The risk of reinfection after *H. pylori* eradication was relatively low in Thai patients after 4-year follow up [123]. Annual reinfection rate was 3.38%. Even if the spouse was infected, 88.89% of patients remained uninfected after 4-years of *H. pylori* eradication. In Singapore, the recurrence of *H. pylori* infection was low at the end of one year after successful eradication therapy in this urban East Asian population [124]. Of

96 consecutive duodenal ulcer patients with biopsy-proven *H. pylori* eradication, recurrence of *H. pylori* infection was detected at 9 and 10 months after confirmation of *H. pylori* eradication in two patients, and at between 13 and 20 months in the remaining four. Besides, following successful *H. pylori* eradication, reinfection with *H. pylori* in patients in Vietnam was found to be higher than in industrialized countries after 1 year [125]. The overall reinfection rate was 23.5%, with 58.8% of the strains being identical to the pre-treatment isolates and 41.2% being different.

The reinfection rate of *H. pylori*, in Korea, was found to be very low, 2.94% per year [126]. The seroreversion rate was 5, 10, and 45% at 2, 10, and 18 months after *H. pylori* eradication, respectively. The recrudescence of *H. pylori* was 3.49%, and the annual reinfection rate was 2.94% per year. However, in subjects after second-line eradication with bismuth-containing quadruple regimens, *H. pylori* reinfection rate of 6.0% per patient-year [127]. No evidence was obtained to indicate that the reinfection rate depended on the age, sex, ulcer location, or eradication regimens. The relapse of dyspeptic symptoms was the only factor predictive *of H. pylori* recurrence.

ACKNOWLEDGEMENT

None declared.

CONFLICT OF INTEREST

The author(s) confirm that this chapter content has no conflict of interest.

REFERENCES

[1] Wong SN, Sollano JD, Chan MM, *et al*. Changing trends in peptic ulcer prevalence in a tertiary care setting in the Philippines: a seven-year study. J Gastroenterol Hepatol 2005; 20: 628-32.

[2] Yim JY, Kim N, Choi SH, *et al*. Seroprevalence of *Helicobacter pylori* in South Korea. Helicobacter 2007; 12: 333-40.

[3] Lee SY, Park HS, Yu SK, *et al*. Decreasing prevalence of *Helicobacter pylori* infection: a 9-year observational study. Hepatogastroenterology 2007; 54: 630-3.

[4] Sasidharan S, Lachumy SJ, Ravichandran M, *et al*. Epidemiology of *Helicobacter pylori* among multiracial community in Northern Peninsular, Malaysia: effect of age across race and gender. Asian Pac J Trop Med 2011; 4: 72-5.

[5] Hoang TT, Bengtsson C, Phung DC, *et al.* Seroprevalence of *Helicobacter pylori* infection in urban and rural Vietnam. Clin Diagn Lab Immunol 2005; 12: 81-5.
[6] Atisook K, Kachinthorn U, Luengrojanakul P, *et al.* Histology of gastritis and *Helicobacter pylori* infection in Thailand: a nationwide study of 3776 cases. Helicobacter 2003; 8: 132-41.
[7] Kim N, Lim SH, Lee KH, *et al.* Seroconversion of *Helicobacter pylori* in Korean male employees. Scand J Gastroenterol 2005; 40: 1021-7.
[8] Goh KL, Chan WK, Shiota S, *et al.* Epidemiology of *Helicobacter pylori* infection and public health implications. Helicobacter 2011; 16(S1): S1-9.
[9] Lee YY, Ismail AW, Mustaffa N, *et al.* Sociocultural and dietary practices among Malay subjects in the north-eastern region of Peninsular Malaysia: a region of low prevalence of *Helicobacter pylori* infection. Helicobacter 2012; 17: 54-61.
[10] Vilaichone RK, Mahachai V, Tumwasorn S, *et al.* Molecular epidemiology and outcome of *Helicobacter pylori* infection in Thailand: a cultural cross roads. Helicobacter 2004; 9: 453-9.
[11] Goh KL, Parasakthi N. The racial cohort phenomenon: seroepidemiology of *Helicobacter pylori* infection in a multiracial South-East Asian country. Eur J Gastroenterol Hepatol 2001; 13: 177-83.
[12] Kang JY, Yeoh KG, Ho KY, *et al.* Racial differences in *Helicobacter pylori* seroprevalence in Singapore: correlation with differences in peptic ulcer frequency. J Gastroenterol Hepatol 1997; 12: 655-9.
[13] Correa P, Piazuelo MB. Evolutionary history of the *Helicobacter pylori* genome: implications for gastric carcinogenesis. Gut Liver 2012; 6: 21-8.
[14] Tay CY, Mitchell H, Dong Q, *et al.* Population structure of *Helicobacter pylori* among ethnic groups in Malaysia: recent acquisition of the bacterium by the Malay population. BMC Microbiol 2009; 9: 126.
[15] Tan TS, Thiberge JM, Vong S, *et al.* Evolutionary history of *Helicobacter pylori* sequences reflect past human migrations in Southeast Asia. PLoS One 2011; 6: e22058.
[16] Goh KL. Epidemiology of *Helicobacter pylori* infection in Malaysia--observations in a multiracial Asian population. Med J Malaysia 2009; 64: 187-92.
[17] Fock KM, Ang TL. Epidemiology of *Helicobacter pylori* infection and gastric cancer in Asia. J Gastroenterol Hepatol 2010; 25: 479-86.
[18] Singh K, Ghoshal UC. Causal role of *Helicobacter pylori* infection in gastric cancer: an Asian enigma. World J Gastroenterol 2006; 12: 1346-51.
[19] Tokudome S, Samsuria Soeripto WD, *et al.* *Helicobacter pylori* infection appears essential for stomach carcinogenesis: observations in Semarang, Indonesia. Cancer Sci 2005; 96: 873-5.
[20] Goh KL, Cheah PL, Md N, *et al.* Ethnicity and *H. pylori* as risk factors for gastric cancer in Malaysia: A prospective case control study. Am J Gastroenterol 2007; 102: 40-5.
[21] Schmidt HM, Ha DM, Taylor EF, *et al.* Variation in human genetic polymorphisms, their association with *Helicobacter pylori* acquisition and gastric cancer in a multi-ethnic country. J Gastroenterol Hepatol 2011; 26: 1725-32.
[22] Schmidt HM, Goh KL, Fock KM, *et al.* Distinct cagA EPIYA motifs are associated with ethnic diversity in Malaysia and Singapore. Helicobacter 2009; 14: 256-63.
[23] Zhu F, Loh M, Hill J, Lee S, *et al.* Genetic factors associated with intestinal metaplasia in a high risk Singapore-Chinese population: a cohort study. BMC Gastroenterol 2009; 9: 76.

[24] Abdullah M, Ohtsuka H, Rani AA, *et al.* *Helicobacter pylori* infection and gastropathy: a comparison between Indonesian and Japanese patients. World J Gastroenterol 2009; 15: 4928-31.

[25] Matsukura N, Yamada S, Kato S, *et al.* Genetic differences in interleukin-1 beta polymorphisms among four Asian populations: an analysis of the Asian paradox between *H. pylori* infection and gastric cancer incidence. J Exp Clin Cancer Res 2003; 22: 47-55.

[26] Yamada S, Matsuhisa T, Makonkawkeyoon L, *et al.* *Helicobacter pylori* infection in combination with the serum pepsinogen I/II ratio and interleukin-1 beta-511 polymorphisms are independent risk factors for gastric cancer in Thais. J Gastroenterol 2006; 41: 1169-77.

[27] Breurec S, Guillard B, Hem S, *et al.* Expansion of European vacA and cagA alleles to East-Asian *Helicobacter pylori* strains in Cambodia. Infect Genet Evol 2011; 11: 1899-905.

[28] Nguyen TL, Uchida T, Tsukamoto Y, *et al.* *Helicobacter pylori* infection and gastroduodenal diseases in Vietnam: a cross-sectional, hospital-based study. BMC Gastroenterol 2010; 10: 114.

[29] Seo TH, Lee SY, Uchida T, *et al.* The origin of non-*H. pylori*-related positive Giemsa staining in human gastric biopsy specimens: A prospective study. Dig Liver Dis 2011; 43: 23-7.

[30] Hirai I, Yoshinaga A, Kimoto A, *et al.* Sequence analysis of East Asian cagA of *Helicobacter pylori* isolated from asymptomatic healthy Japanese and Thai individuals. Curr Microbiol 2011; 62: 855-60.

[31] Cortes MC, Yamakawa A, Casingal CR, *et al.* Diversity of the cagA gene of *Helicobacter pylori* strains from patients with gastroduodenal diseases in the Philippines. FEMS Immunol Med Microbiol 2010; 60: 90-7.

[32] Deankanob W, Chomvarin C, Hahnvajanawong C, *et al.* Enzyme-linked immunosorbent assay for serodiagnosis of *Helicobacter pylori* in dyspeptic patients and volunteer blood donors. Southeast Asian J Trop Med Public Health 2006; 37: 958-65.

[33] Thong-Ngam D, Chayanupatkul M, Vongchampa P, *et al.* An evaluation of a new in-house serum and urine ELISA test for detection of *Helicobacter pylori* infection in Thai population. J Med Assoc Thai 2011; 94: 985-90.

[34] Rahman SH, Azam MG, Rahman MA, *et al.* Non-invasive diagnosis of *H. pylori* infection: evaluation of serological tests with and without current infection marker CIM. World J Gastroenterol 2008; 14: 1231-6.

[35] Lim LG, Yeoh KG, Ho B, *et al.* Validation of four *Helicobacter pylori* rapid blood tests in a multi-ethnic Asian population. World J Gastroenterol 2005; 11: 6681-3.

[36] Kullavanijaya P, Thong-Ngam D, Hanvivatvong O, *et al.* Analysis of eight different methods for the detection of *Helicobacter pylori* infection in patients with dyspepsia. J Gastroenterol Hepatol 2004; 19: 1392-6.

[37] Nguyen LT, Uchida T, Tsukamoto Y, *et al.* Evaluation of rapid urine test for the detection of *Helicobacter pylori* infection in the Vietnamese population. Dig Dis Sci 2010; 55: 89-93.

[38] Choi J, Kim CH, Kim D, *et al.* Prospective evaluation of a new stool antigen test for the detection of *Helicobacter pylori*, in comparison with histology, rapid urease test, 13C-urea breath test, and serology. J Gastroenterol Hepatol 2011; 26: 1053-9.

[39] Yang HR, Seo JK. *Helicobacter pylori* stool antigen (HpSA) tests in children before and after eradication therapy: comparison of rapid immunochromatographic assay and HpSA ELISA. Dig Dis Sci 2008; 53: 2053-8.

[40] Hanvivatvong O, Thong-Ngam D, Kuakarn S, *et al.* Evaluation of *Helicobacter pylori* stool antigen test in Thai patients with upper gastrointestinal bleeding. J Med Assoc Thai 2006; 89(Suppl 3): S98-103.

[41] Yoo JY, Kim N, Park YS, *et al.* Detection rate of *Helicobacter pylori* against a background of atrophic gastritis and/or intestinal metaplasia. J Clin Gastroenterol 2007; 41: 751-5.

[42] Tangmankongworakoon N, Vilaichone RK, Kullavanijaya P, *et al.* The effect of blood on rapid urease test for *Helicobacter pylori* detection: an *in vitro* study. J Med Assoc Thai 2002; 85(Suppl 1): S70-3.

[43] Kim N, Kim JJ, Choe YH, *et al.* Diagnosis and treatment guidelines for *Helicobacter pylori* infection in Korea. Korean J Gastroenterol 2009; 54: 269-78.

[44] Chang YW, Min SK, Kim KJ, *et al.* Delta (13)C-urea breath test value is a useful indicator for *Helicobacter pylori* eradication in patients with functional dyspepsia. J Gastroenterol Hepatol 2003; 18: 726-31.

[45] Oak JH, Chung WC, Jung SH, *et al.* Effect of acid pump antagonist (Revaprazan, Revanex®) on result of 13C urea breath test in patients with *Helicobacter pylori* associated peptic ulcer disease. Korean J Gastroenterol 2011; 57: 8-13.

[46] Kim CG, Choi IJ, Lee JY, *et al.* Biopsy site for detecting *Helicobacter pylori* infection in patients with gastric cancer. J Gastroenterol Hepatol 2009; 24: 469-74.

[47] Shin CM, Kim N, Lee HS, *et al.* Validation of diagnostic tests for *Helicobacter pylori* with regard to grade of atrophic gastritis and/or intestinal metaplasia. Helicobacter 2009; 14: 512-9.

[48] Ottiwet O, Chomvarin C, Chaicumpar K, *et al.* Nested polymerase chain reaction for detection of *Helicobacter pylori* in gastric biopsy specimens. Southeast Asian J Trop Med Public Health 2010; 41: 1423-31.

[49] Kaur G, Madhavan M, Basri AH, *et al.* Rapid diagnosis of *Helicobacter pylori* infection in gastric imprint smears. Southeast Asian J Trop Med Public Health 2004; 35: 676-80.

[50] Hua J, Yeoh KG, Ng HC, *et al.* Improving the success of culturing *Helicobacter pylori* from gastric biopsies. Microbios 1998; 96: 95-101.

[51] Lee SY. Future candidates for indications of *Helicobacter pylori* eradication – do the indications need to be revised? J Gastroenterol Hepatol 2012; 27: 200-11.

[52] Fock KM, Katelaris P, Sugano K, *et al.* Second Asia-Pacific Consensus Guidelines for *Helicobacter pylori* infection. J Gastroenterol Hepatol 2009; 24: 1587-600.

[53] FL, Hu PJ, Liu WZ, *et al.* Third Chinese National Consensus Report on the management of *Helicobacter pylori* infection. J Dig Dis 2008; 9: 178-84.

[54] Asaka M. Guidelines in the management of *H. pylori* infection in Japan. Nihon Rinsho 2009; 67: 2227-32.

[55] Lee SY. Endoscopic gastritis: what does it mean? Dig Dis Sci 2011; 56: 2209-11.

[56] Choi HJ, Lee SY, Lee JH, *et al.* Two atypical cases of nodular gastritis: a poorly differentiated gastric adenocarcinoma and a pseudo-low grade gastric MALT lymphoma. Gastroenterol Res 2010; 3: 41-5.

[57] Stolte M, Bätz CH, Bayerdörffer E, *et al.* *Helicobacter pylori* eradication in the treatment and differential diagnosis of giant folds in the corpus and fundus of the stomach. Z Gastroenterol 1995; 33: 198-201.

[58] Ahn SY, Lee SY, Hong SN, *et al.* Endoscopic diagnosis of open-type atrophic gastritis is related to the histological diagnosis of intestinal metaplasia and Cdx2 expression. Dig Dis Sci 2011; 56: 1119–26.

[59] Gwee KA, Teng L, Wong RK, *et al.* The response of Asian patients with functional dyspepsia to eradication of *Helicobacter pylori* infection. Eur J Gastroenterol Hepatol 2009; 21: 417-24.

[60] Shin A, Park S, Shin HR, *et al.* Population attributable fraction of infection-related cancers in Korea. Ann Oncol 2011; 22: 1435-42.

[61] Gwack J, Shin A, Kim CS, *et al.* CagA-producing *Helicobacter pylori* and increased risk of gastric cancer: a nested case-control study in Korea. Br J Cancer 2006; 95: 639-41.

[62] Nam JH, Choi IJ, Cho SJ, *et al. Helicobacter pylori* infection and histological changes in siblings of young gastric cancer patients. J Gastroenterol Hepatol 2011; 26: 1157-63.

[63] Shin CM, Kim N, Yang HJ, *et al.* Stomach cancer risk in gastric cancer relatives: interaction between *Helicobacter pylori* infection and family history of gastric cancer for the risk of stomach cancer. J Clin Gastroenterol 2010; 44: e34-9.

[64] Chang YW, Han YS, Lee DK, *et al.* Role of *Helicobacter pylori* infection among offspring or siblings of gastric cancer patients. Int J Cancer. 2002; 101: 469-74.

[65] El-Omar EM, Oien K, Murray LS, *et al.* Increased prevalence of precancerous changes in relatives of gastric cancer patients: critical role of *H. pylori*. Gastroenterology 2000; 118: 22-30.

[66] Lee JS, Kwon KA, Jung HS, *et al.* Korea red ginseng on *Helicobacter pylori*-induced halitosis: newer therapeutic strategy and a plausible mechanism. Digestion 2009; 80: 192–9.

[67] Lee WY, Yoon WT, Shin HY, *et al. Helicobacter pylori* infection and motor fluctuations in patients with Parkinson's disease. Mov Disord 2008; 23: 1696-700.

[68] Kim JM, Kim SH, Park KH, *et al.* Investigation of the association between *Helicobacter pylori* infection and normal tension glaucoma. Invest Ophthalmol Vis Sci 2011;52:665-8.

[69] Ki MR, Goo MJ, Park JK, *et al. Helicobacter pylori* accelerates hepatic fibrosis by sensitizing transforming growth factor-β1-induced inflammatory signaling. Lab Invest 2010; 90: 1507-16.

[70] Lee JW, Lee DH, Lee JI, *et al.* Identification of *Helicobacter pylori* in gallstone, bile, and other hepatobiliary tissues of patients with cholecystitis. Gut Liver 2010; 4: 60-7.

[71] Lee SY, Tang SJ, Rockey DC, *et al.* Managing anticoagulation and antiplatelet medications in GI endoscopy: a survey comparing the East and the West. Gastrointest Endosc 2008; 67: 1076-81.

[72] Fock KM, Ng HS, Ng TM, *et al.* A randomised trial of amoxycillin *vs.* clarithromycin in combination with omeprazole for eradication of *Helicobacter pylori* infection in Singapore. Singapore Med J 2000; 41: 482-4.

[73] Kim SY, Jung SW. *Helicobacter pylori* eradication therapy in Korea. Korean J Gastroenterol 2011; 58:67-73.

[74] Qua CS, Manikam J, Goh KL.Efficacy of 1-week proton pump inhibitor triple therapy as first-line *Helicobacter pylori* eradication regime in Asian patients: is it still effective 10 years on? J Dig Dis 2010; 11: 244-8.

[75] Choi KH, Chung WC, Lee KM, *et al.* Efficacy of levofloxacin and rifaximin based quadruple therapy in *Helicobacter pylori* associated gastroduodenal disease: a double-blind, randomized controlled trial. J Korean Med Sci 2011; 26: 785-90.

[76] Kositchaiwat C, Ovartlarnporn B, Kachintorn U, *et al.* Low and high doses of rabeprazole *vs.* omeprazole for cure of *Helicobacter pylori* infection. Aliment Pharmacol Ther 2003; 18: 1017-21.

[77] Chung JW, Lee GH, Han JH, *et al.* The trends of one-week first-line and second-line eradication therapy for *Helicobacter pylori* infection in Korea. Hepatogastroenterology 2011; 58: 246-50.
[78] Goh KL, Manikam J, Qua CS. High-dose rabeprazole-amoxicillin dual therapy and rabeprazole triple therapy with amoxicillin and levofloxacin for 2 weeks as first and second line rescue therapies for *Helicobacter pylori* treatment failures. Aliment Pharmacol Ther 2012; Epub ahead of print.
[79] Lee SK, Lee SW, Park JY, *et al.* Effectiveness and safety of repeated quadruple therapy in *Helicobacter pylori* infection after failure of second-line quadruple therapy: repeated quadruple therapy as a third-line therapy. Helicobacter 2011; 16: 410-4.
[80] Lee BH, Kim N, Hwang TJ, *et al.* Bismuth-containing quadruple therapy as second-line treatment for *Helicobacter pylori* infection: effect of treatment duration and antibiotic resistance on the eradication rate in Korea. Helicobacter 2010; 15: 38-45.
[81] Kang JM, Kim N, Lee DH, *et al.* Second-line treatment for *Helicobacter pylori* infection: 10-day moxifloxacin-based triple therapy *vs.* 2-week quadruple therapy. Helicobacter 2007; 12: 623-8.
[82] Lee SY, Shin YW, Hahm KB. Phytoceuticals: mighty but ignored weapons against *Helicobacter pylori* infection. J Dig Dis 2008; 9: 129-39.
[83] Kim YJ, Chung JW, Lee SJ, *et al.* Progression from chronic atrophic gastritis to gastric cancer; tangle, toggle, tackle with Korea red ginseng. J Clin Biochem Nutr 2010; 46: 195-204.
[84] Suk KT, Kim HS, Kim MY, *et al.* *In vitro* antibacterial and morphological effects of the urushiol component of the sap of the Korean lacquer tree (Rhus vernicifera Stokes) on *Helicobacter pylori.* J Korean Med Sci 2010; 25: 399-404.
[85] Bhamarapravati S, Pendland SL, Mahady GB. Extracts of spice and food plants from Thai traditional medicine inhibit the growth of the human carcinogen *Helicobacter pylori. In Vivo* 2003; 17: 541-4.
[86] Lee JS, Paek NS, Kwon OS, *et al.* Anti-inflammatory actions of probiotics through activating suppressor of cytokine signaling (SOCS) expression and signaling in *Helicobacter pylori* infection: a novel mechanism. J Gastroenterol Hepatol 2010; 25: 194-202.
[87] Ki MR, Ghim SY, Hong IH, *et al.* *In vitro* inhibition of *Helicobacter pylori* growth and of adherence of cagA positive strains to gastric epithelial cells by *Lactobacillus paraplantarum* KNUC25 isolated from kimchi. J Med Food 2010; 13: 629-34.
[88] Vilaichone RK, Mahachai V, Tumwasorn S, *et al.* Inhibitory effect of Lactobacillus acidophilus on *Helicobacter pylori* in peptic ulcer patients: *in vitro* study. J Med Assoc Thai 2002; 85(Suppl 1): S79-84.
[89] Park SK, Park DI, Choi JS, *et al.* The effect of probiotics on *Helicobacter pylori* eradication. Hepatogastroenterology 2007; 54: 2032-6.
[90] Song MJ, Park DI, Park JH, *et al.* The effect of probiotics and mucoprotective agents on PPI-based triple therapy for eradication of *Helicobacter pylori*. Helicobacter 2010; 15: 206-13.
[91] Yoon H, Kim N, Kim JY, *et al.* Effects of multistrain probiotic-containing yogurt on second-line triple therapy for *Helicobacter pylori* infection. J Gastroenterol Hepatol 2011; 26: 44-8.

[92] Park HG, Jung MK, Jung JT, *et al.* Randomised clinical trial: a comparative study of 10-day sequential therapy with 7-day standard triple therapy for *Helicobacter pylori* infection in naïve patients. Aliment Pharmacol Ther 2012; 35: 56-65.

[93] Kim YS, Kim SJ, Yoon JH, *et al.* Randomised clinical trial: the efficacy of a 10-day sequential therapy *vs.* a 14-day standard proton pump inhibitor-based triple therapy for *Helicobacter pylori* in Korea. Aliment Pharmacol Ther 2011; 34: 1098-105.

[94] Kwon JH, Lee DH, Song BJ, *et al.* Ten-day sequential therapy as first-line treatment for *Helicobacter pylori* infection in Korea: a retrospective study. Helicobacter 2010; 15: 148-53.

[95] Sirimontaporn N, Thong-Ngam D, Tumwasorn S, *et al.* Ten-day sequential therapy of *Helicobacter pylori* infection in Thailand. Am J Gastroenterol 2010; 105: 1071-5.

[96] Mahachai V, Sirimontaporn N, Tumwasorn S, *et al.* Sequential therapy in clarithromycin-sensitive and -resistant *Helicobacter pylori* based on polymerase chain reaction molecular test. J Gastroenterol Hepatol 2011; 26: 825-8.

[97] Chang WC, Jo YI, Park HS, *et al.* *Helicobacter pylori* eradication with a 7-day low-dose triple therapy in hemodialysis patients. Clin Exp Nephrol 2010; 14: 469-73.

[98] Jung SW, Lee SW, Hyun JJ, *et al.* Efficacy of *Helicobacter pylori* eradication therapy in chronic liver disease. Dig Liver Dis 2009; 41: 134-40.

[99] Cheon JH, Kim JH, Lee SK, *et al.* *Helicobacter pylori* eradication therapy may facilitate gastric ulcer healing after endoscopic mucosal resection: a prospective randomized study. Helicobacter 2008; 13: 564-71.

[100] Kim JM. Antibiotic resistance of *Helicobacter pylori* isolated from Korean patients. Korean J Gastroenterol 2006; 47: 337-49.

[101] Chung JW, Lee GH, Han JH, *et al.* The trends of one-week first-line and second-line eradication therapy for *Helicobacter pylori* infection in Korea. Hepatogastroenterology 2011; 58: 246-50.

[102] Teo EK, Fock KM, Ng TM, *et al.* Metronidazole-resistant *Helicobacter pylori* in an urban Asian population. J Gastroenterol Hepatol 2000; 15: 494-7.

[103] Ling KL, Luman W, Ho B, *et al.* Efficacy of a nitroimidazole containing triple therapy regime in Singapore. Singapore Med J 2001; 42: 317-21.

[104] Goh KL, Navaratnam P. High *Helicobacter pylori* resistance to metronidazole but zero or low resistance to clarithromycin, levofloxacin, and other antibiotics in Malaysia. Helicobacter 2011; 16: 241-5.

[105] Vilaichone RK, Mahacahai V, Tumwasorn S, *et al.* CagA genotype and metronidazole resistant strain of *Helicobacter pylori* in functional dyspepsia in Thailand. Kachintorn U. J Gastroenterol Hepatol 2011; 26(Suppl 3): S46-8.

[106] Kulsuntiwong P, Chomvarin C, Chaicumpar K, *et al.* Antimicrobial susceptibility of *Helicobacter pylori* isolated from gastric biopsies in dyspeptic patients. Southeast Asian J Trop Med Public Health 2008; 39: 1102-9.

[107] Kumala W, Rani A. Patterns of *Helicobacter pylori* isolate resistance to fluoroquinolones, amoxicillin, clarithromycin and metronidazoles. Southeast Asian J Trop Med Public Health 2006; 37: 970-4.

[108] Ho SL, Tan EL, Sam CK, *et al.* Clarithromycin resistance and point mutations in the 23S rRNA gene in *Helicobacter pylori* isolates from Malaysia. J Dig Dis 2010; 11: 101-5.

[109] Mahachai V, Thong-Ngam D, Noophun P, *et al.* Efficacy of clarithromycin-based triple therapy for treating *Helicobacter pylori*. J Med Assoc Thai 2006; 89(Suppl 3): S74-8.

[110] Hwang TJ, Kim N, Kim HB, *et al.* Change in antibiotic resistance of *Helicobacter pylori* strains and the effect of A2143G point mutation of 23S rRNA on the eradication of *H. pylori* in a single center of Korea. J Clin Gastroenterol 2010; 44: 536-43.
[111] Eun CS, Han DS, Park JY, *et al.* Changing pattern of antimicrobial resistance of *Helicobacter pylori* in Korean patients with peptic ulcer diseases. J Gastroenterol 2003; 38: 436-41.
[112] Kim JM, Kim JS, Kim N, *et al.* Gene mutations of 23S rRNA associated with clarithromycin resistance in *Helicobacter pylori* strains isolated from Korean patients. J Microbiol Biotechnol 2008; 18: 1584-9.
[113] Choi IJ, Jung HC, Choi KW, *et al.* Efficacy of low-dose clarithromycin triple therapy and tinidazole-containing triple therapy for *Helicobacter pylori* eradication. Aliment Pharmacol Ther 2002; 16: 145-51.
[114] Lee JW, Kim N, Nam RH, *et al.* Mutations of *Helicobacter pylori* associated with fluoroquinolone resistance in Korea. Helicobacter 2011; 16: 301-10.
[115] Yoon H, Kim N, Lee BH, *et al.* Moxifloxacin-containing triple therapy as second-line treatment for *Helicobacter pylori* infection: effect of treatment duration and antibiotic resistance on the eradication rate. Helicobacter 2009; 14: 77-85.
[116] Lee YC, Lee SY, Pyo JH, *et al.* Isogenic variation of *Helicobacteral pylori* strain resulting in heteroresistant antibacterial phenotypes in a single host *in vivo*. Helicobacter 2005; 10: 240-8.
[117] Ahmad N, Zakaria WR, Mohamed R. Analysis of antibiotic susceptibility patterns of *Helicobacter pylori* isolates from Malaysia. Helicobacter 2011; 16: 47-51.
[118] Utia K, Syam AF, Simadibrata M, *et al.* Clinical evaluation of dyspepsia in patients with functional dyspepsia, with the history of *Helicobacter pylori* eradication therapy in Cipto Mangunkusumo Hospital, Jakarta. Acta Med Indones 2010; 42: 86-93.
[119] Jang EJ, Park SW, Park JS, *et al.* The influence of the eradication of *Helicobacter pylori* on gastric ghrelin, appetite, and body mass index in patients with peptic ulcer disease. J Gastroenterol Hepatol. 2008; 23(Suppl 2): S278-85.
[120] Kim BC, Kim CG, Nam BH. Effect of *Helicobacter pylori* infection and its eradication on reflux esophagitis and reflux symptoms. Am J Gastroenterol 2010; 105: 2153-62.
[121] Kim N, Park RY, Cho SI, *et al. Helicobacter pylori* infection and development of gastric cancer in Korea: long-term follow-up. J Clin Gastroenterol 2008; 42: 448-54.
[122] Shiotani A, Uedo N, Iishi H, *et al.* Re-expression of sonic hedgehog and reduction of CDX2 after *Helicobacter pylori* eradication prior to incomplete intestinal metaplasia. Int J Cancer 2007; 121: 1182-9.
[123] Thong-Ngam D, Mahachai V, Kullavanijaya P. Incidence of *Helicobacter pylori* recurrent infection and associated factors in Thailand. J Med Assoc Thai 2007; 90: 1406-10.
[124] Khor CJ, Fock KM, Ng TM, *et al.* Recurrence of *Helicobacter pylori* infection and duodenal ulcer relapse, following successful eradication in an urban east Asian population. Singapore Med J 2000; 41: 382-6.
[125] Wheeldon TU, Hoang TT, Phung DC, *et al.* Long-term follow-up of *Helicobacter pylori* eradication therapy in Vietnam: reinfection and clinical outcome. Aliment Pharmacol Ther 2005; 21: 1047-53.
[126] Lee JH, Kim N, Chung JI, *et al.* Long-term follow up of *Helicobacter pylori* IgG serology after eradication and reinfection rate of *H. pylori* in South Korea. Helicobacter 2008; 13: 288-94.

[127] Cheon JH, Kim N, Lee DH, *et al.* Long-term outcomes after *Helicobacter pylori* eradication with second-line, bismuth-containing quadruple therapy in Korea. Eur J Gastroenterol Hepatol 2006; 18: 515-9.

Send Orders for Reprints to reprints@benthamscience.net

Helicobacter Pylori: A Worldwide Perspective 2014, 2014, 130-168

CHAPTER 6

Helicobacter pylori in South America: Epidemiology, Diagnosis and Treatment

Luiz Gonzaga Coelho*

Faculdade de Medicina, Universidade Federal de Minas Gerais, Belo Horizonte, MG, Brasil

Abstract: In most South American countries, *H. pylori* infection prevalence is high, affecting over 70% in populations with precarious living conditions. Due to poor sanitation and low standards of living conditions, the infection is acquired in early childhood. Also, it is estimated that gastric cancer, the main clinical sequela of *H. pylori* infection, has an average incidence rate of 12.4 cases per 100,000 inhabitants (8.4 cases per 100,000 inhabitants for women and 17.3 cases per 100,000 for men) in the continent. It is worth pointing out that there is initial evidence of a decline in prevalence of *H. pylori* infection in some more privileged fragments of the population. The chapter also review the main methods used to diagnosis *H. pylori* infection and their results in South America setting. The management of the infection including anti-*H. pylori* drugs, therapeutic regimes, eradication control, bacterial resistance, relapse and reinfection, and therapy failure is outlined.

Keywords: *Helicobacter pylori*:diagnosis, *Helicobacter pylori*, treatment and antimicrobial resistance, *Helicobacter pylori*: epidemiology, *H. pylori* and gastric cancer, *Helicobacter pylori*, antimicrobial drugs, *Helicobacter pylori*: South America, *Helicobacter pylori*, developing countries.

INTRODUCTION

After *Helicobacter pylori* (*H. pylori*) was identified by Marshall and Warren [1] in 1983 in Australia, this microorganism has been found in different parts of the world in at least 50% of the world population. It is a major, at times dominant, acquired environmental factor in the pathogenesis of a large spectrum of diseases such as acute and chronic gastritis, gastric and duodenal ulcers, gastric carcinoma and lymphoma.

***Address correspondence to Prof. Luiz Gonzaga Coelho:** Rua dos Otoni 705/601 Belo Horizonte 30150-270 Belo Horizonte, MG, Brazil; Tel: +55-31-3222-4641; Fax: +55-31-3226-2866;
E-mail: lcoelho22@gmail.com

Buzás György Miklós (Ed.)

The object of this chapter is to review the main epidemiological, diagnostic and therapeutic aspects of this infection in South America.

EPIDEMIOLOGY

Serological studies carried out in different parts of the world have shown that in developing countries the infection is acquired in early childhood and that most subjects are infected. Conversely, in developed countries, although the infection is uncommon in childhood, there is a progressive increase in its prevalence as people age, and it attacks about 50% of the elderly. The prevalence of *H. pylori* infection in adults in Latin American countries is nearly always higher than 50% of subjects and may vary in any particular country depending on the population studied and the geographical area (Table **1**).

Table 1: *H. pylori* epidemiology in asymptomatic individuals in South America

	Adults (n)	**HP Prevalence**	**Children (n)**	**HP Prevalence**	**Diagnostic Method**
Argentina					
Olmos, 2000. [2]	493	49.1%	261	15.7%	Serology
Santos, 2009. [3]			307	25.0%	Urea breath test
Brazil					
Zaterka, 2007. [4]	993	65.6%	326	35.6%	ELISA
Rodrigues, 2005. [5]	224	80.0%			ELISA
Miranda, 2010. [6]					ELISA
Chile					
Ferreccio, 2007. [7]	2615	73%			ELISA
Colombia					
Campuzano-Maya, 2007. [8]	342	77.2%			Urea breath test
Ecuador					
Gómez, 2004. [9]			257	63%	ELISA
Peru					
Ramirez-Ramos, 2004. [10]	329	48%			Urease, PCR
Uruguay					
González, 2010. [11]	50	70%			Histology, Urease, and Culture
Vazquez Serra, 1997. [12]	720	46%			ELISA
Venezuela					
Chose, 2005. [13]	127	95%	170	78,8%	ELISA
Páez Valery, 2006. [14]					Urea breath test

Table 1: contd...

Bolivia **Friedman, 1997. [15]** **Santos, 2009 [3]**			1392 424	44% 74%	ELISA Urea breath test
Paraguay **Yorg, 2008. [16]**	80	62%			Urea breath test

In populations with precarious living conditions, whether residing in rural or urban areas of the continent, the prevalence of the infection may affect over 70% of the population [5,7,10,11]. Studies conducted in Peru showed similar prevalence for populations at the same socio-economic level among those living on the coast, in the mountains or the Peruvian jungle, with those inhabiting higher altitudes, for unclear reasons, showing more intense histological gastritis than coastal dwellers [10].

Similarly to industrialized nations, *H. pylori* has been associated with chronic gastritis and their consequences such as peptic ulcer disease and gastric cancer. However, accumulating data suggests that, in children, *H. pylori* may produce significant sequelae even before symptoms of gastritis or peptic ulcer develop. In children from poor areas, *H. pylori* can produce rapidly destructive gastric mucosal lesions, which could destroy the gastric acid barrier. This persistent hypochlorhydria may last a long time rendering children more vulnerable to diarrheal diseases and adverse nutritional consequences. However, more importantly, gastric cancer remains a major public health problem in South America [17] (Fig. **1**).

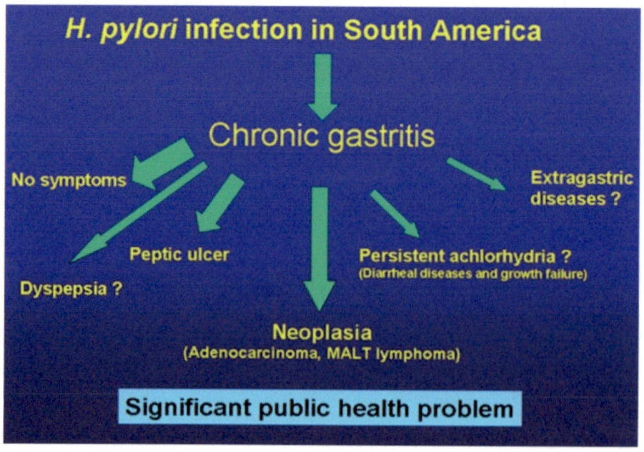

Figure 1: *H. pylori* infection and their consequences in South America.

Fig. **2** shows the estimated incidence rates per 100,000 inhabitants for gastric cancer, the main clinical sequela of infection by *H. pylori*. South America has an average incidence rate for both sexes of 12.4 cases per 100,000 inhabitants, with 8.4 cases per 100,000 inhabitants for women and 17.3 cases per 100,000 for men [18].

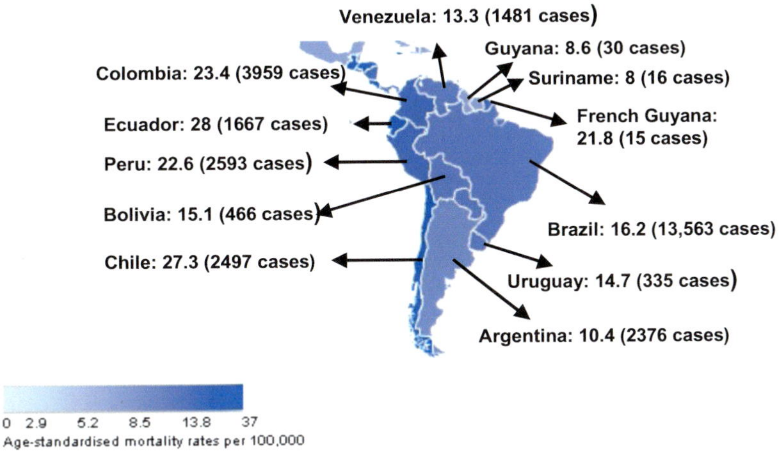

Figure 2. - Estimated Stomach Cancer Incidence in South America in 2008: Men

Source: GLOBOCAN 2008, International Agency for Research on Cancer (18)

The infection is acquired in the first years of life in early childhood, but acquisition among low socio-economic level populations is quicker before they are five years of age [19-21]. Although the exact transmission mechanism remains unclear, person-to-person transmission seems to be the main form of dissemination.

A low socio-economic level with its natural outcomes such as poor hygiene and housing conditions, high agglomeration or household density or living in institutions, improper hygiene habits, an infected family member (especially the mother) is now considered the chief *H. pylori* infection marker. Failure to consistently identify *H. pylori* in any receptor other than man suggests that the microorganism is a strictly human pathogen transmitted directly or indirectly from person to person.

Person to person transmission seems evident from studies with institutionalized children where a high prevalence of infection has been demonstrated in different studies [22,23]. A Brazilian study assessing the role of the mother and siblings in transmitting the infection suggests that *H. pylori* is passed from infected mothers to their children, and that siblings also play an important role in transmitting the disease in the family home [24].

There are doubts as to whether transmission comes about by the oral-oral or the fecal-oral route, or both, or even the gastro-oral route. Epidemiological studies using molecular biology techniques have cleared up some controversial points in this field. So, in favor of oral-oral transmission, we know that gastric mucous has a rapid cell turnover, a continuous desquamation, with the microorganism easily isolated in the gastric juice. The reflux of gastric contents to the oral cavity could allow colonization in the mouth, with saliva as the transmission vehicle. However, although isolated in the gastric juice, the growth of *H. pylori* in the oral cavity has been questioned, as only a few studies have managed to isolate it in the mouth (saliva and dental plaque). Most of the studies using molecular biology studies have as yet been insufficient to assure with certainty that it was *H. pylori* in the oral cavity and not other microorganisms. Other evidences from experiments with animals as well as studies in Africa, where pre-chewing of food by the mother was a risk factor for infection by *H. pylori,* suggest that the oral-oral route may be involved in transmitting the disease. Conversely, in favor or the fecal-oral route it is known that *H. pylori* is isolated in the gastric acid and is continuously eliminated by the intestines. Studies using a polymerase chain reaction (PCR) have shown that *H. pylori* is eliminated in the stools and, in at least one study, viable microorganisms were identified [25] that were able to survive and be eliminated into the environment, thus feces or any matter contaminated by the feces could possibly constitute a transmission vehicle. On the Latin American continent, studies conducted in Peru [26] have shown that water can be the transmission vehicle, while two studies, one done in Chile [27] and the other in Columbia [28], suggest that using uncooked vegetables irrigated with water possibly contaminated by human waste are a risk factor for *H. pylori* infection. In

Brazil it has been proven that samples of *H. pylori* artificially inoculated into lettuce and carrots exposed in normal atmospheric conditions and modified manage to survive for 120 hours, and therefore may be one way the infection propagates [29]. The role of dental plaque acting as a habitual receptor of *H. pylori* infection has provided differing results in studies done in Brazil and Venezuela [30,31].

In conclusion, and in the light of current knowledge, it seems that both the oral-oral and gastro-oral routes may be responsible for transmitting the disease. The fecal-oral route would be dominant in populations in which infection in childhood and a low socio-economic level is highly prevalent, while the oral-oral route would predominate in populations with more favorable socio-economic indicators, and, therefore, low possibilities of fecal contamination; in these circumstances, even transitory colonization in the oral cavity would be an obligatory stage, and would be explained because *H. pylori* infection has been decreasing progressively in developed countries. It is worth pointing out that even on the Latin American continent there is initial evidence of a decline in prevalence of *H. pylori* infection at least in some fragments of the population. In Peru, Ramirez-Ramos has reported an 80 to 45% reduction in the high to middle socioeconomic level, with a sustained reduction in associated diseases such as gastroduodenal ulcer and gastric adenocarcinoma. Such findings, however, are not observed in low level socioeconomic populations [10]. In Argentina, Janjetic *et al.* studying 1030 children in Buenos Aires, using the 13C urea breath test, demonstrated a reduction in *H. pylori* infection prevalence from 41.2% in the 2002-2004 period to 26% in the 2007-9 period [32]. In Brazil, Kawakami *et al.* assessed *Helicobacter pylori* infection prevalence over a 10-year period in children submitted to upper digestive endoscopy, and demonstrated 60.5% *H. pylori* prevalence in the first year of the study and 30.4% in the last year [33]. Using the urea breath test, Coelho *et al.* also demonstrated a declining *H. pylori* infection rate among medical students in Brazil from 42% in 1993 to 21% in 2007 [34].

DIAGNOSIS

The main diagnosis methods used to detect *H. pylori* (Fig. **3**) and its peculiarities in South America will be reviewed.

Histology - Staining methods
Culture
Urease test
Breath test with carbon-13 labeled urea
Serological tests
Determination of fecal antigens
Molecular tests

Figure 3: *H. pylori* infection: main diagnostic methods.

H. pylori is detected in the gastric mucosa by different methods, either in fragments removed during endoscopy (invasive tests) and used for histopathological, microbiological, biochemical and molecular studies, or by non-endoscopic techniques (non-invasive tests) that include searching for *H. pylori* anti-antibodies in the blood and sometimes in the urine and saliva, by breath tests using carbon-13 labeled urea, and by investigating fecal antigens.

Histology - Staining Methods

Histology is a reliable method for diagnosing the presence of this microorganism. *H. pylori* can be identified in hematoxylin-eosin (H&E) stained histological sections, Giemsa, Warthin-Starry, Gram, carbolfuchsin or Gimenez, among others. There are limitations to this technique. Firstly, gastric fragments obtained may contain few epithelial surfaces to be examined, so collecting two fragments of the antrum and two from the gastric body for study is recommended. Secondly, the number of bacteria with typical morphology may be too small to afford a definitive conclusion as to its presence. Thirdly, the prior use of antimicrobials (in the last 30 days) or proton pump inhibitors (in the last seven to ten days) diminishes the bacterial density impairing the accurate identification. And finally histological diagnosis depends on the pathologist's expertise and the time they devote to identifying the microorganism. In summary, histology may, in ideal conditions, reach nearly 95% sensitivity and specificity in identification the bacteria. It is important to remember that the presence of inflammatory activity (presence of polymorphonuclears in the lamina propria) suggests the presence of the bacteria and requires it be carefully researched into. The presence of other bacteria or staining artifacts in the mucosa may give rise to false-positive results when bacteria density is small and morphology is atypical. When necessary, molecular or immuno-histochemical methods may confirm the presence of *H. pylori* in the tissue [35].

Another deeply rooted practice in most South American pathology laboratories (outside the universities and centers of excellence) is the use of routine staining by H&E alone, which often does not allow *H. pylori* infection to be reliably identified. Inclusion of easy, low cost, easy to perform additional staining, such as Giemsa and carbofuchsin [36] described in Brazil in 1989, must be encouraged in the continent's pathology laboratories' routine.

Culture

H. pylori can be grown from fragments removed endoscopically and transported to the laboratory in various apparatus: a sterile recipient, either dry or with hypertonic glucose, saline solution, and sterile agar or thioglycolate preservatives as a base. The fragments obtained can be kept in different media at +4°C for up to five hours prior to processing without losing viability. They can also be kept, perhaps indefinitely, when frozen at -70°C. The microorganism is identified based on the presence of typical colonies (punctiform, circular, convex and non-hemolytic), in the bacteria's Gram morphology, the urease-positive test and the oxidasis and catalysis reactions. In 1987 in Brazil, Queiroz *et al.* described the inclusion of the triphenyltetrazolium chloride growth medium (Belo Horizonte medium) which made the bacteria more easily recognizable [37]. Besides providing a definite diagnosis of the infection, it enables the sample's susceptibility to antimicrobials, as well as the presence of pathogenicity factors, to be studied. Compared to other diagnosis methods, the culture shows variable sensitivity (82-98%), depending on experience with the technique. Due to technical performance difficulties, it is not commonly used in daily practice [35].

Urease Test

Due to the *H. pylori's* high urease enzyme production, different indirect tests can be carried out in the endoscopy room to confirm the presence of the microorganism in biopsy fragments. The urease present in the gastric fragments unfolds the urea present in the medium used as a test as follows:

$$\begin{array}{c} NH_2 \\ | \\ \text{urease} \\ C = O + H_20 \longrightarrow 2NH_4^+ + HCO_3 \\ | \\ NH_2 \end{array}$$

The ammonia formed (reducing acidity) raises the pH, which can be detected by an indicator, usually phenol red, altering the color of the medium from yellow to pink. The change rate will depend on the urease activity present, which is ultimately fairly dependent on the number of bacteria, although there may be differences from one strain to another in the ability to produce urease. The test can become positive within minutes and is taken as positive if the color turns in up to 24 hours.

The use of histamine H_2 receptor antagonists and proton pump inhibitors affect the accuracy of the urease test and a two weeks interval between suspending the drugs and holding the test is recommended. As a test requiring high bacteria density (10^3 to 10^4 microorganisms, at least, for a positive test), the previous use of bismuth or antimicrobials reducing the bacteria load even temporarily may also give rise to false-negative results. The presence of active or recent gastrointestinal hemorrhage can interfere in the urease test [38].

It should be remembered that the test is based on the fact that *H. pylori* is the only microorganism present in the stomach that produces urease. So, exceptionally, patients infected with *Helicobacter heilmanni*, or densely colonized by other urease producers, may also test positive for urease.

Breath Test with Carbon-13 Labeled Urea

As with the urease test, the breath tests are based on urease activity. However in this instance what matters is the CO_2 produced and not the ammonia released. Urea can be labeled on the carbon atom with the stable, non-radioactive, 13C isotope. Breath tests consist of making the urease produced by the *H. pylori* unfold the labeled urea ingested during the test forming HCO_3^- and NH_4^+. As the solubility of $C0_2$ in the gastric juice is low, the $^{13}C0_2$ soon goes through the gastric mucosa and reaches the blood stream. In this way, the expired $^{13}C0_2$ is easily detected by a mass spectrometer, or, more recently, by an infrared analyzer, which is easy to use and reasonably inexpensive. The carbon-13 test is absolutely safe and non-radioactive and may be performed on children and pregnant women. It is carried out after an 8 hour overnight fast. First of all, the patient blows into a small balloon to collect and test their pre-test expired air. Next, they take 75 mg of carbon-13 labeled urea added to a glass of orange juice. Thirty minutes later a further collection of expired air is carried out and the material is analyzed in an infrared spectrophotometer. Results are obtained on a delta basis per absolute mil or as DOB "*delta over baseline*", which indicates the change in the $^{13}CO_2/^{12}CO_2$ ratio from the metabolic activity induced by administering the labeled urea.

Proton pump inhibitors and H_2 receptor antagonists as well as antibiotics can induce false-negative results, and it is recommended they be suspended two and four weeks respectively prior to the test. False-positive results are seldom observed, and may occur in patients who underwent gastric resection surgery or individuals with oral flora rich in urease producing microorganisms which retain the ingested urea in the mouth for a long time before it is swallowed. It is now universally accepted as a gold standard method for *H. pylori* infection diagnosis and treatment control in adults and children over six years old, with sensitivity and specificity always above 95% [39]. Although an Italian study [40] has suggested that doses of 13C-urea of up to 10mg are capable of keeping the test highly accurate, a study done in Brazil using 25mg of 13C-urea showed a decrease in the test's accuracy to 92.9% [41].

Breath tests initially using carbon-14 [42] and carbon-13 since 1999, were validated for adults [43], adolescents and children [44] in South America. Although highly accurate, simple and relatively low-cost, the test has not yet been incorporated into daily gastroenterological practice, and use is confined to large urban centers and for epidemiological studies [3,8,14]. The relatively low cost of the endoscopic test and the respective histopathological study in South America relative to North America and Europe, and difficulties in obtaining spectrometers and the 13C urea substrate, are factors that have been making it difficult for its use in South America to spread.

Serological Tests

H. pylori infected subjects develop specific antibodies in the serum against this microorganism. Besides being non-invasive and relatively economical, serological tests indicate the presence of the bacillus in the stomach as a whole, not just in one or more fragments of the organ as in the endoscopic methods. Several tests have been described, including complement fixation, agglutination, hemagglutination, indirect immune-fluorescence, ELISA and Immunoblot. In general, ELISA tests have been used the most. But, although very useful in epidemiological studies, they are not useful for diagnosing active infection, since patients who have had the bacteria eradicated may remain seropositive for years. In a Brazilian study, 83/130 (64%) patients with peptic ulcers remained seropositive 6.4 years after the microorganism had been eradicated [45]. Therefore, serological tests have been recommended in situations of equivocal results of other diagnostic methods such as recent use of antimicrobial and/or antisecretory drugs, bleeding peptic ulcers, atrophy and gastric malignancies [38]. The presence of specific anti-*H. pylori* antibodies may also be shown in other organic fluids, such as urine and saliva. Most serological tests provide specificity higher than 90%, but sensitivity ranging from 60 to 90%. Overall, diagnostic accuracy is low at approximately 80–84%, and they should be validated locally [35,46]. In South America, validation studies of different serological tests using IgC have been done in Argentina [47,48], Brazil [49,50], Chile [51], Ecuador [52] and Venezuela [53]. Less used in daily practice, research into serum antibodies reacting to the CagA protein may be applied to detect samples of bacteria with the CagA gene. After becoming commercially available early in 2000 [54,55], it was validated in Brazil in 2004 [56]. Because *H. pylori,* especially anti-CagA, antibodies detected by immunoblotting, can remain in the plasma longer than antibodies identified by enzyme immunoassays, and even for years after successful eradication therapy, immunoblotting seems to be the most sensitive method for detecting a past *H. pylori* infection [57,58] and the immunoblotting technique is the serologic test gold standard [59].

Determination of Fecal Antigens

Although *H. pylori* culture is seldom made from stools, the presence of antigens in fecal material may be determined by immunoenzimatic tests using monoclonal antibodies. The recently published Maastricht IV Consensus [38] recognized the role of tests to detect fecal antigens in diagnosing the infection and its usefulness in cure control, but only in those tests based on the ELISA method. A Brazilian study showed that the monoclonal stool antigen test is accurate for diagnosing *H. pylori* in children under 7, but it must be validated locally in order to find the best cutoff for each population [60]. The easy-to-perform rapid immunochromatographic tests on stool samples in studies conducted in Europe and Asia proved to be limited in accuracy, particularly because of the low positive predictive values [61,62]. However, the predictive values of the tests depend both on sensitivity and specificity (characteristics inherent in the tests) and the disease's prevalence in the population studied. The studies assessing the predictive values of the rapid immunochromatographic tests in the context of controlling *H. pylori* infection treatment were conducted on populations in which *H. pylori* infection prevalence was lower than that found in South America. Two studies in South America using different rapid immunochromatographic tests have been carried out. In Brazil, Silva *et al.* [63] assessed patients not submitted to treatment for *H. pylori* infection and found a positive predictive value of 88% (IC 95%: 75.7-95.5) and a negative predictive value of 87,5% (CI95%: 74.7-95.3), while in Venezuela Contreras *et al.* [64] found a positive predictive value of 78% (CI: 95%: 58-91) and a negative predictive value of 86% (CI: 95%: 68-96). New studies using the immunochromatographic method, before and after treatment for *H. pylori* infection, are needed to determine its real accuracy in South America. Difficulties in conducting the test and collecting the stools, a moderately high cost and questionable acceptability by patients [65] have hampered its use.

Molecular Tests

Molecular methods, particularly the PCR, have been increasingly used in diagnosing different aspects of *H. pylori* infection. PCR is a DNA amplification procedure resulting in rapid production of multiple copies of a DNA "target" sequence. The technique may be applied on material from gastric biopsies or any organic fluids (stools, saliva and gastric juice). Its extreme sensitivity and specificity enable a single DNA copy of the microorganism in the examined material to be identified. This property, on the other hand, also increases the odds of false-positives occurring, either because of the presence of residues of the microorganism in the material or their presence in the set of instruments used in the endoscopy and their occasionally not being properly sterilized and cleaned. Very contaminated materials, with mixed flora, may also contain bacteria with a gene sequence similar to those of *H. pylori* and also lead to false-positive results. Nevertheless, the PCR sensitivity and specificity for the *H. pylori* infection range from 90 to 100%.

More recently, molecular methods, especially PCR, have been increasingly used to detect bacteria and identify mutations associated with development of resistance to clarithromycin e fluoroquinolones, directly from the gastric fragment with no need for prior culture of the microorganism [35, 66-71]. Mutation points located in the bacteria's 23S rRNA gene, in the 2142 (A2142G e A2142C) e 2143 (A2143G) nucleotide positions, reduce affinity between ribosomes and clarithromycin, causing the microorganism to resist the drug [35]. The fluoroquinolones inhibit the DNA gyrase A subunit, codified by the GYRA gen, which is located in an area called a determining region of resistance to quinolone, and the mutations observed in the *H. pylori* infection are most commonly found in codons 87 and 91 [35,71,72]. Studies comparing the performance of molecular tests with growth of the microorganism have shown 100% specificity in detecting the bacteria [70], 96-100% concordance in identifying resistance to clarithromycin and 94% in identifying resistance to fluoroquinolones [66-69].

Additionally, the PCR may be used to detect bacteria genes associated with virulence factors in epidemiological studies and in retrospective analyses using material previously fixed in paraffin. This property of the technique is particularly useful for studies involving the association of MALT lymphoma and *H. pylori*. The lack of response to eradication of *H. pylori* in patients with low grade MALT lymphoma is usually due to the presence of a high grade component unidentified in the histological study, or to the existence of certain cytogenetic changes, among which are chromosomal translocations, especially t(11;18)(q21;q21), which would condition an independence of the lymphoma cells to antigenic stimulus with the resulting non-regression of the lymphoma after eradication of *H. pylori*. Determination of the presence of these changes may be conducted in molecular biology laboratories, even in paraffin-embedded material, and has highly significant clinical implications. So, patients with a low grade MALT lymphoma, after proven to carry the translocation t(11;18)(q21;q21), in addition to effecting eradication of *H. pylori*, should be promptly referred to another therapy type, considered effective and suitable (surgery, chemotherapy and/or radiotherapy), and not have to wait, as they do now, for the tumor's histological response to bacterial eradication, since that may take some months to be determined [73,74].

In 2009 in Peru, Ramírez-Ramos & Sánchez-Sánchez [75] described the main molecular studies conducted in Latin America from 2003 to 2008 regarding the expression frequency of the cagA, vacA, babA2, oipA e cagE genotypes in different diseases associated with *H. pylori* infection. Bacterial virulence factors such as CagA increase the risk of gastric cancer. It has been shown that CagA has variability in its C-terminal region, which includes a Glu-Pro-Ile-Tyr-Ala (EPIYA) sequence that is present in variable numbers in CagA from different strains. On the basis of sequences flanking the EPIYA motifs, four distinct segments have been described: EPIYA-A, -B, -C and –D. Most strains have EPIYA-A and EPIYA-B motifs. The EPIYA-C motif is characteristic of the Western strains, whereas the EPIYA-D segment characterizes East Asian strains. These motifs are geographically diverse and become tyrosine phosphorylated when they enter epithelial cells in the host, presumably starting off the chain of events that may eventually result in neoplastic transformation [76]. Studies performed in Brazil and Chile found that strains harboring a higher number of *Helicobacter pylori* CagA EPIYA C phosphorylation sites were associated with higher risk of gastric cancer and more severe histopathological findings in the gastric mucosa [77,78].

TREATMENT

Who to Treat?

In 2000, the Latin-American Consensus Conference on *Helicobacter pylori* infection [79] considered agreed indications for *H. pylori* therapy patients with gastric or duodenal ulcers (active or past history), low grade gastric MALT-type lymphoma, and patients with early gastric cancer, after endoscopic or surgical resection. Situations where indications of treatment were considered debatable included patients with functional dyspepsia, a family history of gastric cancer, gastroesophageal reflux disease requiring long-term use of proton pump inhibitors, and severe gastritis diagnosed by endoscopy and histology. Table **2** shows the indications for treatment of infection in *Helicobacter pylori*-positive patients by the recent World Gastroenterology Organisation Global Guideline: *Helicobacter pylori* in developing countries [80]. Regarding *H. pylori* eradication for gastric cancer prevention, the Asian-Pacific consensus has already recommended a policy of *H. pylori* eradication in regions at high risk for gastric cancer (age-standardized incidence rate greater than 20 per 100.000 inhabitants). This approach has not yet been considered in South America [81].

Table 2: Indications for treatment of infection in *Helicobacter pylori*-positive patients*

1. Past or present duodenal and/or gastric ulcer, with or without complications
2. Following resection of gastric cancer
3. Gastric mucosa-associated lymphoid tissue (MALT) lymphoma
4. Atrophic gastritis
5. Dyspepsia
6. Patients with first-degree relatives with gastric cancer
7. Patient's wishes

*Source: World Gastroenterology Organisation Global Guideline *Helicobacter pylori* in Developing Countries [80]

How to Treat

Although *H. pylori in vitro* is sensitive to a broad range of antimicrobials, and temporary suppression of the microorganism right after therapy ends is easily obtained, its actual eradication – herein defined as the absence of the microorganism in tests conducted at least a month after the end of the treatment, is not easily obtained. It may be said that practically all antimicrobials have already been tested as monotherapy against the microorganism with unsatisfactory results, with eradication rates mostly between 20 and 40% of cases. In addition to the primary or secondary resistance of *H. pylori* to antimicrobials, other factors have been implicated in the discrepancy between the results obtained *in vitro* and those observed *in vivo*. The microorganism has a thick glycocalyx that functions as a partial barrier to antimicrobials. Moreover, being firmly stuck to the epithelium, it limits the action of the antimicrobials.

Also of importance is the intragastric activity of antimicrobials, in particular for those acting topically against the microorganism and making up the largest contingent among available drugs, as we will see. They need to dissolve rapidly and disperse well in the stomach. They must be stable and active in a broad pH range, particularly in low pH environments. It is also necessary for the biologically active compound particles to have the proper size and ionic load to penetrate the mucus layer lining the stomach and reach the gastric mucosa. For drugs of systemic action, absorption by the stomach and the small intestine and subsequent secretion by the gastric mucosa is required. Therefore, many anti-*H. pylori* therapy failures are due to decreased activity by antimicrobials used in the gastric microenvironment, resulting in sub-inhibitory concentrations at the gastric mucosa level.

Although practically all the antimicrobials available on the world market have already been tested against *H. pylori*, only eight of them (one of which is not marketed in South America) are now used to treat this infection and will be discussed here (Fig. **4**).

Clarithromycin
Amoxicillin
Bismuth salts
Nitroimidazoles
Tetracyclines
Furazolidone
Levofloxacin
Rifabutin

Figure 4: Anti-*H. pylori* agents.

Anti-*H. Pylori* Drugs

Clarithromycin

This is to date the most used antimicrobial in first-line *H. pylori* eradication schemes. A bacteriostatic macrolide, a semi-synthetic analogue of erythromycin – it exerts its antibacterial action by binding to the microorganisms' 50S ribosomal subunits, suppressing their proteic synthesis – it presents a broad spectrum of *in vitro* action against anaerobic and aerobic bacteria, both Gram-positive and Gram-negative, and is highly effective against *H. pylori*. It is stable in an acid medium, and its half-life is 1 hour if the pH of the gastric juice is around 2, but when pH rises to 7, its half-life may last as long as about 70 hours [82]. The most common adverse reactions are nausea, diarrhea and a sour taste in the mouth. Development of resistance after use results essentially from two chromosomal mutations located in the 23S rRNA gene, nucleotides 2146 and 3147, which diminishes affinity between ribosomes and clarithromycin, and produces the microorganism's resistance to the drug [35]. Indeed, the eradication rates of *H. pylori* with the classic triple therapy (proton pump inhibitor, clarithromycin and amoxicillin) go from 87%, when the bacteria is sensitive to clarithromycin, to 17% when it is resistant. The rate of secondary resistance, *i.e.* resistance observed after treatment failure, usually reaches 60% or more, which means that repeating treatment with clarithromycin must be avoided, unless antimicrobial sensitivity tests are available [82,83].

In South America, studies done in Argentina [84], Brazil [85-88], Chile [89], Columbia [90], Paraguay [91] and Uruguay [92] to assess its resistance, showed resistance rates to clarithromycin of between 2 and 24%. The lowest values were observed in Paraguay (2%) and Columbia (3%) and the highest in Argentina (24%), Uruguay (12%), Chile (20%) and Brazil (between 9 and 16.5%) which showed intermediate resistance rates.

Amoxicillin

Amoxicillin – a semi-synthetic penicillin that interferes in the synthesis of the peptidoglycans in the bacterial cell wall – is highly active against *H. pylori* and presents a CIM_{90} of 0.12mg/1. Being trivalent, it becomes lipophilic, facilitating its penetration into the stomach's mucous and epithelial layers. It works at different pH values, and is quite stable in an acid medium even with gastric pH close to 2, and may also present antimicrobial activity when intragastric pH approaches 7 [93]. Well absorbed by the gastroduodenal and intestinal mucosa, it becomes highly concentrated in the gastric juice and mucosa 30 minutes after oral administration, with a plasmatic half-life of about 15 hours [94]. Intravenous administration of amoxicillin results in undetectable levels in the gastric mucosa, suggesting that systemic absorption is of little importance. Its most common side effects are allergic reaction, diarrhea, candidiasis and less commonly pseudomembranous colitis. Although extremely used for years by the population, *H. pylori* strains resistant to amoxicillin are highly uncommon.

Bismuth Salts

The compounds used the most are bismuth subsalicylate and colloidal bismuth subcitrate, both spreading evenly throughout the gastric mucosa. It is estimated that minimum quantities are absorbed (1 to 2%) and over 99% of the bismuth ingested shows up in the stools, and only small quantities are detected in the blood stream [95]. Although a study suggests that co-administration of omeprazole, by raising gastric pH, may increase absorption of salt and, consequently its toxic potential [96], Vieira *et al.* [97], among us in Brazil, demonstrated that the use of conventional doses of colloidal bismuth subcitrate associated with the proton pump inhibitor (lansoprazole) prescribed for seven to fourteen days, does not determine potentially toxic plasmatic concentrations of bismuth, and may be used safely in anti-*H. pylori* therapies. It is excreted by the kidneys and may persist for up to 12 weeks after therapy is discontinued. The serum concentrations of bismuth increase in the presence of severe renal insufficiency (creatinine clearance ≤ 20ml/min) and it is prudent to lower the dose in such a condition. In the colon, bismuth salts are converted into bismuth sulfide, which is responsible for the blackish coloring in the stools of patients. Exactly how the bismuth salts mechanism works is unknown. In the 70s high doses of bismuth were used for long periods and associated with neurotoxicity, and to this day its use is banned in several countries such as France, for example. A recent meta-analysis involving 35 studies with 4763 patients showed that bismuth salts on their own or associated with other antimicrobials in eradicating *H. pylori* are safe and well tolerated [98].

Nitroimidazoles

Nitroimidazoles - metronidazole, tinidazole and, less commonly, secnidazole - are widely used in anti-*H. pylori* therapy regimens and there seems to be a cross-resistance between them [99]. They are actively secreted into the gastric juice and saliva, and only differ from each other because of the dosages used and their plasmatic half-life. Metronidazole is more commonly used due to its excellent *in vitro* activity against *H. pylori*. Its antimicrobial activity is independent of gastric pH, as its CIM is close to 2mg/1 and its half-life is 8-12 hours. Nitroimidazoles are given as a prodrug that needs to be activated within the target cell by one or two electron transfer processes. This reduction leads to the formation of nitro-anion radicals and imidazole intermediates that cause lethal damage to subcell structures and DNA [100]. Their most common side effects are a metallic taste in the mouth, sickness, loss of appetite, a coated tongue and diarrhea in up to 20% of cases. Due to their disulfiram-like effect, abstinence from alcohol must be recommended while they are used. A relevant restriction placed on their use is the high rate of primary or secondary resistance to *H. pylori*, reaching rates of up to 82% in South America [80]. Some studies suggest that increasing the metronidazole dose and prolonging the treatment may partially overcome any resistance [38].

Tetracyclines

Tetracycline acts by reversibly binding itself to the 30S ribosomal subunits. This process blocks the ribosomal RNA inhibiting synthesis of bacterial polypeptides. *H. pylori* is quite sensitive to *in vitro* tetracycline with a CIM ranging from 0.12 to 1.2mg/l, and the latter is stable and active in an acid pH medium. Milk and antacids hamper its absorption because, on combining with metallic ions, calcium, magnesium or aluminum, formation of inactive chelates is facilitated. The most common adverse reactions are dose-dependent and include sickness, vomiting and epigastric pain, although hypersensitivity reactions such as urticaria, rash and anaphylaxis may occur. Resistance to tetracycline is seldom described. Although tetracycline HCL is the most commonly used, in Brazil results using doxycycline in association with other anti-*H. pylori* drugs have been good [101].

Furazolidone

Furazolidone is a synthetic derivative of nitrofurans effective against a broad spectrum of bacteria and parasites. The bactericide activity of furazolidone is the result of its ability to inhibit various bacterial enzymes, particularly those involved in the Krebs cycle. Studies on healthy adults show that furazolidone appears in the plasma 1 hour after ingestion, with maximum absorption peaking in the first 4 hours. It is the least costly of all anti-*H. pylori* drugs. One restriction against using it is the high rate of adverse, chiefly gastrointestinal, effects. Like metronidazol, it also has a disulfiram-like effect, and abstinence from alcohol is recommended while using it. Records of furazolidone resistant strains are rare. Although recommended as an alternative therapy by the Latin American in 2000 [79], Brazilian in 2005 [102], and Chinese Consensus in 2008 [103], as well as the

World Gastroenterology Organization in 2011 [80], it is not available on the European and North American markets, because of genotoxic and carcinogenetic effects in animals [104-106]. In a pooled-data analysis, Zullo *et al.* have expressed concerns over its use [107]. The International Agency for Research on Cancer (IARC), in 1997, classified furazolidone as a type 3 carcinogen (unclassifiable as to carcinogenicity in humans) [108], and both the European Agency for the Evaluation of Medical Products in 1999 and the US Food and Drug Administration agency in 2002 banned its use in animals, in order to avoid the presence of residues in meat-derived foods. Furazolidone is not approved by the European Medicines Agency (EMA) either as a human medicine or for animal use, [109-111]. It is commercialized in many countries of Latin America, China and Iran. In an editorial reviewing Zullo´s pooled-data analysis [107], Graham & Lu consider furazolidone to be an unfairly maligned and underutilized drug, and especially useful in areas where resistance is widespread and multiple [112].

Levofloxacin

This is a broad spectrum fluoroquinolone, more effective against Gram-negatives, and widely used for urinary tract, pelvic and respiratory infections. As a bactericide agent, it acts by inhibiting bacterial DNA synthesis. It shows good oral absorption and is not much affected when taken with meals. The drug is well tolerated, adverse reactions are uncommon but gastrointestinal effects may exist. It has a long half-life and may be taken once daily. It has recently been used as a second or third line therapy to eradicate *H. pylori* in patients resistant to schemes classically used to treat the infection. An emerging problem is the rising occurrence of resistant strains. A recent study in Peru found 36.9% of strains to be resistant to levofloxacin [113].

Rifabutin

Derived from rifamicin, it is habitually used for *Mycobacterium avis* infections on patients with immunodeficiency. Its potential usefulness against *H. pylori* is because of its high *in vitro* sensitivity and it does not share resistance to clarithromycin [114]. Primary resistance to rifabutin is rare, lower than 1.5% [115]. Some studies suggest cross resistance with rifampicin to be possible [116]. Adverse effects are modest and may nevertheless cause leucopenia and plaquetopenia, which are reversible by stopping the medication. It is costly and not yet available in South America. Infectious disease control agencies argue that its use be reserved for treating patients with *M. tuberculosis* multiresistant strains. When associated with amoxicillin and proton pump inhibitors, it has shown encouraging results in eradicating *H. pylori* in patients with multiple therapy failure after using classical antibiotics such as amoxicillin, clarithromycin, metronidazol and levofloxacin [115].

Table **3** illustrates the antimicrobial resistance rates from *H. pylori* isolates observed in South America.

Table 3: Antibiotic Resistance in *H. pylori* isolates from South America

Country, Year (REF)	Number Tested	Antibiotic Resistance (%)					
		Amox	Metro	Clar	Quino	Fura	Tetra
Argentina, 2006 [84]	242			24			
Brazil, 2002 [85]	202		53	9			
Brazil, 2003 [86]	155	13	55	16		13	13
Brazil, 2009 [87]	53		54	8	15		
Brazil, 2010 [88]				16.5			
Chile, 2007 [89]	50		27	20			27
Colombia, 2009 [90]	106	1.9	82	3.8			0
Paraguay, 2007 [91]	54	2.0	33	2			
Peru, 2011 [107]					36.9		
Uruguay, 2009 [92]	79	0	36	12	3.5		0

THERAPY REGIMES

First-Line Therapies

Proton pump inhibitor (PPI) in a standard dose (omeprazole 20 mg, lansoprazole 30 mg, pantoprazole 40 mg, rabeprazole 20 mg or esomeprazole 40%), + AMOXICILLIN 1.0g + CLARITHROMICIN 500mg, twice a day, for seven days.

This is still the most used and recommended regimen worldwide and in South America also [79,80]. Its effectiveness depends basically on resistance rates to clarithromycin, and is not recommended for populations in areas where rates exceed 20%. Although not excellent, in the last ten years this regimen has shown eradication rates greater than 80% in Argentina [117], Brazil [118-120], Columbia [121] and Peru [75,122]. These results have also been recently described by a Spanish group in treating the *H. pylori* infection for twelve years [123]. A recent randomized trial involving seven Latin American countries, including Chile and Columbia, obtained 82.2% eradication of *H. pylori* with the triple classic scheme during 14 days, this regimen being preferable to 5-day concomitant or 10-day sequential four-drug regimens [124].

Most of the recommendations by consensus groups recommend seven days' duration, mainly because of the cost factor. In fact, meta-analysis studies show a gain of 4% when the period is extended to 10 days and 5% when extended to 14 days [125-128]. Indiscriminate use of other macrolides, such as azithromycin, because of a cross resistance mechanism, may hamper eradication rates [129,130].

For patients with a possible or proven history of allergy to penicillin, the regimen described above is recommended, replacing amoxicillin with furazolidone 200mg, twice a day [80,102,131]. Other options include using metronidazole or levofloxacin instead of amoxicillin, or adopting regimens using tetracycline e metronidazole and bismuth salts [132-134].

SEQUENTIAL TREATMENT SCHEME: PPI in a standard dose + AMOXICILLIN 1.0g, twice a day during the first five days, followed by: PPI in a standard dose + CLARITHROMYCIN 500mg + TINIDAZOLE 500mg, twice a day for five more days.

A ten day treatment regimen, developed by Italian investigators, consists of administering a proton pump inhibitor in a standard dose and amoxicillin 1.0g twice a day in the first five days, followed by administration of a proton pump inhibitor in a standard dose, clarithromycin 500 and tinidazole 500 mg, administered twice a day for five more days. Although most of the studies are still limited to a single country, initial results show eradication rates of about 90% [135-137], with some Asian studies showing less significant results [138]. The precise mechanism of this association is still unknown. It is speculated that, by reducing bacterial density, amoxicillin (against which resistance seldom exists) favors the effectiveness of the drugs administered subsequently (clarithromycin and tinidazole). As previous studies have already shown that bacteria are able to develop outflow channels for clarithromycin, transferring it rapidly out of the bacterial wall and preventing it from binding to the ribosomes, it is accepted that amoxicillin administered previously, on acting on the cell wall by weakening it, would prevent these outflow channels from developing, making the action of the antibiotics more effective when administered in the second stage of the treatment [139]. Studies confirming the effectiveness of this scheme in South America are lacking. In a recent randomized Latin American trial in which 486 patients received the sequential scheme, *H. pylori* eradication rates reached 76.5% [124].

QUADRUPLE TREATMENT: PPI in a standard dose + COLLOIDAL BISMUTH SUBCITRATE 120mg, four times a day + TETRACYCLINE HYDROCHLORIDE 500mg, four times a day + METRONIDAZOLE 250mg four times a day for 7-10 days.

It represents a scheme recommended in areas with resistance rates to clarithromycin higher than 20%. It has recently been provided in kits in the USA and Europe. A randomized clinical trial involving 39 European centers, compared the classical triple scheme for 7 days, with quadruple therapy containing tetracycline, metronidazole and bismuth salt in a single formulation (Pylera ®) and a proton pump inhibitor, administered for 10 days to 440 patients submitted to anti-*H. pylori* treatment for the first time. Eradication rates were 55% for the triple scheme and 80% for the quadruple scheme ($p<0.0001$). It should be pointed out that 70% of the strains were resistant to metronidazole and 20% to clarithromycin [140]. Recent meta-analysis showed that quadruple therapy provides eradication rates similar to those observed with classical triple therapy [141]. Its drawback is the need to take a large number of tablets per day, compromising compliance with the treatment.

CONCOMITANT TREATMENT (WITHOUT BISMUTH): PPI + AMOXICILLIN + TETRACYCLINE HYDROCHLORIDE + METRONIDAZOLE, for 7-14 days.

Concomitant (non-bismuth) therapy (PPI-amoxicillin- clarithromycin-nitroimidazole for 7-14 days) appears to be an effective, safe, and a well-tolerated alternative for countries where bismuth salts are not available or the effectiveness of triple therapy is unacceptably low. It also seems to be less complex than sequential therapy. Recent meta-analysis showed superiority of concomitant therapy over triple therapy; with intention-to-treat eradication rate of 89.7% (95% CI: 86.8–92.1%) [141]. Clarithromycin resistance may reduce the effectiveness of concomitant therapy, although the decrease in eradication rates seems to be far lower than in standard triple therapy. Experience with non-bismuth quadruple therapy in patients with metronidazole-resistant strains is still very limited. A recent Columbian randomized clinical trial found similar results for a 14-day regimen with 500 mg clarithromycin b.i.d., 500 mg metronidazole t.i.d., and 500 mg amoxicillin t.i.d. (with and without a proton pump inhibitor) (86.8% eradication rate), and a 10-day triple therapy (85.3% eradication rate) [142].

FURAZOLIDONE-CONTAINING REGIMENS

Regimens using furazolidone associated with an antimicrobial (amoxicillin, clarithromycin or tetracycline) as a first line of treatment for *H. pylori* infection has been used in adults and children in Brazil with eradication rates of 79.1% (95% CI: 74.1-84.2%). Treatment is carried out for seven days, furazolidole doses used range from 100mg (children) to 400mg/day and adverse, especially gastrointestinal, effects occur frequently [131,143-147]. Furazolidole in association with bismuth salt and tetracycline or amoxicillin has been used in Peru and Columbia with eradication rates of 83% and 86% respectively [148,149].

A systematic review and meta-analysis of the effect of furazolidole- and nitrofurantoin-based regimens in the eradication of infection showed that the side-effects of the regimens containing furazolidole were significantly more frequent than in standard therapies. Primary triple regimens containing furazolidole are slightly less efficient than the standard primary combinations [150].

Eradication Control

Infection cure control must be carried out in a period no less than a month after the treatment ends, preferably two to three months after the treatment ends, to avoid occurrence of false-negatives. The breath test with carbon 13 labeled urea is the ideal non-invasive method for carrying out eradication control. It is highly sensitive and specific, of moderate cost, and is gradually becoming available in South America. To avoid the possibility of false-negatives, patients must abstain from antisecretors (two weeks) and antimicrobials (four weeks) before the test is done. Fecal antigen testing has also been used with excellent results. Should the fecal antigen test not be available, eradication control may be done by digestive endoscopy, searching for the bacteria in histological cuts and by the urease test, using antrum and body gastric fragments. Quantitative serology is not an established method for confirming eradication of the bacteria.

Relapse and Reinfection

Since patients may not respond to treatment at the outset, and even because it is just possible for the bacteria to relapse, cure control must be done. In developed countries, where the microorganism is less prevalent, relapse seems to be related to the reappearance of the original bacterial strain rather than to actual reinfections. Studies in South America point to infection recurrence rates of 2.9% in Argentina [151], 4.2% in Chile [152] and between 2 and 7% in Brazil [45,153]. *H. pylori* recurrence one year after eradication treatment in a recent large population randomized trial in seven Latin American countries was 11.5% [154].

Table 4: Risk factors for failure of *H. pylori* eradication therapy

Compliance [155]
Cag-negative strains [156]
CYP2C19 genetic polymorphisms [157]
Smoking [158]
Altered immunity
Elevated bacterial load
Hyperacidity
Associated-disease [159]
Presence of intracellular bacteria [160]
Antimicrobial resistance [metronidazole and clarithromycin] [38]

Therapy Failure

Nowadays it is considered that a therapy regimen is clinically relevant and acceptable, if the eradication rate is higher than 80% or, preferably, 90%. The eradication rate of a first line of treatment based on triple therapy with a proton pump inhibitor and two antimicrobials varies from 80 to 90%. When a second line of treatment is used on these 10 to 20% of patients who present a therapy failure at the first attempt of eradication, its effectiveness varies between 70 and 80%. Thus about 5 to 20% of the patients will remain infected after two courses of treatment. Although different factors may contribute to therapy failure (Table **4**), the main factor, as already discussed, is bacterial resistance, especially to clarithromycin and metronidazole.

Second-Line Therapies - After Failure of Clarithromycin-Containing Regimens:

QUADRUPLE THERAPY: A standard dose of PPI + COLLOIDAL BISMUTH SUBCITRATE 120mg, four times a day + TETRACYCLIN HYDROCHLORIDE 500mg, four times a day + METRONIDAZOLE 250mg, four times a day, for 10 -14 days.

Three European reviews show that this alternative is able to further eradication after failure of the classical triple regimen around 80% [161-163]. Due to the high rates of primary resistance to metronidazole on the Latin American continent, few studies exist [75]. However, some studies suggest that primary resistance to imidazoles may perhaps be overcome by increasing the dose and/or the duration of the treatment [140,141,164]. It must also be considered that, when metronidazole resistance is assessed using the E-test, its prevalence tends to be overestimated [165]. In South America, use of the quadruple scheme, replacing metronidazole for furazolidone, is a frequent option (see below).

PPI in a standard dose, twice a day + AMOXICILLIN 1.0g, twice a day + LEVOFLOXACIN 500mg, once a day, for 10 days.

This is one of the most used anti-*H. pylori* regimens used throughout the world in re-treating *H. pylori* infection, with two recent meta-analysis studies showing eradication rates close to 80% [166,167]. It is well tolerated, and adverse effects, when present, are of low intensity and usually gastrointestinal. Its cost is accessible and in some South American countries it has recently been provided in kits, enhancing compliance with treatment. A drawback is that recent studies call attention to *H. pylori's* increasing resistance to quinolones, especially in areas where its use among the population is more widespread [168,169].

FURAZOLIDONE-CONTAINING REGIMENS

Quadruple therapy regimens where metronidazole is replaced by furazolidone have been used in South America, especially in Peru, Columbia and Brazil, to treat patients resistant to the classical triple scheme [75,101,170,171]. In Brazil the quadruple scheme for retreatment recommended by the Brazilian Consensus on *H. pylori* [102] consists of administering a standard dose of a proton pump inhibitor + amoxicillin 1.0g (or doxycycline 100mg) + furazolidone 200 mg + colloidal bismuth subcitrate 240 mg (2 tablets), administered twice a day (after lunch and dinner) for 10 days. A study showed that with this therapy regimen eradication in Brazil reached 80% [101]. As suggested earlier by Graham *et al.*, by using two daily intakes [172], compliance seems to increase while this regimen's adverse effects diminish.

Triple therapy regimens using furazolidone once or twice a day, in association with levofloxacin and a proton pump inhibitor during seven to ten days have also been used as rescue therapy in Brazil [101,173,174]. Another retreatment option recommended by the Brazilian Consensus on *H. pylori* is the use of a standard dose of proton pump inhibitor + levofloxacin 500 mg + furazolidone 200mg (2 tablets), with all the medications being administered in a single daily dose for 10 days with eradication rates close to 80% [101,102].

Third-Line Therapies

A standard PPI dose, twice a day + AMOXICILLIN 1.0g twice a day + RIFABUTIN 150mg once a day for 10 days.

This retreatment option is not yet easily available in South America. Although rifabutin is highly effective against *H. pylori*, it is expensive and may give rise to leucopenia and thrombocytopenia, which are reversible after suspending the medication. Derived from rifampicin, it is used to treat Mycobacterium infections in patients with immunodeficiency, and recommended to be set aside for treating multiresistant mycobacteria [175]. A recent review showed resistance rates to *H.*

pylori of only 1.3% (95% CI = 0.9-1.7%). The average eradication rate of regimes containing rifabutin as a second line of treatment was 79% (67-92%), third line 66% (55-77%), and, as a fourth or fifth line, 70% (60-79%) [115].

As already discussed, tests for sensitivity to antimicrobials, obtained by culture or molecular tests, should be used to guide immune cases and determine new therapy alternatives.

ACKNOWLEDGEMENT

None Declared.

CONFLICT OF INTEREST

The author(s) confirm that this chapter content has no conflict of interest.

REFERENCES

[1] Marshall BJ, Warren JR. Unidentified curved bacilli in the stomach of patients with gastrits and peptic ulceration. Lancet 1984; i: 1311-15.

[2] Olmos JA, Rios H, Higa R. Prevalence of *Helicobacter pylori* infection in Argentina: results of a nationwide epidemiologic study. J Clin Gastroenterol 2000;31:33-37.

[3] Santos IS, Boccio J, Davidsson L, *et al. Helicobacter pylori* is not associated with anaemia in Latin America: results from Argentina, Brazil, Bolivia, Cuba, Mexico and Venezuela. Public Health Nutrition 2009: 12, 1862–70.

[4] Zaterka S, Eisig JN, Chinzon D, Rothstein W. Factors Related to *Helicobacter pylori* Prevalence in an Adult Population in Brazil. Helicobacter 2007;12: 82–88.

[5] Rodrigues MN, Queiroz DM, Rodríguez RT, Rocha AMC, Carlos RL, Braga LLBC. Prevalence of *Helicobacter pylori* infection in Fortaleza, Northeastern Brazil. Rev Saude Publica 2005;39:847-49.

[6] Miranda AC, Machado RS, Silva EM, Kawakami E. Seroprevalence of *Helicobacter pylori* infection among children of low socioeconomic level in São Paulo Sao Paulo Med J. 2010;128187-91.

[7] Ferreccio C, Rollán A, Harris PR, Serrano C, Gederlini A, Margozzini P, *et al.* Gastric cancer is related to early *Helicobacter pylori* infection in a high-prevalence country. Cancer Epidemiol Biomarkers Prev 2007; 16: 662-67.

[8] Campuzano-Maya G, Hoyos-Castaño D, Calvo-Betancur VD, Suárez-Ramírez OA, Lizcano-Cardona D, Rojas-Arbeláez CA. Prevalence of *Helicobacter pylori* infection in physicians in Medellín, Colômbia. Acta Gastroenterol Latinoam. 2007;3799-103.

[9] Gómez NA, Salvador A, Vargas PE, Zapatier JA, Alvarez J. Seroprevalencia de *Helicobacter pylori* en la población infantil ecuatoriana. Rev Gastroenterol Peru 2004; 24 230-33.

[10] Ramírez Ramos A, Gilman R, Watanabe-Yanamoto J, Rosas-Aguirre A. Estudio de la Epidemiología de la infección por el *Helicobacter pylori* en el Perú: 20 años después. Acta Gastroenterol Latinoam 2004; 34; 69-79.

[11] González N, Fernández L, Pérez Pérez G, *et al.* Infección por *Helicobacter pylori* en pacientes uruguayos de origen africano: características clínicas, endoscópicas y genéticas. Acta Gastroenterol Latinoam 2010;40:206-10.

[12] Vazquez Serra G, Fazzio Rolleri S, Velázque-García MS, *et al.* Prevalence study of Helicobacter infection in a Montevideo population. Arch. Med. Interna (Montevideo) 1997;19:95-99.

[13] Chose C, Jerez-Pérez G, van Doorn LJ, Domínguez-Bello MG, Blaser MJ. High Frequency of Gastric colonization with multiple *Helicobacter pylori* Stains in Venezuela Subjects. J Clin Microb 2005; 43: 2635-41.

[14] Páez Valery MC, Barón MA, Solano L, Nadaff G, Boccio J, Barrado A. *Helicobacter pylori* infection (13C-UBT), and its relationship with nutritional and socioeconomic factors in low income school children from Valencia, Venezuela. Arch Latinoam Nutr. 2006; 56:342-49.

[15] Friedman CR, Quick R, Khanna B, Salcido A, lihoshi N, Gironaz M, Ganzales O, Hutwagner L, Tauxe R, Mintz E, Gold BD. Epidemiology of *Helicobacter pylori* Infection in Rural Bolivian Children. J Pediat Gastroenterol Nutr 1997; 25: 466.

[16] Yorg JA. Prevalencia de *Helicobacter pylori* por el método del aliento (Ureasa) en el Paraguay. XXI Congreso de ALASBIMN Santa Cruz, Bolivia. Alasbimn Journal 2008;10: 22-25.

[17] Mandeville KL, Krabshuis J, Ladep NG, Mulder CJ, Quigley EM, Khan SA. Gastroenterology in developing countries: Issues and advances. World J Gastroenterol 2009;15: 2839-54.

[18] Ferlay J, Shin HR, Bray F, Forman D, Mathers C and Parkin DM. GLOBOCAN 2008 v1.2, Cancer Incidence and Mortality Worldwide: IARC CancerBase No. 10 [Internet] Lyon, France: International Agency for Research on Cancer; 2010. Available from: http://globocan.iarc.fr, accessed on 17/July/2012.

[19] Escobar-Pardo ML, de Godoy AP, Machado RS, *et al.* Prevalence of *Helicobacter pylori* infection and intestinal parasitosis in children in Xingu Indian Reservation. J Pediatr (Rio J)2011;87:393-98.

[20] Parente JM, da Silva BB, Palha Dias MP, Zaterka S, Nishimura N, Zeitune JM. *Helicobacter pylori* infection in children of low and high socioeconomic status in northeast Brazil. Am J Trop Med Hyg 2006;75:509-12.

[21] Glynn MK, Friedman CR, Gold BD, *et al.* Seroincidence of *Helicobacter pylori* infection in a cohort of rural Bolivian children: acquisition and analysis of possible risk factors. Clin Infect Dis 2002;35:1059-65.

[22] Nessa J, Chart H, Owen RJ, Drasar B. Human serum antibody response to *Helicobacter pylori* whole cell antigen in an institutionalized Bangladeshi population. J Appl Microbiol 2001;90:68-72.

[23] Morad M, Merrick J, Nasri Y. Prevalence of *Helicobacter pylori* in people with intellectual disability in a residential care center in Israel. J Intell Disabil Res 2002;46:141-143.

[24] Fialho AM, Braga AB, Braga Neto MB, *et al.* Younger siblings play a major role in *Helicobacter pylori* transmission among children from a low-income community in the Northeast of Brazil. Helicobacter 2010;15:491-96.

[25] Thomas JE, Gibson GR, Darboe MK, Dale A, Weaver LT. Isolation of *Helicobacter pylori* from human faeces. Lancet 1992;340:1194-95.

[26] Klein PD, Graham DY, Gaillour A, Opekun AR, Smith EO. Water source as risk factor for *Helicobacter pylori* infection in Peruvian children. Gastrointestinal Physiology Working Group. Lancet 1991;337:1503-06.

[27] Hopkins RJ, Vial PA, Ferreccio C, *et al.* Seroprevalence of *Helicobacter pylori* in Chile: vegetables may serve as one route of transmission. J Infect Dis 1993;168:222-26.

[28] Goodman KJ, Correa P, Aux HJT, *et al. Helicobacter pylori* infection in the Colombian Andes: a population-based study of transmission pathways. Am J Epidemol 1996;144:290-99.

[29] Gomes B, Martinis E. Fate of *Helicobacter pylori* artificially inoculated in lettuce and carrot samples. Braz J Microbiol 2004;35:145-50.

[30] Kignel S, de Almeida Pina F, André EA, Alves Mayer MP, Birman EG. Occurrence of *Helicobacter pylori* in dental plaque and saliva of dyspeptic patients. Oral Dis. 2005;11:17-21.

[31] Berroterán A, Perrone M, Correnti M, Cavazza ME, Tombazzi CV, Goncalvez R. Prevalencia de *Helicobacter pylori* en muestras de placa dental de un grupo de pacientes venezolanos mediante la técnica de reacción en cadena de la polimerasa. Acta Odontol Venez 2002;40:45-51.

[32] Janjetic MA, Goldman CG, Barrado DA, *et al.* Decreasing trend of *Helicobacter pylori* infection in children with gastrointestinal symptoms from Buenos Aires, Argentina. Helicobacter 2011;16:316-19.

[33] Kawakami E, Machado RS, Ogata SK, Langner M. Decrease in prevalence of *Helicobacter pylori* infection during a 10-year period in Brazilian children. Arq Gastroenterol. 2008;45:147-51.

[34] Coelho MC, Bomfim IN, Moreira MR, Santa-Cecilia EV, Oliveira SM, Trindade OR, Coelho LG. Infection by *Helicobacter pylori* among medical students in Brazil. Helicobacter 2007;12: 454.

[35] Mégraud F, Lehours P. *Helicobacter pylori* detection and antimicrobial susceptibility testing. Clin Microbiol Rev 2007;20:280-322.

[36] Rocha GA, Queiroz DM, Mendes EM, Lage AP, Barbosa AJ. Simple carbolfuchsin staining foe showing C. *pylori* and other spiral bacteria in gastric mucosa. J Clin Pathol 1989;42:1004-05.

[37] Queiroz DMM, Mendes EN, Rocha GA. Indicator medium for isolation of *Campylobacter pylori*. J Clin Microbiol 1987;25:2378-79.

[38] Malfertheiner P, Megraud F, O'Morain CA, *et al.* Management of *Helicobacter pylori* infection—the Maastricht IV/ Florence Consensus Report. Gut. 2012; 61:646-64.

[39] Gisbert JP, Pajares JM. ^{13}C-urea breath test in the diagnosis of *Helicobacter pylori* infection- a critical review. Aliment Pharmacol Ther 2004;20:1001-17.

[40] Gatta L, Ricci C, Tampieri A, *et al.* Accuracy of breath test using low doses of ^{13}C-urea to diagnose *Helicobacter pylori* infection: randomized controlled trial. Gut. 2006;55:457-62.

[41] Coelho LG, Silva-Jr AE, Coelho MC, *et al.* Does low dose 13C-urea breath test maintain a satisfactory accuracy in diagnosing *Helicobacter pylori* infection? Arq Gastroenterol 2011; 48: 104-08.

[42] Coelho LG, Chausson Y, Passos MC, *et al.* 14C-urea breath test to diagnose gastric *Helicobacter pylori* colonization. Gastroenterol Clin Biol. 1990;14:801-05.

[43] Coelho LG, Reber M, Passos MC, *et al.* Application of isotopeselective non-dispersive infrared spectrometry for the evaluation of the 13C-urea breath test: comparison with three concordant methods. Braz J Med Biol Res 1999; 32: 1493–97.

[44] Kawakami E, Machado RS, Reber M, Patricio FR. 13C-urea breath test with infrared spectroscopy for diagnosing *Helicobacter pylori* infection in children and adolescents. J Pediatr Gastroenterol Nutr 2002; 35: 39–43.

[45] Coelho LGV, Passos MCF, Cunha FAF, *et al. Helicobacter pylori* reinfection rates and serological evaluation in a 6,4 years follow-up study from an emerging country. Gut 1999;45(Suppl 111):A110.

[46] Selgrad M, Kandulski A, Malfertheiner P. *Helicobacter pylori*: diagnosis and treatment. Curr Opin Gastroenterol. 2009;25:549-56.

[47] Fazzio S, Vázquez G, Ardao G, *et al. Helicobacter pylori*: estúdio comparativo de diferentes técnicas diagnósticas. Acta Gastroenterol Latinoam 1995;25:269-76.

[48] Doweck J, Quintana C, Barrios A, *et al.* Evaluación de sensibilidad, especificidad y valor predictivo de seis métodos serológicos cualitativo para la detección de anticuerpos contra el *Helicobacter pylori*. Acta Gastroenterol Latinoam 1997;27:259-61.

[49] Rocha GA, Oliveira AMR, Queiroz DMM, *et al.* Serodiagnosis of *Helicobacter pylori* intection by Cobas Core ELISA in adults from Minas Gerais, Brazil. Braz J Med Biol Res 1998;31:1263-68.

[50] Monici LT, Nishimura NF, Hara NH, Zeitune JMR. Validação de um método imunoenzimático para detecção da infeção pelo *Helicobacter pylori*. J Bras Patol 1999;35:65-70.

[51] González CG, Serrano C, Harris PR. Diagnóstico de la infección por *Helicobacter pylori* en niños mediante la detección de antígenos en deposiciones. Rev Med Chile 2007;135:182-188.

[52] Zapatier JA, Gómez NA, Vargas PE, Maya SV. Valoración de la serología como método diagnóstico de *Helicobacter pylori* en la población local de la ciudad de Guayaquil. Acta Gastroenterol Latinoam 2007;37:104-09.

[53] Urrestarazu M, Serrano N, Uzcátegui A, Díaz L, Ávila M, Lunar M, Pinero R, Cavazza M. Evaluación de un ensayo inmunoenzimático para la detección de *Helicobacter pylori*en muestras de heces. Rev Soc Venez Microbiol 2001;21:23-5.

[54] Monteiro, L., Bergey B, Grãs N, Megraud F. Evaluation of the performance of the Helico Blot 2.1 as a tool to investigate the virulence properties of *Helicobacter pylori*. Clin. Microbiol. Infect. 2002;8:676–79.

[55] Park, C. Y., Cho YK, Kodama T, El-Zimaity HM, Osato MS, Graham DY, Yamaoka Y. New serological assay for detection of putative *Helicobacter pylori* virulence factors. J. Clin. Microbiol. 2002;40:4753–56.

[56] Rocha AM, Rocha GA, Leite JL, Lisboa RLL, Silva PVO, Queiroz DMM. Inmunoblotting for the serodiagnosis of *Helicobacter pylori* infection in Brazilian patients with and without gastric carcinoma. Mem Inst Oswaldo Cruz 2004;99:189-93.

[57] Ekstrom AM, Held M, Hansson LE, Engstrand L, Nyren O. *Helicobacter pylori* in gastric cancer established by CagA immunoblot as a marker of past infection. Gastroenterology 2001;121:784-89.

[58] Ramos AP, De Fuccio MB, Moretzsohn LD, *et al.* Cystic fibrosis, *H. pylori* infection and gastroduodenal abnormalities. Helicobacter 2011;16(suppl.1):128.

[59] Ho B, Marshall BJ. Accurate diagnosis of *Helicobacter pylori*. Serologic testing. Gastroenterol Clin North Am. 2000;29:853-62.

[60] Raguza D, Machado RS, Ogata SK, Patrício FR, Kawakami E. Validation of a monoclonal stool antigen test for diagnosing *Helicobacter pylori* infection in young children. J Ped Gastroenterol Nutrition 2010;50:400-403.

[61] Calvet X, Lario S, Ramirez-Lazaro MJ, *et al.* Accuracy of monoclonal stool tests for determining cure of *Helicobacter pylori* infection after treatment. Helicobacter 2010; 15:201-205.

[62] Schwarzer A, Lottspeich C, Russmann H, *et al.* Evaluation of a novel rapid one-step monoclonal chromatographic immunoassay for detection of *Helicobacter pylori* in stool from children. Eur J Clin Microbiol Infect Dis 2007;26:475-80.

[63] Silva JMK, Villares CA, Monteiro MS, Colaúto C, Santos AF, Mattar R. Validation of a rapid stool antigen test for diagnosis of *Helicobacter pylori* infection. Rev. Inst. Med. Trop. Sao Paulo 2010; 52125-28.

[64] Contreras M, García MA, Rodríguez MJ, *et al.* Validez de un test inmunocromatográfico rápido para la detección de *Helicobacter pylori* en heces. Interciencia 2006;31:136-39.

[65] Cullen KP, Broderick BM, Jayaram J, Flynn B, O'Connor HJ. Evaluation of the *Helicobacter pylori* stool antigen (HpSA) test in routine clinical practice: is it patient-friendly? Ir Med J 2002;95:305–06.

[66] Cambau E, Allerheiligen V, Coulon C *et al.* Evaluation of a new test, genotype HelicoDR, for molecular detection of antibiotic resistance in *Helicobacter pylori.* J Clin Microbiol 2009;47: 3600-07.

[67] Glocker E, Kist M. Rapid detection of point mutations in the gyrA gene of *Helicobacter pylori* conferring resistance to ciprofloxacin by a fluorescence resonance energy transfer-based real-time PCR approach. J Clin Microbiol 2004;42:2241-46.

[68] Woo HY, Park DI, Park H *et al.* Dual-priming oligonucleotide-based multiplex PCR for the detection of *Helicobacter pylori* and determination of clarithromycin resistance with gastric biopsy specimens. Helicobacter 2009;14:22-8.

[69] Wüppenhorst N, Hobmaier B, Kist M. Evaluation of Genotype HelicoDR for molecular detection of *H. pylori* and its resistance against clarithromycin and fluoroquinolones. Helicobacter 2010;15: 387.

[70] Deye VYM, Burette A, Bentatou Z, *et al.* Practical use of GenoType® HelicoDR, a molecular test for *Helicobacter pylori* detectionand susceptibility testing. Diag Microbiol Infect Dis 2011;70:557-60.

[71] Moore, RA., Beckthold B, Wong S, Kureishi A, Bryan LE. Nucleotide sequence of the *gyrA* gene and characterization of ciprofloxacin resistant mutants of *Helicobacter pylori.* Antimicrob Agents Chemother 1995; 39:107–11.

[72] Tankovic J, Lascols C, Sculo Q, Petit JC, Soussy CJ. Single and double mutations in *gyr*A but not in *gyr*B are associated with low- and high-level fluoroquinolone resistance in *Helicobacter pylori*. Antimicrob Agents Chemother 2003; 47:3942–44.

[73] Liu H, Ye H, Ruskone-Fourmestraux A, *et al.* T(11;18) is a marker for all stage gastric MALT lymphomas that will not respond to *H. pylori* eradication. Gastroenterology. 2002;122:1286-94.

[74] Ruskoné-Fourmestraux A, Fischbach W, Aleman BM, *et al.* EGILS consensus report. Gastric extranodal marginal zone B-cell lymphoma of MALT Gut. 2011;60:747-58.

[75] Ramírez-Ramos A, Sánchez-Sánchez R. Contribución de Latinoamérica al estudio del *Helicobacter pylori*. Acta Gastroenterol Latinoam 2009;39:197-18.

[76] Hatakeyama M. Anthropological and clinical implications for the structural diversity of the *Helicobacter pylori* CagA oncoprotein. Cancer Sci 2011;102:36-43.

[77] Batista SA, Rocha GA, Rocha AM, *et al.* Higher number of *Helicobacter pylori* CagA EPIYA C phosphorylation sites increases the risk of gastric cancer, but not duodenal ulcer. BMC Microbiol. 2011;Mar 24;11:61.

[78] González I, Romero J, Rodríguez B, *et al.* High prevalence of virulence-associated genotypes in *Helicobacter pylori* clinical isolates in the Region del Maule, Chile. Scand J Infect Dis. 2011;43:652-55.

[79] Coelho LG, Leon-Barua R, Quigley EM, *et al.* Latin-American consensus conference on *Helicobacter pylori* infection. Am J Gastroenterol 2000;95:2688-91.

[80] Hunt RH, Xiao SD, Megraud F, *et al.* World Gastroenterology Organisation Global Guideline *Helicobacter pylori* in Developing Countries. J Clin Gastroenterol 2011;45:383-88.

[81] Fock KM, Talley N, Moayyedi P, *et al.* Asia-Pacific consensus guidelines on gastric cancer prevention. J Gastroenterol Hepatol 2008;23:351-65.

[82] Mégraud F, Lamouliatle H, Delchier JC, *et al.* *Helicobacter pylori* resistance to antimicrobial agents after failure of an initial treatment and impact on results of second-line treatment strategies: a multicenter prospective study. Gastroenterology 2001;120(Suppl 1):A15.

[83] Heep M, Kist M, Strobel S, Beck D, LehnN. Secondary resistance among 554 isolates of *Helicobacter pylori* after failure of therapy. Eur J Clin Microbiol Infect. Dis 2000;19:538–41.

[84] Stege PW, Veja AE. Analysis of resistance to clarithromycin and *iceA* status in *Helicobacter pylori* isolates from San Luis, Argentina. Int J Antimicrob Agents 2006;28: 477–78.

[85] Prazeres-Magalhães P, Queiroz DM, Campos DVB, *et al. Helicobacter pylori* primary resistance to metronidazole and clarithromycin in Brazil. Antimicrob. Agents Chemother 2002; 46:2021-23.

[86] Godoy AP, Ribeiro ML, Benvengo YH, *et al.* Analysis of antimicrobial susceptibility and virulence factors in *Helicobacter pylori* clinical isolates. BMC Gastroenterol 2003; 3(8):20.

[87] Jaime Natan E, Silva FM, Barbuti RC, Navarro-Rodrigues T, Moraes-Filho JP, Pedrazzoli J Jr. *Helicobacter pylori* antibiotic resistance in Brazil: clarithromycin is still a good option. Arq Gastroenterol 2011;48:261-64.

[88] Lins AK, Lima RA, Magalhães M. Clarithromycin-resistant *Helicobacter pylori* in Recife, Brazil, directly identified from gastric biopsies by polymerase chain reaction. Arq Gastroenterol 2010;47:379-82.

[89] Vallejos C, Garrido L, Cáceres D, *et al.* Prevalence of metronidazole, claritromycin and tetracycline resistance in *Helicobacter pylori* isolated from Chilean patients. Rev Med Chile 2007;135:287-93.

[90] Alvarez A, Moncayo JI, Santacruz JJ, Santacoloma M, Corredor LF, Reinosa E. Antimicrobial susceptibility and mutations involved in clarithromycin resistance in *Helicobacter pylori* isolates from patients in the western central region of Colombia. Antimicrob Agents Chemother. 2009;53:4022-24.

[91] Fariña N, Kasamatsu E, Samudio M, Morán M, Sanabria R, Laspina F. Antimicrobial susceptibility of *H. pylori* strains obtained from Paraguayan patients. Rev Med Chil. 2007;135:1009-14.

[92] Torres-Debat ME, Pérez-Pérez G, Olivares A, *et al.* Antimicrobial susceptibility of *Helicobacter pylori* and mechanisms of clarithromycin resistance in strains isolated from patients in Uruguay. Rev Esp Enferm Dig. 2009;101:757-62.

[93] Tytgat GNJ, Noach LA. *H. pylori* eradication. In: R.H. Hunt & G.N.J. Tytgat, editors. *Helicobacter pylori.* Basic mechanisms to clinical cure. London: Kluwer Academic Publishers; 1994. p. 550-69.

[94] Veldhuyzen van Zanten SJO, Goldie J, Hollingworth K, Silleti CF, Richardson H, Hunt RH. Secretion of intravenously administered antibiotics in gastric juice: implicationsfor management of *Helicobacter pylori*. J Clin Pathol 1992;245:225-27.

[95] Nwokolo CU, Lewin JF, Hudson M, Pounder RE. Transmucosal penetration of bismuth particles in the human stomach. Gastroenterology 1992; 102:163-67.

[96] Treiber G, Walker S, Klotz U. Omeprazole-induced increase in the absorption of bismuth from tripotassium dicitrate bismuthate. Clin Pharmacol Ther 1994;55:486-91.

[97] Vieira WL, Coelho LG, Rocha OG, *et al.* Blood and urine level of bismuth in patients on *H. pylori* therapy. Can J Gastroenterol 1999;13(Suppl.B):156B.

[98] Ford AC, Malfertheiner P, Giguère M, Santana J, Khan M, Moayyedi P. Adverse events with bismuth salts for *Helicobacter pylori* eradication: Systematic review and meta-analysis. World J Gastroenterol 2008; 14: 7361-70.

[99] Glupczynski Y, Megraud F, Lopez-Brea M, Andersen LP. European multicentre survey of *in vitro* antimicrobial resistance in *Helicobacter pylori*. Eur J Clin Microbiol Infect Dis 2001; 20:820–23.

[100] Sisson G, Jeong JY, Goodwin A, *et al.* Metronidazole activation is mutagenic and causes DNA fragmentation in *Helicobacter pylori* and in *Escherichia coli* containing a cloned *H. pylori* RdxA(+) (nitroreductase) gene. J Bacteriol 2000;182: 5091–96.

[101] Sanches BSF, Coelho LGV, Moretzsohn LD, Vieira-Jr G. Failure of *Helicobacter pylori* treatment after regimes containing clarithromycin: new practical therapeutic options. Helicobacter 2008;13: 572–76.

[102] Coelho LG, Zaterka S. II Consenso Brasileiro sobre *Helicobacter pylori*. Arq Gastroenterol 2005;42:128-32.

[103] Hu FL, Hu PJ, Liu WZ, *et al.* Third Chinese National Consensus Report on the management of *Helicobacter pylori* infection. J Dig Dis 2008; 9:178–84.

[104}. Tatsuta M, Iishi H, Baba M, Taniguchi H. Attenuating effect of the monoamine oxidase inhibitor furazolidone on the anti-carcinogenetic effect of cysteamine on gastric carcinogenesis induced by N-methyl-N′-nitro-N-nitrosoguanidine in Wistar rats. Int J Cancer. 1991;48:605–08.

[105] Ahmed HH, El-Aziem SH, Abdel-Wahhab MA. Potential role of cysteine and methionine in the protection against hormonal imbalance and mutagenicity induced by furazolidone in female rats. Toxicology. 2008;243:31–42.

[106] http://www.fda.gov/OHRMS/DOCKETS/98fr/05-4158.htm, accessed at 15 June 2012.

[107] Zullo A, Ierardi E, Hassan C, De Francesco V. Furazolidone-based therapies for *Helicobacter pylori* infection: A pooled-data analysis. Saudi J Gastroenterol 2012;18:11-17.

[108] IARC Monographs on the evaluation of carcinogenic risks to humans. Furazolidone. 1998;31.

[109] The European Agency for the Evaluation of Medicinal Products. Veterinary Medicines Evaluation Unit. Annex IV. 1999 Oct;:14.

[110] FDA Prohibits Nitrofuran Drug Use. Veterinarian Newsletter. 2002;17(2).

[111] Available from: http://www.ema.europa.eu/. Last accessed on 2011 Oct 12]

[112] Graham D & Lu H. Furazolidone in *Helicobacter pylori* Therapy: Misunderstood and Often Unfairly Maligned Drug Told in A Story of French Bread. Saudi J Gastroenterol. 2012;18:1-2.

[113] Tamayo HM, Noriega-Aldave AP. Determinación de la susceptibilidad de cepas de *Helicobacter pylori* a levofloxacino en formato pequeño y método de difusión en disco usando agar yema de huevo. Rev Gastroenterol Peru. 2011; 31-3: 224-29.

[114] Megraud F. Basis for the management of drug-resistant *Helicobacter pylori* infection. Drugs 2004; 64: 1893–1904.

[115] Gisbert JP, Calvet X. Review article: rifabutin in the treatment of refractory *Helicobacter pylori* infection. Aliment Pharmacol Ther. 2012;35:209-21.

[116] Suzuki S, Suzuki H, Nishizawa T, *et al.* Past rifampicin dosing determines rifabutin resistance of *Helicobacter pylori*. Digestion 2009;79: 1-4.

[117] Antelo P, Almuzara M, Avagnina A, *et al.* Diagnóstico y tratamiento de la infección por Hp: su relación con la úlcera gastrointestinal y la resistencia a los antimicrobianos. Medicina (B. Aires) 2001;61:545-51.

[118] Coelho LG, Mattos AA, Francisconi CF, Castro LP, André SB. Efficacy of the dosing regimen of pantoprazole 40 mg, amoxicillin 1000 mg and clarithromycin 500 mg, twice daily for 7 days, in the eradication of *Helicobacter pylori* in patients with peptic ulcer. Arq Gastroenterol. 2004;41:71-6.

[119] Felga G, Silva FM, Barbuti RC, Navarro-Rodriguez T, Zaterka S, Eisig JN. Clarithromycin-based triple therapy for *Helicobacter pylori* treatment in peptic ulcer patients. J Infect Dev Ctries. 2010;4:712-16.

[120] Mazzoleni LE, Sander GB, Francesconi CF, *et al. Helicobacter pylori* eradication in functional dyspepsia: HEROES trial. Arch Intern Med. 2011;171:1929-36.

[121] Otero W, Gutierrez O, Quintero F, Orozco C, Ibañez M. Eficacia de pantoprazol combinado con claritromicina y amoxicilina para la erradicación de *Helicobacter pylori* en pacientes con úlcera duodenal o dispepsia no ulcerosa. Rev Colomb Gastroenterol 2000;15:247-51.

[122] Ramírez-Ramos A, Sánchez-Sánchez R. *Helicobacter pylori* 25 años después (1983 -2008): epidemiología, microbiología, patogenia, diagnóstico y tratamiento. Rev Gastroenterol Perú. 2009;29:158-70.

[123] Gisbert JP, McNicholl AG. Maintenance of *Helicobacter pylori* eradication rates with triple therapy over 12 years in a Spanish hospital. Helicobacter. 2012;17:160-61.

[124] Greenberg ER, Anderson GL, Morgan DR, *et al.* 14-day triple, 5-day concomitant, and 10-day sequential therapies for *Helicobacter pylori* infection in seven Latin American sites: a randomised trial. Lancet. 2011;378:507-14.

[125] Calvet X, Garcia N, Lopez T, *et al.* A meta-analysis of short *vs.* long therapy with a proton pump inhibitor, clarithromycin and either metronidazole or amoxicillin for treating *Helicobacter pylori* infection. Aliment Pharmacol Ther 2000;14:603-09.

[126] Ford A, Moayyedi P. How can the current strategies for *Helicobacter pylori* eradication therapy be improved? Can J Gastroenterol 2003;17(Suppl B):36B-40B.
[127] Fuccio L, Minardi ME, Zagari RM, *et al.* Meta-analysis: duration of first-line proton pump inhibitor based triple therapy for *Helicobacter pylori* eradication. Ann Intern Med 2007;147:553-62.
[128] Haydee B, Salvana A, Ang ELR, *et al.* Duration of proton-pump inhibitor-based triple therapy for *Helicobacter pylori* eradication: a meta-analysis. Gastroenterology 138:5 (Suppl.1):S-340.
[129] Osato MS, Reddy SG, Piergies AA, Bochenek WJ, Testa RT, Graham DY. Comparative efficacy of new investigational agents against *Helicobacter pylori.* Aliment Pharmacol Ther. 2001;15:487-92.
[130] Kato S, Fujimura S, Udagawa H, *et al.* Antibiotic resistance of *Helicobacter pylori* strains in Japanese children. J Clin Microbiol. 2002;40:649-53.
[131] Dani R, Queiroz DM, Dias MG, *et al.* Omeprazole, clarithromycin and furazolidone for the eradication of *Helicobacter pylori* in patients with duodenal ulcer. Aliment Pharmacol Ther 1999;13:1647-52.
[132] Gisbert JP, Gisbert JL, Marcos S, *et al. Helicobacter pylori* first-line treatment and rescue options in patients allergic to penicillin. Aliment Pharmacol Ther 2005;22:1041-46.
[133] Rodriguez-Torres M, Salgado-Mercado R, Rios-Bedoya CF, *et al.* High eradication rates of *Helicobacter pylori* infection with first- and second-line combination of esomeprazole, tetracyclin and metronidazole in patients allergic to penicillin. Dig Dis Sci 2005;50:634-9.
[134] Gisbert JP, Perez-Aisa A, Castro-Fernandez M, *et al. Helicobacter pylori* first-line treatment and rescue option containing levofloxacin in patients allergic to penicillin. Dig Liver Dis 2010;42:287-90.
[135] Zullo A, Vaira D, Vakil N, *et al.* High eradication rates of *Helicobacter pylori* with a new sequential treatment. Aliment Pharmacol Ther 2003;17:719–26.
[136] Focareta R, Forte G, Forte F, *et al.* Could the 10-days sequential therapy be considered a first choice treatment for the eradication of *Helicobacter pylori* infection? Dig Liver Dis 2003;35(Suppl 4):S33.
[137] Vaira D, Zullo A, Vakil N, *et al.* Sequential therapy *vs.* standard triple-drug therapy for *Helicobacter pylori* eradication: a randomized trial. Ann Intern Med 2007;146:556–63.
[138] Choi WH, Park DI, Oh SJ, *et al.* Effectiveness of 10 day-sequential therapy for *Helicobacter pylori* eradication in Korea. The Korean Journal of Gastroenterology. 2008;5:280-84.
[139] De Francesco V, Margiotta M, Zullo A, *et al.* Clarithromycin-resistant genotypes and eradication of *Helicobacter pylori.* Ann Intern Med 2006;144:94–100.
[140] Malfertheiner P, Bazzoli F, Delchier JC, *et al. Helicobacter pylori* eradication with a capsule containing bismuth subcitrate potassium, metronidazole, and tetracycline given with omeprazole *vs.* clarithromycin-based triple therapy: a randomised, open-label, non-inferiority, phase 3 trial. Lancet. 2011;377:905-13.
[141] Luther J, Higgins PD, Schoenfeld PS, Moayyedi P, Vakil N, Chey WD. Empiric quadruple *vs.* triple therapy for primary treatment of *Helicobacter pylori* infection: Systematic review and meta-analysis of efficacy and tolerability. Am J Gastroenterol. 2010;105:65-73.
[142] Fischbach LA, Bravo LE, Zarama GR, *et al.* A randomized clinical trial to determine the efficacy of regimens containing clarithromycin, metronidazole, and amoxicillin among

histologic subgroups for *Helicobacter pylori* eradication in a developing country. Helicobacter. 2009;14:100-108.

[143] Machado RS, Silva MR, Viriato A. Furazolidone, tetracycline and omeprazole: A low-cost alternative for *Helicobacter pylori* eradication in children. J Pediatr (Rio J) 2008;84:160–65.

[144] Coelho LG, Passos MC, Martins GM, Bueno ML, Gomes BS, Lopes LG, *et al.* Once-daily *Helicobacter pylori* treatment to family members of gastric cancer patients. Am J Gastroenterol. 2000;95:832–33.

[145] Kawakami E, Machado RS, Ogata SK, Langner M, Fukushima E, Carelli AP, *et al.* Furazolidone-based triple therapy for *H. pylori* gastritis in children. World J Gastroenterol. 2006;12:5544–549.

[146] Frota LC, da Cunha Mdo P, Luz CR, de Araujo-Filho AH, Frota LA, Braga LL. *Helicobacter pylori* eradication using tetracycline and furazolidone *vs.* amoxicillin and azithromycin in lansoprazole based triple therapy: An open randomized clinical trial. Arq Gastroenterol. 2005;42:111–15.

[147] De Idiáquez D, Bussalleu A, Rodrigo I, Cabello J, Caviedes G, Cok J, *et al. Helicobacter pylori* infection eradication in dyspeptic patients with and without peptic ulcer. Rev Gastroenterol Peru. 1999;19:179–94.

[148] Araujo Castillo R, Pinto Valdivia JL, Ramírez D, Cok García J, Bussalleu Rivera A. New ultrashort scheme for *Helicobacter pylori* infection eradication using tetracyline, furazolidone and colloidal bismuth subcitrate in dyspeptic patients with or without peptic ulceration in the National Hospital Cayetano Heredia. Rev Gastroenterol Peru. 2005;25:23–41.

[149] Segura AM, Gutiérrez O, Otero W, Angel A, Genta RM, Graham DY. Furazolidone, amoxycillin, bismuth triple therapy for *Helicobacter pylori* infection. Aliment Pharmacol Ther. 1997;11:529–532.

[150] Buzás GM, Józan J. Nitrofuran-based regimens for the eradication of *Helicobacter pylori* infection. J Gastroenterol Hepatol. 2007;22:1571-81.

[151] Giordano-Romano A, Améndola R, Racca J, *et al.* Tasa de reinfeción al año de erradicación esitosa del *Helicobacter pylori*. Acta Gastroenterol Latinoamer. 2001;4:16.

[152] Figueroa G, Acuna R, Troncoso M, *et al. H. pylori* reinfection rate after triple therapy in Chilean duodenal ulcer patients. Am J Gastroenterol 1996;91:1395-99.

[153] Eisig J, Zaterka S, Silva FM, *et al. Helicobacter pylori* recurrence in patients with duodenal ulcer: Clinical, endoscopic, histologic, and genotypic aspects. A 10-year Brazilian series. Helicobacter 2006;11:431-35.

[154] Morgan DR, Torres X, Greenberg ER, *et al. H. pylori* recurrence one year after eradication treatment in a population randomized trial in seven Latin American sites. Gastroenterology 2012; 142 (Suppl. 1):S-478-79.

[155] Graham DY, Lew GM, Malaty HM, *et al.* Factors influencing the eradication of *Helicobacter pylori* with triple therapy. Gastroenterology 1992; 102:493-96.

[156] Gisbert JP, Hermida C, Pajares JM. Are twelve days of omeprazole, amoxicillin and clarithromycin better than six days for treating *H. pylori* infection in peptic ulcer and in nonulcer dyspepsia? Hepatogastroenterology 2001;48:1383–88.

[157] Zhao F, Wang J, Yang Y, *et al.* Effect of CYP2C19 genetic polymorphisms on the efficacy of proton pump inhibitor-based triple therapy for *Helicobacter pylori* eradication: a meta-analysis. Helicobacter 2008;13:532-41.

[158] Suzuki T, Matsuo K, Ito H, *et al.* Smoking increases the treatment failure for *Helicobacter pylori* eradication. Am J Med 2006;119:217-24.

[159] Broutet N, Tchamgoué S, Pereira E, Lamouliatte H, Salamon R, Mégraud F. Risk factors for failure of *Helicobacter pylori* therapy--results of an individual data analysis of 2751 patients. Aliment Pharmacol Ther. 2003;17:99-109.

[160] Dubois A & Borén T. *Helicobacter pylori* is invasive and it may be a facultative intracellular organism. Cell Microbiol 2007;9(5):1108–16.

[161] Lee JM, Breslin NP, Hyde DK, *et al.* Treatment options for *Helicobacter pylori* infection when proton pump inhibitor-based triple therapy fails in clinical practice. Aliment Pharmacol Ther 1999;13:489-96.

[162] Gisbert JP, Gisbert JL, Marcos S, *et al.* Empirical rescue therapy after *Helicobacter pylori* treatment failure: a 10-year single-centre study of 500 patients. Aliment Pharmacol Ther 2008;27:346-54.

[163] Rokkas T, Sechopoulos P, Robotis I, *et al.* Cumulative *H. pylori* eradication rates in clinical practice by adopting first and second-line regimens proposed by the Maastricht III consensus and a third-line empirical regimen. Am J Gastroenterol 2009;104:21-25.

[164] Laine L, Hunt R, El-Zimaity H, Nguyen B, Osato M, Spénard J. Bismuth-based quadruple therapy using a single capsule of bismuth biskalcitrate, metronidazole, and tetracycline given with omeprazole *vs.* omeprazole, amoxicillin, and clarithromycin for eradication of *Helicobacter pylori* in duodenal ulcer patients: a prospective, randomized, multicenter, North American trial.Am J Gastroenterol. 2003;98:562-67.

[165] Osato MS, Reddy R, Reddy SG, Penland RL, Graham DY. Comparison of the Etest and the NCCLS-approved agar dilution method to detect metronidazole and clarithromycin resistant *Helicobacter pylori.* Int. J. Antimicrob. Agents 2001;17:39-44.

[166] Gisbert JP, Morena F. Systematic review and meta-analysis: levofloxacin-based rescue regimens after *Helicobacter pylori* treatment failure. *Aliment Pharmacol Ther* 2006;23:35–44.

[167] Saad RJ, Schoenfeld P, Kim HM, *et al.* Levofloxacin-based triple therapy *vs.* bismuth-based quadruple therapy for persistent *Helicobacter pylori* infection: a meta-analysis. Am J Gastroenterol 2006;101:488–96.

[168] Perna F, Zullo A, Ricci C, Hassan C, Morini S, Vaira D. Levofloxacin-based triple therapy for *Helicobacter pylori* re-treatment: role of bacterial resistance. Dig Liver Dis. 2007;39:1001-05.

[169] Marzio L, Coraggio D, Capodicasa S, Grossi L, Cappello G. Role of the preliminary susceptibility testing for initial and after failed therapy of *Helicobacter pylori* infection with levofloxacin, amoxicilin, and esomepraole. Helicobacter 2006;11:237-42.

[170] Gutierrez O, Otero W, Cardona H, Quintero F, Orozco C, Sanchez L. Terapia cuádruple con furazolidona como tratamiento de rescate para la infección de *Helicobacter pylori.* Rev Colomb Gastroenterol 2003;18:222-24.

[171] Eisig JN, Silva FM, Rodriguez TN, Hashimoto CL, Barbuti RC. A furazolidone-based quadruple therapy for *Helicobacter pylori* retreatment in patients with peptic ulcer disease. Clinics (Sao Paulo). 2005;60:485-8.

[172] Graham DY, Belson G, Abudayyeh, Osato MS, Dore MP, El-Zimaity HM. Twice daily (mid-day and evening) quadruple Therapy for *H. pylori* infection in the United States. Dig Liver Dis 2004;36:384-7.

[173] Coelho LG, Moretzsohn LD, Vieira WL, *et al.* New once-daily, highly effective rescue triple therapy after multiple *Helicobacter pylori* treatment failures: a pilot study. Aliment Pharmacol Ther 2005, 21:783-87.

[174] Eisig JN, Silva FM, Barbuti RC, *et al.* Efficacy of a 7-day course of furazolidone, levofloxacin, and lansoprazole after failed *Helicobacter pylori* eradication. BMC Gastroenterol. 2009;26;9:38.

[175] Brogden RN, Fitton A. Rifabutin. A review of its antimicrobial activity, pharmacokinetic properties and therapeutic efficacy. Drugs 1994; 47: 983-1009.

Send Orders for Reprints to reprints@benthamscience.net
Helicobacter Pylori: A Worldwide Perspective 2014, 2014, 169-182

CHAPTER 7

Helicobacter pylori in Israel: Epidemiology, Pathophysiology, Diagnosis, Management and Resistance to Therapy

Haim Shmuely and Yaron Niv*

Department of Gastroenterology, Rabin Medical Center, Tel Aviv University 39 Jabotinski Street, 49100 Petach Tikva, Israel

Abstract: In Israel, there is a 60% prevalence of *H. pylori* infection in the adult population. The annual incidence of gastric cancer is approximately 15 per 100,000 population. The male/female ratio for a positive ^{13}C urea breath test (UBT) in diagnosing *H. pylori* infection is 1:1.77. Women have significantly higher UBT results than men. *H. pylori* infection is associated with a more severe inflammatory reaction, decreased gastric acid secretion and increased mucin secretion in relatives of patients with gastric cancer. Primary resistance to clarithromycin and metronidazole has been reported as 8.2% and 38.2%, respectively. Secondary resistance of clinical isolates from previously treated adults to clarithromycin, metronidazole, and levofloxacin is 65.7%, 57.1%, and 18.6%, respectively. Resistance to both clarithromycin and metronidazole is 32.8%, and to clarithromycin, metronidazole, and levofloxacin, 12.8%. All isolates are sensitive both to amoxicillin and tetracycline. In untreated children, the rate of resistance to metronidazole is 19%, and to clarithromycin, 25%. Corresponding rates among the isolates from children previously treated for *H. pylori* are 52% and 42%. No resistance is found to amoxicillin, tetracycline or levofloxacin in either group. Sequential regimen, used as primary therapy, attained significantly higher eradication rates than the standard triple therapy. The addition of cranberry to triple therapy improves the rate of *H. pylori* eradication in females. Susceptibility-guided retreatment is associated with better eradication rates than empiric treatment. The annual recurrence rate of *H. pylori* after successful eradication in Israel is 0.37% to 0.55%.

Keywords: Helicobacter, Israel, recurrence, recrudescence, reinfection, developed countries, developing countries, clarithromycin, metronidazole, amoxicillin, tetracycline, sequential therapy, concomitant therapy, urea breath test, rapid urease test, stool antigen test, gastroscopy, gastric cancer, peptic ulcer, maltoma.

***Address correspondence to Yaron Niv:** Department of Gastroenterology, Rabin Medical Center, Petach Tikva, Israel; Tel: 972-504065401; Fax: 972-39210313; Email: yniv@clalit.org.il

EPIDEMIOLOGY

The Israeli population is comprised of two major ethnic groups: the Jewish population (80%) of which 11% -13.9% are estimated as religious ultra-orthodox, and the Israeli Arab population (20%) [1-3]. The Arab population resides mainly in rural areas in towns or neighborhoods separated from the Jewish population. A recent study [4] examined the prevalence, correlates and trends of *H. pylori* infection in Israel using residual sera obtained during 2007-2008 from 1466 Jewish subjects aged 0-77 years and 897 Arabs aged 0-19 years, and during 2000-2001 from 627 Jewish and 575 Arab subjects aged 0-19 years. Age-adjusted *H. pylori* seroprevalence was 45.2% for the Jewish participants. Seropositivity increased with age, reaching 60% at age ≥50 years and ranged from 24.3% in subjects originating from North America/Western Europe/Australia to 63.2% in those from Asia/Africa/South America. Among Arabs, *H. pylori* seroprevalence was 42.1%, reaching 65% in adolescents. No significant change was observed in seroprevalence between 2000-2001 and 2007-2008. High prevalence of *H. pylori* was found in Arabs and Jews originating from countries of high *H. pylori* endemicity. These findings are characteristic of countries with a diverse ethnic structure and recent immigration.

The age-adjusted prevalence of *H. pylori* infection in the Jewish population was 45.2%. The prevalence of *H. pylori* infection increases significantly with age. *H. pylori* infection is acquired in childhood [5, 6]; therefore, the increasing infection prevalence between preschool age, school age and adolescence possibly reflects the acquisition of the infection, while the increase between adolescence and adulthood possibly results from a birth cohort effect. This pattern of rising *H. pylori* infection prevalence with age has been observed in previous studies [7, 8]. The population groups are distinguished by socioeconomic status (SES), demographic and social features.

Recently, Muhsen *et al.* [9] reported that *H. pylori* seropositivity was 22.9%, 25.2%, and 45.6% among Jewish, ultra-orthodox Jewish and Arab children, respectively. *H. pylori* seroprevalence increased significantly with age in the three study groups, but remained consistently higher in Arab children. CagA seropositivity was 40.8% and 45.0% among Jewish and Arab children, respectively, and the highest among subjects of lower SES.

Most *H. pylori* infections are acquired at preschool age. Transient infection beyond this age is uncommon in this population. *H. pylori* -infected siblings are the major reservoir of *H. pylori* in early and late childhood, demonstrating sustained intra-familial transmission of *H. pylori.* The prevalence of *H. pylori* infected Israeli Arabs increased from 49.7% in 2004 to 58.9% in 2007. The approximate annual incidence of infection during 2004-2009 was 5%. Sibling's *H. pylori* positivity at baseline increased the risk for late acquisition of *H. pylori* infection, while maternal education lowered the risk. In a multivariate analysis, sibling's *H. pylori* positivity was the only significant variable associated with early and persistent *H. pylori* infection.

There is a constant declining rate of infection with *H. pylori* in the general population, associated with a decreased chance of developing peptic ulcer disease and its complications [10, 11]. This trend in *H. pylori* acquisition is most probably the underlying explanation of the birth-cohort pattern of ulcer disease. The risk of developing a peptic ulcer increased among birth-cohorts born during the 19th century, peaked among those born at the end of the 19th century, and then decreased in all subsequent generations [12]. This decreased rate of *H. pylori* infection may be ascribed to both improved hygienic conditions, leading to a reduction in the rate of acquisition, and the eradication of this pathogen in patients. The reduction of *H. pylori* infection in Israel is well documented. At the beginning of the 1990's, the estimated prevalence of *H. pylori* infection was 65% in urban [13] and 72% in rural populations [2], subsequently decreasing to 53% [14] after implementation of eradication therapy.

Data obtained from the National Hospital Discharge Database of the Israeli Ministry of Health from January 1, 1996 through December 31, 2007 [15] confirmed that the overall rates of hospital admissions for acute non-variceal bleeding decreased significantly from 29.3 to 16.8 cases/10^5 population/year. The decreased rates were similar in both genders due to lower rates of bleeding from duodenal (13.6 to 5 cases/10^5 population/year) and gastric ulcers (4.3 to 2.4 cases/10^5 population/year). The rates of bleeding from other causes remained unchanged. The rates of surgical interventions for bleeding control decreased significantly (from 11 to 4%). The decline in the overall incidence of acute non-variceal bleeding during the study period was due to a significant decrease in the rate of bleeding peptic ulcers.

PATHOPHYSIOLOGY

The mucous barrier plays an important role in protecting the gastrointestinal tract from mechanical and chemical damage. Mucins, the major component of mucus, are high-molecular-weight glycoproteins synthesized by epithelial cells. Normal gastric mucus expresses the mucins MUC1, MUC5AC, and MUC6. The development of gastric carcinoma is associated with changes in mucin expression, namely a decrease in MUC5AC and MUC6 and aberrant *de novo* expression of MUC2, MUC3, and MUC4 [16]. *H. pylori* infection associated with the development of gastric carcinoma induces a wide range of changes in the gastric mucus. A reversible alteration of mucins glycosylation occurs which affects the protective function of the gastric mucus [17]. *H. pylori* may inhibit the synthesis of gastric mucin, but not its secretion or degradation [18]. CagA-positive strains of *H. pylori* cause a significantly stronger inhibition of mucus synthesis than CagA-negative strains [19]. In addition, *H. pylori* infection causes an aberrant MUC6 expression, with a reduction in MUC1 and MUC5AC expression, reverting after elimination of the infection [20]. First-degree relatives of patients with gastric cancer have a 1.5-fold to 3-fold increased risk of developing gastric cancer [21]. Relatives of gastric cancer patients, who are also carriers of a CagA-positive strain of *H. pylori*, have an 8-fold risk of developing gastric cancer [22]. Mucosal atrophy, hypochlorhydria, high lymphoid follicle density, pangastritis, and interleukin 1β polymorphism are frequently observed in family members of gastric cancer patients and are associated with an increased risk of the disease [23,24].

A recent study [25] compared gastric acid and mucin secretion in dyspeptic Israeli patients, with and without a family history of gastric cancer and *H. pylori* infection. Twenty-six dyspeptic patients underwent esophago-gastro-duodenoscopy, gastric biopsies, and acid and mucin secretory tests. The sample was stratified according to the family history of gastric cancer and *H. pylori* status. Neither cases nor controls, who were negative for *H. pylori* infection, demonstrated any change in gastric acid and mucin expression. *H. pylori* infection resulted in the same inflammatory score in both groups, however, only the patients with a family history of gastric cancer developed hypochlorhydria. Patients infected with *H. pylori* had a significantly higher degree of inflammation than uninfected patients. *H. pylori*-positive patients with a positive family history had a lower basal and maximal gastric acid output than infected patients with no family history and noninfected controls, and a higher basal and maximal mucin output than infected patients with no family history. MUC5AC was the major mucin species expressed in gastric juices. *H. pylori* infection is associated with a more severe inflammatory reaction consisting of decreased gastric acid secretion and increased mucin secretion in relatives of Israeli patients with gastric cancer.

DIAGNOSIS

Urea Breath Test

In Israel, the ^{13}C urea breath test (UBT) is widely used in diagnosing *H. pylori* infection for all age groups. UBT remains the most reliable noninvasive method for diagnosing *H. pylori* infection and eradication following treatment in adults [26] and children [27]. Testing is performed with carbon 13-urea, which has the highest reported sensitivity among the available noninvasive tests for *H. pylori* [28] and is the best for validation of *H. pylori* eradication [29].

Several large studies of Israeli populations were performed using the databases of the two largest health management organizations in Israel. The first study [30] used the database of Maccabi Health Care Services (MHS), the second largest health management organization in Israel, with 1.6 million insured members (27% of the total population). The MHS [^{13}C]-UBT computerized database was assessed to identify the UBT delta values of all individuals tested for *H. pylori* infection for the first time by UBT, between 1999 and 2001. A total of 7,373 patients with a UBT test of ≥2 ppm during the study period were identified (4,531 females and 2,842 males). For ages 10-80 years, a significantly higher mean UBT value was recorded for females (24.7 ppm) compared with males (17.6 ppm). This study provides an additional factor of maternal transmission of *H. pylori.* A higher female gastric active and viable bacterial load may facilitate oral-oral and gastric-oral mother-to-child transmission. Whatever the mechanism may be, this analysis demonstrated quantitatively, for the first time, gender-associated differences in *H. pylori* host interaction.

A very recent study [31] characterized both the age- and gender-based trends of UBT results from early childhood through late adulthood. This study used the database of the largest central *H. pylori* laboratory of Clalit Health Services, the largest health management organization in Israel, with over 3.8 million insured members (53% of the total population). All positive UBTs during 2007-2008 were analyzed as to age and gender. Overall, 24,237 tested positive (DOB $\geq$ 3.5), 2,470 were repeated positives, consequently, 21,767 positive UBT values were available for the initial analysis. In both males and females, 41% of the initial UBTs were positive. Once again females had significantly higher results than males in early childhood and throughout old age. There appears to be an association between high UBT values and female gender among Israeli patients with *H. pylori* infection. *H. pylori* is most commonly transmitted from person to person, as suggested by the high prevalence of interfamilial clustering. Mothers apparently play a key role in the transmission of the infection to their children [32].

The prognostic factors for successful eradication of *H. pylori* in the Israeli population were assessed from the central *H. pylori* laboratory of Clalit Health Services. To test the success of *H. pylori* eradication, Niv *et al.* [33] studied 5,885 consecutive patients who had undergone 13C-UBT test. The patients were grouped according to the number of total treatment regiments provided prior to the test: 5,442 received one course of treatment (Group I), 380 received two courses (Group II), and 63 three courses (Group III). The 13C-UBT was positive in 27.8%, 37.4%, and 47.6% of patients, groups I, II, and III, respectively. A combination of omeprazole, amoxicillin, and clarithromycin was used in 31.3%, 27.4%, and 7.9% in groups I, II, and III, respectively, and a combination of omeprazole, amoxicillin, and metronidazole in 15.2%, 28.9%, and 28.6%, respectively. Regimens that contained clarithromycin were used in decreasing order in groups I, II, and III, and regimens containing metronidazole, bismuth, or tetracycline, in increasing order. The only good prognostic factor for successful eradication was Israeli origin, while European-American and Asian-African origin, recurrence of symptoms, history of duodenal ulcer, and chronic proton pump inhibitor (PPI) use did not favor successful eradication. These results suggest that origin, history of peptic disease, and chronic PPI use are predictors of eradication failure.

In developing countries, the recurrence rate of *H. pylori* after successful eradication is up to 42%, while in developed countries it is estimated to be less than 3% [34]. Recurrence after successful eradication may be due to a flare up of the same bacterium (recrudescence) or to a new contamination with similar or different species (re-infection) [35]. Studies using PCR have revealed that most recurrences are in fact recrudescence: the same bacterium has been able to survive the treatment as a coccoid form, subsequently undetected in the [^{13}C]-UBT carried out after eradication. In 2000, Cohen *et al.* [36] assessed the recurrence rate of *H. pylori* in dyspeptic patients who had undergone [^{13}C]-UBT at the central *H. pylori* laboratory of Clalit Health Services and for whom the results were negative (successful eradication). In 2007, these patients were requested to fill out a questionnaire as to their symptoms and then undergo a second [^{13}C]-UBT. In total, 65 patients participated. Twenty-six out of the 65 (Group A) had undergone the first test for validation of the successful eradication of *H. pylori*, and 39 (Group B) had done so for dyspepsia. One patient in each group had a positive [^{13}C]-UBT (3.84% in Group A and 2.56% in Group B; non-significant difference (NS)). The mean annual *H. pylori* recurrence rate was calculated as 0.55% and 0.37% in Group A and Group B patients, respectively (NS). These results demonstrate a very low re-infection or new infection rates in Israeli adults and are in line with other trials in developed countries, although they do not support a retesting program for patients after successful eradication therapy. However, this rate of re-infection, although low, is clinically important since the definitive cure of peptic disease and prevention of ulcer complications as well as the cure for MALT lymphoma, are dependent on the successful eradication of *H. pylori* infection.

Antimicrobial Resistance

Children

High *H. pylori* resistance rates in children are of concern since the antimicrobial treatments approved for the treatment of *H. pylori* infection in this age group, are more limited than in adults. Tetracycline and levofloxacin, generally recommended as second-line or rescue therapies after treatment failure in adults, are generally not used in children because of the risk of side effects. Tetracycline is limited to children over 8 years of age to prevent enamel staining, although it remains a therapeutic option for older adolescents. Quinolones are suspected of causing cartilage aberrations and are currently FDA-approved for use only in patients older than 18 years.

In a recent prospective study [37], 55 *H. pylori* isolates cultured from 53 patients (36 naïve and 19 previously treated patients; median age-13 years; range 2-17 years) were tested for antibiotic susceptibility by the E-test. The isolate resistance rates from the naïve patients were 19% and 25% to metronidazole and clarithromycin, respectively. Corresponding rates among the isolates from patients previously treated for *H. pylori* were 52% and 42%. No resistance was found to amoxicillin, tetracycline or levofloxacin. Of the 53 patients, 22 (40%) reported amoxicillin treatment for *H. pylori* or other indications in the year prior to culture; 13 (20%) reported metronidazole therapy, and 12 (23%) an intake of clarithromycin or azithromycin. Resistance of *H. pylori* to clarithromycin was significantly associated with previous macrolide usage. There was no correlation between *H. pylori* resistance to metronidazole and previous use of metronidazole. In two patients, each of the gastric biopsies yielded a strain of *H. pylori* with a different resistance pattern. The isolates also differed in resistance to metronidazole. *H. pylori* resistance rate to clarithromycin and metronidazole is high in Israeli children, particularly in those previously treated for *H. pylori* infection, in which culture-based treatment should be considered. The simultaneous colonization of multiple strains in a minority of patients needs to be further characterized.

Adults

The resistance rates of *H. pylori* isolates to metronidazole, clarithromycin, tetracycline, amoxicillin and cefixime was tested [38] in 138 clinical isolates of *H. pylori* isolated from antral biopsy specimens of 138 dyspeptic adults (71 females, 67 males; median age 55 years), one isolate from each patient, at the Rabin Medical Center, a major tertiary hospital in central Israel. Primary *H. pylori* resistance rates to clarithromycin and metronidazole in naïve patients were 8.2% and 38.2%, respectively. Corresponding resistance rates for isolates of *H. pylori* from treated patients were significantly higher: 46.4% and 60.7%. Dual resistance was found in 5.5% of untreated patients and 32.1% of treated patients. In eight of the nine isolates from the treated patients, dual resistance was found to metronidazole and clarithromycin. No resistance to tetracycline was detected. Resistance to amoxicillin was found in only one isolate (MIC = 1.5 mg/L) from an untreated patient.

Levofloxacin, the l-form of the fluoroquinolone ofloxacin is a broad-spectrum antibiotic [39]. High eradication rates were reported [40, 41] with levofloxacin-based triple therapy. The *in vitro* activity of levofloxacin, amoxicillin, clarithromycin, metronidazole, and tetracycline was tested against 70 clinical isolates of *H. pylori* recovered from 70 Israeli dyspeptic patients [42]. All patients had previously failed 2 treatment regimens: first-line triple therapy with omeprazole, amoxicillin, and clarithromycin and second-line quadruple therapy with omeprazole, metronidazole, tetracycline, and bismuth. Resistance to clarithromycin, metronidazole, and levofloxacin was found in 65.7%, 57.1%, and 18.6% of isolates, respectively. Resistance to both clarithromycin and metronidazole was found in 32.8%, and to clarithromycin, metronidazole, and levofloxacin in 12.8%. Only 4 of the isolates were resistant to both clarithromycin and levofloxacin, and none were resistant to levofloxacin alone or to metronidazole and levofloxacin. In Israel, physicians should consider triple therapy with omeprazole, levofloxacin, and amoxicillin in patients unsuccessfully treated with first- and second-line regimens

TREATMENT

Sequential Therapy

A combination of a proton pump inhibitor (PPI) together with two antibiotics has been recognized in Israel as the first-line therapy of choice for *H. pylori* eradication since the publication of a randomized controlled trial in 1996 [43]. Indeed during the early years of treatment, standard triple therapy produced cure rates of at least 90%. However, during the last decade, the eradication rates in many countries decreased dramatically to approximately 70% [44]. In Israel, cure rates as low as 57% have been reported, [45] which have been related to antibiotic resistance, mainly clarithromycin.

In a recent prospective study [46], 124 Israeli naïve *H. pylori* infected patients, diagnosed by both UBT and rapid urease test, were treated with a sequential therapy protocol which included omeprazole 20 mg bid and amoxicillin 1 g bid for 5 days, followed by omeprazole 20 mg bid, clarithromycin 500 mg bid and tinidazole 500 mg bid for the next 5 days. The eradication rate was 95.8% per protocol analysis and 92.7 by intention to treat analysis. Side effects were reported in 21 patients (16.9%). The sequential regimen attained significantly higher eradication rates in naive patients than usually reported for conventional triple therapy. Sequential therapy may be an alternative first-line therapy in eradicating *H. pylori* in Israel.

Susceptibility-Guided *vs.* Empiric Retreatment

Bacterial resistance to clarithromycin or metronidazole significantly increased in isolates from Israeli patients who failed previous eradication treatments. An increase in clarithromycin and metronidazole -resistant strains from 8.2% and 38.2% in untreated patients to 46.4% and 60.7%, respectively, was reported after treatment failure [38]. This finding suggests that previous treatment failure is a significant contributing factor to acquired bacterial resistance to both clarithromycin and metronidazole.

The efficacy of susceptibility-guided *vs.* empiric retreatment for *H. pylori,* after at least one treatment failure, was reported in 49 Israeli patients in whom at least one treatment regimen for *H. pylori* eradication had failed [47]. All 49 patients underwent gastric biopsy and culture and were retreated according to the *in vitro* susceptibility results. Findings were compared with those of 49 control patients referred for a [^{13}C]-UBT after empiric treatment. Eradication was significally successful in 42 patients in the guided-therapy group (86%) and 31 in the empiric-therapy group (63%). Susceptibility-guided therapy was associated with a significantly higher eradication success. This study suggests that in Israeli patients, susceptibility-guided retreatment appears to be significantly more effective than empiric retreatment in eradicating *H. pylori* after at least one previous treatment failure.

Cranberry

In vitro studies have shown that cranberry juice constituents inhibit the adhesion of *H. pylori* to gastric cells [48]. Antiadhesion agents may be considered antimicrobial agents, albeit they do not act to kill or arrest the growth of the target bacteria, but rather impair their ability to gain a foothold in the host. As these agents are not bactericidal, their use lessens the selective propagation and spread of strains resistant to them. One such agent is a high-molecular-weight, nondialysable material (NDM) found in cranberries [49]. Based on these findings, together with studies showing that NDM inhibited the adhesion of two-thirds of tested clinical isolates of *H. pylori*, including bacteria expressing sialic acid-specific adhesion, suggested that cranberry juice may have the ability to eradicate *H. pylori in vivo* [50]. In a randomized controlled study, cranberry juice alone accounted for a 15% rate of *H. pylori* eradication, compared to 5% for placebo [51].

In a clinical study conducted in Israel [52], 177 patients with *H. pylori* infection treated with OAC for 1 week were randomly allocated to receive 250 mL of either cranberry juice or a placebo beverage, twice daily and only cranberry juice or a placebo beverage for the next 2 weeks. Treatment outcome was determined by the UBT. An additional control group consisted of patients, referred to the same center during the same period, who were treated only with OAC for 1 week. Overall, the rate of *H. pylori* eradication was 82.5%, with no statistically significant difference among the groups. Analysis by gender revealed that for female subjects, the eradication rate was higher in the cranberry-OAC group (95%) than in the placebo-OAC group (87%) and significantly higher than in the non-placebo-OAC group (80%). For males, the rate was not significantly lower in the cranberry-OAC group (74%) *vs.* the placebo-OAC group (80.0%) and non-placebo-OAC group (85%). These results suggest that the addition of cranberry to triple therapy improves the rate of *H. pylori* eradication in females.

ACKNOWLEDGEMENT

None Declared.

CONFLICT OF INTEREST

The author(s) confirm that this chapter content has no conflict of interest.

REFERENCES

[1] Gdalevich M, Cohen D, Ashkenazi I, Mimouni D, Shpilberg O, Kark JD. *Helicobacter pylori* infection and subsequent peptic duodenal disease among young adults. Int. J. Epidemiol. Central Bureau of Statistics. Statistical abstracts of Israel 2010. Publication number 61. Jerusalem: State of Israel, 2011. Available from http://www.cbs.gov.il/reader/shnatonhnew_site.htm.

[2] Gilboa S, Gabay G, Zamir D, Zeev A, Novis B. *Helicobacter pylori* infection in rural settlements (Kibbutzim) in Israel. Int J Epidemiol 1995;24:232-37.

[3] Gurovich N, Cohen-Kastro E. Ultra-orthodox Jews geographic distribution and semographic, social and economic characteristics of the ultra-orthodox Jewish population in Israel 1996-2001. Central Bureau of Statistics; 2004.

[4] Muhsen K, Cohen D, Spungin-Bialik A, Shohat T. Seroprevalence, correlates and trends of *Helicobacter pylori* infection in the Israeli population. Epidemiol Infect 2011;21:1-8.

[5] Malaty, HM, El-Kasabany A, Graham DY *et al.* Age at acquisition of *Helicobacter pylori* infection: a follow-up study from infancy to adulthood. Lancet 2002; 359:931-35.

[6] Rowland, M, Daly L, Vaughan M *et al.* Age-specific incidence of *Helicobacter pylori*. Gastroenterology 2006;130:65-72.

[7] Anonymous. Epidemiology of, and risk factors for, *Helicobacter pylori* infection among 3194 asymptomatic subjects in 17 populations. The EUROGAST Study Group. Gut 1993;34:1672-76.

[8] Vyse AJ, Gay NJ, Hesketh LM *et al.* The burden of *Helicobacter pylori* infection in England and Wales. Epidemiol. Infect. 2002;128:411-17.

[9] Muhsen K, Nir A, Spungin-Bialik A, Bassal R, Goren S, Cohen D. Interaction among ethnicity, socioeconomic status, and *Helicobacter pylori* seroprevalence in Israeli children and adolescents. J Pediatr Gastroenterol Nutr 2011;53:524-27.

[10] Sonnenberg A. Time trends of ulcer mortality in Europe. Gastroenterology 2007;132:2320-27.

[11] Van der Hulst RW, Rauws EA, Koycu B *et al.* Prevention of ulcer recurrence after eradication of *Helicobacter pylori*: a prospective long-term follow-up study. Gastroenterology 1997;113:1082-86.

[12] Sonnenberg A. Causes underlying the birth-cohortphenomenonof peptic ulcer:analysis of mortality data 1911-2000, England and Wales. Int J Epidemiol 2006;35:1090-97.

[13] Novis BH, Gabay G, Naftali T. *Helicobacter pylori*: the Middle East scenario. Yale J Biol Med 1998;71:135-41.

[14] Birkenfeld S, Keter D, Dikman R *et al.* Prevalence of *Helicobacter pylori* infection in health-care personnel of primary care and gastroenterology clinics. J Clin Gastroenterol 2004; 38:19-23.

[15] Hershcovici T, Haklai Z, Gordon ES, Zimmerman J. Trends in acute non-variceal bleeding in Israel in 1996-2007: a significant decrease in the rates of bleeding peptic ulcers. Dig Liver Dis 2010;42:477-81.

[16] Ota H, Nakayama J, Momosse M *et al. Helicobacter pylori* infection produces reversible glycostlation chages to gastric mucins. Virchows Arch 1998;433:419-26.

[17] Byrd JC, Yunker CK, Xu Q *et al.* Inhibition of gastric mucin synthesis by *Helicobacter pylori*. Gastroenterology 2000;118:1072-1079.

[18] Beil W, Enss ML, Muller S *et al.* Role of vacA and cagA in *Helicobacter pylori* inhibition of mucin synthesis in gastric mucous cells. J Clin Microbiol 2000;38:2215-18.

[19] Morgenstern S, Koren R, Moss SF *et al.* Does *Helicobacter pylori* affect gastric mucin expression? Relationship between gastral antral mucin expression and *Helicobacter pylori* colonization. Eur J Gastroenterol Hepatol 2001;13:19-23.

[20] Byrd JC, Yan P, Sternberg LR *et al.* Aberrant expression of gland-type gastric mucin in the surface epithelium of *Helicobacter pylori*-infected patients. Gastroenterology 1997;113:455-64.

[21] La Vecchia C, Negri E, Franceschi S *et al.* Family history and the risk of stomach and colorectal cancer. Cancer 1992;70:50-55.

[22] Brenner H, Arndt V, Sturmer T *et al.* Individual and joint contribution of family history and *Helicobacter pylori* infection to the risk of gastric carcinoma. Cancer 2000;88:274-79.

[23] El-Omar EM, Oien K, Murray LS *et al.* Increased prevalence of precancerous changes in relatives of gastric cancer patients: critical role of *H. pylori*. Gastroenterology 2000;118:22-30.

[24] Sepulveda A, Peterson LE, Shelton J *et al.* Histological patterns of gastritis in *H. pylori*-infected individuals with a family history of gastric cancer. Am J Gastroenterol. 2002;97:1365-70.

[25] Vilkin A, Levi Z, Morgenstern S *et al.* Higher gastric mucin secretion and lower gastric acid output in first-degree relatives of gastric cancer patients. J Clin Gastroenterol. 2008;42:36-41.

[26] Chey WD, Wong BC. American College of Gastroenterology Guidelines on the Management of *Helicobacter pylori* infection. Am J Gastroenterol 2007;102:1808-25.

[27] Bourke B, Ceponis P, Chiba N *et al.* Canadian Helicobacter Study Group Consensus Conference: update on the approach to *Helicobacter pylori* infection in children and adolescents – an evidence-based evaluation. Can J Gastroenterol 2005;19:399-408.

[28] Hino B, Eliakim R, Levine A *et al.* Comparison of invasive and non-invasive tests diagnosis and monitory of *Helicobacter pylori* infection in children. J Pediatr Gastroenterol Nutr 2004;39:519-23.

[29] Sherman P, Czinn S, Drumm B *et al.* *Helicobacter pylori* infection in children and adolescents: working group report of the First World Congress of Pediatric Gastroenterology, Hepatology and Nutrition. J Pediatr Gastroenterol Nutr 2002;2:128-133.

[30] Shmuely H, Yahav J, Samra Z *et al.* Elevated 13C urea breath test values females infected with *Helicobacter pylori*. Dig Dis Sci 2007;52:402-04.

[31] Zevit N, Niv Y, Shirin H, Shamir R. Age and gender differences in urea breath test results. Eur J Clin Invest 2011;41:767-72.

[32] Weyermann M, Adler G, Brenner H, Rothenbacher D. The mother as a source of *Helicobacter pylori* infection. Epidemiol. 2006;17:332-34.

[33] Niv Y, Koren R. 13C-urea breath test for success of *Helicobacter pylori* eradication: study of 5885 Israeli patients. Dig Dis Sci 2005;50:1513-16.

[34] Gisbert JP. The recurrence of *Helicobacter pylori* infection: incidence and variables influencing it. A critical review. Am J Gastroenterol 2005; 100:2083-99.

[35] Xia HX, Talley NJ, Keane CT *et al.* Recurrence of *Helicobacter pylori* infection after successful eradication: nature and possible causes. Dig Dis Sci 1997;42:1821-34.

[36] Cohen M, Sapozinikov B, Niv Y. *Helicobacter pylori* recurrence and infection rate in Israeli adults. Dig Dis Sci 2008;53:1211-14.

[37] Zevit N, Levy I, Shmuely H, Samra Z, Yahav J. Antibiotic resistance of *Helicobacter pylori* in Israeli children. Scand J Gastroenterol 2010;45:550-55.

[38] Samra Z, Shmuely H, Niv Y *et al.* Resistance of *Helicobacter pylori* isolated in Israel to metronidazole, clarithromycin, tetracycline, amoxicillin and cefixime. J Antimicrob Chemother 2002;49:1023-26.

[39] Davis R, Bryson HM. Levofloxacin. A review of its antibacterial activity, phamacokinetics and therapeutic efficacy. Drugs 1994;47:677-700.

[40] Zullo A, Hassan C, De Francesco *et al.* A third-line levofloxacin-based rescue therapy for *Helicobacter pylori* eradication. Dig Liver Dis 2003;35:232-36.

[41] Cammarota G, Cianci R, Cannizzaro O *et al.* Efficacy of two one-week rabeprazole/levofloxacin-based triple therapies for *Helicobacter pylori* infection. Aliment Pharmacol Ther 2000;14:1339-43.

[42] Yahav J, Shmuely H, Niv Y, Bechor J, Samra Z. *In vitro* activity of levofloxacin against *Helicobacter pylori* isolates from patients after treatment failure. Diagn. Microbiol. Infect. Dis. 2006;55:81-83.

[43] Bertoni G, Sassatelli R, Nigrisoli E *et al.* Triple therapy with azithromycin, omeprazole and amoxicillin is highly effective in the eradication of *Helicobacter pylori*: a controlled trial *vs.* omeprazole plus amoxicillin. Am J Gastroenterol 1996;91:258-63.

[44] O'Connor A, Gisbert J, O'Morain C. Treatment of Helicobacter infection. Helicobacter 2009;14:46-51.

[45] Niv Y, Abuksis G, Koren R. 13C-urea breath test, referral patterns and results in children. J Clin Gastroenterol 2003;3:142-46.

[46] Schmilovitz-Weiss H, Shalev T, Chechoulin Y *et al.* High eradication rates of *Helicobacter pylori* infection following sequential therapy: the Israeli experience treating naïve patients. Helicobacter 2011;16:229-33.

[47] Yahav J, Samra Z, Niv Y *et al.* Susceptibility-guided *vs* empiric retreatment of *Helicobacter pylori* infection after treatment failure. Dig Dis Sci 2006;51:2316-21.

[48] Ofek I, Goldhar J, Zafriri D, Lis H, Adar R, Sharon N. Anti-*Escherichia coli* adhesion activity of cranberry and blueberry juices. N Engl J Med 1991;324:1599.

[49] Burger O, Ofek I, Tabak M *et al.* A high molecular mass constituent of cranberry juice inhibits *Helicobacter pylori* adhesion to human gastric mucus. FEMS Immunol Med Microbiol. 2000;29:295-301.

[50] Burger O, Weiss E, Sharon N *et al.* Inhibition of *Helicobacter pylori* adhesion to human gastric mucus by a high-molecular-weight constituent of cranberry juice. Crit Rev Food Sci Nutr 2002;42:279-84.

[51] Zhang L, Ma J, Pan K *et al.* Efficacy of cranberry juice on *Helicobacter pylori* infection: a double-blind, randomized placebo-controlled trial. Helicobacter 2005;10:139-45.

[52] Shmuely H, Burger O, Neeman I *et al.* Susceptibility of *Helicobacter pylori* isolates to the antiadhesion activity of a high-molecular-weight constituent of cranberry. Diagn Microbiol Infect Dis 2004;50:231-35.

Send Orders for Reprints to reprints@benthamscience.net
Helicobacter Pylori: A Worldwide Perspective 2014, **2014, 183-201**

CHAPTER 8

Helicobacter pylori in Romania: Epidemiology, Diagnosis and Treatment

Lidia Ciobanu[1], Marian Taulescu[2] and Dan Lucian Dumitraşcu[3,*]

[1]University of Medicine and Pharmacy, 3rd Medical Clinic, Regional Institute of Gastroenterology and Hepatology, Cluj-Napoca, Romania; [2]University of Agricultural Sciences and Veterinary Medicine, Pathology Department, Cluj-Napoca, Romania and [3]University of Medicine and Pharmacy, 2nd Medical Clinic, Cluj-Napoca, Romania

Abstract: In the last two decades, Romanians dealt with post-revolution economic problems and extensive reforms. In this context we analyzed the prevalence trends of *Helicobacter pylori* (*H. pylori*) infection in symptomatic and asymptomatic patients, focused more on northwestern region of our country. An interesting part of our report describes the prevalence of *Helicobacter* species in pets; coinfection with different strains of *Helicobacter* such as *H. pylori, H. felis* and *H. heilmannii* being identified in dogs and cats. Specific risk factors were analyzed, like intrafamilial transmission, occupational exposure and zoonotic transmission, as *H. pylori* was proved to be a pathogenic factor in cats and dogs. Diagnostic methods used for clinical and research purposes are comparative debated in humans and animals. Original Romanian research about *H. pylori* involvement in gastro-duodenal pathology is also presented. Our studies focused both on human and animal pathology, in functional and organic disorders (from chronic gastritis till carcinogenesis). Some remarks are done about clinical and experimental treatment. The efficacy of actual treatment in use is debated as the eradication rates are very low using first line therapy.

Keywords: *Helicobacter pylori*, *Helicobacter* species infection, epidemiology, lifestyle, seroprevalence, zoonotic risk, intrafamilial transmission, virulence factor, pathogenesis, chronic gastritis, carcinogenesis, pathology, premalignant gastric lesions, diagnostic methods, eradication therapy, pets.

PREVALENCE DATA IN SYMPTOMATIC AND ASYMPTOMATIC PATIENTS - EPIDEMIOLOGICAL TRENDS IN THE LAST 20 YEARS

Romania is the only Latin country in Eastern Europe, on the Lower Danube,

[*]**Address correspondence to Dan Lucian Dumitraşcu:** 2nd Medical Clinic, Cluj-Napoca, Romania; Tel: +40-722-756475; Fax: +40-264-593355; E-mail: ddumitrascu@umfcluj.ro

Buzás György Miklós (Ed.)

within and outside the Carpathian arch, bordering on the Black Sea. Romania shares a border with Hungary and Serbia to the west, Ukraine and Moldova to the northeast and east, and Bulgaria to the south. After the Revolution from 1989, Romania began its transition from communism towards democracy and a capitalist market economy. In the last two decades, Romanians dealt with post-revolution economic problems and extensive reforms. Romania is now a middle-income country with high human development.

Socioeconomic status and sanitation are responsible for differences in the prevalence of *Helicobacter pylori* (*H. pylori*) around the world, being higher in developing countries [1]. Also, time trends were investigated both in developed and in developing countries [2 - 8]. In these studies it was observed a reduction of prevalence more important in developed countries, being correlated with improvements in socioeconomic status and followed by decreasing in the incidence of gastric cancer [5, 6].

Our actual report is focused on epidemiology and diagnosis methods of *H. pylori* in human and pets in Romania. Based on our experimental studies with different positive genes of *H. pylori* in Wistar rats and guinea pigs we also looked for new eradication therapies of this infection.

First report about prevalence of *H. pylori* infection in Romania was published in 1990s [9]. The authors reported the prevalence of this infection in symptomatic patients addressed to a gastroenterological ambulatory from northwestern region and also in a group of asymptomatic patients (healthy controls). Using histological staining from antral gastric mucosa, *Helicobacter*-like organisms were identified. Tissue samples were stained by the Wayson technique in 509 subjects and found that 72.8% of patients with gastric ulcer were infected, 69.6% with duodenal ulcer, 69.2% with bulbitis, 61% with chronic gastritis, 50% with gastric cancer. Using the histological method, they found a low prevalence of infection in healthy controls: 34.3%. These data do not reflect the prevalence in general population. Also, they found that age and sex had no significance influence on the prevalence of *Helicobacter*-like organisms found in symptomatic patients. The histological studies are biased by the sampling error and by the presence of atrophic gastritis.

In 1994, a comprehensive book was published regarding the involvement of *H. pylori* in gastric and duodenal pathologies, containing some studies from north-western Romanian population [10]. The authors investigated the infection using the urease test from antral biopsies. A previous studied had been performed in order to determine the accuracy of this urease "home-made" test, positivity at two hours corresponding to more than 30 bacteria on microscopic field. The authors reported an increased prevalence with age: for less than 20 years - 50%; between 21-30 years old - 78.1%; between 31-40 years old – 85.9%; between 41-50 years old - 80.3%, between 51-60 years old 81.4%; between 61-70 years old – 74.6% and between 71-80 years old 61.5%. For that period (1990s) it was noticed an increased prevalence of infection in symptomatic patients in the northwestern part of Romania.

An epidemiological study on asymptomatic subjects, from western part of our country, using serological test, found high rates of infection in adult population, in 2003 [11]. The study population consists of 960 employees and it was standardized for age and gender distribution of the Western regional population. The prevalence of infection in the adult population was 68.5%. In the aged group 18-30 years - 65.3%, in group 31 - 40 years - 71.6%, in group 41 - 50 years - 75%, and in group 51 - 60 years - 88.7% [11].

In the same year, an interesting study was published in 2003 regarding the seroprevalence of antibodies to *H. pylori* in Romanian adopted children, with age between 4 month and 16 years old [12]. For Romanian children a high prevalence was noted: 20%. The authors also reported that previous residence in an orphanage (compared with foster care), older age at adoption, and coinfection with intestinal parasites were more common among children seropositive for anti-*H. pylori* antibodies [12]. In the same year, another epidemiological study performed on dyspeptic children, from northwestern region found a higher prevalence of infection: 40% [58]. This research included 267 subjects, aged between 5-18 years and the presence of infection was considered if both, urease test and histological staining revealed infection [13].

In recent years, our data concerning the epidemiology of *H. pylori* infection, revealed still high percentages in symptomatic and asymptomatic outpatients from north-western part: 55,9% *vs* 60,83% (p=0.3). We investigated 855 dyspeptic patients and 120 asymptomatic subjects using ^{14}C-urea breath test [14].

As Romanian is facing improvements on socio-economic status in recent years, with better sanitation and easily access to medical care, we compared data on *H. pylori* epidemics in order to see if there is a tendency of decreasing. Even methods used in these studies are not homogenous, compared data from the northwestern dyspeptic patients (Table **1**), exposed to the same socio-economic conditions, could suggest some epidemiological trends.

First comparison was made on the same category of age, in different periods of time. Second comparison followed the prevalence trends over 15 years in the same population. In the children group it was noticed a decreased prevalence with 10% from 1994 to 2003. Also in young adults from 1994 until 2009, the prevalence dropped significantly from 78.1% until 51.7%. Similar prevalence is seen in the youngest group, followed over time: 50% in 1994, without a significant increased in 2009: 51.71%. For this age group, the rate of infection in adult life is very little. These data may reflect first epidemiological trends of decreasing the prevalence of infection in Romania. As expected, these changes affects younger population, so no important changes were noticed in the mortality rate from gastric cancer in the last years in Romania: 17.54 in 1992% and 17.74% in 2003 [14].

Table 1: Epidemiological trends of *H. pylori* prevalence in symptomatic patients in Northwestern part of Romania.

Population Age	**Prevalence**	**Reported Year**	**Reference**	**Methodology**
Less than 20 years	50 %	1994	[10]	Urease test
21-30 years	78.1%	1994	[10]	Urease test
31-40 years	71.6%	1994	[10]	Urease test
5-18 years	40 %	2003	[13]	Urease test and histology
21-30 years	51.71 %	2009	[15]	^{14}C- Ureea Breath test

Different gastric *Helicobacter* species are frequently found in animals, especially in dogs and cats, being present in both asymptomatic (60-100%) and those with chronic vomiting (74-90%). In dogs the gastric *Helicobacter* infection is produces by *H. felis, H. bizzozeronii, H. salomonis* and *H. heilmannii.* Coinfection with one or more bacterial species, usually *H. bizzozeronii* and *H. heilmannii* occurs in 15-20% of dogs [16, 17]. All those bacteria in domestic carnivores are referred as gastric *Helicobacter*-like organisms (GHLO). They are microaerophilic, gram negative spiral bacteria with numerous flagella and which enables them to survive in an acid environment [18]. Natural infection with *H. pylori* in dogs is disputed, but there are authors who have identified this bacteria by PCR method [19]. In cats, gastric infection with *Helicobacter* species is also common, ranging between 86-100%, being identified *H. felis, H. heilmannii, H. pamatensis* and *H. pylori* [16, 20, 21].

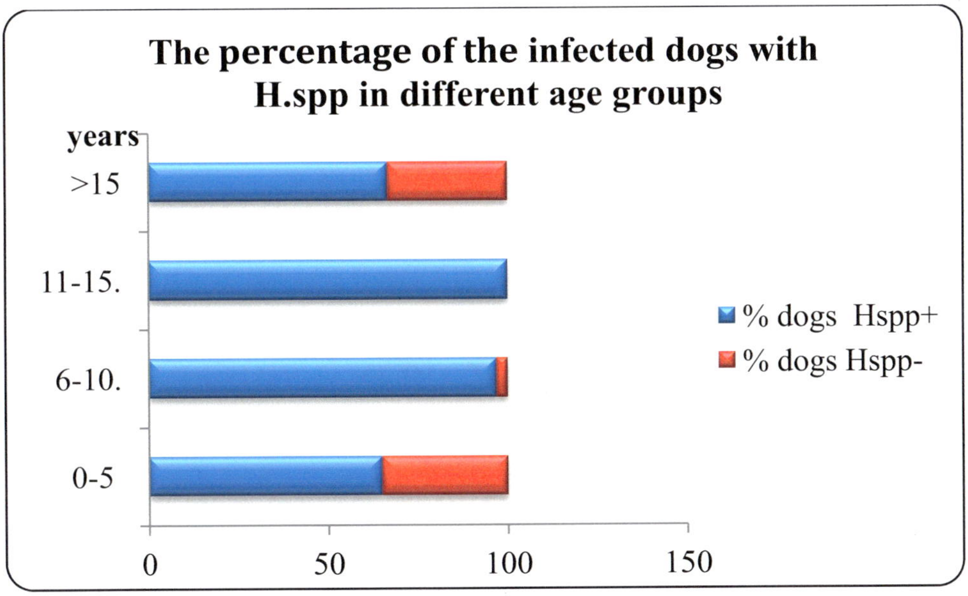

Figure 1: The age distribution of *Helicobacter* species infection in dogs from Northwestern region of Romania [22].

In Romania, a currently epidemiological study showed an increased number of infected animals with *Helicobacter* species, 62/71 dogs (87.32%) and 23/25 (92%) cats (Figs. **1** and **2**), which have developed numerous gastropathies [22], similar data has been reported by some researchers [23, 24]. A coinfection with several species of *Helicobacter* such as *H. pylori, H. felis* and *H. heilmannii* was also identified in dogs and cats. Gastric helicobacters were identified in all regions of the stomach, but in dogs these bacteria were found more frequently in the *pyloric* area (58/71, 81.69%), and in cats in the corpus (23/25, 92%). In both dogs and cats gastric infection with *Helicobacter* species was found in older animals.

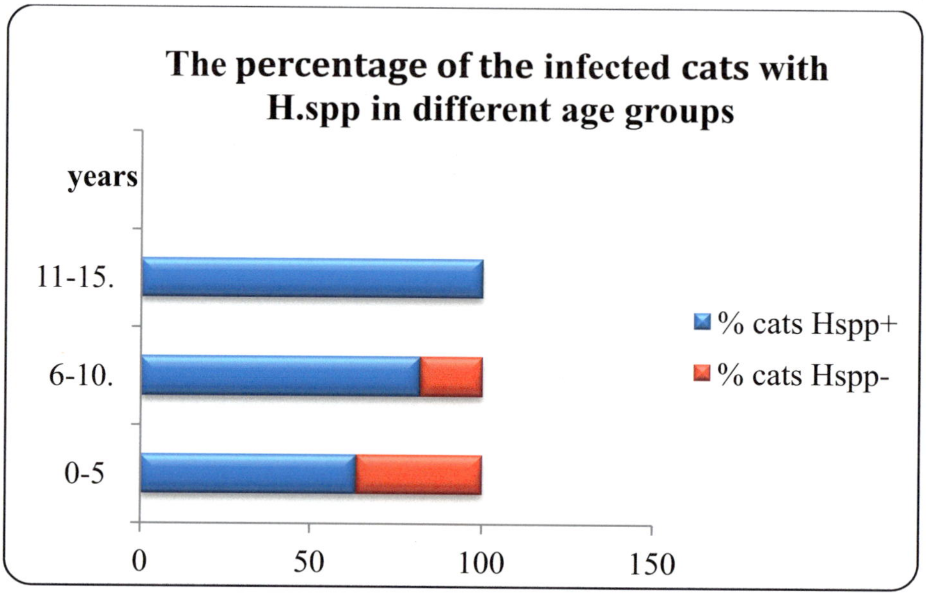

Figure 2: The age distribution of *Helicobacter* species infection in cats from Northwestern region of Romania [22].

RISK FACTORS (INCLUSIVE ZOONOTIC TRANSMISSION)

The major determinants of prevalence of *H. pylori* in developing countries are socioeconomic status factors, density of living and sanitation conditions [25]. Routes of transmission are considered: direct contact between subjects [25], contaminated water, sources or food [26, 27, 28], zoonotic transmission [26] and iatrogenic transmission during endoscopies and dental care [29].

Romanian researcher reports some studies on this subject. Intrafamilial transmission reported in 1994 was 77% in 10 families (33 members) with dyspeptic symptoms, intraspousal transmission being of 60%. Two cases of *H. pylori* - associated gastric cancer in a husband-wife pair from Romanian immigrants were described [30].

Occupational exposure was studied. In literature, conflicting data are reported, regarding the prevalence of infection in endoscopy stuff. Some studies performed in Australia and China found higher prevalence in this category [31, 32], but other studies from Germany and Japan did no confirm this observation [33, 34]. In Romania using serological test. Ten years ago, a serological studied performed in northwestern Romanian city, Cluj-Napoca, found 66% of gastroenterologists infected, 66% of general surgeons and 100% of pediatrics [35].

Zoonotic transmission of infection was also incriminated as *H. pylori* was isolated from non-human primates and domestic cats [36, 37]. Other evidences of transmission from animals to humans *via* fecal-oral transmission were higher prevalence of infection among people exposed to sheep [38]. Gnotobiotic pigs and dogs have been successfully infected with *H. pylori* [37, 39, 40]. In pets, gastric infection with *H. pylori* was identified in multiple studies by immunohistochemistry [41] and PCR [22, 42] from gastric samples. Because of the discovery of *H. pylori* in cats harboring in a research colony [20, 21] as well as in dogs [19], these pets may be a potential natural reservoir of *H. pylori* and could pose a zoonotic risk.

DIAGNOSTIC METHODS

Romanian Societies of Gastroenterology have published consensus reports serving as recommendations for the management of patients with *H. pylori* [43, 44]. The recommended tests by Romanian guidelines actually include the recommendations of the Maastricht consensus. In a study performed in 2002, Romanian trainees proved to have good theoretical knowledge about diagnosis method for *H. pylori* infection [45].

In recent years, the most used noninvasive method for *H. pylori* diagnosis in gastroenterological departments is antigen *H. pylori* from stools. Only a few centers use respiratory tests, based on ^{13}C, for economic reasons. General practitioners have a long experience with serological test in patients without alarms symptoms and frequently recommend treatment based on clinic symptoms and positivity for antibodies.

Upper digestive endoscopy in human (Fig. **3**) and necropsy exam (Fig. **4**) in animals allow lesions detection and biopsies sampling for urease test, microbiology, histopathology, immunohistochemistry and PCR methods.

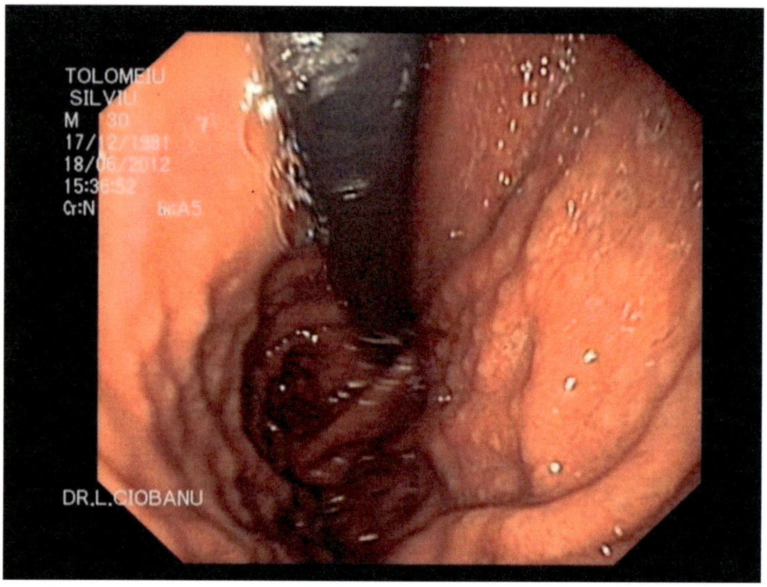

Figure 3: Stomach, upper digestive endoscopy (UDE) exam; man, 30 years old. Diffuse chronic gastritis, valioliforme type (Dr. Lidia Ciobanu).

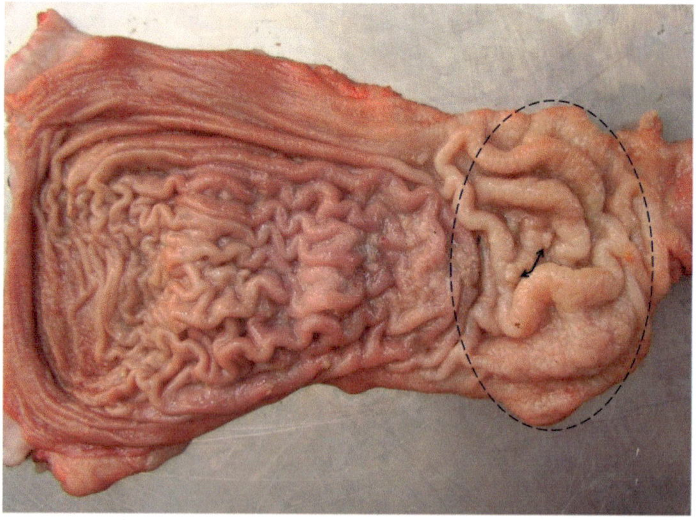

Figure 4: Stomach, necropsy exam; dog, 11 years old. Hypertrophic chronic gastritis (marked area) and two polypoid structures (black arrow) in the *pyloric* region (Dr. M. Taulescu).

In Romania, for the evaluation of *Helicobacter* spp. gastric infection in dogs and cats only invasive methods have been used, which required the removal of the gastric mucosa [22, 41, 42].

The cytological exam isn't usually used in human patients mainly because in clinical practice is rather preferred the urease test. On the contrary, in dogs and cats the cytopathological exam could be considered the "gold standard".

Touch cytology with Gram or Diff Quick staining is a simple, rapid, and sensitive diagnostic test for diagnosing infection with GHLO [46, 47]. Through this test Taulescu *et al.* in 2011 identified gastric helicobacters in dogs in a proportion of 92, 95% and in cats 84%. A higher incidence of *Helicobacter* infection has been identified in the antrum part of the stomach were, the length of bacteria ranging between 3-7 micrometers (μm) [22].

In dogs and cats, compared to the cytology exam, the urease test has an excellent sensitivity, but lower specificity (55.55% at the antrum, 96, 96% at the cardia). In human patients the specificity of rapid urease test has a high sensitivity and specificity [22] whereas in dogs and cats there are other urease-producing bacteria in the gastric mucosa (eg, *Proteus* spp.) which can give a false positive results [48].

In Romania, the bacteriological exam for *H. pylori* (culture and antibiogram) is not routinely performed. Using different commercial medium for *H. pylori* culture, multiple colonies were obtained after 24 hours by Muller - Hinton and Columbia agar, while by *H. pylori* selective agar, the colonies were obtained after 7 days [22].

The histological exam evaluates gastric injuries and detects *Helicobacter* organisms in stained slides from gastric biopsies. Different strains, such as silver stains, Giemsa [49], toluidine blue [50], Warthin Stary, Hematoxylin and eosin and immunohistochemistry based on anti-*Helicobacter pylori* polyclonal antibody were already used. Identification of *H. pylori* from gastric biopsies using Hematoxylin and eosin stain is extremely difficult. Special stains, such as Giemsa and/or immunohistochemistry (IHC) using anti - *H. pylori* antibodies [51] improve the sensitivity and specificity of this method.

In Romania, *H. pylori* infection was confirmed in gastric biopsies from human patients by indirect immunohistochemistry using polyclonal antibodies (Ab) anti - *H. pylori* (Fig. **5** and **6**) and PCR method using specific nucleotide sequences for *H. pylori* [22]. Immunohistochemistry for *H. pylori* is considered an useful diagnostic tool in human pathology [52], but has been infrequently used as a diagnostic assay for gastric *Helicobacter* species infection in veterinary medicine [53]. Using the PCR technique on the gastric biopsies permits diagnosis, as well as identification of the *Helicobacter* species. Primers are mostly derived from either the urease gene or from the 16S rRNA gene [47].

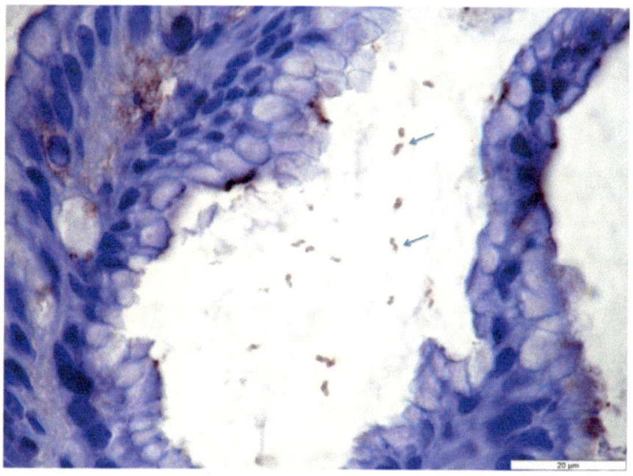

Figure 5: Gastric mucosa biopsy from human, immunohistochemistry method. Positive reaction for *H. pylori* using anti-*Helicobacter pylori* polyclonal antibody, characteristic shape - crane wings (see the arrows), Haematoxylin and eosin counterstaining, bar = 20μm. (Dr. M. Taulescu).

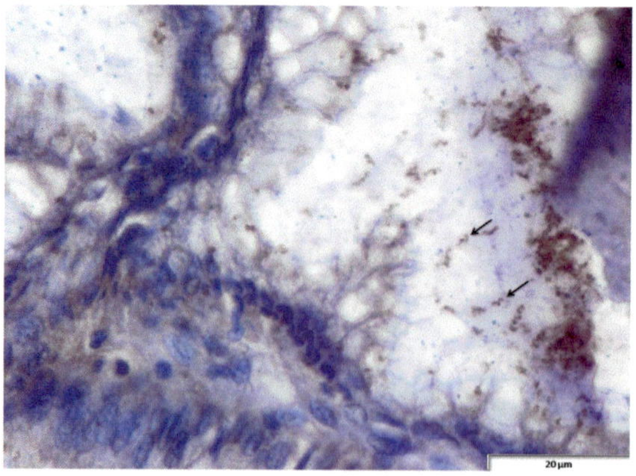

Figure 6: Gastric mucosa biopsy from a dog, immunohistochemistry method. Positive reaction for *H. pylori* using anti-*Helicobacter pylori* polyclonal antibody, characteristic shape - crane wings (see the arrows). Hematoxylin and eosin counterstaining, bar =20μm. (Dr. M. Taulescu).

An important virulence factor it is considered to be the product of the *vacA* gene, the vacuolated cytotoxin, which causes the vacuolation of the target cells' cytoplasma both *in vivo* and *in vitro*. Although all the strains have this gene, only 50% are capable to cause the vacuolation of the epithelial cells' cytoplasma [54]. Another virulence factor is the *CagA* protein (protein associated with the citotoxicity), which is codified by the *cagA* gene, found in 50-60% from the *H. pylori* strains [55].

Our genetic analysis of *cagA* and *vacA* genes, from *H. pylori* cultures revealed all samples positive for *cagA s2* and ¾ positive for *vacA* (Fig. **7**) [22].

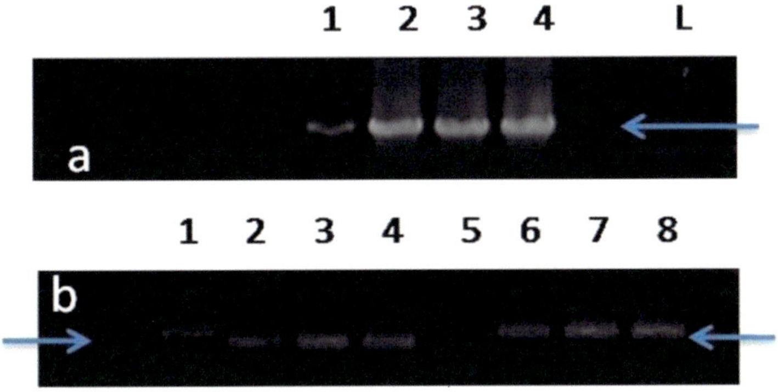

Figure 7*:* Human gastric tissue DNA analysis. Products from PCR performed with specific primers for *H. pylori* (a) at 1700 bp (right arrow) were detected by electrophoresis. Lanes 1, 2, 3 and 4 are positives, L - ladder; (b) Products from PCR, performed with primers for *vacA* at 259 bp (right arrow) and *cagA* at 297 bp (left arrow). Lanes 2, 3,4 are positives at 259 pb; lanes 1, 6, 7,8 are positives at 297 pb (Dr. M. Taulescu).

HELICOBACTER PYLORI INVOLVEMENT IN THE GASTRO-DUODENAL PATHOLOGY

H. pylori is strongly associated with chronic active gastritis, peptic ulcers, gastric adenocarcinoma and MALT lymphoma (MALToma) [56, 57]. In dogs, the naturally infection with *Helicobacter* spp. have been associated with lymphoid nodules hyperplasia, mild and diffuse inflammatory infiltrate with lymphocytes, plasma cell and eosinophils, glandular degeneration with atrophy and fibrosis. Generally, no correlation has been found between the level of bacterial colonization and the severity of gastritis [50, 57].

A recent pathological study of canine gastric lesions, revealed different changes, such as active chronic gastritis with foveolar hyperplasia (Fig. **9**), fibrous tissue proliferation, multiple foci of intestinal metaplasia and dysplasia, these being similar to the patterns of *H. pylori* gastritis in humans. In humans, commonly *H. pylori* gastric infection results in active chronic gastritis (Fig. **8**), while in dogs and cats the inflammatory lesions associated with *Helicobacter* species varied [22]. According with other studies [23], the *Helicobacter* species infection in dogs and cats is associated with several gastric mucosa injuries, characterized by both foveolar and glandular epithelial changes, mononuclear and neutrophils infiltrate, lymphoid follicles hyperplasia, especially in cats, and fibrous tissue proliferation in the lamina propria [22].

Some Romanian researchers described several experimental gastric infections with *H. pylori* strains in guinea pigs [22], rats [58] and dogs [40]. They showed a progressive evolution of *H. pylori* gastritis. In the acute phase, various histological features such as a superficial and deep necrosis of the epithelium, hyperemia, edema, hemorrhages and inflammatory infiltrate consisted of neutrophils were identified, while in the chronic infection, mononuclear cells (lymphocytes and plasma cells) infiltrate in the lamina propria, lymphoid follicle hyperplasia and fibrous tissue proliferation were seen. These aspects are similar to *Helicobacter* active chronic gastritis which have been found in human patients [59]. *H. pylori* is believed to be the most important risk factor for the gastric cancer. *H. pylori* is associated with a higher risk of cancer by inducing different progressive premalignant lesions such as atrophic pangastratis, body predominant pattern and impairment of gastric secretory function [60]. Some researchers from Romania focused on the involvement of this pathogen in gastric carcinogenesis. The authors identified the presence of intestinal metaplasia in 61.60% of patients with chronic gastritis, mostly with complete metaplasia. They have concluded the importance of chronic gastritis, intestinal metaplasia, and *H. pylori* infection in the pathogenic mechanism of the gastric cancer [61]. In dogs, foci of preneoplastic lesions, like glandular atrophy and epithelial dysplasia were found in both hyperplastic and inflammatory gastric polyps, while intestinal metaplasia occurred only in hyperplastic ones. Adenomatous polyps revealed both intestinal metaplasia and epithelia dysplasia, but no glandular atrophy was identified. *Helicobacter* species infection was found in all cases [22].

A debated problem is the involvement of *H. pylori* infection in the functional pathology. In Romania a paper looked for the effect of *H. pylori* infection on gastric emptying and found no effect for the emptying of a semi-fluid meal [62].

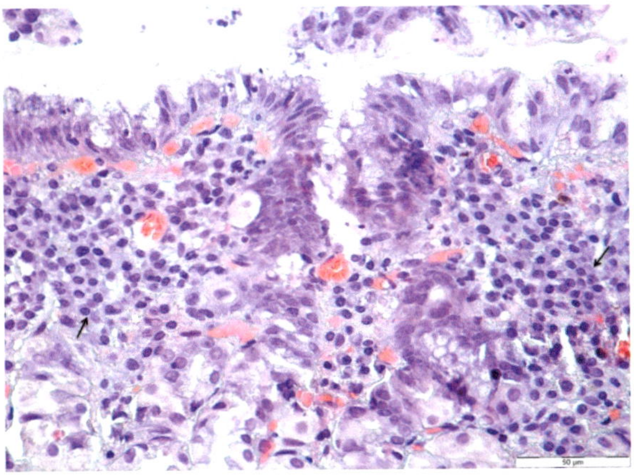

Figure 8: The histologic examination of the gastric corpus showing a chronic, severe and superficial active chronic gastritis, characterized by mononuclear cells (plasma cells - arrows and lymphocytes) and mild neutrophil infiltration of the lamina propria; man, 50 years old. Hematoxylin and eosin stain, bar = 50 µm. (Courtesy dr. C. Catoi, Pathology Department, Faculty of Veterinary Medicine Cluj-Napoca, Romania).

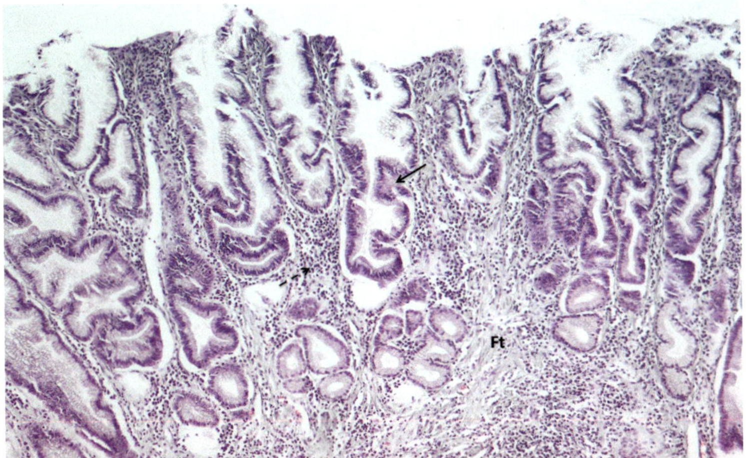

Figure 9: The histologic examination of the gastric antrum showing a chronic hypertrophic gastritis, characterized by diffuse mononuclear cells infiltration of the lamina propria (interrupted arrow), fibrous tissue proliferation (Ft), lymphoid follicle hyperplasia (Lf), glandular atrophy, foveolar hyperplasia and branched crypts (arrow); dog, 11 years old. Masson Trichrome stain, bar = 100 µm. (Dr. M. Taulescu).

TREATMENT IN USE AND EFFICACY

As *H. pylori* infections is very frequent among general and dyspeptic Romanian population with significant involvement in the pathogenesis of different gastro-duodenal disorders are we efficient in treating the infection?

An interesting study reported the results about the knowledge of Romanian medical trainees towards the *H. pylori* infection and its therapy [44]. The preferred therapy regiment is proton pump inhibitor (PPI) + clarithromicine + amoxiciline, for 7 days, since it is well known from clinical experience about the high rates of metronidazol resistance [44].

Using this approach only 58.9% obtained the eradication, in a urea breath test study performed on northwestern 214 subjects [15]. This high rate of treatment failure is in part due to claritromicine resistance that reaches 32% in a studied performed on isolated strains cultures [63]. In the same studied that investigated 100 Romanians patients from southern regions high resistance rates were also reported for metronidazole: 92.8% and amoxicillin: 50% [44]. Interesting, in this study the isolated strains proved to be sensitive to ciprofloxacin and levofloxacin [44]. In Europe recent large studies reported resistance rates were 17.5% for clarithromycin, 14.1% for levofloxacin and 34.9% for metronidazole, and were significantly higher for clarithromycin and levofloxacin in Western/Central and Southern Europe (>20%) than in Northern European countries (<10%) [64]. In this study a significant association was found between outpatient quinolone use and the proportion of levofloxacin resistance ($p=0.0013$) [64]. As in Romania quinolone is an extensively use antibiotic, it is assumed that *H. pylori* rapidly develop resistance to these agents. Because the antibiotic resistance is not routinely done, the accuracy of testing quinolone resistance has to be improved.

A second line therapy is based on bismuth association, but without metronidazol. A third line therapy eradication associated levofloxacin to amoxiciline and PPI.

Compared with other countries were some authors have obtained good results using a combination of amoxicillin, metronidazole, and famotidine for *Helicobacter* infection treatment in dogs and cats [65] in Romania there are no studies about eradication of spontaneous infection in pets.

Our research focused on the experimental evaluation of a new eradication therapy of *H. pylori cagA/vacA+* genes infection through the administration of a triple medication (omeprazole, rifaximin, amoxicillin) and probiotics (Enterolactis). By this protocol the eradication of *H. pylori* infection in gastric mucosa was obtained in 80% and the gastric inflammation was markedly reduced [22].

In respect to the preventive strategy of gastric cancer by eradicating *H. pylori* infection, the problem is still debated and no consensus was issued yet [66].

ACKNOWLEDGEMENT

None Declared.

CONFLICT OF INTEREST

The autors declared no potential conflicts of interest with respect to the research, authorship, and/or publication of this article.

REFERENCES

[1] Graham DY, Adam E, Reddy GT, *et al.* Seroepidemiology of *Helicobacter pylori* infection in India. Comparison of developing and developed countries. Dig Dis Sci 1991; 36: 1084-8.

[2] Apostolopoulos P, Vafiadis-Zouboulis I, Tzivras M, *et al. Helicobacter pylori* infection in Greece: the changing prevalence during a ten-year period and its antigenic profile. BMC Gastroenterol 2002; 16: 2:11.

[3] Asaka M, Kimura T, Kudo M, *et al.* Relationship of *Helicobacter pylori* to serum pepsinogens in an asymptomatic Japanese population. Gastroenterology 1992; 102:760-6.

[4] Chen J, Bu XL, Wang QY *et al.* Decreasing seroprevalence of *Helicobacter pylori* infection during 1993-2003 in Guangzhou, southern China. Helicobacter 2007; 12: 164-9.

[5] Kato M, Asaka M, Shimizu Y *et al.* Relationship between *Helicobacter pylori* infection and the prevalence, site and histological type of gastric cancer, Aliment Pharmacol Ther 2004; 20 (Suppl 1): 85-9.

[6] Rehnberg-Laiho L, Rautelin H, Koskela P, *et al.* Decreasing prevalence of helicobacter antibodies in Finland, with reference to the decreasing incidence of gastric cancer. Epidemiol Infect 2001; 126: 37-42.

[7] Tkachenko MA, Zhannat NZ, Erman LV. Dramatic changes in the prevalence of *Helicobacter pylori* infection during childhood: a 10-year follow-up study in Russia. J Pediatr Gastroenterol Nutr 2007; 45: 428-32.

[8] Yim JY, Kim N, Choi SH *et al.* Seroprevalence of *Helicobacter pylori* in South Korea. *Helicobacter* 2007; 12: 333-40.

[9] Andreica V, Dumitraşcu D, Saşcă N, *et al. Helicobacter* - like organisms in gastroduodenal diseases. Gastroenterol Clin Biol 1990; 14:437-41.

[10] Andreica V, Andreica M. Infectia cu *Helicobacter pylori* în bolile stomacului şi duodenului. Editura Hippocrate, Sibiu, Romania, 1994.
[11] Sporea I, Popescu A, van Blankenstein M, *et al.* The prevalence of *Helicobacter pylori* infection in western Romania. Rom J Gastroenterol 2003; 12: 15-8.
[12] Miller LC, Kelly N, Tannemaat M, Grand RJ. Serologic prevalence of antibodies to *Helicobacter pylori* in internationally adopted children. *Helicobacter* 2003; 8: 173-8.
[13] Serban R, Grigorescu-Sido P, Gheban D, Kiss E. *Helicobacter pylori* gastritis in children: endoscopical and histological aspects. Rom J Gastroenterol 2002; 11: 297-301.
[14] Valean S, Mircea PA, Oprea L, *et al.* Trends of mortality rates from gastric cancer and colorectal cancer in Romania, 1955-2003. J Gastrointestin Liver Dis 2006; 15: 111-5.
[15] Ciobanu L, Prundus RC, Diaconu B, *et al.* Epidemiological Trends of *Helicobacter pylori* prevalence in central-western part of Romania. J Gastrointestin Liver Dis 2009;18 (Supplement 1):17.
[16] Jalava K, On SLW, Vandamme P, *et al.* Isolation and identification of *Helicobacter* spp. from canine and feline gastric mucosa. Appl Environ Microbiol 1998; 64: 3998–06.
[17] Kenneth W, Strauss-Ayali D, McDonough PL, *et al.* Gastric Function in Dogs and Felis with Naturally Acquired Gastric *Helicobacter* spp. Infection. J Vet Intern Med 1999; 13: 507-15.
[18] Lecoindre P, Chevallier M, Peyrol S, *et al.* Gastric helicobacters in cats. J Feline Med Surg 2000; 2: 19-27.
[19] Buczolits S, Hirt R, Rosengarten R, Busse HJ. PCR-based genetic evidence for occurrence of *Helicobacter pylori* and novel *Helicobacter* species in the canine gastric mucosa. Vet Microbiol 2003; 95, 259-70.
[20] Handt LK, Fox JG, Stalis IH, *et al.* Characterization of feline *Helicobacter pylori* strains and associated gastritis in a colony of domestic cats. J Clin Microbiol 1995; 33: 2280.
[21] Handt LK, Fox JG, Dewhirs FE, *et al. Helicobacter pylori* isolated from the domestic cat: public health implication. Infect Immun1994; 62: 2367-74.
[22] Taulescu M, "Gastric pathology associated with different species of *Helicobacter* in pets ", M.S. thesis, University of Agricultural Sciences and Veterinary Medicine, Cluj-Napoca, Romania, 2011.
[23] Eaton KA, Dewhist FE, Paster BJ, *et al.* Prevalence and varietis of *Helicobacter* species in dogs from random sources and pet dogs: animal and public health implications. J Clin Microbiol 1996; 34: 3165- 70.
[24] Henry GA, Long PH, Burns J L, Charbonneau DL. Gastric spiriliosis in beagles. Am J Vet Res 1987; 48: 831-36.
[25] Cheng H, Hu F, Zhang L, *et al.* Prevalence of *Helicobacter pylori* infection and identification of risk factors in rural and urban Beijing, China. Helicobacter 2009; 14: 128-33.
[26] Goodman KJ, Correa P, Tenganá Aux HJ, *et al. Helicobacter pylori* infection in the Colombian Andes: a population-based study of transmission pathways. Am J Epidemiol 1996;144: 290-9.
[27] Hopkins RJ, Vial PA, Ferreccio C, *et al.* Seroprevalence of *Helicobacter pylori* in Chile: vegetables may serve as one route of transmission. J Infect Dis 1993;168: 222-6.
[28] Klein PD, Graham DY, Gaillour A, *et al.* Water source as risk factor for *Helicobacter pylori* infection in Peruvian children. Gastrointestinal Physiology Working Group Lancet 1991; 337:1503-6.

[29] Brown LM. *Helicobacter pylori*: epidemiology and routes of transmission. Epidemiol Rev 2000; 22: 283-97.

[30] Dasanu CA, Rathmann J, Alexandrescu DT. *H. pylori*-associated gastric cancer in a husband-wife pair: a veritable family affair. South Med J 2009; 102: 1158-60.

[31] Mitchell H, Lee A, Carrick J. Increased incidence of *Campylobacter pylori* infection in gastroenetrologists: further evidence to support person-to-person transmission of *C. pylori*. Scand J Gastroenterol 1989; 24: 396-400.

[32] Su YC, Wang WM, Chen LT, *et al.* High prevalence of IgG against *Helicobacter pylori* infection among endoscopists in Taiwan. Dig Dis Sci 1996; 44: 1571-6.

[33] Braden B, Duan LP, Caspary WF, *et al.* Endoscopy is not a risk factor for *Helicobacter pylori* infection - but medical practice is. Gastrointest Endosc 1997;46: 305-10.

[34] Nishikawa J, Kawai H, Takahashi A, *et al.* Seroprevalence of immunoglobulin G antibodies against *Helicobacter pylori* among endoscopy personnel in Japan. Gastrointest Endosc 1998; 48: 237-43.

[35] Andreica V, Pascu O, Georoceanu A, *et al.* The prevalence of *Helicobacter pylori* infection in medical staff. Rom J Gastroenterol 1998; 4:243-48.

[36] Dubois A, Berg DE, Incecik ET, *et al.* Transient and persistent experimental infection of humans primates with *Helicobacter pylori*: implication for human disease. Infect Immun 1996; 62: 2885-91.

[37] Fox LK. Non-human reservoirs of *Helicobacter pylori*. Aliment Pharmacol Ther, 1995; 9(suppl 2): 93-103.

[38] Dore MP, Sepulveda AR, El-Zimaiti H, *et al.* Isolation of *Helicobacter pylori* from sheep implications for transmision to humans. Am J Gastroenterol 2001; 96: 1396-1401.

[39] Catoi C, Andreica V, Gal A, Catoi AF. Experimental and spontaneous infection with *Helicobacter pylori* in dogs, München, Germany 2007; p.76.

[40] Cătoi C, Baba AI, Dombay E, *et al.* Experimental infection with *Helicobacter pylori* in dogs. Bulletin UASVM, Veterinary Medicine 2003; 60: 52-7.

[41] Taulescu M, Gal A, Bolfa P, *et al.* Identification of *Helicobacter pylori* infection from the gastric samples of dogs with gastritis lesions by immnunohistochemical method. Bulletin UASVM, Veterinary Medicine 2010; 67: 337-41.

[42] Taulescu M, Catoi C, Gal A, *et al.* Diagnosis of spontaneous gastric infection with *Helicobacter* species in dogs using PCR method. Scientific Papers - Veterinary Medicine UASMV Iasi 2009; 52: 304-10.

[43] Acalovschi M, Chira C, Andreica V. Consensus conference of the National Societies of Gastroenterology and Digestive Endoscopy, Bucharest, Romania, 3 November 2000. Rom J Gastroenterol 2001; 10:259-62.

[44] Oproiu A, Acalovschi M, Oproiu C. *Helicobacter pylori* in benign gastro-duodenal diseases. Rom J Gastroenterol 1996; 5:147-58.

[45] Dumitraşcu DL, Popescu M. The attitude of Romanian medical trainees towards the eradication of *H. pylori*. Rom J Gastroenterol 2002; 11: 291-6.

[46] Happonen I, Linden J, Saari S, *et al.* Detection and effects of H*elicobacter*s in healthy dogs and dogs with signs of gastritis. J Am Vet Med Assoc 1998; 213: 1767-74.

[47] Neiger R, Dieterich C, Burnens AP, *et al.* Detection and prevalence of *Helicobacter* infection in pet cats. J Clin Microbiol 1998; 36: 634-37.

[48] Eaton KA, Brooks CL, Morgan DR, Krakowka S. Essential role of urease in pathogenesis of gastritis induced by *Helicobacter pylori* in gnotobiotic piglets. Infect Immun 1991; 59: 2470–2475.
[49] Hermanns W, Kregel K, Breuer W, Lechner J. *Helicobacter*-like organisms: Histopathological examination of gastric biopsies from dogs and cats. J Comp Pathol 1995; 112: 307-18.
[50] Happonen I, Saari S, Castren L, *et al.* Occurrence and topographical mapping of gastric *Helicobacter*-like organisms and their association with histological changes in apparently healthy dogs and cats. J Vet Med A 1996; 43: 305-15.
[51] Marzio L, Angelucci D, Grossi L, *et al.* Anti - *Helicobacter pylori* specific antibody immunohistochemistry improves the diagnostic accuracy of *Helicobacter pylori* in biopsy specimen from patients treated with triple therapy. Am J Gastroenterology 1998; 93: 223-26.
[52] Jonkers D, Stobberingh E, de Bruine A, *et al.* Evaluation of immunohistochemistry for the detection of *Helicobacter pylori* in gastric mucosal biopsies 1997; J Infect 35: 149-54.
[53] Jakob W, Stolte M, Valentin A, Schroder HD. Demonstration of *Helicobacter pylori*-like organisms in the gastric mucosa of captive exotic carnivores. J Comp Pathol 1997; 116: 21-33.
[54] Jakob W, Stolte M, Valentin A, Schroder HD. Demonstration of *Helicobacter pylori*-like organisms in the gastric mucosa of captive exotic carnivores. J Comp Pathol 1997; 116: 21-33.
[55] Covacci A, Censini S, Bugnoli M, *et al.* Molecular characterization of the 128-kDa immunodominant antigen of *Helicobacterpylori* associated with cytoxicity and duodenal ulcer. Proc Natl Acad Sci 1993; 90: 5791-95.
[56] Blaser MJ. The bacteria behind ulcers. Sci Am 1996; 274:104-7.
[57] Lee A, Fox JC, Hazell S. Pathogenecity of *Helicobacter pylori:* a perspective. Infect Immun 1993; 61: 1601-10.
[58] Cătoi C, Gal A, Dombay E, *et al.* Experimental Infection with *Helicobacter pylori* in rats. Bulletin UASVM, Veterinary Medicine 2006; 63: 34-8.
[59] El-Omar EM. The importance of interleukin 1β in *Helicobacter pylori* associated disease. Gut 2001; 48:743-47.
[60] El-Omar EM, Carrington M, Chow WH, *et al.* Increased prevalence of precancerous changes in relatives of gastric cancer patients: critical role of *H. pylori*. Gastroenterol 2000; 118: 22-30.
[61] Dirnu R, Secureanu FA, Neamțu C, *et al.* Chronic gastritis with intestinal metaplasia: clinico-statistical, histological and immunohistochemical study. Rom J Morphol Embryol 2012; 53: 293-7.
[62] Dumitrascu DL, Pascu O, Drãghini A, *et al. Helicobacter pylori* infection does not influence the gastric emptying of a semisolid meal. Rom J Gastroenterol 1996; 5: 167-74.
[63] Ilie M, Popa M, Chifiriuc MC, *et al. Helicobacter pylori* cultivation from gastric biopsies and susceptibility to antibiotics used in empirical therapy. Roum Arch Microbiol Immunol. 2011; 70: 60-4.
[64] Ruiz J. Mechanisms of resistance to quinolones: target alterations, decreased accumulation and DNA gyrase protection. J Antimicrob Chemother 2003; 51: 1109-17.
[65] DeNovo RC, Magne ML. Current concepts in the management of *Helicobacter* associated gastritis. 13th ACVIM Forum, Lake Buena Vista, Florida: USA, 1995.

[66] Leja M, Dumitrascu DL. Should We Screen for *Helicobacter pylori* to Prevent Gastric Cancer? Dig Dis 2007; 25: 218-21.

CHAPTER 9

Helicobacter pylori in Greece: Epidemiology, Diagnosis, and Treatment

Theodore Rokkas*

Henry Dunant Hospital, Athens, Greece

Abstract: This article reviews aspects concerning *Helicobacter pylori* (*H. pylori*) epidemiology, diagnosis and treatment in Greece. As in most countries *H. pylori* is the cause of most peptic ulcer disease and a primary risk factor for gastric cancer. Eradication of the organism results in ulcer healing and reduces the risk of ulcer recurrence and complications. Testing and treatment have no clear value in patients with documented nonulcer dyspepsia; however, a strategy of testing and treating is preferred in non-differentiated dyspepsia patients without endoscopy. In the office setting, initial serology testing is practical and affordable, with endoscopy reserved for use in patients with alarm symptoms for ulcer complications, cancer or those who do not respond to treatment. Treatment involves 10- to 14-day multidrug regimens including antibiotics and acid suppressants, combined with education about avoidance of other ulcer-causing factors and close follow-up. Follow-up testing (*i.e.*, urea breath or stool antigen test) is recommended for patients who do not respond to therapy or those with a history of ulcer complications or cancer.

Keywords: *Helicobacter pylori*, epidemiology, diagnosis, treatment, eradication, Greece, Maastricht IV consensus, peptic ulcer, non-ulcer dyspepsia.

INTRODUCTION

Helicobacter pylori (H. pylori) is recognized as the most frequent chronic human bacterial infection, present in nearly 50% of the world's population. *H. pylori* (originally named *Campylobacter pyloridis*) and its link with gastritis was discovered in the early 80's [1-4]. It is widely believed that the discovery of *H. pylori* and the acknowledgement of its impact on upper gastrointestinal (GI) diseases is one of the most important medical developments of the last century. *H. pylori* is crucial in the pathogenesis of upper GI diseases with include gastritis,

***Address correspondence Theodore Rokkas:** Henry Dunant Hospital, Athens, Greece; Tel: +30-210-6431334; Fax: +30-210-6431442, E-mail: sakkor@otenet.gr peptic ulcer disease (PUD) and gastric cancer. *H. pylori* eradication may result in reduced PUD and may prevent gastric cancer. However, concern has been shown over failure of eradicatoin treatment and increasing resistance to antimicrobials. Nowadays the guidelines on *H. pylori* infection are given by various consensus reports with the Maastricht IV consensus report [5] being the most widely accepted.

REVIEW AIMS AND METHODOLOGY

Since the discovery of *H. pylori*, research on the bacterium in Greece has flourished and the establishment of the Hellenic *Helicobacter pylori* Study Group (HHPSG) has positively influenced this. Thus many publications by Greek researchers have appeared in peer review journals, concerning both clinical and basic aspects of this infection. The aim of this article therefore, is to review aspects concerning *H. pylori* epidemiology, diagnosis and treatment in Greece. To achieve this, extensive English-language, computer-aided medical literature searches of the PubMed/MEDLINE and Embase databases for human studies were performed to find relevant publications. The following search terms were used: ("*Helicobacter pylori*" OR "helicobacter"AND "*pylori*" OR "*H. pylori*" AND "epidemiology" OR "diagnosis" OR "therapy" OR "treatment" AND "Greece".

This search yielded 101 suitable publications for review [6-107].

H. pylori Epidemiology in Greece

Thirty five papers [6-40] provided information on *H. pylori* epidemiology in Greece and this information is summarized as follows: The prevalence of *H. pylori* infection varies widely by geographic area, age, race, and socioeconomic status. Because it is not possible to ascertain when infection occurs clinically, most of the information on the rates of *H. pylori* in geographically and demographically diverse populations comes from seroprevalence studies. Based on serological studies in Greece, that were performed in healthy adults and children at the beginning of the 90's and were repeated at the end of the decade, it appears that the prevalence of *H. pylori* infection is decreasing. The most likely explanation does not differ from that reported for developing and developed countries. The economic development of this country has gradually and steadily resulted in an improvement of certain socioeconomic parameters and most importantly in living conditions. This, along with improvement of the level of education in the general population, information programs on the hygienic handling, preparation and preservation of food and water have had an enormous impact on the epidemiology of *H. pylori* infection. Intrafamily transmission has been successfully shown in spouses of infected Greek individuals whereas almost all first degree relatives of infected children are heavily colonized by *H. pylori.* Improvement of these parameters has been shown to prevent massive person-to-person and possibly environment-to-person transmission of the infection. As a result, significantly fewer Greek children and adolescents are now being infected during this crucial period of life. The pace of the socioeconomic and environmental change is faster for urban than rural areas and this is actually mirrored by the increased incidence and prevalence of the infection as well as the slower rate at which the prevalence of the infection is declining in the rural population. Because *H. pylori* infection follows the pattern of a cohort phenomenon, dramatic changes are expected in the epidemiology of *H. pylori* associated diseases. In fact, all practicing gastroenterologists in urban areas and especially in referral centers face the decline of non-NSAID related duodenal ulcer disease and a steadily rising incidence of *H. pylori* negative/non-hiatal hernia associated reflux oesophagitis. Furthermore, it seems that the incidence of the *H. pylori* positive functional dyspepsia is declining. *H. pylori* infection prevalence is much higher in patients with functional dyspepsia aged over 50 years than in the younger age group. It is, however, very interesting that despite the decline in acquisition of *H. pylori* infection, the prevalence of cagA+ and vacA+ *H. pylori* strains isolated in the Greek population is still quite high and may predict underlying peptic ulcer disease. This interesting observation in a country with a low incidence of gastric cancer raises several challenging hypotheses, such as that the Mediterranean diet enriched with fresh fruits is protective against the development of atrophic gastritis despite the presence of *H. pylori*. This is further supported by the findings in the Eurogast study where the population of Crete had a very low prevalence of non-cardia gastric cancer in view of a high prevalence of *H. pylori* infection[42]. Excluding gastric cancer, the pattern of *H. pylori* infection in the Greek population and the course of its associated diseases does not differ from that found in western European countries. Thus, the prevalence of *H. pylori* in peptic ulcer disease is in the expected prevalence range. In addition, cagA+ *H. pylori* strains are most likely to be protective against the development of reflux oesophagitis and induce gastric atrophy and/or low grade MALT lymphomas. However, Greek patients with newly diagnosed Crohn's disease or ulcerative colitis had a significantly higher rate of *H. pylori* infection compared with their western Europeans counterparts. Disease associations with *H. pylori* infection are also quite similar in the native Greek population to those reported in Western European countries. This applies to *H. pylori* infection prevalence in patients with diabetes mellitus, chronic renal failure, colon polyps, duodenogastric reflux, coronary artery disease, neurological disease, acne rosacea, children with recurrent abdominal pain, *etc.*

DIAGNOSIS

Forty two papers [42-83] provided information on *H. pylori* diagnosis and this information is summarized as follows: Because acute infection with *H. pylori* is generally asymptomatic, it is not possible to ascertain when infection occurs on the basis of symptoms or clinical findings. Most epidemiologic studies of the prevalence of *H. pylori* infection in Greece usually use serologic tests. Biopsy-based diagnostic methods are often used in hospital settings. Non-invasive tests for the diagnosis of *H. pylori* infection are the C-urea breath test (UBT) and monoclonal stool antigen tests. The most accurate test for diagnosing *H. pylori* infection is the UBT, especially for patients who do not require endoscopy. It is preferable not to use serology in clinical practice because the antibodies are detectable for several months after successful treatment of *H. pylori.* When testing for *H. pylori,* especially after treatment, it is recommended that patients should stop taking anti-secretory drugs (*i.e.*, PPIs or H2 receptor antagonists for at least two weeks and antibiotics for at least four weeks) prior to testing so as to avoid *H. pylori* suppression and reduction of test sensitivity. Endoscopy is required when there is a suspicion of serious underlying conditions such as bleeding, anaemia, weight loss, dysphagia, persistant vomiting *etc.* In biopsies taken during endoscopy, detection of *H. pylori* can be achieved with several methods, such as the rapid urea test, which is adequately accurate. When eradication fails repeatedly, endoscopy is required to obtain gastric mucosa samples for determining antibiotic sensitivity and resistance.

TREATMENT

Twenty four papers [84-107] provided information on *H. pylori* treatment in Greece and this information is summarized as follows.

General Aspects

In all *H. pylori* treatments, proton pump inhibitors (PPIs) are an integral constituent of therapy and are generally regarded as equivalent in efficacy. Even though there are pharmacokinetic differences between the PPIs, there is no evidence of a clinically significant difference in *H. pylori* eradication rates when different PPIs are used in first-line triple therapy regimens. It is recommend [5] that in populations with clarithromycin resistance of more than 15%, antibiotic susceptibility should be tested before treatment is started. Greece is among the European countries with the highest *in vitro* resistant strains to metronidazole. There have been very few reports for amoxil-resistance of *H. pylori* but resistance to clarithromycin is steadily rising. Widespread abuse, misuse and inappropriate use of antibiotics is responsible for increasingly recognized resistant strains to *H. pylori* infection. Resistance to metronidazole, is considered of secondary importance compared to clarithromycin concerning eradication failure. Resistance to fluoroquinolones is increasing. As in other populations, in the Greek population, the immediate and long-term outcome of treatment may be influenced by various factors. Among significant predictors of treatment failure antibiotic resistance and poor compliance to treatment are the most important. Other factors include duration of therapy, patients' old age, non-ulcer dyspepsia and smoking. Adherence to treatment is a multifactorial process and non-adherence is a major cause of treatment failure. Some studies of treatment regimens suggest compliance rates of >95%, while other studies suggest that 10% of patients prescribed eradication therapy will fail to take even 60% of medicines. Adverse events, most notably diarrhoea and taste disturbance are relatively frequent with current eradication regimens, and may lead to treatment discontinuation. In addition, patients may find eradication regimens complex and the importance of good compliance needs to be emphasised to patients. Enhanced compliance programmes are labour intensive but may be worthwhile; evidence suggests that when patients are given greater knowledge of their illness and the importance of compliance stressed, this results in significantly greater levels of both compliance and eradication.

Indications and Applied Therapies

Regarding therapeutic issues in Greece, the main indications for *H. pylori* treatment are shown in Table **1**. In brief, treatment for *H. pylori* is based on the Maastricht IV consensus report [5].

Table 1: Main indications for treatment for *H. pylori* infection in Greece (based on the Maastricht IV guidelines [5]).

• Peptic ulcer disease
• Gastric MALT lymphoma
• Atrophic gastritis status
• Non-ulcer dyspepsia "Test and treat" strategy
• After resection of gastric cancer
• Gastric cancer patient's first degree relatives
• Patient's wishes
• Iron deficiency anaemia not explained by other tests
• Idiopathic thrombocytopenic purpura
• Patients in need of long-term NSAIDs

In children, recurrent abdominal pain is not considered an indication for application of the "test and treat" plan for *H. Pylori* treatment. Instead the aim of a diagnostic approach in recurrent abdominal pain should be to determine the cause of GI symptoms and not the detection of *H. pylori* infection. However children with upper GI symptoms should be tested for *H. pylori* and treated in case of *H. pylori* positivity after excluding other causes of their symptoms

First-Line Therapy: It appears that so far the combination of a proton pump inhibitor with clarithromycin 500mg and amoxicillin 1g twice a day is the first line treatment of choice for the Greek population. The duration of treatment has not been extensively studied but there is inconclusive evidence that 10-day regimens may be superior to 7-day regimens. Very recently, proton pump inhibitor-based quadruple therapies and sequential therapies [5] are increasingly being used as first line therapies, mainly because resistance to clarithromycin is steadily rising.

Second-Line Therapy: Therapy with levofloxacin, amoxicillin and a PPI has been shown to be suitable for second-line treatment. Due to the increasing rate of resistance of fluoroquinolones, and the increasing rate of tendonitis some concerns have been expressed. PPI based quadruple or sequential therapies should be used as salvation therapies in patients who have failed to eradicate *H. pylori* infection with triple therapy. This regimen should be given for at least 10 and preferably 14-days.

Patients with allergy to penicillin are a challenging group. In such patients a combination of PPI, levofloxacin and clarithromycin showed good results as second line treatment.

Rescue Therapy: For rescue therapy (after failure of second-line therapy) patients should be referred for endoscopy and treatment should be based on susceptibility testing. For infected children the therapeutic regimens in use are essentially similar to those for adults.

Confirmation of Eradication

It is important to confirm eradication of *H. pylori*, particularly in patients who have had treatment for gastric MALT lymphoma, or those who have undergone resection for gastric cancer and in patients whose symptoms persist after eradication treatment for dyspepsia. The use of UBT or a monoclonal stool antigen test is recommended, except in cases where repeat endoscopy is indicated *e.g.* gastric ulcer. UBT is the best option to confirm eradication; there is no role for the use of serology in eradication. Successful treatment should be confirmed four weeks or more after the end of treatment.

ACKNOWLEDGEMENT

None Declared.

CONFLICT OF INTEREST

The author(s) confirm that this chapter content has no conflict of interest.

REFERENCES

[1] Marshall BJ, Warren JR. Unidentified curved bacilli in the stomach of patients with gastritis and peptic ulceration. Lancet 1984; 1: 1311-1315.
[2] McColl K. *Helicobacter pylori* infection, N Engl J Med 2010; 362:1597-604.
[3] Tan V, Wong B, *Helicobacter pylori* and gastritis: untangling a complex relationship 27 years on. Journal of Gastroenterology and Hepatology 2011;26, Suppl 1:42-45
[4] Yeomans N. The ulcer sleuths: the search for the cause of peptic ulcers, Journal of Gastroenterology and Hepatology, 2011;26, Suppl 1:35-41
[5] Malfertheiner P, Megraud F, O'Morain CA, Atherton J, Axon AT, Bazzoli F, Gensini GF, Gisbert JP, Graham DY, Rokkas T, El-Omar EM, Kuipers EJ; European Helicobacter Study Group. Management of *Helicobacter pylori* infection--the Maastricht IV/ Florence Consensus Report. Gut. 2012; 61: 646-64.
[6] Altman E, Chandan V, Harrison BA, *et al. Helicobacter pylori* isolates from Greek children express type 2 and type 1 Lewis and α1,6-glucan antigens in conjunction with a functional type IV secretion system. J Med Microbiol. 2012; 61:559-66.
[7] Apostolopoulos P, Vafiadis-Zouboulis I, Tzivras M, *et al. Helicobacter pylori* (*H. pylori*) infection in Greece: the changing prevalence during a ten-year period and its antigenic profile. BMC Gastroenterol. 2002 May 16; 2:11.
[8] Archimandritis A, Bitsikas J, Tjivras M, *et al. Helicobacter pylori* infection in Greece in healthy people and in patients with peptic ulcer and with dyspepsia without ulcer. J Clin Gastroenterol. 1993;16:257-8.
[9] Archimandritis AJ, Chronaki M, Kalogeras D, *et al.* The incidence of *Helicobacter pylori* is not increased in obese people, but the risk of duodenal ulcer is higher in *H. pylori*-positive people of high obesity. J Clin Gastroenterol. 2003; 36:184-5.
[10] Christodoulou DK, Milionis HJ, Pappa P, *et al.* Association of *Helicobacter pylori* infection with cardiovascular disease--is it just a myth? Eur J Intern Med. 2011; 22:191-4.
[11] Diamantidis MD, Ioannidou-Papagiannaki E, Kountouras J, *et al.* High prevalence of *Helicobacter pylori* infection in Greek patients with myelodysplastic syndromes. Acta Haematol. 2010;124:141-9.
[12] Kamberoglou DK, Savva SC, Kalapothakos PN, *et al.* Prevalence and risk factors associated with specialized intestinal metaplasia at the esophagogastric junction. Hepatogastroenterology. 2002; 49: 995-8.
[13] Katsanos KH, Tatsioni A, Tsakiris V, *et al. Helicobacter pylori* is a major public health priority in western Balkans: an endoscopy referral center experience. Eur J Intern Med. 2010; 21: 306-9.
[14] Katsinelos P, Tziomalos K, Chatzimavroudis G, *et al.* Eradication therapy in *Helicobacter pylori*-positive patients with halitosis: long-term outcome. Med Princ Pract. 2007; 16: 119-23.
[15] Kountouras J, Zavos C, Katsinelos P, *et al.* Greek and Israeli patterns of *Helicobacter pylori* infection and their association with glaucoma: similarities or diversities? J Glaucoma. 2008;17: 503-4.

[16] Kountouras J, Tsolaki M, Boziki M, *et al.* Association between *Helicobacter pylori* infection and mild cognitive impairment. Eur J Neurol. 2007; 14: 976-82.

[17] Kountouras J, Tsolaki M, Gavalas E, *et al.* Relationship between *Helicobacter pylori* infection and Alzheimer disease. Neurology. 2006;66: 938-40.

[18] Kountouras J, Deretzi G, Zavos C, *et al.* Association between *Helicobacter pylori* infection and acute inflammatory demyelinating polyradiculoneuropathy. Eur J Neurol. 2005;12: 139-43.

[19] Kyriazanos I, Ilias I, Lazaris G, *et al.* A cohort study on *Helicobacter pylori* serology before and after induction in the Hellenic Navy. Mil Med. 2001; 166: 411-5.

[20] Kyriazanos ID, Sfiniadakis I, Gizaris V, *et al.* The incidence of *Helicobacter pylori* infection is not increased among obese young individuals in Greece. J Clin Gastroenterol. 2002; 34: 541-6.

[21] Kyriazanos LD, Ilias L, Gizaris V, *et al.* Seroepidemiology of *Helicobacter pylori* infection in hellenic navy recruits. Eur J Epidemiol. 2001;17(6):501-4.

[22] Lazaridou E, Apalla Z, Sotiraki S, *et al.* Clinical and laboratory study of rosacea in northern Greece. J Eur Acad Dermatol Venereol. 2010; 24: 410-4.

[23] Mentis A, Blackwell CC, Weir DM, *et al.* ABO blood group, secretor status and detection of *Helicobacter pylori* among patients with gastric or duodenal ulcers. Epidemiol Infect. 1991; 106: 221-9.

[24] Moschovi M, Menegas D, Stefanaki K, *et al.* Primary gastric Burkitt lymphoma in childhood: associated with *Helicobacter pylori*? Med Pediatr Oncol. 2003; 41: 444-7.

[25] Nikolopoulou A, Tousoulis D, Antoniades C, *et al.* Common community infections and the risk for coronary artery disease and acute myocardial infarction: evidence for chronic over-expression of tumor necrosis factor alpha and vascular cells adhesion molecule-1. Int J Cardiol.;130: 246-50.

[26] Panos GZ, Xirouchakis E, Tzias V, *et al. Helicobacter pylori* infection in symptomatic HIV-seropositive and -seronegative patients: a case-control study. AIDS Res Hum Retroviruses. 2007; 23: 709-12.

[27] Pateraki E, Mentis A, Spiliadis C, *et al.* Seroepidemiology of *Helicobacter pylori* infection in Greece. FEMS Microbiol Immunol. 1990; 2: 129-36.

[28] Philippou N, Koursarakos P, Anastasakou E, *et al. Helicobacter pylori* seroprevalence in patients with lung cancer. World J Gastroenterol. 2004; 10:3342-4.

[29] Rigopoulos D, Katsambas A, Karalexis A, Papatheodorou G, Rokkas T. No increased prevalence of *Helicobacter pylori* in patients with alopecia areata. J Am Acad Dermatol. 2002; 46:141.

[30] Rokkas T, Sechopoulos P, Pistiolas D, Margantinis G, Koukoulis G. *Helicobacter pylori* infection and gastric histology in first-degree relatives of gastric cancer patients: a meta-analysis. Eur J Gastroenterol Hepatol. 2010; 22: 1128-33.

[31] Rokkas T, Pistiolas D, Sechopoulos P, Robotis I, Margantinis G. Relationship between *Helicobacter pylori* infection and esophageal neoplasia: a meta-analysis. Clin Gastroenterol Hepatol. 2007; 5:1413-1417.

[32] Rokkas T, Liatsos C, Karameris A, *et al.* Proliferating cell nuclear antigen (PCNA) immunostaining in *Helicobacter pylori* infection: impact of eradication. Pathol Oncol Res. 1999; 5:304-8.

[33] Roma E, Panayiotou J, Pachoula J, Kafritsa Y, *et al.*. Intrafamilial spread of *Helicobacter pylori* infection in Greece. J Clin Gastroenterol. 2009; 43:711-5.

[34] Roma-Giannikou E, Shcherbakov PL. *Helicobacter pylori* infection in pediatrics. Helicobacter. 2002;7 Suppl 1:50-5.

[35] Roussos A, Philippou N, Mantzaris GJ, Gourgoulianis KI. Respiratory diseases and *Helicobacter pylori* infection: is there a link? Respiration. 2006; 73:708-14.

[36] Roussos A, Tsimpoukas F, Anastasakou E, *et al.*. *Helicobacter pylori* seroprevalence in patients with chronic bronchitis. J Gastroenterol. 2002; 37:332-5.

[37] Triantafillidis JK, Gikas A, Hyphantis T, *et al. Helicobacter pylori* infection in hospital workers over a 5-year period: correlation with demographic and clinical parameters. J Gastroenterol. 2002; 37:1005-13.

[38] Tzathas C, Triantafyllou K, Mallas E, Triantafyllou G, Ladas SD. Effect of *Helicobacter pylori* eradication and antisecretory maintenance therapy on peptic ulcer recurrence in cirrhotic patients: a prospective, cohort 2-year follow-up study. J Clin Gastroenterol. 2008 Jul; 42:744-9.

[39] Yiannopoulou KG, Efthymiou A, Karydakis K, *et al. Helicobacter pylori* infection as an environmental risk factor for migraine without aura. J Headache Pain. 2007; 8:329-33.

[40] Zervas A, Katopodi A, Protonotariou A, Tolis G, Zouridakis S. The incidence of *Helicobacter pylori* infection in Greek female patients with autoimmune hypothyroidism: is there a relationship? J Clin Gastroenterol. 2002; 35:413-4.

[41] Epidemiology of, and risk factors for, *H. pylori* infection among 3194 asymptomatic subjects in 17 populations. The Eurogast study group. Gut 1993; 34:1672-1676.

[42] Adamopoulos AB, Stergiou GS, Sakizlis GN, *et al.* Diagnostic value of rapid urease test and urea breath test for *Helicobacter pylori* detection in patients with Billroth II gastrectomy: a prospective controlled trial. Dig Liver Dis. 2009; 41: 4-8.

[43] Adamopoulos AB, Efstathiou SP, Tsioulos DI, *et al.* Bleeding duodenal ulcer: comparison between *Helicobacter pylori* positive and *Helicobacter pylori* negative bleeders. Dig Liver Dis. 2004; 36: 13-20.

[44] Albanidou-Farmaki E, Giannoulis L, Markopoulos A, *et al.* Outcome following treatment for *Helicobacter pylori* in patients with recurrent aphthous stomatitis. Oral Dis. 2005; 11: 22-6.

[45] Angelidis AS, Tirodimos I, Bobos M, *et al.* Detection of *Helicobacter pylori* in raw bovine milk by fluorescence *in situ* hybridization (FISH). Int J Food Microbiol. 2011 2151: 252-6.

[46] Archimandritis A, Apostolopoulos P, Sougioultzis S, *et al.*. The CLO test is unreliable in diagnosing *H. pylori* infection in post-surgical stomach; is there any role of *H. pylori* in peptic ulcer recurrence? Eur J Gastroenterol Hepatol. 2000;12: 93-6.

[47] Aroni K, Tsagroni E, Kavantzas N, Patsouris E, Ioannidis E. A study of the pathogenesis of rosacea: how angiogenesis and mast cells may participate in a complex multifactorial process. Arch Dermatol Res. 2008; 300: 125-31.

[48] Gatopoulou A, Mimidis K, Giatromanolaki A, *et al.* Impact of *Helicobacter pylori* infection on histological changes in non-erosive reflux disease. World J Gastroenterol. 2004; 10: 1180-2.

[49] Georgopoulos SD, Triantafyllou K, Fameli M, *et al.* Molecular analysis of B-cell clonality in *Helicobacter pylori* gastritis. Dig Dis Sci. 2005; 50: 1616-20.

[50] Kapsoritakis AN, Potamianos S, Matrella E, *et al. Helicobacter pylori*-associated protein-losing hypertrophic gastropathy with hypercholesterolemia. Dig Dis Sci. 1999; 44: 1843-7.

[51] Kostaki M, Fessatou S, Karpathios T. Refractory iron-deficiency anaemia due to silent *Helicobacter pylori* gastritis in children. Eur J Pediatr. 2003; 162: 177-9.

[52] Koumi A, Filippidis T, Leontara V, Makri L, Panos MZ. Detection of *Helicobacter pylori*: A faster urease test can save resources. World J Gastroenterol. 2011; 17: 349-53.
[53] Kountouras J, Boziki M, Gavalas E, *et al.* Five-year survival after *Helicobacter pylori* eradication in Alzheimer disease patients. Cogn Behav Neurol. 2010; 23: 199-204.
[54] Kountouras J, Boziki M, Gavalas E, *et al.* Eradication of *Helicobacter pylori* may be beneficial in the management of Alzheimer's disease. J Neurol. 2009; 256: 758-67.
[55] Kountouras J, Zavos C, Chatzopoulos D. A concept on the role of *Helicobacter pylori* infection in autoimmune pancreatitis. J Cell Mol Med. 2005; 9: 196-207.
[56] Kyriazanos ID, Sfiniadakis I, Dimakos P, *et al.* Impact of body mass index on fasting blood glucose concentration among Helicobater *pylori* carriers. Dig Dis. 2003; 21: 262-5.
[57] Kyrlagkitsis I, Ladas SD, Mallass EG, *et al.* Evaluation of a conventional ELISA (Novitec) and a near patient immunochromatographic test (Stick H. pyl) for *Helicobacter pylori* antigen detection in stool. Hepatogastroenterology. 2007; 54: 799-802.
[58] Ladas SD, Malamou H, Triantafyllou K, *et al.* Performance of two immunosorbent assay kits for the detection of serum immunoglobulin G to *Helicobacter pylori* in untreated greek patients. Scand J Gastroenterol. 2002; 37: 512-6.
[59] Ladas SD, Varzakakos I, Malamou H, *et al.* Evaluation of a single-step serological assay for laboratory diagnosis of *Helicobacter pylori* infection. Eur J Clin Microbiol Infect Dis. 2002; 21: 56-9.
[60] Ladas SD, Malamou H, Giota G, *et al.* Prospective evaluation of a whole-blood antibody test (FlexPack HP) for in-office diagnosis of *Helicobacter pylori* infection in untreated patients. Eur J Gastroenterol Hepatol. 2000; 12: 727-31.
[61] Ladas SD, Rokkas T, Georgopoulos S, *et al.* Predictive factors and prevalence of follicular gastritis in adults with peptic ulcer and nonulcer dyspepsia. Dig Dis Sci. 1999; 44: 1156-60.
[62] Ladas SD, Katsogridakis J, Malamou H, *et al.*. *Helicobacter pylori* may induce bile reflux: link between *H. pylori* and bile induced injury to gastric epithelium. Gut. 1996; 38: 15-8.
[63] Lazaraki G, Kountouras J, Metallidis S, *et al.* Endothelial nitric oxide synthase (eNOS) is not upregulated in gastric mucosa of *Helicobacter pylori* (*H. pylori*)-positive patients with type 2 diabetes mellitus. Dig Liver Dis. 2009; 41: 253-62.
[64] Leontiadis GI, Minopoulos GI, Maltezos E, *et al.* Effects of *Helicobacter pylori* infection on gastric emptying rate in patients with non-ulcer dyspepsia. World J Gastroenterol. 2004; 10: 1750-4.
[65] Mentis A, Tzouvelekis L, Spiliadis C, Blackwell CC, Weir DM. Inhibition of *Helicobacter pylori* haemagglutination activity by human salivary mucins. FEMS Microbiol Immunol. 1990; 2: 125-7.
[66] Panayotopoulou EG, Sgouras DN, Papadakos KS, *et al.* CagA and VacA polymorphisms are associated with distinct pathological features in *Helicobacter pylori*-infected adults with peptic ulcer and non-peptic ulcer disease. J Clin Microbiol. 2010; 48: 2237-9.
[67] Papamichael KX, Papaioannou G, Karga H, Roussos A, Mantzaris GJ. *Helicobacter pylori* infection and endocrine disorders: is there a link? World J Gastroenterol. 2009; 15: 2701-7.
[68] Pavlidis TE, Atmatzidis KS, Papaziogas BT, *et al. Helicobacter pylori* infection in patients undergoing appendectomy.Swiss Surg. 2002; 8: 110-2.
[69] Rokkas T, Pistiolas D, Sechopoulos P, Robotis I, Margantinis G. The long-term impact of *Helicobacter pylori* eradication on gastric histology: a systematic review and meta-analysis. Helicobacter. 2007; 12 Suppl 2: 32-8.

[70] Rokkas T, Ladas SD, Triantafyllou K, *et al.* The association between CagA status and the development of esophagitis after the eradication of *Helicobacter pylori*. Am J Med. 2001; 110: 703-7.

[71] Rokkas T, Ladas SD, Liatsos C, *et al.* Effectiveness of acid suppression in preventing gastroesophageal reflux disease (GERD) after successful treatment of *Helicobacter pylori* infection. Dig Dis Sci. 2001; 46: 1567-72.

[72] Rokkas T, Liatsos C, Karameris A, *et al.* Serologic detection of CagA positive *Helicobacter pylori* strains predicts the presence of peptic ulcer in young dyspeptic patients. Gastrointest Endosc. 1999;50: 511-5.

[73] Rokkas T, Ladas S, Liatsos C, *et al.* Relationship of *Helicobacter pylori* CagA status to gastric cell proliferation and apoptosis. Dig Dis Sci. 1999; 44: 487-93.

[74] Roma E, Panayiotou J, Kafritsa Y, *et al.* Upper gastrointestinal disease, *Helicobacter pylori* and recurrent abdominal pain. Acta Paediatr. 1999;88: 598-601.

[75] Roma-Giannikou E, Roubani A, Sgouras DN, *et al.* Endoscopic tests for the diagnosis of *Helicobacter pylori* infection in children: Validation of rapid urease test. Helicobacter. 2010; 15: 227-32.

[76] Roussos A, Philippou N, Krietsepi V, *et al.* *Helicobacter pylori* seroprevalence in patients with chronic obstructive pulmonary disease. Respir Med. 2005; 99: 279-84.

[77] Sgouras D, Maragkoudakis P, Petraki K, *et al.* *In vitro* and *in vivo* inhibition of *Helicobacter pylori* by *Lactobacillus casei* strain Shirota. Appl Environ Microbiol. 2004; 70: 518-26.

[78] Sgouras DN, Panayotopoulou EG, Papadakos K, *et al.* CagA and VacA polymorphisms do not correlate with severity of histopathological lesions in *Helicobacter pylori*-infected Greek children. J Clin Microbiol. 2009; 47: 2426-34.

[79] Sgouras DN, Panayotopoulou EG, Martinez-Gonzalez B, *et al.* Lactobacillus johnsonii La1 attenuates *Helicobacter pylori*-associated gastritis and reduces levels of proinflammatory chemokines in C57BL/6 mice. Clin Diagn Lab Immunol. 2005; 12: 1378-86.

[80] Skopelitou AS, Mitselou A, Katsanos KH, Alexopoulou V, Tsianos EV. Immunohistochemical expression of Fhit protein in *Helicobacter pylori* related chronic gastritis, gastric precancerous lesions and gastric carcinoma: correlation with conventional clinicopathologic parameters. Eur J Gastroenterol Hepatol. 2003; 15: 515-23.

[81] Tsamakidis K, Panotopoulou E, Dimitroulopoulos D, *et al.* Herpes simplex virus type 1 in peptic ulcer disease: an inverse association with *Helicobacter pylori*. World J Gastroenterol. 2005; 11: 6644-9.

[82] Tsami A, Petropoulou P, Kafritsa Y, Mentis YA, Roma-Giannikou E. The presence of *Helicobacter pylori* in dental plaque of children and their parents: is it related to their periodontal status and oral hygiene? Eur J Paediatr Dent. 2011; 12: 225-30.

[83] Anagnostopoulos GK, Tsiakos S, Margantinis G, Kostopoulos P, Arvanitidis D. Esomeprazole *vs.* omeprazole for the eradication of *Helicobacter pylori* infection: results of a randomized controlled study. J Clin Gastroenterol. 2004; 38: 503-6.

[84] Anagnostopoulos GK, Kostopoulos P, Margantinis G, Tsiakos S, Arvanitidis D. Omeprazole plus azithromycin and either amoxicillin or tinidazole for eradication of *Helicobacter pylori* infection. J Clin Gastroenterol. 2003; 36: 325-8.

[85] Archimandritis A, Balatsos V, Delis V, Manika Z, Skandalis N. "Reappearance" of *Helicobacter pylori* after eradication: implications on duodenal ulcer recurrence: a prospective 6 year study. J Clin Gastroenterol. 1999; 28: 345-7.

[86] Georgopoulos S, Papastergiou V, Xirouchakis E, *et al.* Evaluation of a four-drug, three-antibiotic, nonbismuth-containing "concomitant" therapy as first-line *Helicobacter pylori* eradication regimen in Greece. Helicobacter. 2012; 17: 49-53.

[87] Georgopoulos SD, Ladas SD, Karatapanis S, *et al.* Effectiveness of two quadruple, tetracycline- or clarithromycin-containing, second-line, *Helicobacter pylori* eradication therapies. Aliment Pharmacol Ther. 2002; 16: 569-75.

[88] Georgopoulos SD, Ladas SD, Karatapanis S, *et al.* Factors that may affect treatment outcome of triple *Helicobacter pylori* eradication therapy with omeprazole, amoxicillin, and clarithromycin. Dig Dis Sci. 2000; 45: 63-7.

[89] Kamberoglou D, Polymeros D, Sanidas I, *et al.* Comparison of 1-week *vs.* 2- or 4-week therapy regimens with ranitidine bismuth citrate plus two antibiotics for *Helicobacter pylori* eradication. Aliment Pharmacol Ther. 2001; 15: 1493-7.

[90] Karatapanis S, Georgopoulos SD, Papastergiou V, *et al.* "7, 10 and 14-days rabeprazole-based standard triple therapies for *H. pylori* eradication: are they still effective? A randomized trial". Acta Gastroenterol Belg. 2011; 74: 407-12.

[91] Krystallis C, Kamberoglou D, Pistiolas D, *et al.* A new second-line sequential regimen for *Helicobacter pylori* eradication based on levofloxacin: a pilot study. Dig Dis Sci. 2010; 55: 3630-1.

[92] Ladas SD, Malamou-Lada H, Economou G, Tassios PS, Raptis SA. A three-day octreotide-containing *Helicobacter pylori* eradication therapy for cure of peptic ulcers. Hepatogastroenterology. 1998; 45: 761-4.

[93] Ladas SD, Tassios PS, Malamou HC, Protopapa DP, Raptis SA. Omeprazole induces a long-term clinical remission of protein-losing gastropathy of Ménétrier's disease. Eur J Gastroenterol Hepatol. 1997; 9: 811-3.

[94] Mantzaris GJ, Petraki K, Archavlis E, *et al.* Omeprazole triple therapy *vs.* omeprazole quadruple therapy for healing duodenal ulcer and eradication of *Helicobacter pylori* infection: a 24-month follow-up study. Eur J Gastroenterol Hepatol. 2002; 14: 1237-43.

[95] Mantzaris GJ, Hatzis A, Tamvakologos G, *et al.* Prospective, randomized, investigator-blind trial of *Helicobacter pylori* infection treatment in patients with refractory duodenal ulcers. Healing and long-term relapse rates. Dig Dis Sci. 1993; 38: 1132-6.

[96] Michopoulos S, Tsibouris P, Bouzakis H, *et al.* Randomized study comparing omeprazole with ranitidine as anti-secretory agents combined in quadruple second-line *Helicobacter pylori* eradication regimens. Aliment Pharmacol Ther. 2000; 14: 737-44.

[97] Papadaki HA, Skordilis P, Minadakis G, *et al.* Complete regression of primary gastric plasmacytoma following *Helicobacter pylori* eradication. Ann Hematol. 2003; 82: 589-92.

[98] Papatheodoridis GV, Archimandritis AJ. Role of *Helicobacter pylori* eradication in aspirin or non-steroidal anti-inflammatory drug users. World J Gastroenterol. 2005; 11: 3811-6.

[99] Paraschos S, Magiatis P, Mitakou S, *et al. In vitro* and *in vivo* activities of Chios mastic gum extracts and constituents against *Helicobacter pylori*. Antimicrob Agents Chemother. 2007; 51: 551-9.

[100] Rokkas T, Sechopoulos P, Robotis I, Margantinis G, Pistiolas D. Cumulative *H. pylori* eradication rates in clinical practice by adopting first and second-line regimens proposed by the Maastricht III consensus and a third-line empirical regimen. Am J Gastroenterol. 2009; 104: 21-5.

[101] Rokkas T, Simsek I, Ladas S. *Helicobacter pylori* and non-malignant diseases. Helicobacter. 2007; 12 Suppl 1: 20-2.

[102] Rokkas T. Impact of *H. pylori* infection on the management of dyspepsia. Dig Dis. 2001; 19: 123-6.

[103] Rokkas T, Mavrogeorgis A, Liatsos C, Rallis E, Kalogeropoulos N. Optimal dose of omeprazole in combination with amoxicillin in eradicating *H. pylori* and preventing relapses in duodenal ulcer patients. Hepatogastroenterology. 1995; 42: 842-6.

[104] Rokkas T, Papatheodorou G, Karameris A, *et al. Helicobacter pylori* infection and gastric juice vitamin C levels. Impact of eradication. Dig Dis Sci. 1995; 40: 615-21.

[105] Rokkas T, Karameris A, Mavrogeorgis A, Rallis E, Giannikos N. Eradication of *Helicobacter pylori* reduces the possibility of rebleeding in peptic ulcer disease. Gastrointest Endosc. 1995; 41: 1-4.

[106] Tzivras M, Balatsos V, Souyioultzis S, *et al.* High eradication rate of *Helicobacter pylori* using a four-drug regimen in patients previously treated unsuccessfully. Clin Ther. 1997; 19: 906-12.

[107] Tzivras M, Archimandritis A, Balatsos V, *et al.* One-week therapy with omeprazole, clarithromycin and metronidazole or ornidazole, followed by 3 weeks' treatment with omeprazole, eradicates *Helicobacter pylori* equally and heals duodenal ulcer. Eur J Gastroenterol Hepatol. 1997; 9: 1185-9.

Send Orders for Reprints to reprints@benthamscience.net
Helicobacter Pylori: A Worldwide Perspective 2014, **2014, 216-233**

CHAPTER 10

Helicobacter pylori Infection in Iran: Epidemiology, Treatment and Diagnosis

Amin Talebi Bezmin Abadi and Johannes G. Kusters*

Department of Medical Microbiology, University Medical Center Utrecht, Utrecht, The Netherlands

Abstract: *Helicobacter pylori* infection contributes to the development of various gastroduodenal disorders. Clinical manifestation after *H. pylori* infection is an important issue for gastroenterologist. Design and optimizing usage of new drugs against *H. pylori* has always been a major topic in *Helicobacter pylori* (*H. pylori*) research. There are many articles published over the last decade on *H. pylori* treatment and diagnosis. Since the incidence, virulence, and resistance of *H. pylori* are different for each region diagnosis and treatment require a local approach. Iran is a country with a high rate of *H. pylori* infection and consequently a huge number of patients suffer from *H. pylori* induced digestive diseases. In this chapter we will present a comprehensive summary on *H. pylori* epidemiology, diagnosis and treatment in Iran over the last years.

Keywords: *Helicobacter pylori*, Iran, prevalence.

OVERVIEW

Until some thirty years ago it was commonly believed that no bacteria could colonize the stomach because of the harsh acidic condition. This concept has radically changed after Marshall & Warren's discovery in 1983 when they showed that *H. pylori* was able to infect the human stomach [1]. Eventually, their concept that *H. pylori* was a gastric colonizer and pathogen responsible for a wide range gastroduodenal disorders, resulted in the abandonment of old theories such as association between stress and gastric ulcers. It is now commonly accepted that within a few weeks upon the initial infection by *H. pylori* a superficial gastritis will develop [2]. Unless treated, the infection will last for life and thus result in a chronic gastritis and may ultimately progress in ulceration and possibly even

***Address correspondence to Johannes G. Kusters:** Department of Medical Microbiology, University Medical Center Utrecht, The Netherlands; Tel: +31 88 7553687; Fax: + 31 88 75 55426;
E-mail: h.kusters@umcutrecht.nl

stomach cancer. The *H. pylori* infection occurs worldwide and an estimated 3.5 billion individuals of world population [3], are thought to carry this bacterium in their stomach. Moreover, three quarters of the gastric cancer cases and 90% of individuals with duodenal ulcer have been identified as *H. pylori* positive [4], but major regional differences exist in infection rates and *H. pylori* related pathology [5]. Soon after the discovery of *H. pylori* as a gastric pathogen it was found that eradication significantly decreased the risk of gastric malignancy [6], and hence the World Health Organization (WHO) has been categorized *H. pylori* as class-I carcinogen agent attributing to the genesis of gastric cancer [7].

Actually, after this statement by WHO, scientists became eager to conduct research on *H. pylori* and its likely association with gastric cancer; especially in regions such Iran where the rate of gastric cancer reported is relatively high [8, 9]. Recent studies showed that *H. pylori* is a relatively high diverse microorganism [10, 11] and this results in major differences in virulence factors between the various isolates. Not only do these strain differences affect the efficacy of treatment regimens on the prevention of ulcers and gastric malignancies [3, 12] they also affect finding the suitable treatment formula to deal with *H. pylori.* With approximately 76 million inhabitants Iran is one of the most populated countries in Mid-East. Its relative high ulcer and gastric cancer rate has been a major trigger to perform local studies on *H. pylori* pathogenesis, treatment, prevalence, *etc.* In this chapter, we aim to present a comprehensive overview of the investigated topics over the past 17 years. Starting in 1995, approximately three hundred Pubmed indexed papers have been published which all had been conducted on the subject of *H. pylori* in Iranians with upper abdominal complaints (Pubmed keywords: *Helicobacter pylori*, year, virulence factors, treatment, Metronidazole, Clarithromycin, diagnostic tests). The majority of these papers (~32%) were on pathogenesis and 85 papers (~28%) were on the treatment of *H. pylori* infection in Iran (Fig. **1**).

When comparing Iran with its neighbouring countries, there is no significant differences between the dominant topics that have been investigated ($P>0.05$), but Iranian researchers seem to have published more PubMed indexed papers; (See Fig. **2**). This is probably the result of the increase by Iranian government in the budget for research on gastric cancer and related subjects. Hence we expect to see much more published papers in the next couple of years.

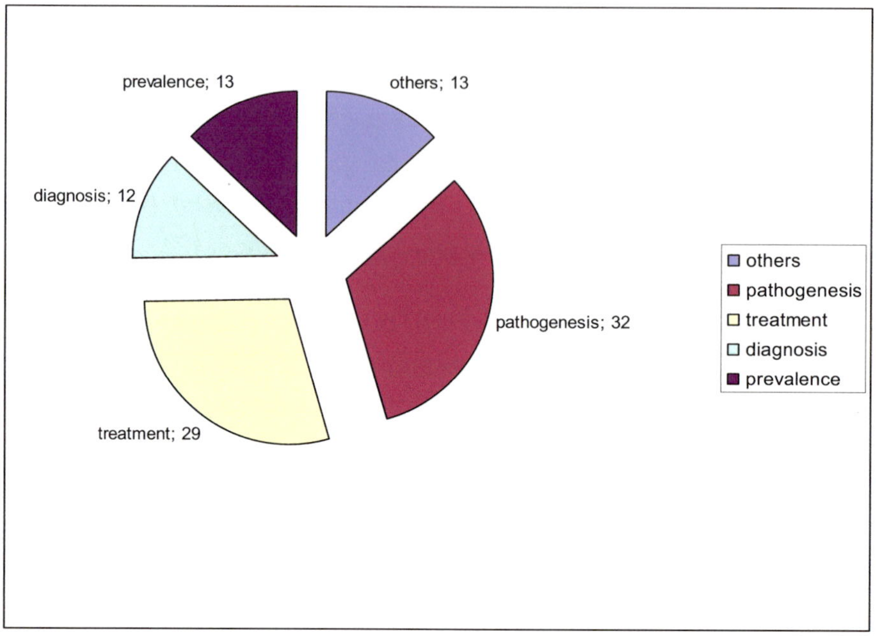

Figure 1: Distribution of PubMed indexed papers on *H. pylori* research in Iran over the last 17 years (1995-2012).

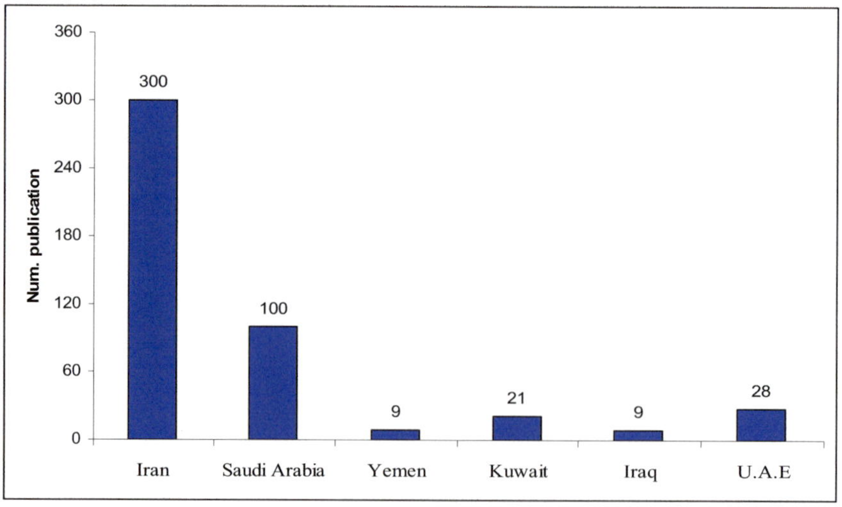

Figure 2: Comparison of the number of PubMed indexed *H. pylori* related papers from Iran and its neighbouring countries published between 1995 and 2012.

When analysing the Iranian *H. pylori* related papers there is a strong increase after 2006 (Fig. **4**). Perhaps the award of the Nobel prize to Marshall and Warren in 2005 has triggered researchers in Iran to enhance their efforts in this area [13]. Strikingly, 10% of the *H. pylori* related papers are from a small are within the North of country where only 9% of the Iranian population resides (Fig. **3**). This is probably explained by the high infection rate of *H. pylori* in the people this area and the high number of patients with gastrointestinal complaints thus creating a strong patient population to perform research [14-16].

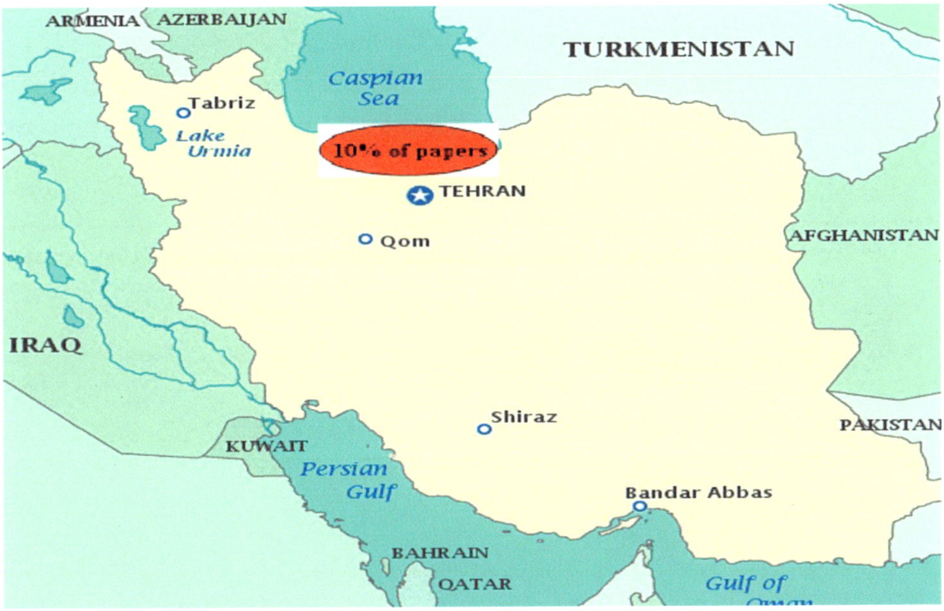

Figure 3: High percentage of conducted research at the small region in north of Iran.

Pathogenesis of *H. pylori*

Large part of the papers from Iran focuses on *H. pylori* virulence. Iran has a high prevalence of *H. pylori* infection [17] especially in the Mazandaran province where the infection rate exceeds 90% [15]. This high prevalence of infection facilitates the collection of a large number of *H. pylori* strains from a narrow geographical region in order to perform comprehensive studies on the putative association between the association of bacterial virulence factors and clinical outcome of *H. pylori* infection. Although the clinical outcome of the infection is thought to be determined by host, bacterial and environmental factors [18], the exact mechanisms that determine the clinical outcome of the infection are not clear. On the host site the immune status [19] and host acid secretion seem critical determinants in this process [20]. On the bacterial side virulence factors like *dupA*, *babA*$_2$, *oipA*, *homB, cagA, VacA* and *iceA* have been shown to affect the development of post-infection disorders [21]. Since there is specialized chapters on virulence we restrict our discussion her to some relevant findings from Iran. The incidence of gastric cancer in Iran is relatively high making it easy to collect sufficiently large cohorts to study links between bacterial virulence factors and cancer. In our former study, the prevalence of *cagA* among the gastritis, MALT Lymphoma and gastric cancer were 85,% 19% and 57%, respectively [22]. Thus we had a significant link between cancer and the presence of *cagA* in the infecting strains but note that only strains were collected in a relatively small area of Iran

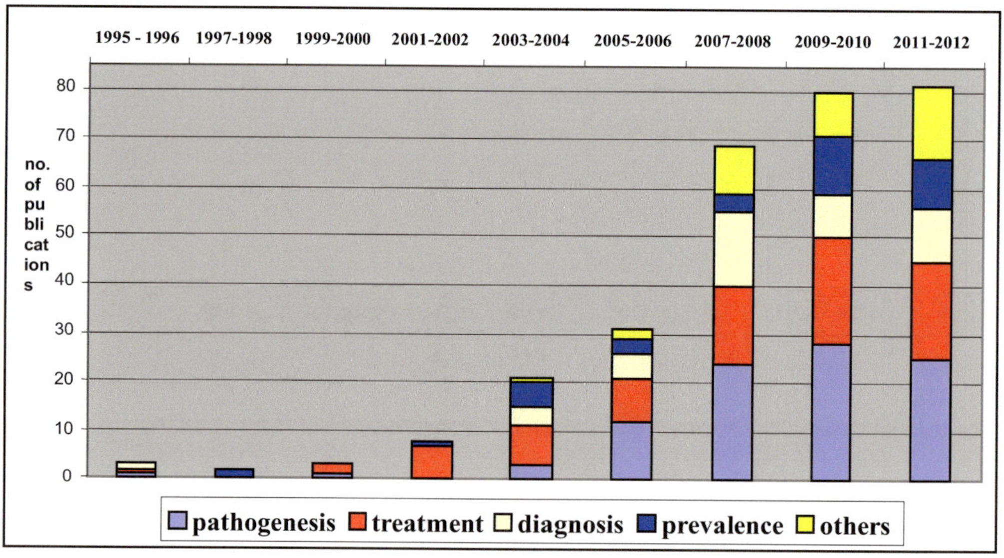

Figure 4: Distribution of Medline cited papers related to *H. pylori* infections in Iran published between 1995 and 2012.

and it is not clear if our findings may be generalized for the whole of Iran. In an other study, the prevalence of homB of *H. pylori* isolated from patients from northern Iran was found to be significantly higher in gastric cancer patients (78%) than in patients suffering from peptic ulcers (20%) or gastritis (43%) (P<0.0001) [23]. From this it was concluded that presence of *homB* seems to be associated with gastric cancer and gastritis rather than DU [23]. Interestingly the duodenal ulcer promoting gene (*dupA*) has a reverse association. The DupA has been proposed as a novel *H. pylori* virulence factor associated with an increased rate for occurrence of duodenal ulcer [DU] and a decreased risk for gastric cancer (GC) [23, 24]. The biological function of DupA has thus far not been identified, but *in vitro* studies indicate that DupA induces interleukin-8 production [24] thereby affecting the inflammation. Using a set of strains isolated from Iran it was shown that DupA is associated with an enhanced capability to survive and at low pH [23, 24] This enhanced ability to withstand low pH may affect the preferential colonization in the stomach (antrum *vs.* corpus) thus affecting the disease outcome [23, 24]. Undoubtedly many more studies will come from this region as the high prevalence of *Helicobacter* and associated disease facilitates the collection of large study populations from a small and homogeneous area needed to perform such association studies.

DIAGNOSIS

Different approaches for diagnoses of *Helicobacter* have been introduced in literature, and while some of them seem rather successful others probably need to be adapted. Certainly, a first condition in the management of *H. pylori* infection is the proper detection of the infection [4, 5, 25]. Interestingly, it has been demonstrated that different methods for the diagnosis of the infection result in diverse outcomes on *H. pylori* incidence within the same regions of a country [26-28]. Here we will briefly focus on recent advances in detection and diagnosis of *H. pylori* in different human resources in order to allow a better discussion on the current status of *H. pylori* infection and diagnosis in Iran. Not only in Iran, but also in other countries, antibiotic resistance is the foremost problem when trying to manage infections. It poses a big challenge when designing rational eradication therapies that on needs to consider it carefully. So next to its prevalence, we will also discuss here the antibiotic resistance and the consequences this has for treatment of Iranian *Helicobacter* strains.

PREVALENCE

Even though there is no evidence for a zoonotic transmission of *H. pylori*, it is believed that the ancestral *H. pylori* strain was living in gastric epithelium of vertebrates [7, 12, 29]. While *H. pylori* has no other known niche than the human stomach its high prevalence among the population results in a steady transmission between infected and uninfected individuals. Several studies have investigated the possible role of *H. pylori* in oral cavity and dental plaque but they mostly just confirmed the presence of bacterium in oral secretions and not actual colonisation of the oral cavity. While it is thus not sure how *H. pylori* can be transmitted, it is thought to occur by direct contact (Human-to-human) or indirectly through food or water [7, 30-32]. The initial acquisition is thought mostly to occur during the early childhood and most children are infected by their parents [7]. Generally, the prevalence of *H. pylori* in world is around the 40-50%, but this rate is relatively higher in developing countries [33, 34]. In developing countries like Iran, infection with *H. pylori* usually occurs during early childhood [33]. In spite of the fact that the majority of new infections is during childhood there is also an increase in incidence with increasing age in adults. In the recent past there was a high percentage of *H. pylori* infection that was probably due to lesser socioeconomic status and reduced hygiene [31, 35]. This, combined with several studies that indeed confirm that the acquisition of *H. pylori* infection occurs during the childhood [36]; suggests that the observed age related increase is most likely due to the age cohort effect rather than a gradual increase in the numbers of newly infected subjects.

Incidence of *H. pylori* Infection in Iran

The prevalence of *H. pylori* infections can differ drastically both within and between countries and Iran is not an exception to this. Mikaeli *et al.* [29] claimed that the prevalence of *H. pylori* in Yazd and Ardebil are 30% and 47%, respectively and there is a significant association between occurrence of gastric cancer and high prevalence of *H. pylori*. Different environmental factors, dietary habits and life style might be an acceptable explanation for this difference. While these factors all contribute to the cancer incidence infection *H. pylori* infection is a prerequisite as is clear from the many report that show a significant association between an increased *H. pylori* prevalence and an increase in gastric cancer cases [16, 37, 38]. In Iran there is indeed a high overall prevalence of *H. pylori* (Table **1**) but clearly local differences in the infection rate seem to exist that cannot be explained by methodological differences. Most likely the observed differences reflect better diagnostic/therapeutic approaches and improvements in hygiene and life style.

Table 1: An Overview of studies evaluating the prevalence of *H. pylori* in Iran

Authors	**State/Province**	**Prevalence of *H. pylori* [%]**	**Year**	**Reference**
Mikaeli *et al.*	Yazd	30	1999	[29]
Mikaeli *et al.*	Ardebil	47	1999	[29]
Moghaddam	Mashhad	85	2010	[39]
Moghaddam *et al.*	Mashhad	62	2005	[40]
Mansour-Ghanei *et al.*	Rasht	40	2009	[41]
Metanat *et al.*	Zahedan	34	2010	[42]
Nasrolahi *et al.*	Mazandaran	46	2008	[43]
Talebi *et al.*	Mazandaran	88	2011	[17]
Talebi *et al.*	Mazandaran	93	2012	[11]
Milani *et al.*	Tabriz	28	2012	[44]
Khameneh *et al.*	Urmia	47	2011	[45]
Rasmi *et al.*	Urmia	65	2011	[46]

The highest infection rates for *H. pylori* are reported in the North of Iran [State of Mazandaran] where in a recent paper it was estimated to be 93% (Table **1**). The prevalence of *H. pylori* is much less in southern Iran (34%) [28].

Prevalence of *H. pylori* Among the Immigrants

It has been shown that the prevalence of *H. pylori* varies between the different ethnic groups in a given geographical distinct. Iran is a country where many Afghan immigrants are living and they represent the main group of immigrants in Iran. The latest reports are indicating that approximately one million Afghans immigrants moved into Iran in the last decades. Most of them are living in the north of Iran as this seems to offer better job opportunities for them there. Interestingly as explained above the Northern parts of Iran also seem to have highest *H. pylori* infection rates. Unfortunately, data regarding the *H. pylori* status among the Afghan immigrants is currently not available.

TREATMENT

It has been shown that successful eradication of *H. pylori* infection prevents the recurrence of duodenal ulcer and other disorders but it is still under debate if eradication will also reduce the genesis of gastric carcinoma [47]. In spite of all the efforts to create an optimal treatment protocol the normal cure rate of *H. pylori* infections are still much lower than those for most other bacterial infections. Due to increasing levels of antimicrobial resistance there even seems to be a global decline in the rate of successful treatment over the last years [48-51]. The existing guidelines suggest to only use therapeutic regimens that result in an *H. pylori* infection eradication rate up to 80-90%, but mostly only efficacy data for western countries are available [52-54]. Treatment usually consist of a combination of two antibiotics and a proton pump inhibitor [47]. Most of these therapeutic failures are reported in the first-line treatment against *H. pylori*. Often here empirical/standard regimes of antibiotics are used that have not been adapted to the antibiotic resistance of the infecting strains. In addition given to the severe side effect of these combination therapies consumptions [25, 55] patients are often not motivated enough to complete the cure. The resulting poor compliance not only result in therapy failure, it also a major factor in the induction of antibiotic resistance [4, 5]. Given the high level of antibiotic resistance against metronidazole, clarithromycin and furazolidone in Iran [56-59] the generic western therapeutic protocols might need some tweaking but to our knowledge no optimal therapeutic regimen for Iran has been reported thus far. Below will briefly discussed the various generic treatment options for *H. pylori*, and while these are mostly based on data from Western countries we will wherever possible elaborate on the local situation in Iran.

Antibiotic Therapy Against *H. pylori*

Having treatment protocol consisting of a single drug sounds attractive and indeed for most bacterial infections mono therapies provides an efficient way of dealing with them. For *H. pylori* infections the efficacy of various drugs in monotherapy has been accessed. Only for clarithromycin reasonable results have been obtained, but these are not good enough to eradicate *H. pylori* [60, 61] and thus not much further research on mono therapies is performed. Since usage of a single antibiotic for eradicating the *H. pylori* was not successful, combinations of different antibiotic formulas have been initiated [25, 55, 62, 63]. Eventually, numerous different regimens against *H. pylori* infection have been tested and efficacy differs due to local resistance status [17, 25, 44, 47, 54, 55, 63]. Obviously, the selection of antibiotics for the optimal therapeutic regimen is further complicated by factors such as patient compliance, cost, drug side effects, and non-determined status of antibiotic resistance. However, in here we described the situation of different combination regimens (dual, triple, and quadruple therapy) against *H. pylori* infections in Iran.

Dual/ Triple Therapy

The combination of a proton pump inhibitor [64, 65] with one or two antibiotics (clarithromycin & amoxicillin) has been suggested as the best first line therapy to eradicate *H. pylori* infections [4, 25, 52, 62, 66, 67]. The efficacy for dual therapy in Iran was tested in two studies [68, 69]. Both studies found that the rate of clearance was not acceptable (<50%) but at least symptoms decreased. As previously described [64] the best results were obtained with the combination of a proton pump inhibitor and clarithromycin. It is to be expected however that due to the increase in clarithromycin usage [and hence the expected induction of resistance against clarithromycin] the efficacy of this regime might rapidly decrease. Obviously, dual therapy is more prone to small changes in resistance levels than triple therapies. In addition the efficacy rate of dual therapy is ~30% less than triple therapy among the symptomatic and asymptomatic Iranian populations [69]. The first findings with triple therapy were satisfactory, although some small differences were observed between these studies [70-72]. As expected from other studies [14, 17, 69] also in Iranian patients there is a higher efficacy of triple therapy when compared to dual therapy [15, 17, 62, 72, 73]. Bahremand *et al.* [74] suggested (PPI+AMX+CLR) as first line treatment and achieved as acceptable eradication rate (92%). The combination of proton pump inhibitor [64] with amoxicillin and clarithromycin is the most used triple therapy [47, 66, 75] and this combination also seemed to work well in Iran [72, 75] However recent studies indicate a drastic decrease in eradication rate when using this regime [76, 77]. As with all therapies the efficacy of triple therapy is highly dependent on the primary resistance of the strains present in the patients treated. It was shown that eradication rates are relatively high (88%) if strains are clarithromycin sensitive but decrease significantly (down to 19%) if strains were clarithromycin resistant [78]. Gisbert and Calvet reported that triple therapy can be still be used provided some modifications are applied [79]. Another important contributor to the efficacy of the therapy is the optimal duration of treatment. In a meta-analysis from Calvet *et al.* [80] it was shown that two weeks therapy resulted in a 10% better eradication than a 7 days therapy. While longer regimens are more beneficial from the eradication perspective, they also result in more pronounced side effects for the patients treated. Also studies in Iran show that 2 weeks treatment are more effective for *H. pylori* eradication than shorter treatment periods [77, 81]. In a study by Najafi *et al.* [82], furazolidone plus amoxicillin with a proton-pump inhibitor showed high eradication rate among Iranian children. Especially for therapeutic regimens for children special care should be taken to keep the treatment as short as possible [83]. However, Najafi *et al.* only examined this with a treatment period of two weeks, and hence they could not draw any conclusion on the effect of the much propagated one-week duration of this formula on Iran children. Treatment lasting longer than strictly necessary not only enhances any putative adverse effects for the patient, it also promotes the induction of resistance in the infecting *H. pylori* strain. The usage of furazolidone in Iran has recently been significantly increased due to the lower price than clarithromycin [84] and increased usage will also promote the resistance. Thus shortening the duration of the therapy is of utmost importance in order to avoid over exposure and to minimize the induction of resistance. Hence the advise to use furazolidone with caution as the induction of significant resistance levels in *H. pylori* may render furazolidone therapy less efficient in the near future [85].

Quadruple Drug Therapy

Quadruple therapy regimens consist of a H_2 receptor blocker, or a proton pump inhibitor, combined with three antimicrobial agents [62] thus rendering it more effective than triple therapy. Most Iranian studies who examined the effect of quadruple therapy used a two week treatment regime and found it to be very effective, [86, 87]. However the complex composition of Quadruple therapy often requires up to four doses a day that each have different compositions. A problem with this is that patient compliance is often lower than with dual and triple therapies [25, 75, 80]. Recently several simplified Quadruple therapies with twice-daily regimens have been tested in Iran. The compositions of these regimens were bismuth subcitrate plus amoxicillin, or tetracycline, and metronidazole, or furazolidone, and clarithromycin or azithromycin [72, 73] and both studies show that these simplified Quadruple therapies have better patient compliance without losing their effectiveness. Conclusively, quadruple therapies can be an effective regimen *vs. H. pylori* infection in Iran.

Helicobacter pylori & Probiotics: A Potential for New Treatment Options?

"Live microorganisms which when administered in a proper way confer a health benefit on the human" is the comprehensive definition for probiotic described by FAC/WHO [88]. It has been shown that consumption of probiotics can contribute to the resistance against some infectious agents including Helicobacter [89, 90]. Although a clear inhibitory effect of Lactobacillus on the growth of *H. pylori* is not always evident, it offers a potential novel additive to intervention that reduces the adverse effect of treatment among the patients [91]. Given the high incidence of *H. pylori* in Iran [11], it is worthwhile to expand research on the putative beneficial effect of combining antimicrobial treatment with probiotics.

CONCLUSION

Several *H. pylori* studies have been initiated in Iran over the past decade and the experience of working with this fastidious microorganism is now present in many local laboratories. This combined with the high prevalence of *Helicobacter* in Iran facilitates the collection of large study populations from a small and homogeneous area needed to perform even more exiting studies.

ACKNOWLEDGEMENT

None Declared.

CONFLICT OF INTEREST

The author(s) confirm that this chapter content has no conflict of interest.

REFERENCES

[1] Megraud F. A humble bacterium sweeps this year's Nobel Prize. Cell. 2005; 123:975-6.

[2] van Vliet AHM, Bereswill S, Kusters JG. Ion Metabolism and Transport, in: *Helicobacter pylori.* Physiology and genetics, eds. Mobley HLT, Mendz GL, Hazell SL, ASM Press, Washington. 2001; pp. 193-206

[3] Atherton JC. The pathogenesis of *Helicobacter pylori*-induced gastroduodenal diseases. Annu Rev Pathol. 2006;1:63–96.

[4] Malfertheiner P, Megraud F, O'Morain CA, Atherton J, Axon AT, Bazzoli F, *et al.* Management of *Helicobacter pylori* infection--the Maastricht IV/ Florence Consensus Report. Gut. 2012;61:646-64.

[5] Graham DY, Dore MP. *Helicobacter pylori* therapy demystified. Helicobacter. 2011;16:343-5.

[6] Peterson WL, Graham DY, Marshall B, Blaser MJ, Genta RM, Klein PD, *et al.* Clarithromycin as monotherapy for eradication of *Helicobacter pylori*: a randomized, double-blind trial. Am J Gastroenterol. 1993;88:1860-4.

[7] Kusters JG, van Vliet AH, Kuipers EJ. Pathogenesis of *Helicobacter pylori* infection. Clin Microbiol Rev. 2006;19:449-90.

[8] Yamaoka Y, Osato MS, Sepulveda AR, Gutierrez O, Figura N, Kim JG, *et al.* Molecular epidemiology of *Helicobacter pylori*: separation of *H. pylori* from East Asian and non-Asian countries. Epidemiol Infect. 2000;124:91-6.

[9] Asaka M, Kimura T, Kato M, Kudo M, Miki K, Ogoshi K, *et al.* Possible role of *Helicobacter pylori* infection in early gastric cancer development. Cancer. 1994;73:2691-4.

[10] Salama NR, Gonzalez-Valencia G, Deatherage B, Aviles-Jimenez F, Atherton JC, Graham DY, *et al.* Genetic analysis of *Helicobacter pylori* strain populations colonizing the stomach at different times postinfection. J Bacteriol. 2007;189:3834-45.

11] Talebi Bezmin Abadi A, Taghvaei T, Wolfram L, Kusters JG. Infection with *Helicobacter pylori* strains lacking dupA is associated with an increased risk of gastric ulcer and gastric cancer development. J Med Microbiol. 2012;61:23-30.

[12] Basso D, Plebani M, Kusters JG. Pathogenesis of *Helicobacter pylori* infection. Helicobacter. 2010;15 Suppl 1:14-20.

[13] Lopez Vidal Y, Ponce de Leon S. [Reflections on the Nobel prize, the *Helicobacter pylori*, the peptic ulcer and the scientific paradigms]. Rev Invest Clin. 2006;58:6-8.

[14] Rezaii J, Tavakoli H, Esfandiari K, Ashegh H, Hasibi M, Ghanei G, *et al.* Association between *Helicobacter pylori* infection and laryngo-hypopharyngeal carcinoma: a case-control study and review of the literature. Head Neck. 2008;30:1624-7.

[15] Talebi Bezmin Abadi A, Taghvaei T, Mobarez AM, Carpenter BM, Merrell DS. Frequency of antibiotic resistance in *Helicobacter pylori* strains isolated from the northern population of Iran. J Microbiol. 2011;49:987-93.

[16] Siavoshi F, Malekzadeh R, Daneshmand M, Ashktorab H. *Helicobacter pylori* endemic and gastric disease. Dig Dis Sci. 2005;50:2075-80.

[17] Talebi Bezmin Abadi A, Ghasemzadeh A, Taghvaei T, Mobarez AM. Primary resistance of *Helicobacter pylori* to levofloxacin and moxifloxacine in Iran. Intern Emerg Med. 2011; 25.

[18] HL. M. *Helicobacter pylori* factors associated with disease development. Gastroenterology. 1997;113:s21-8.

[19] Robinson K, Argent RH, Atherton JC. The inflammatory and immune response to *Helicobacter pylori* infection. Best Pract Res Clin Gastroenterol. 2007;21:237-59.

[20] Sobala GM, Crabtree JE, Dixon MF, Schorah CJ, Taylor JD, Rathbone BJ, *et al.* Acute *Helicobacter pylori* infection: clinical features, local and systemic immune response, gastric mucosal histology, and gastric juice ascorbic acid concentrations. Gut. 1991;32:1415-8.

[21] Atherton JC. The pathogenesis of *Helicobacter pylori*-induced gastro-duodenal diseases. Annu Rev Pathol. 2006;1:63-96.

[22] Talebi Bezmin Abadi A, Ghasemzadeh A, Mohabati Mobarez A. Low frequency of cagA-positive *Helicobacter pylori* strains isolated from Iranian patients with MALT lymphoma. Intern Emerg Med. 2011 Apr 2, DOI 10.1007/s11739-011-0579-6.

[23] Talebi Bezmin Abadi A, Rafiei A, Ajami A, Hosseini V, Taghvaei T, Jones KR, *et al.* *Helicobacter pylori* homB, but not cagA, is associated with gastric cancer in Iran. J Clin Microbiol. 2011;49:3191-7.

[24] Lu H, Hsu PI, Graham DY, Yamaoka Y. Duodenal ulcer promoting gene of *Helicobacter pylori*. Gastroenterology. 2005;128:833-48.

[25] Graham DY, Shiotani A. New concepts of resistance in the treatment of *Helicobacter pylori* infections. Nat Clin Pract Gastroenterol Hepatol. 2008;5:321-31.

[26] Megraud F, Lehours P. *Helicobacter pylori* detection and antimicrobial susceptibility testing. Clin Microbiol Rev. 2007;20:280-322.

[27] Cambau E, Allerheiligen V, Coulon C, Corbel C, Lascols C, Deforges L, *et al.* Evaluation of a new test, genotype HelicoDR, for molecular detection of antibiotic resistance in *Helicobacter pylori*. J Clin Microbiol. 2009;47:3600-7.

28] Megraud F. Detection of *Helicobacter pylori* and its sensitivity to antibiotics. A step forward in the use of molecular methods. Gastroenterol Clin Biol. 2007 31:790-1.

[29] Mikaeli J, Malekzadeh, R, Ziad Alizadeh, b, Nasseri Mogaddam, s, *et al.* Prevalence of *Helicobacter pylori* in two Iranian provinces with high and low Incidence of Gastric Carcinoma. AIM. 1999.

[30] Schwarz S, Morelli G, Kusecek B, Manica A, Balloux F, Owen RJ, *et al.* Horizontal *vs.* familial transmission of *Helicobacter pylori*. PLoS Pathog. 2008;4:e1000180.

[31] Lee YY, Ismail AW, Mustaffa N, Musa KI, Majid NA, Choo KE, *et al.* Sociocultural and dietary practices among Malay subjects in the north-eastern region of Peninsular Malaysia: a region of low prevalence of *Helicobacter pylori* infection. Helicobacter. 2012;17:54-61.

[32] Al-Ahmad A KA, Weckesser S, Wittmer A, Rauberger H, Jakob T, Hellwig E, Kist M, Waidner B. Is *Helicobacter pylori* a resident or a transient germ in human oral cavity? J Med Microbiol. 2012;61:1146-52.

[33] Nouraie M, Latifi-Navid S, Rezvan H, Radmard AR, Maghsudlu M, Zaer-Rezaii H, *et al.* Childhood hygienic practice and family education status determine the prevalence of *Helicobacter pylori* infection in Iran. Helicobacter. 2009;14:40-6.

[34] Latifi-Navid S, Ghorashi SA, Siavoshi F, Linz B, Massarrat S, Khegay T, *et al.* Ethnic and geographic differentiation of *Helicobacter pylori* within Iran. PLoS One. 2010;5:e9645.

[35] Kalach N, Bontems P, Koletzko S, Mourad-Baars P, Shcherbakov P, Celinska-Cedro D, *et al.* Frequency and risk factors of gastric and duodenal ulcers or erosions in children: a

prospective 1-month European multicenter study. Eur J Gastroenterol Hepatol. 2010;22:1174-81.

[36] Mitchell H, Mégraud F. Epidemiology and diagnosis of *Helicobacter pylori* infection. Helicobacter. 2002;7:8-16.

[37] Blaser MJ, Kuipers EJ, Ernst P, Axon A, Megraud F. Panel discussion: breaking the link--clinical options to minimize risk. Aliment Pharmacol Ther. 1999;13 Suppl 1:19-23.

[38] Yamaoka Y, Kodama T, Kita M, Imanishi J, Kashima K, Graham DY. Relation between cytokines and *Helicobacter pylori* in gastric cancer. Helicobacter. 2001;6:116-24.

[39] Nakhaei Moghaddam M. Prevalence of *Helicobacter pylori* Infection in Patients with Digestive Complaints Using Urea Breath Test in Mashhad, Northeast Iran. JRHS. 2010;10:77-80.

[40] Nakhaei Moghaddam M K-KM, Malekzadeh F, Fumani A. Prevalence of *H. pylori* in biopsy specimens and determination of sensitivity and specificity of its diagnostic methods. Journal of Gonabad University of Medical Sciences and Health Services. 2005;11:37-40.

[41] Mansour-Ghanaei F, Yousefi Mashhour, M, Joukar, F, Sedigh, M, Bagher-Zadeh,ah, Jafarshad, R. Prevalence of *Helicobacter pylori* Infection among Children in Rasht, Northern Iran. Middle East Journal of Digestive Diseases. 2009;2:84-8.

[42] Metanat M, sharifi-mood, B, Izadi, SH. Prevalence of *Helicobacter pylori* infection in healthcare workers. Turk J Med ScI. 2010;40:965-9.

[43] Nasrolahei M S, M, Ahanjan, M, Daryani, A. Prevalence of *Helicobacter pylori* in gastric mucosa and dental plaque in Sari northern Iran. Journal of Chineese Medicine. 2008;3:83-8.

[44] Milani M GR, Akhi MT, Nahaei MR, Hasani A, Somi MH, Rafeey M, Sharifi Y. The status of antimicrobial resistance of *Helicobacter pylori* in Eastern Azerbaijan, Iran: comparative study according to demographics. J Infect Chemother. 2012; 18: 848-852.

[45] Khameneh ZR SN, Hatami S, Afshari AT. The seroprevalence of *Helicobacter pylori* infection in renal transplant recipients. Transplant Proc. 2011;43:3720-2.

[46] Rasmi Y MK, Farshid S, Kheradmand F. Seroprevalence of anti-*Helicobacter pylori* and anticytotoxin-associated gene A antibodies [corrected] according to ABO blood groups and rhesus status among hemodialysis patients. Iran J Kidney Dis. 2011;5:110-3.

[47] O'Connor A, Gisbert JP, McNamara D, O'Morain C. Treatment of *Helicobacter pylori* infection 2011. Helicobacter. 2011;16:53-8.

[48] Gisbert JP, Perez-Aisa A, Bermejo F, Castro-Fernandez M, Almela P, Barrio J, *et al.* Second-line Therapy With Levofloxacin After Failure of Treatment to Eradicate *Helicobacter pylori* Infection: Time Trends in a Spanish Multicenter Study of 1000 Patients. J Clin Gastroenterol. 2012 29.

[49] Sanches B, Coelho L, Moretzsohn L, Vieira G, Jr. Failure of *Helicobacter pylori* treatment after regimes containing clarithromycin: new practical therapeutic options. Helicobacter. 2008;13:572-6.

[50] Gisbert JP, Gisbert JL, Marcos S, Jimenez-Alonso I, Moreno-Otero R, Pajares JM. Empirical rescue therapy after *Helicobacter pylori* treatment failure: a 10-year single-centre study of 500 patients. Aliment Pharmacol Ther. 2008;27:346-54.

[51] Delchier JC. *Helicobacter pylori* infection: what to do after first intent treatment failure?. Rev Prat. 2008;58:1442-4.

[52] Gisbert JP, Pajares R, Pajares JM. Evolution of *Helicobacter pylori* therapy from a meta-analytical perspective. Helicobacter. 2007;12 Suppl 2:50-8.

[53] Graham DY, Fischbach L. *Helicobacter pylori* treatment in the era of increasing antibiotic resistance. Gut. 2010;59:1143-53.

[54] Graham DY, Fischbach L. Sequential therapy for *Helicobacter pylori* infection: ethical considerations revisited. J Clin Gastroenterol. 2010;44:523.

[55] Vakil N, Megraud F. Eradication therapy for *Helicobacter pylori*. Gastroenterology. 2007;133:985-1001.

[56] Amin Talebi Bezmin Abadi TT, Dino Vaira. Considerable use of furazolidone in Iran. Saudi J Gastroenterol. 2010;4:308-9.

[57] Daghaghzadeh H, Emami MH, Karimi S, Raeisi M. One-week *vs.* two-week furazolidone-based quadruple therapy as the first-line treatment for *Helicobacter pylori* infection in Iran. J Gastroenterol Hepatol. 2007;22:1399-403.

[58] Rafeey M, Ghotaslou R, Nikvash S, Hafez AA. Primary resistance in *Helicobacter pylori* isolated in children from Iran. J Infect Chemother. 2007;13:291-5.

[59] Fallahi GH, Maleknejad S. *Helicobacter pylori* culture and antimicrobial resistance in Iran. Indian J Pediatr. 2007;74:127-30.

[60] Graham DY, Opekun AR, Klein PD. Clarithromycin for the eradication of *Helicobacter pylori*. J Clin Gastroenterol. 1993;16:292-4.

[61] Peterson WL GD, Marshall B, Blaser MJ, Genta RM, Klein PD, Stratton CW, Drnec J, Prokocimer P, Siepman N. Clarithromycin as monotherapy for eradication of *Helicobacter pylori*: a randomized, double-blind trial. Am J Gastroenterol. 1993;88:1160-4.

[62] Megraud F. *Helicobacter pylori* and antibiotic resistance. Gut. 2007;56:1502.

[63] Salles N, Megraud F. Current management of *Helicobacter pylori* infections in the elderly. Expert Rev Anti Infect Ther. 2007;5:845-56.

[64] Sappington PL, Cruz RJ, Jr., Harada T, Yang R, Han Y, Englert JA, *et al.* The ethyl pyruvate analogues, diethyl oxaloproprionate, 2-acetamidoacrylate, and methyl-2-acetamidoacrylate, exhibit anti-inflammatory properties *in vivo* and/or *in vitro*. Biochem Pharmacol. 2005;70:1579-92.

[65] Mégraud F DH. Clinical relevance of resistant strains of *Helicobacter pylori*: a review of current data. Gut. 1998;43:1:S61-5.

[66] O'Connor A, Gisbert J, O'Morain C. Treatment of *Helicobacter pylori* infection. Helicobacter. 2009;14 Suppl 1:46-51.

[67] Bazzoli Franco ZRM, Fossi Stefania, Pozzato Paolo, Alampi Giulia, Simoni Patrizia,Sottiliv Sandra, Roda Aldo, Roda Enrico. Short-term low-dose triple therapy for the eradication of *Helicobacter pylori*. European Journal of Gastroenterology & Hepatology. 1994;6:757-846.

[68] Saberi-Firoozi M, Massarrat S, Zare S, Fattahi M, Javan A, Etaati H, *et al.* Effect of triple therapy or amoxycillin plus omeprazole or amoxycillin plus tinidazole plus omeprazole on duodenal ulcer healing, eradication of *Helicobacter pylori*, and prevention of ulcer relapse over a 1-year follow-up period: a prospective, randomized, controlled study. Am J Gastroenterol. 1995;90:1419-23.

[69] Alizadeh-Naeeni M, Saberi-Firoozi M, Pourkhajeh A, Taheri H, Malekzadeh R, Derakhshan MH, *et al.* Effect of *Helicobacter pylori* eradication or of ranitidine plus metoclopramide on *Helicobacter pylori*-positive functional dyspepsia. A randomized, controlled follow-up study. Digestion. 2002;66:92-8.

[70] Uygun A KA, Yesilova Z, Safali M, Ilgan S, Karaeren N. Comparison of sequential and standard triple-drug regimen for *Helicobacter pylori* eradication: a 14-day, open-label,

randomized, prospective, parallel-arm study in adult patients with nonulcer dyspepsia. Clin Ther. 2008;30:528-34.

[71] Archimandritis A BV, Delis V, Mentis A, Kastanas K, Scandalis N. Triple therapy eradicated *H. pylori* equally in patients pretreated with omeprazole or ranitidine. A 12-month follow-up. J Clin Gastroenterol. 1995;20:12-6.

[72] Reza Malekzadeh MM, Farideh Siavoshi, Sadegh Massarrat. Treatment of *helicobacter pylori* infection in iran: low efficacy of recommended western regimens. Arch Iranian Med. 2004;7:1-8.

[73] Saberi-Firoozi M, M. Experiences with *Helicobacter pylori* Treatment in Iran. Iran J Med Sci December. 2006;31:181-5.

[74] Malfertheiner P MF, O'Morain C, Bazzoli F, El-Omar E, Graham D, Hunt R, Rokkas T, Vakil N, Kuipers EJ. Current concepts in the management of *Helicobacter pylori* infection: the Maastricht III Consensus Report. GUT. 2007;56:772-81.

[76] Saad RJ CW. Treatment of *Helicobacter pylori* infection in 2006. Gastroentrol Hepatol Annu Rev 2006;1:30-5.

[77] Kadayifci A BH, Cemil Savas M, Simsek I. Eradication of *Helicobacter pylori* with triple therapy: an epidemiologic analysis of trends in Turkey over 10 years. Clin Ther. 2006;28:1960-6.

[78] Megraud F. *H. pylori* antibiotic resistance: prevalence, importance, and advances in testing. Gut 2004;53:1374–84.

[79] Gisbert JP CX. Review article: the effectiveness of standard triple therapy for *Helicobacter pylori* has not changed over the last decade, but it is not good enough. Aliment Pharmacol Ther. 2011;31:1255-68.

[80] Calvet X GN, López T, Gisbert JP, Gené E, Roque M. A meta-analysis of short *vs.* long therapy with a proton pump inhibitor, clarithromycin and either metronidazole or amoxycillin for treating *Helicobacter pylori i*nfection. Aliment Pharmacol Ther. 2000;14:603-9.

[81] Fuccio L MM, Zagari RM, Grilli D, Magrini N, Bazzoli F. Meta-analysis: duration of first-line proton-pump inhibitor based triple therapy for *Helicobacter pylori* eradication. Ann Intern Med. 2007;147:553-62.

[82] Mehri Najafi AK, Gholamhossein Fallahi, Fatemeh Farahmand, Farzaneh Motamed, Mohammad Sobhani. Success Rate of furazolidone-based triple therapy for eradication of *Helicobacter Pylori* in children. Iranian Journal of Pediatrics. 2009;19:244-8.

[83] Khor CJ FK, Ng TM, Teo EK, Sim CS, Tan AL, Ng A. Recurrence of *Helicobacter pylori* infection and duodenal ulcer relapse, following successful eradication in an urban east Asian population. Singapore Med J. 2000;41:382-6.

[84] Fakheri H, Taghvaei T, Hosseini V, Bari Z. A comparison between sequential therapy and a modified bismuth-based quadruple therapy for *Helicobacter pylori* eradication in Iran: a randomized clinical trial. Helicobacter. 2012;17:43-8.

[85] Talebi Bezmin Abadi A, Tarang Taghvaei, Vaira D. Considerable use of furazolidone in Iran. Saudi J Gastroenterol. 2010;4:308-9.

[86] Fakheri H, Merat S, Hosseini V, Malekzadeh R. Low-dose furazolidone in triple and quadruple regimens for *Helicobacter pylori* eradication. Aliment Pharmacol Ther. 2004;19:89-93.

[87] Malekzadeh R, Ansari R, Vahedi H, Siavoshi F, Alizadeh BZ, Eshraghian MR, *et al.* Furazolidone *vs.* metronidazole in quadruple therapy for eradication of *Helicobacter pylori* in duodenal ulcer disease. Aliment Pharmacol Ther. 2000;14:299-303.

[88] FAO/WHO Report o[1]n Joint FAO/WHO Expert Consultation on Evaluation of Health and Nutritional Properties of Probiotics in Food Including Powder Milk with Live Lactic Acid Bacteria. 2001.

[89] Gill HS GF. Probiotics and human health: a clinical perspective. Postgrad Med J. 2004;80:516–26.

[90] Ullivan A NC. Probiotics and gastrointestinal diseases.. J Intern Med 2005;256:78–92.

[91] Saneeyan H, Layeg, S. Effectiveness of Probiotic on treatment of *Helicobacter pylori* infection in children. JIMS. 2011;11: 882-9

CHAPTER 11

Current Methods Used for the Diagnosis of *Helicobacter pylori* Infection

Francis Mégraud[1,2,*], Emilie Bessède[1,2] and Philippe Lehours[1,2]

[1]INSERM U853, 33076 Bordeaux, [2]Université de Bordeaux, National Reference Center for Helicobacters, Bacteriology laboratory, 33076 Bordeaux, France

Abstract: A number of methods have been proposed to diagnose *Helicobacter pylori* infection. In this chapter, each method is presented and the critical aspects are highlighted. It is common practice to distinguish the methods which necessitate an endoscopy and obtention of biopsy specimens, the so-called invasive methods, from the methods which are performed on blood, stools, air, *etc.*, the so-called non-invasive methods. Among the invasive methods, histology is probably the most commonly used worldwide, and has been recently completed by the use of the OLGA or OLGIM system to evaluate the gastric cancer risk. Culture is demanding for transport but there has been a renewed interest because of the increase in *H. pylori* antimicrobial resistance. The rapid urease test, while not as sensitive, has the great advantage of providing a quick result allowing to prescribe immediately a treatment. Molecular methods are developing, especially real-time PCR for which kits are now available, detecting *H. pylori* and its resistance to clarithromycin, and allowing standardization. An advantage of this method is the possibility to apply it to stools, rendering it non-invasive. However, at this stage, DNA extraction is still a problem. The best method to be used in such specimens is a stool antigen test using an ELISA with monoclonal antibodies. However, many still prefer the urea breath test which has become a standard in the field. Finally ELISA serological tests have also experienced a revival since they are the only tests to be used on patients taking proton pump inhibitors, nowadays a common situation.

Keywords: Histology, culture, rapid urease test, standard PCR, real-time PCR, urea breath test, stool antigen test, serology, ELISA, immunoblot, pepsinogen, sensitivity, specificity, OLGA, *Helicobacter heilmannii.*

INTRODUCTION

Thirty years after the discovery of *Helicobacter pylori*, the diagnosis of this

[*]**Address correspondence to Francis Mégraud:** Laboratoire de Bactériologie, Hospital Pellegrin 33076, Bordeaux, France; Tel: +33-(0)55-6795977; Fax: +33 (0)55-6796018; E-mail: francis.megraud@chu-bordeaux.fr

Buzás György Miklós (Ed.)

bacterium still remains difficult. The reason is essentially due to the difficulty in accessing the stomach, or the stomach content, in comparison to other organs. An endoscopy is needed to obtain biopsies, which is an invasive procedure, unpleasant for the patient and which cannot be repeated as much as sometimes needed. Furthermore, the niche of *H. pylori* is at the surface of the mucosa and therefore biopsies are preferred to gastric juice which could be obtained by nasogastric aspiration. Histology, culture, rapid urease test (RUT) and PCR are the methods used on gastric biopsies. Other methods have been applied allowing a non-invasive diagnosis: serology, detection of *H. pylori* antigens in stools (stool antigen test, SAT) and the original urea breath test (UBT), the first method based on a non-radioactive isotope (^{13}C) developed in human medicine [1].

A problem still remaining is also the lack of a true gold standard to get insight into the real performances of a diagnostic method. Histology is too dependent on the observer, and culture on the transport and laboratory conditions. UBT, despite the fact that it is an indirect method, does not have these limitations and could be considered for this purpose but it does not have an optimal sensitivity. Therefore, the best reference used for a positive biopsy is usually a combination of tests, *e.g.* 1) positive culture and 2) in the case of a negative culture, histology or RUT (or UBT) both of which must be positive.

There has also been lengthy discussion on the interest of performing *H. pylori* serology these last years. The reason is mainly due to the variety of tests present on the market with very heterogeneous accuracy (from 75 to 95%). Since there is not enough data to compile for each individual kit, the systematic reviews pooled the results of all of the kits together and ended up, as expected, with a poor result. A recent comparison of tests did, nevertheless, show good performances of some serological tests which could compete with the other *H. pylori* tests [2]. The evolution of medical care, *i.e.* free access to proton pump inhibitors (PPI) which are now consumed by many patients, leads to temporary negativity of all diagnostic tests with the exception of serology, because the antibodies remain for months. Therefore, this is the only technique which should be employed in such case if an accurate kit is available.

In this chapter, the technical aspects and the advantages and limits of the different tests will be presented, according to the classical division between invasive tests and non-invasive tests.

Invasive Tests

The invasiveness is due to the need to perform a fiberoptic endoscopy in order to get biopsies.

Despite the development of magnifying endoscopic procedures, it is still not possible to visualize *H. pylori* directly at the mucosal level. However, these techniques (magnifying Narrow Band Imaging (NBI), confocal laser endomicroscopy and endocytoscopy) offer more information on the status of the mucosa.

NBI, for example, allows the identification of mucosal patterns and predicting intestinal metaplasia or *H. pylori* infection [3]. Confocal laser endomicroscopy was able to predict *H. pylori* gastritis with a 92% accuracy [4].

Above all, these methods allow to obtain targeted biopsies.

1. Histology

Histology is the most frequently used invasive test all over the world, possibly because gastroenterologists are used to dealing with pathologists in other aspects of their specialty.

Method: The obtention of gastric biopsies must follow the Sydney system [5, 6], *i.e.* 2 antral and 2 corpus biopsies. The biopsies are immediately introduced into 10% formaldehyde used as a fixative. In the lab the biopsy specimens are paraffin embedded if possible after orientation, and thin 3 to 5 μm sections are cut at different levels. The standard hematoxylin–eosin stain allows a visualization of the bacteria but is not the best suited for detection because of the weak contrast between the bacteria and the mucus.

Several special stains which are not specific can be used. The Giemsa stain is probably one of the most frequently used because it is simple and allows a good contrast [7]. The Warthin Starry stain offers the best contrast; historically is was the stain which allowed R. Warren to detect the bacteria [8], however it is time consuming and technically costly and therefore is not commonly used.

The final step, the macroscopic observation, is very critical. The typical morphology of *H. pylori* is a comma or S-shaped bacillus observed on the epithelial surface under high magnification. The bacteria can be seen adhering to epithelial cells in the crypts or in the mucus but not in areas of intestinal metaplasia. They can be clustered in some areas of the mucosa.

Critical Aspects: The advantages of the histology technique are:

I. The fixation enables transportation without special conditions.

II. A semi-quantitative evaluation is possible.

III. The slides can be re-read, if necessary.

IV. The presence of active gastritis, a surrogate marker of *H. pylori*, may lead to a more meticulous observation in the case of the absence of the bug. This situation is more frequent now that PPIs are taken more systematically before an endoscopy is performed.

V. *Helicobacter heilmannii*, a non-culturable bacterium of zoonotic origin which is sometimes present and induces gastritis, can be detected.

VI. In the case of doubtful results, an *H. pylori* specific immunohistochemistry can be used or alternatively a fluorescent *in situ* hybridization (FISH) test [9]. These methods would allow for example to identify coccoidal forms.

The FISH method can also detect clarithromycin resistance using oligonucleotides from 23S rDNA labelled with a different fluorochrome than that used for *H. pylori* detection based on 16S rDNA (SeeFast *H. pylori* Combi Kit, SeaPro Theranostics, Lelystad, The Netherlands). PCR can be performed on archival material with the limitation that fixation may break DNA into small fragments only detectable with primers targeting short DNA fragments.

An important added value of histological observation is the capacity to describe the characteristics of the gastric mucosa in terms of inflammation, activity, atrophy, intestinal metaplasia, dysplasia, and eventually malignancy. The Sydney System originally developed for this purpose has now been completed by the OLGA [10] or OLGIM [11] system, allowing a more operational approach since combining the observations of the antrum and corpus enables an appreciation of the risk of malignancy. This allows a further decision concerning an eventual follow-up of the lesions [12].

There are, however, limits to this technique. It is crucial that the surface of the mucosa be present on the slides, because it is mainly there that the bacteria are present. The expertise of the pathologist and the time devoted to the diagnosis are also key elements. Several interobserver reproducibility tests have been published. In two series the kappa value was 0.69 and 0.74 while it was 0.39 to 0.39 in another, a value of 0.75 corresponds to an excellent reproducibility [13, 14].

Under the best conditions, the sensitivity and specificity of histology is in the range of 95%.

2. Culture

While culture is currently the most frequent method used to detect bacterial infectious diseases, this is not the case with *H. pylori*. However, historically this method led to the beginning of the story of this peculiar bacterium when it grew for the first time over the Easter weekend of 1982 [15].

Method: As for histological diagnosis, gastric biopsies are obtained during endoscopy.

The endoscope disinfection is critical, but current procedures are satisfactory. Usually only one biopsy from the antrum and one from the fundus are requested. They must be obtained before the biopsies for histology in order to avoid a possible transfer of fixative to the bacteriology container. To maintain the bacteria viable, it is important to avoid desiccation and room temperature, so the biopsies must be introduced into a transport medium usually a semi solid agar (Portagerm *pylori*, bioMérieux) and maintained at 4°C in a cool transport container. This procedure allows a delay of 24h. In the event of a longer delay before plating, freezing in a dry tube at -80°C or in liquid nitrogen are the best options.

If there is enough material it is recommended to prepare a slide to be Gram stained. It may allow to see bacteria with the typical shape of *H. pylori*.

The biopsies must be ground before plating. Indeed, the biopsies are not distributed homogeneously and grinding will increase the number of colonies to grow. The best method is to grind them in disposable rather than reusable grinders to totally eliminate the risk of contamination from patient to patient (especially with DNA if PCR has to be performed).

Only freshly prepared plates should be used in order to get the best growth potential. Different medium bases can be used, *e.g.* brucella agar, Wilkins Chalgren agar, Columbia agar, or brain heart agar with a growth supplement, either blood or serum and preferably 10% [16]. Human blood appears to give a slight advantage [17]. Numerous other growth supplements have been proposed: egg yolk, charcoal, starch, bovine serum albumin, cyclodextrin, mucins, *etc.*

In order to detect the colonies more easily, it is possible to add 2, 3, 5 triphenyltetrazolium chloride to the medium. *H. pylori* will reduce it to insoluble formazan complexes resulting in pigmented golden colonies [18].

The addition of selective supplements is also important to inhibit possible contaminating flora, either from the oral cavity or from the intestine in the case of duodenal reflux or bacterial overgrowth.

Studies of the gastric microbiota have indeed shown that bacteria other than Helicobacters can be present in the stomach including Firmicutes, Bacteroidetes, Actinobacteria and other Proteobacteria [19].

The selective supplements usually include vancomycin to inhibit gram positive bacteria; polymyxin, nalidixic acid, trimethoprim, cefsulodin to inhibit gram negative bacteria; and amphotericin to inhibit fungi.

Once plated with the ground biopsy suspension, the agar plate must be incubated quickly in a microaerobic atmosphere at 37°C. There are different ways to obtain a microaerobic atmosphere which we will not be discussed here. It must also be noted that *H. pylori* is also a capnophilic bacteria and that it can grow well in an incubator containing 10% CO_2.

At primary culture, *H. pylori* leads to small colonies after 3 days of incubation. It is important not to wait too long before subculturing because the colonies can evolve rapidly to non-viable coccoidal forms. A late subculture is often the reason for the lack of *H. pylori* growth on secondary culture for bacteriologists who are beginners in this field. In the case of a lack of growth, it is necessary to wait 10 days before concluding that the culture is negative.

Under proper conditions, subcultures grow after 2 days. This will allow further identification and antimicrobial susceptibility testing. The strains can be kept by freezing them at -80°C or in liquid nitrogen after preparing a heavy suspension in 20% glycerol broth.

When isolated from gastric biopsies, given the rare presence of other bacteria of this type, the identification is easy and includes urease, catalase and oxidase tests (all positive) in addition to microscopic examination which shows gram negative rods, not always quite curved and not very mobile. The identification can be substantiated by other enzymatic tests.

When isolated from a more complex source, *e.g.* stools or the environment, the problem is very different. The identification must be confirmed by a molecular method, *e.g.* PCR.

Besides gastric biopsies, gastric juice obtained *via* a nasogastric tube or a string test (Enterotest) has been used. These procedures are less invasive but lead to a lower sensitivity (87% *vs.* 100% for gastric biopsy culture) [20]. *H. pylori* appears to survive in gastric juice for less than 2 hours.

Culture of other Helicobacters such as *Helicobacter cinaedi* [21] or even *H. heilmannii* [22] once has been possible. Campylobacters can also be found. A special subspecies of *Campylobacter jejuni* was indeed identified for the first time in gastric biopsies. In a Japanese survey, *Campylobacter hyointestinalis*, a pig bacterium, was found in a few cases [23].

Critical Aspects: The advantages of this technique are:

1. The ability to identify a bacterium with the greatest precision.

2. The best specificity of all of the techniques currently available, allowing even whole genome sequencing if needed.

3. The possibility of performing susceptibility testing to all antibiotics which is the main added value.

4. The possibility of performing all the molecular typing methods.

5. The ability to keep the strain frozen over a long time period.

6. The possibility of having an absolute quantification of the bacteria according to the biopsy weight.

However, the limits of this technique are the stringent transport conditions and the necessity to have dedicated personnel in the bacteriology lab. These are reasons for the limited sensitivity of the technique which ideally should permit the growth of a single bacterium per specimen.

3. Rapid Urease Test (RUT)

Soon after the discovery that *H. pylori* produces urease with a high specific activity and in abundance, a test using this property was proposed and now serves as a rapid diagnostic test [24].

Method: A gastric biopsy is introduced into a special urea-rich medium. The strong urease breaks down the urea into carbon dioxide and ammonia. The ammonium ion increases the pH which leads to the change in color of the pH indicator. The first medium used was an agar based medium and the pH indicator was phenol red which changed from yellow at an acidic pH to red at a higher pH. This procedure has been marketed as the CLO test (Kimberly-Clark, Neenah, WI, USA). Among others there is a strip based test with two areas separated by a microporous membrane, one where the urease hydrolyzes urea and the other where NH_3 is trapped and changes the pH (*Pylori*Tek, Serim, Elkhart, IN, USA).

Other kits are commercially available and testing can also be performed using in-house media.

Critical Aspects: The advantages of the RUT are:

1. It is a simple method and cheap compared to the other invasive methods.

2. A quick result (2 hours for the new generation tests) can be obtained while the previously cited tests require 24 hours before concluding to negativity.

3. It is specific and allows the administration of an empiric treatment when positive.

4. A rough quantification of the bacteria present may be deduced from the time of the color change but without any great precision.

5. The RUT may also detect the urease produced by *H. heilmannii* when present in a sufficient quantity.

The main limit of this technique is its sensitivity. It appears that at least 10^5 bacteria are necessary to get a color change. The sensitivity as a primary diagnostic test may be in the range of 90% but it decreases if the test is performed one month after therapy because the bacterial load is most likely lower.

Attempts in increasing sensitivity by increasing the urea concentration, avoiding the buffer, increasing the size and number of biopsies were not successful.

Indeed, the progress of the last generation tests essentially concerned the delay in positivity.

The use of this test must definitely be restricted to gastric biopsies because in other niches, for example, the oral cavity, there are urease positive bacteria and so a positive urease test does not mean anything.

4. Molecular Methods

The method essentially used is PCR. It was developed at the time of the discovery of *H. pylori* and therefore the detection of this bacterium followed the different steps of the evolution of the method.

Standard PCR

Method: The standard method to detect *H. pylori* in gastric biopsies necessitates the design of primers targeting a gene of this bacterium in an area as specific as possible. This can be done by sequence alignment but also necessitates controlling with all of the related bacteria.

For *H. pylori* the main target genes which have been used concern the genes of the urease operon: *urea*A [25], *glm*M [26], but also the 16S rDNA gene [27], the *tsa*A gene [28] or random sequences. Previous studies show that the 16S rRNA gene is not very good for the detection of *H. pylori.* A comparison of 26 sets of primers used to detect *H. pylori* showed that all produce some false positive results [29].

PCR is performed on gastric biopsy extracts obtained by various means, either simple boiling in a lysis buffer, phenol extraction, extraction using kits (Qiagen) or apparati (MagnaPur, Arrow).

The amplicons obtained are detected by electrophoresis which shows a band at the expected molecular weight (MW). Confirmation can be obtained either by hybridization or sequencing.

The possibility to detect several targets in one reaction (multiplex PCR) allows a simultaneous diagnosis of both *H. pylori* and its eventual resistance to several antibiotics. In this respect, a kit was developed in order to detect resistance to macrolides and fluoroquinolones by strip hybridization (GenoType Helico DR, Hain Lifescience, Nehren, Germany) [30]. Another method, namely the DPO-PCR, for Dual Priming Oligonucleotide is a new PCR format that increases sensitivity and specificity by eliminating imperfect primers annealing by using primers of a special structure [31].

Standard PCR has also been used in many laboratories to detect pathogenic factors of *H. pylori*: genes of the *cag* pathogenicity island (*cag* PAI), *e.g. cag*A and *cag*E, as well as *oip*A, *dup*A, and *ice*A, genes involved in adherence (*bab*A2, *sab*A) or polymorphisms of the *vac*A gene. Multiplex PCR has also been performed for this purpose. However, the positive predictive value of the presence of these factors is not high enough to recommend performing these tests in routine.

Critical Aspects: The advantages of PCR are:

1) DNA is relatively stable and therefore, biopsies do not need special transport conditions (the PCR can even be performed on urease tests sent by post).

2) A precise quantification of the number of bacteria present can be made [32].

3) The possibility of using typing methods based on a given gene, including the CagA EPIYA phosphorylation motifs which allow to identify the East Asian strains.

4) As mentioned above, detection of resistance to certain antibiotics can be carried out as well as the detection of genes potentially involved in pathogenicity.

PCR can also be used to detect Helicobacters other than *H. pylori* and, as stated before, *H. heilmannii*. Indeed, *H. heilmannii* organisms are comprised of 2 types: *H. heilmannii* I which is a bacterium of porcine origin and is now named "candidatus *Helicobacter suis*" [33] and *H. heilmannii* II corresponding to 3 species usually present in the stomach of cats and dogs: *H. felis*, *Helicobacter salomonis* and *Helicobacter bizzozeronii*.

A multiplex PCR based on the tRNA intergenic spacers and on the urease gene has been developed to discriminate between these 3 species [34]. It can combine with a 16S rRNA gene PCR to detect "*candidatus H. suis*".

The limits of PCR lie first in the fact that Taq polymerase inhibitors can be present in the biopsy material. Fortunately it is not common. Some authors propose to include an internal control amplified by the same primers but leading to an amplicon of different size [35]. Despite this potential risk, the sensitivity of standard PCR is close to that of culture and histology.

More challenging is the risk of contamination of the environment with amplicons. This major risk explains the necessity to use different rooms to perform the different steps of the PCR and to take rigorous measures to avoid such contamination. One of the measures is to avoid carrying out nested PCR. Despite taking these precautions into account, the main risk of standard PCR is nevertheless that of false positive results altering the specificity.

Real-Time PCR

Method: The introduction of this technique has been a breakthrough in the field.

The principle is to follow the increase in amplicons formed in real time. It can be done either by using an intercalating agent, *e.g.* SYBR green I dye, or labelled probes such as those used in fluorescence resonance energy transfer (FRET) [36] or by hydrolysis of a special probe after hybridization.

For the FRET, in addition to primers which are specific to the target gene, a biprobe is also designed which binds to the amplicon. It includes 1) an acceptor probe (sensor probe) 5' labelled with LC-Red 640 designed to bind in a given area, for example, where an eventual mutation to be detected is located, and 2) a donor probe (anchor probe) 3' labelled with fluorescein, hybridizing 3 to 5 nucleotides upstream. When the anchor probe fluorophore is excited, it transfers the energy to the sensor probe fluorophore, which emits a signal. When the amplification step is finished, it is possible to perform a melting curve analysis which can show the presence of a mutation. Given that most antimicrobial resistances in *H. pylori* are the consequence of mutations it is a way to predict resistance.

The Taqman assay uses a special hybridization probe labelled with 2 fluorochromes at the 5’ end (reporter) and 3’end (quencher). The reporter signal emission is inhibited by the quencher. When the probe will hybridize, the Taq polymerase will move and hydrolyse the probe due to its 5' exonuclease activity liberating the reporter, there will be a progressive increase in fluorescence, proportionally to the amount of probe hydrolysed.

Another approach combining primer and probe in the same molecule (scorpion primers) was also developed and turned out to be highly sensitive and specific [37].

Critical Aspects: The advantages of real-time PCR are the following:

1) As with a standard PCR, this method can lose sensitivity because of the presence of Taq polymerase inhibitors. However, this is not as critical because the sensitivity of real-time PCR is higher than that of standard PCR.

2) Another big advantage of real-time PR lies in the specificity. Because all of the steps are performed in the same tube which will never be opened, the risk of amplicon contamination is low.

3) It is a quick procedure which usually can be performed within 2 to 3 hours.

4) Kits have been developed which allow a standardized procedure to be carried out (Table **1**).

5) It is a very efficient procedure for quantification of *H. pylori* in gastric biopsies with the possibility of standardization on a eucaryotic gene, *e.g.* GPDH [38].

6) It allows the detection of clarithromycin resistance and performs better than culture to detect heteroresistance.

7) Real-time PCR can be performed on other specimens than gastric biopsies, *e.g.* gastric juice or feces. The problem with feces is the low amount of *H. pylori* DNA present and the usual presence of Taq

polymerase inhibitors, *e.g.* complex polysaccharides originating from vegetable sources in the diet [39]. The DNA extraction procedure becomes crucial and even so, the sensitivity is usually lower than that on gastric biopsies.

Table 1: Molecular tests commercially available to detect *H. pylori* and its resistance to antibiotics

Test	Principle	Company
- **For Clarithromycin Resistance only**		
ClariRes assay	FRET-PCR-MCA	Engenetix, Vienna, Austria
MutaREAL *Helicobacter pylori*	FRET-PCR-MCA	Immundiagnostik AG, Bensheim, Germany
Seeplex ClaR *H. pylori* ACE Detection	DPO-PCR	Seegene, Seoul, Korea
SeaFAST *H. pylori* Combi Kit	FISH	SeaProTheranostics, Lelystad, The Netherlands
- **For Clarithromycin and Fluoroquinolone Resistance**		
GenoType HelicoDR	DNA striptest	Hain Life Science, Nehren, Germany

With regard to the oral cavity, PCR detection of *H. pylori* must be performed with at least 2 PCRs using different gene targets [40, 41]. The presence of other Epsilonproteobacteria in this only partially explored microbiota may lead to false positives if only one target, such as the urease gene, is used. The same may be true for specimens from the environment.

There are few limits to this method, one being the cost of the special thermocycler necessary to carry out the procedure, and to a small extent, a continuing risk of false positive results.

Non-Invasive Tests

1. Urea Breath Test

Method: As with the RUT, the urea breath test (UBT) is also based on the presence of a strong and abundant urease produced by *H. pylori*. This test was proposed in 1987 by Graham *et al.* using a non-radioactive isotope ^{13}C to detect *H. pylori* in humans [42].

A solution of ^{13}C labelled urea ingested by the patient is rapidly hydrolyzed by *H. pylori* urease if this bacterium is present in the stomach, labelled CO_2 is absorbed by the blood and exhaled in the expired air.

Given that the ^{13}C isotope is present at a low but variable rate in different foods, it is recommended to perform a control and so the collection of breath samples occurs before ^{13}C-urea ingestion (T_0) and usually 30 minutes after ingestion (T_{30}). The $^{13}C/^{12}C$ ratio is measured in both specimens and the result is expressed as the difference (delta over baseline (DOB) per 1,000) between the 2 measurements.

Several critical parameters have been standardized to obtain the best results. First it is advised to perform the test on an empty stomach and to ingest citric acid, used as a test meal to delay the gastric emptying [43]. It appears that citric acid may also sensitize the test *via* a direct effect on UreI, a proton-gated urea channel which makes urea more accessible to the urease [44]. Orange juice can be used as an alternative, especially in children, but does not seem to be as good [45].

Second, the dose of labelled urea has been standardized at 75 mg for an adult. This dose appears to be sufficient with regard to the urease K_{max}.

Third, the breath collection is performed after 30 minutes. This delay has been fixed to ensure avoiding the small peaks of $^{13}CO_2$ which could result from the presence of urease positive oral bacteria, and which occurs earlier. During this 30 minute delay, the patient must remain seated quietly and must not eat, drink or smoke.

Fourth, the determination of the $^{13}C/^{12}C$ ratio can be performed either on an isotope ratio mass spectrometer, requiring only a few ml of expired air (collected by blowing in a tube with a straw) [46] or on an isotope-selective non-dispersive infrared spectrometer requiring a greater amount of expired air (collected by filling a special bag) [47].

Fifth, the cut-off to define a positive sample has been drawn at 4 DOB per 1,000. According to the method used to determine the cut-off, different values are obtained, ranging from 3 to 4.9 per 1,000. The recommendation is not to consider a grey zone, rather to take the value in between. Indeed there are very few cases falling in this range of values and it is advisable to perform another test after some delay. A cut-off of 3 DOB per 1,000 has been proposed when UBT is used for treatment follow-up.

Despite this standardization, some companies are proposing tests with different quantities of labelled urea and different detection times. Examples are 100 mg urea and detection after 20 minutes (Otsuka) either in solution or as a tablet [48, 49].

It must be noted that an apparatus allowing the on-line follow-up of a $^{13}C/^{12}C$ ratio has been developed which leads to a result in a maximum of 20 minutes (Breath ID, Oridion, Israel) [50].

Another test proposed in some countries consists of the ingestion of ^{14}C-labelled urea, a radioactive isotope. There is no need for a control specimen but the volume of expired air is critical. The collection is made with a special breath card and analyzer (Heliprobe, Noster System AB, Stockholm, Sweden) [51]. The dose of ^{14}C administered is 1 μCi. Collection occurs 20 minutes after ingestion. The cut-off value to define a positive sample is 2% of the administered dose. This test cannot be used on children and pregnant women.

Critical Aspects: The advantages of the UBT are:

1) The air specimens can be transported easily and at room temperature, especially for the tubes, while the volume of the bags may be a problem.

2) The measurement is objective, *i.e.* independent of the observer.

3) The test allows a second measurement on the same tube or another tube.

4) It is very reproducible.

5) The sensitivity is good, in the range of 95% and similar to the best invasive tests. Only a few cases with a limited number of bacteria present in the stomach are missed. It gives the higher accuracy among the noninvasive tests in the systematic review of Nocon *et al.* [52].

6) The UBT also has a good specificity. Only urease positive bacteria, *e.g. H. heilmannii* can give a positive result and more seldomly other bacteria, *e.g.* Proteus, in the case of an atrophic stomach and bacterial overgrowth.

7) A semi-quantitative evaluation of the bacterial load in the stomach can be obtained and eventually predict the risk of treatment failure when the load is very high. In addition, a marked tendency to increased UBT values after failure of second line or third line therapy was noted [53].

There are, however, a few drawbacks. This test has been found to lack specificity when used in children younger than 2 years old. It can also lead to false positive results in case of bleeding.

As all of the other tests except serology, PPI consumption can negativate the test in up to 20% of the cases [54]. Therefore, PPI must be stopped during 2 weeks before performing the test [55]. It has been claimed that using a modified test meal may allow the use of a UBT even when PPI are being consumed, but these data have not been confirmed.

2. Stool Antigen Test

Method: Antigens specific to *H. pylori* can be detected in stools by using immunologic methods, especially ELISAs. The stool antigen test (SAT) is indeed a direct test in contrast to the other non-invasive tests. Culture cannot be used because, if present, *H. pylori* is not viable. PCR in stools is possible but may have a limited sensitivity due to the difficulty in DNA extraction, as indicated in the section on PCR.

The first generation of tests used polyclonal antibodies prepared against specific *H. pylori* antigens, coated on microwells and peroxidase-conjugated polyclonal antibodies to detect the immune complex.

The good results obtained initially in terms of sensitivity and specificity [56] were not confirmed in the following studies and the test was considered to be inferior to the UBT [57]. However, a new generation of SAT appeared, using monoclonal antibodies against specific *H. pylori* antigens, which led to a better accuracy and a constant quality of the reagents [58].

Attempts have also been made to develop rapid tests based on immunochromatography. While there is great interest in such tests, their accuracy is not yet sufficient to recommend their use [59].

The results of meta-analyses definitely favor the use of monoclonal antibody-based ELISAs [60]. More recently a comparison of 6 kits before and after eradication concluded that the Hp StAR EIA had the best agreement with the UBT [61].

Critical Aspects: These tests have been used essentially on patients with normal bowel movements. The impact of a short transit time should theoretically favor elimination of unaltered antigens unless there is an important dilution factor. In contrast, constipation should lead to degradation of the antigens and a lower sensitivity. This situation may be common in elderly patients and is a reason for caution when using this test in these patients.

It is also possible theoretically that enteric *Helicobacter* species, which may eventually be present in stools, share the same antigens as *H. pylori* and may therefore be detected, leading to false positive results.

Another limit in this method lies in the fact that, for cultural reasons, people may not like to give stool samples for analysis when other possibilities exist. This particular problem does not occur with children who are used to providing stools.

3. Detection of H. pylori Antibodies

Method: As with any infectious agent, *H. pylori* induces a specific systemic immune response which can be used for the diagnosis of this infection.

The method essentially employed is ELISA and its derivatives, *e.g.* rapid immunochromatographic method and immunoblotting: the former is not recommended because of its lack of accuracy [55] while the latter can be considered as a confirmatory test.

Their performances are dependent on the antigens used which vary from one kit to another. A mixture of antigens appears to be the most suitable.

The best antibodies to be looked for are IgG because *H. pylori* infection is a chronic infection. IgM may be present in the early stages but this situation is seldomly encountered. Systemic IgA may also be elevated but rarely without the presence of IgG. The IgG may take several weeks to appear after a primo infection. In contrast, after *H. pylori* eradication therapy, they may remain elevated for months or even years [62].

Critical Aspects: As stated before, the nature of the antigens used in the ELISA is important for the sensitivity of the test. A comparison of the ELISAs commercially available in France was performed and showed that only 3 kits had an accuracy in the range of 95%: *Pylori*set EIA-G (Orion Diagnostics, Espoo, Finland), *Helicobacter pylori* IgG (BioHit, Helsinki, Finland), and Enzygnost (Siemens, Eschborn, Germany) [2]. The poor reputation of serology in terms of specificity relates to the fact that 1) in some studies the reference test itself performed poorly and 2) the meta-analyses carried out included studies performed with all of the kits and not only those which are the most accurate.

Antibodies in infants and children can be at low level with the risk of false negative reactions. The same can be true in the case of an Ig deficiency.

It has been shown that antibodies against the CagA protein indeed persist for a very long time, even after the disappearance of *H. pylori* and of *H. pylori* antibodies tested globally. Veijola *et al.* using an immunoblot (Helicoblot 2.1) could still detect CagA antibodies in 87% of the patients 10 years or more after successful eradication [63]. Serology can be useful to prove the etiology of a gastric carcinoma in cases where the bacteria which initiated the process are no longer present.

The *H. pylori* antigens may vary between strains questioning the value of using the same kits worldwide. Indeed, it seems to be essentially true for the East Asian strains compared to the others, leading to the use of special kits in this area. The kits developed in Europe do not need to have a special validation when used in Europe.

Other tests which detect *H. pylori* antibodies in urine or saliva have also been proposed but their accuracy is not high enough to recommend them [55].

Serology is, in fact, a good test when proper kits are used. It is especially of interest when other tests fail because of antibiotics or PPI consumption, when there is a gastric hemorrhage, or in the event of malignancies, *e.g.* gastric MALT lymphoma or gastric adenocarcinoma [55].

"Serologic Biopsy"

Studies from Japan have highlighted the interest of measuring pepsinogen I (PGI) and II (PGII) and the PGI/II ratio in serum samples using ELISAs, in addition to *H. pylori* antibodies.

The rate of PGI and the PGI/II ratio decreases (≤70ng/ml and ≤3.0 respectively) when premalignant lesions are present in the stomach, *i.e.* atrophy and intestinal metaplasia, and can be a way to detect these lesions and follow their evolution. In combination with *H. pylori* antibodies, Miki proposed 4 categories (Table **2**) [64]. The risk of gastric cancer increases in a stepwise manner from group A to D [65]. The most alarming group corresponds to those with a low PgI/II ratio with no detectable *H. pylori* antibodies. According to the MAPS guidelines, these subjects must be followed by endoscopy every 3 years [12];

Table 2: Definition of the risk groups for precancerous conditions according to *Helicobacter pylori* serology and pepsinogen I/II ratio determination [64]

	***H. pylori* Serology**	**PG I/II Ratio**	**Risk Group**
A	Negative	Normal	None
B	Positive	Normal	*H. pylori* infection without severe atrophy
C	Positive	Decreased	*H. pylori* infection with severe atrophy
D	Negative	Decrease	Severe atrophy with extensive intestinal metaplasia

In conclusion, the diagnosis of *H. pylori* infection, while remaining difficult, has made progress this last decade, especially by the introduction of molecular methods allowing to test clarithromycin susceptibility. The use of such tests in stools is also promising but is still faced with the problem of PCR inhibitors. In addition, UBT has been confirmed as a reference test and its use has spread in most countries. Furthermore, serology, using certain kits, has been rehabilitated since we are faced with patients taking PPI.

ACKNOWLEDGEMENT

None Declared.

CONFLICT OF INTEREST

The author(s) confirm that this chapter content has no conflict of interest.

REFERENCES

[1] Megraud F, Lehours P. *Helicobacter pylori* detection and antimicrobial susceptibility testing. Clin Microbiol Rev. 2007;20:280-322.

[2] Burucoa C, Delchier JC, Courillon-Mallet A, de Korwin JD, Mégraud F, Zerbib F, Raymond J, Fauchère JL. Comparative evaluation of 29 commercial *Helicobacter pylori* serological kits. Helicobacter. 2013;18(3):169-79.

[3] Alaboudy AA, Elbahrawy A, Matsumoto S, Yoshizawa A. Conventional narrow-band imaging has good correlation with histopathological severity of *Helicobacter pylori* gastritis. Dig Dis Sci. 2011;56:1127-30.

[4] Tahara T, Shibata T, Nakamura M, Yoshioka D, Okubo M, Arisawa T, *et al.* Gastric mucosal pattern by using magnifying narrow-band imaging endoscopy clearly distinguishes histological and serological severity of chronic gastritis. Gastrointest Endos. 2009;70:246-53.

[5] Dixon MF, Genta RM, Yardley JH, Correa P. Classification and grading of gastritis. The updated Sydney System. International Workshop on the Histopathology of Gastritis, Houston 1994. Am J Surg Pathol 1996;201161-81.

[6] Price AB. The Sydney System: histological division. J Gastroenterol Hepatol 1991;6209-22.

[7] Kolts BE, Joseph B, Achem SR, Bianchi T, Monteiro C. *Helicobacter pylori* detection: a quality and cost analysis. Am J Gastroenterol 1993;88:650-5.

[8] Warren JR, Marshall B. Unidentified curved bacilli on gastric epithelium in active chronic gastritis. Lancet. 1983;i:1273-5.

[9] Trebesius K, Panthel K, Strobel S, Vogt K, Faller G, Kirchner T, *et al.* Rapid and specific detection of *Helicobacter pylori* macrolide resistance in gastric tissue by fluorescent *in situ* hybridisation. Gut. 2000;46:608-14.

[10] Rugge M, Meggio A, Pennelli G, Piscioli F, Giacomelli L, De Pretis G, *et al.* Gastritis staging in clinical practice: the OLGA staging system. Gut. 2007;56:631-6.

[11] Capelle LG, de Vries AC, Haringsma J, Ter Borg F, de Vries RA, Bruno MJ, *et al.* The staging of gastritis with the OLGA system by using intestinal metaplasia as an accurate alternative for atrophic gastritis. Gastrointest Endos. 2010;71:1150-8.

[12] Dinis-Ribeiro M, Areia M, de Vries AC, Marcos-Pinto R, Monteiro-Soares M, O'Connor A, *et al.* Management of precancerous conditions and lesions in the stomach (MAPS): guideline from the European Society of Gastrointestinal Endoscopy (ESGE), European Helicobacter Study Group (EHSG), European Society of Pathology (ESP), and the Sociedade Portuguesa de Endoscopia Digestiva (SPED). Endoscopy. 2012;44:74-94.

[13] Christensen AH, Gjorup T, Hilden J, Fenger C, Henriksen B, Vyberg M, *et al.* Observer homogeneity in the histologic diagnosis of *Helicobacter pylori*. Latent class analysis, kappa coefficient, and repeat frequency. Scand J Gastroenterol 1992;27:933-9.

[14] Santucci R, Amorosi S, Pileri S, Terranova A, Morselli AM. Observer variation in the histological assessment of *Helicobacter pylori* on gastric biopsies. Gastroenterology. 1994;106(A172).

[15] Marshall B, Warren JR. Unidentified curved bacilli on gastric epithelium in active chronic gastritis. Lancet. 1983;i:127.-1275.

[16] Megraud F, Bonnet F, Garnier M, Lamouliatte H. Characterization of "*Campylobacter pyloridis*" by culture, enzymatic profile, and protein content. J Clin Microbiol 1985;22:1007-10.

(17] Westblom TU, Madan E, Riff BR. Improved growth of *Helicobacter pylori* using a liquid medium supplemented with human serum. Ital J Gastroenterol. 1991;29((suppl. 2)):48.

[18] Queiroz DM, Mendes EN, Rocha GA. Indicator medium for isolation of *Campylobacter pylori*. J Clin Microbiol 1987;25:2378-9.

[19] Bik EM, Eckburg PB, Gill SR, Nelson KE, Purdom EA, Francois F, *et al.* Molecular analysis of the bacterial microbiota in the human stomach. Proc Nat Acad Sci USA 2006;103:732-7.

[20] Leodolter A, Wolle K, von Arnim U, Kahl S, Treiber G, Ebert MP, *et al.* Breath and string test: a diagnostic package for the identification of treatment failure and antibiotic resistance of *Helicobacter pylori* without the necessity of upper gastrointestinal endoscopy. World J Gastroenterol. 2005;11(4):584-6.

[21] Pena JA, McNeil K, Fox JG, Versalovic J. Molecular evidence of *Helicobacter cinaedi* organisms in human gastric biopsy specimens. J Clin Microbiol 2002;40:1511-3.

[22] Andersen LP, Norgaard A, Holck S, Blom J, Elsborg L. Isolation of a "*Helicobacter heilmannii*"-like organism from the human stomach. Eur J Clin Microbiol Infect Dis. 1996;15:95-6.

[23] Seo TH, Lee SY, Uchida T, Fujioka T, Jin CJ, Hwang TS, *et al.* The origin of non-*H. pylori*-related positive Giemsa staining in human gastric biopsy specimens: A prospective study. Dig Liver Dis. 2011;43:23-7.

[24] McNulty CA, Dent JC, Uff JS, Gear MW, Wilkinson SP. Detection of *Campylobacter pylori* by the biopsy urease test: an assessment in 1445 patients. Gut. 1989;30(8):1058-62

[25] Clayton C, Kleanthous K, Tabaqchali S. Detection and identification of *Helicobacter pylori* by the polymerase chain reaction. J Clin Pathol 1991;44:515-6.

[26] De Reuse H, Labigne A, Mengin-Lecreulx D. The *Helicobacter pylori ure*C gene codes for a phosphoglucosamine mutase. J Bacteriol 1997;179(11):3488-93.

[27] Hoshina S, Kahn SM, Jiang W, Green PH, Neu HC, Chin N, *et al.* Direct detection and amplification of *Helicobacter pylori* ribosomal 16S gene segments from gastric endoscopic biopsies. Diagn Microbiol Infect Dis. 1990;13:473-9.

[28] Hammar M, Tyszkiewicz T, Wadstrom T, O'Toole PW. Rapid detection of *Helicobacter pylori* in gastric biopsy material by polymerase chain reaction. J Clin Microbiol 1992;30:54-8.

[29] Sugimoto M, Wu JY, Abudayyeh S, Hoffman J, Brahem H, Al-Khatib K, *et al.* Unreliability of results of PCR detection of *Helicobacter pylori* in clinical or environmental samples. J Clin Microbiol 2009 Mar;47:738-42.

[30] Cambau E, Allerheiligen V, Coulon C, Corbel C, Lascols C, Deforges L, *et al.* Evaluation of a new test, genotype HelicoDR, for molecular detection of antibiotic resistance in *Helicobacter pylori*. J Clin Microbiol 2009;47:3600-7.

[31] Lehours P, Siffre E, Megraud F. DPO multiplex PCR as an alternative to culture and susceptibility testing to detect *Helicobacter pylori* and its resistance to clarithromycin. BMC Gastroenterology. 2011;11:112.

[32] Monteiro L, Hua J, Birac C, Lamouliatte H, Megraud F. Quantitative polymerase chain reaction for the detection of *Helicobacter pylori* in gastric biopsy specimens. Eur J Clin Microbiol Infect Dis. 1997;16):143-9.

[33] De Groote D, van Doorn LJ, Ducatelle R, Verschuuren A, Haesebrouck F, Quint WG, *et al.* '*Candidatus Helicobacter suis*', a gastric helicobacter from pigs, and its phylogenetic relatedness to other gastrospirilla. Int J Systematic Bacteriol 1999;49 Pt 4:1769-77.

[34] Baele M, Van den Bulck K, Decostere A, Vandamme P, Hanninen ML, Ducatelle R, *et al.* Multiplex PCR assay for differentiation of *Helicobacter felis*, *H. bizzozeronii*, and *H. salomonis*. J Clin Microbiol 2004;42:1115-22.

[35] Thoreson AC, Borre M, Andersen LP, Jorgensen F, Kiilerich S, Scheibel J, *et al.* *Helicobacter pylori* detection in human biopsies: a competitive PCR assay with internal control reveals false results. FEMS Immuno Med Microbiol. 1999;24:201-8.

[36] Wittwer CT, Ririe KM, Andrew RV, David DA, Gundry RA, Balis UJ. The LightCycler: a microvolume multisample fluorimeter with rapid temperature control. BioTechniques. 1997;22:176-81.

[37] Burucoa C, Garnier M, Silvain C, Fauchere JL. Quadruplex real-time PCR assay using allele-specific scorpion primers for detection of mutations conferring clarithromycin resistance to *Helicobacter pylori*. J Clin Microbiol. 2008;46:2320-6.

[38] Roussel Y, Harris A, Lee MH, Wilks M. Novel methods of quantitative real-time PCR data analysis in a murine *Helicobacter pylori* vaccine model. Vaccine. 2007;25:2919-29.

[39] Monteiro L, Bonnemaison D, Vekris A, Petry KG, Bonnet J, Vidal R, *et al.* Complex polysaccharides as PCR inhibitors in feces: *Helicobacter pylori* model. J Clin Microbiol. 1997;35:995-8.

[40] Cirak MY, Ozdek A, Yilmaz D, Bayiz U, Samim E, Turet S. Detection of *Helicobacter pylori* and its CagA gene in tonsil and adenoid tissues by PCR. Arch Otolaryngol Head Neck Surg 2003;129:1225-9.

[41] Chaudhry S, Idrees M, Izhar M, Butt AK, Khan AA. Simultaneous amplification of two bacterial genes: more reliable method of *Helicobacter pylori* detection in microbial rich dental plaque samples. Curr Microbiol. 2011;62:78-83.

[42] Graham DY, Klein PD, Evans DJ, Jr., Evans DG, Alpert LC, Opekun AR, *et al.* *Campylobacter pylori* detected noninvasively by the 13C-urea breath test. Lancet. 1987;1:1174-7.

[43] Dominguez-Munoz JE, Leodolter A, Sauerbruch T, Malfertheiner P. A citric acid solution is an optimal test drink in the 13C-urea breath test for the diagnosis of *Helicobacter pylori* infection. Gut. 1997;40:459-62.

[44] Shiotani A, Saeed A, Yamaoka Y, Osato MS, Klein PD, Graham DY. Citric acid-enhanced *Helicobacter pylori* urease activity *in vivo* is unrelated to gastric emptying. Aliment Pharmacol Ther. 2001;15:1763-7.

[45] Leodolter A, Dominguez-Munoz JE, Von Arnim U, Malfertheiner P. Citric acid or orange juice for the 13C-urea breath test: the impact of pH and gastric emptying. Aliment Pharmacol Ther. 1999;13:1057-62.

[46] Braden B, Duan LP, Caspary WF, Lembcke B. More convenient 13C-urea breath test modifications still meet the criteria for valid diagnosis of *Helicobacter pylori* infection. Z Gastroenterol. 1994;32:198-202.

[47] Koletzko S, Haisch M, Seeboth I, Braden B, Hengels K, Koletzko B, *et al.* Isotope-selective non-dispersive infrared spectrometry for detection of *Helicobacter pylori* infection with 13C-urea breath test. Lancet. 1995;345:961-2.

[48] Ohara S, Kato M, Saito M, Fukuda S, Kato C, Hamada S, *et al.* Comparison between a new 13C-urea breath test, using a film-coated tablet, and the conventional 13C-urea breath test for the detection of *Helicobacter pylori* infection. J Gastroenterol. 2004;39:621-8.

[49] Peng NJ, Lai KH, Liu RS, Lee SC, Tsay DG, Lo CC, *et al.* Capsule 13C-urea breath test for the diagnosis of *Helicobacter pylori* infection. World J Gastroenterol. 2005;11:1361-4.

[50] Israeli E, Ilan Y, Meir SB, Buenavida C, Goldin E. A novel 13C-urea breath test device for the diagnosis of *Helicobacter pylori* infection: continuous online measurements allow for faster test results with high accuracy. J Clin Gastroenterol. 2003;37:139-41.

[51] Hegedus O, Ryden J, Rehnberg AS, Nilsson S, Hellstrom PM. Validated accuracy of a novel urea breath test for rapid *Helicobacter pylori* detection and in-office analysis. Eur J Gastroenterol Hepatol. 2002;14:513-20.

[52] Nocon M, Kuhlmann A, Leodolter A, Roll S, Vauth C, Willich SN, *et al.* Efficacy and cost-effectiveness of the 13C-urea breath test as the primary diagnostic investigation for the detection of *Helicobacter pylori* infection compared to invasive and non-invasive diagnostic tests. GMS health technology assessment. 2009;5:Doc14.

[53] Buzás GM, Széles I. Interpretation of the 13C-urea breath test in the choice of second- and third-line eradication of *Helicobacter pylori* infection. J Gastroenterol. 2008;43:108-14.

[54] Leal YA, Flores LL, Fuentes-Panana EM, Cedillo-Rivera R, Torres J. 13C-urea breath test for the diagnosis of *Helicobacter pylori* infection in children: a systematic review and meta-analysis. Helicobacter. 2011;16:327-37.

[55] Malfertheiner P, Megraud F, O'Morain CA, Atherton J, Axon AT, Bazzoli F, *et al.* Management of *Helicobacter pylori* infection--the Maastricht IV/ Florence Consensus Report. Gut. 2012;61:646-64.

[56] Vaira D, Malfertheiner P, Megraud F, Axon AT, Deltenre M, Hirschl AM, *et al.* Diagnosis of *Helicobacter pylori* infection with a new non-invasive antigen-based assay. HpSA European study group. Lancet. 1999 1 3;354:30-3.

[57] Perri F, Manes G, Neri M, Vaira D, Nardone G. *Helicobacter pylori* antigen stool test and 13C-urea breath test in patients after eradication treatments. Am J Gastroenterol. 2002;972756-62.

[58] Makristathis A, Barousch W, Pasching E, Binder C, Kuderna C, Apfalter P, *et al.* Two enzyme immunoassays and PCR for detection of *Helicobacter pylori* in stool specimens

from pediatric patients before and after eradication therapy. J Clin Microbiol. 2000;383710-4.

[59] Gisbert JP, Pajares JM. Stool antigen test for the diagnosis of *Helicobacter pylori* infection: a systematic review. Helicobacter. 2004;9347-68.

[60] Gisbert JP, de la Morena F, Abraira V. Accuracy of monoclonal stool antigen test for the diagnosis of *H. pylori* infection: a systematic review and meta-analysis. Am J Gastroenterol. 2006;1011921-30.

[61] Blanco S, Forne M, Lacoma A, Prat C, Cuesta MA, Latorre I, *et al.* Comparison of stool antigen immunoassay methods for detecting *Helicobacter pylori* infection before and after eradication treatment. Diagn Microbiol Infect Dis. 2008;61150-5.

[62] Kosunen TU, Seppala K, Sarna S, Sipponen P. Diagnostic value of decreasing IgG, IgA, and IgM antibody titres after eradication of *Helicobacter pylori*. Lancet. 1992 11;339):893-5.

[63] Veijola L, Oksanen A, Sipponen P, Rautelin H. Evaluation of a commercial immunoblot, Helicoblot 2.1, for diagnosis of *Helicobacter pylori* infection. Clin Vaccine Immunol. 2008;15:1705-10.

[64] Miki K. Gastric cancer screening by combined assay for serum anti-*Helicobacter pylori* IgG antibody and serum pepsinogen levels - "ABC method". Proceedings of the Japan Academy. 2011;87:405-14.

[65] Watabe H, Mitsushima T, Yamaji Y, Okamoto M, Wada R, Kokubo T, *et al.* Predicting the development of gastric cancer from combining *Helicobacter pylori* antibodies and serum pepsinogen status: a prospective endoscopic cohort study. Gut. 2005;54:764-8.

Send Orders for Reprints to reprints@benthamscience.net
Helicobacter Pylori: A Worldwide Perspective 2014, 2014, 259-275

CHAPTER 12

Towards an Individualised Treatment of *Helicobacter pylori* Infection

Akiko Shiotani[1] and David Y. Graham[2,*]

[1]Department of Internal Medicine, Kawasaki Medical School, Okayama, Japan and [2]Department of Medicine, Michael E. DeBakey VAMC and Baylor College of Medicine, Houston, Texas, USA

Abstract: Optimal treatment of *H. pylori* should produce cure rates of at least 90%, preferably 94% or greater per protocol. Initially, 14-day triple therapy was highly successful but clarithromycin resistance led to a fall in cure rates to 80% or less. Intelligent choice of empiric therapy requires knowledge of the local or regional patterns of drug resistance and monitoring the outcome of therapy to provide early warning of development of resistance.

We recommend the following general rules 1) Do not use legacy triple therapy consisting of a PPI, clarithromycin and amoxicillin unless it has been proven to be highly effective locally; 2) Do not reduce the doses of commonly used antibiotics unless it has been shown that lower doses reliably produce eradication rates of 90% or greater; 3) The duration of therapy should be 14 days unless a shorter duration has been shown locally to produce equally high treatment success; 4) Following treatment failure avoid reuse clarithromycin or fluoroquinolones as resistance had likely developed and cannot be overcome by increasing the dose or duration of therapy; and 5) Avoid clarithromycin and fluoroquinolones in first line therapy if either has been used in the past even for a different indication. We recommend using four drug combinations as first line (*i.e.*, concomitant, hybrid, or bismuth-containing regimens). Second-line therapy should consist of antimicrobials that have not been used previously. Salvage therapy (*i.e.*, after 2 or more failures) should be chosen on the basis of the results of antimicrobial susceptibility testing.

Keywords: MALT, mucosa-associated lymphoid tissue, ITP, immune thrombocytopenic purpura, PPI, proton pump inhibitor, *H. pylori, Helicobacter pylori,*ITT, intention to treat, bLf, bovine lactoferrin*, S. boulardii, Saccharomyces boulardii.*

*Address correspondence to David Y. Graham:** Michael E. DeBakey Veterans Affairs Medical Center, Houston, USA; Tel: +1-713-795-0232; Fax: +1-713-790-1040; E-mail: dgraham@bcm.tmc.edu

BACKGROUND

Helicobacter pylori (H. pylori) is an important common human pathogen that causes acute-on-chronic progressive gastric mucosal inflammation. Progressive *H. pylori*-induced inflammation is etiologically related to chronic atrophic gastritis and its associated diseases, such as peptic ulcer, gastric cancer and gastric mucosa-associated lymphoid tissue (MALT) lymphoma, atrophic gastritis is associated with vitamin B12, iron deficiency, and reduced absorption of L-DOPA and L-thyroxine oral thyroid hormone replacement therapy [1]. The infection is also associated with other extradigestive diseases such as chronic immune thrombocytopenic purpura (ITP) [2,3].

H. pylori, like other common bacterial infections can be cured using relatively short courses of antimicrobial therapy. Although *H. pylori* is susceptible to a wide variety of antimicrobial agents *in vitro*, clinical studies have shown that, while resistance as assessed in the laboratory is associated with treatment failure, susceptibility does not always equate with treatment success. Most current anti-*H. pylori* therapies were developed by gastroenterologists and not be specialists in infectious diseases and employ a wide variety of antimicrobials and what may appear to be a random assortment of doses, dosing intervals, and treatment durations. Importantly, most common treatment regimens have never been optimized in terms of parameters such as dose or duration, susceptibility testing is infrequently available, and until recently testing for cure was not considered necessary all of which resulted in confusion regarding the best therapy(s) or the appropriate measure of treatment.

As other common treatable bacterial infections, optimized therapy of patients with susceptible organisms should reliable produce cure rates of 95% or greater per protocol. The best results have been obtained with combinations of 3 or more antimicrobial agents plus an antisecretory drug [4]. Treatment failures with of *H. pylori* infections using optimized regimens (defined as reliably yielding 95% or greater cures with susceptible organisms) can be linked to failure to take the drugs properly (poor compliance), the presence of resistance, or inappropriate alterations in the regimen such as different formulations, doses, dosing intervals, relation of dosing with meals, or duration of therapy. Because a therapy is multiantimicrobial complicates assessing the results of the effects of the presence of resistance. Susceptible bacteria interact with all of the antibiotics (*e.g.*, both amoxicillin and clarithromycin in a triple therapy) whereas resistant bacteria may interact with only one (*e.g.*, amoxicillin and not clarithromycin in clarithromycin resistance in triple therapy). For a clinical example, it was noted that the efficacy of 7 day triple therapy consisting of a proton pump inhibitor (PPI), clarithromycin and amoxicillin averaged 88% in patients with clarithromycin sensitive bacteria but was only 18% in the presence of clarithromycin resistance. Superficially, clarithromycin resistance appears to decrease the treatment success by 70% [4]. However, the effectiveness of clarithromycin in those with clarithromycin resistant strains was actually 0%. The mechanism of action of clarithromycin requires the antimicrobial bind to the organisms' ribosomes; resistance is associated with changes in the binding site such that binding is prevented or impaired and it has no effect on bacterial growth [5]. This changes the PPI, clarithromycin, amoxicillin triple therapy into a dual, PPI – amoxicillin therapy. The treatment success for the dual combination given for 7 days is approximately 20% (*i.e.*, the outcome of the triple therapy trial above). Increasing the duration of therapy of triple therapy to 14 days in the same population would have increased the treatment success to approximately 50% [6] and thus appear to reduce the adverse effects of clarithromycin resistance. One might even conclude that extending the duration of therapy would appear to have a successful strategy to partially overcome resistance. In reality, the outcome for those with clarithromycin resistant *H. pylori* would have been the same whether or not clarithromycin was included in the regimen as both triple therapy and PPI-amoxicillin dual therapy would give essentially identical results (see below for discussion of predicting the outcome in the presence of resistance).

History of Effective *H. pylori* Therapy

The first truly successful therapy (defined as reliably yielding 90% or greater) eradication consisted of the combination of a bismuth, tetracycline, and metronidazole [7]. However, that regimen proved to have reduced effectiveness in the presence of metronidazole resistance and an enhanced version consisting of the addition of a PPI, an increase in the total daily dose of metronidazole to 1,500 to 1,600 mg and a duration of 14 days resulted in a high rate of success despite the presence of metronidazole resistance [7,8]. Despite the high rate of success, widespread acceptance of bismuth-containing therapy was not forthcoming. Reservations included the requirement for dosing three or preferably four times daily, the large number of pills required, lack of availability of bismuth in many areas, and perhaps most importantly, until recently, the absence of a pharmaceutical sponsor to assist in marketing of the regimen. In contrast, triple therapy consisting of a PPI, clarithromycin, and amoxicillin (triple therapy) offered twice daily dose and major pharmaceutical support for marketing. Marketing efforts also included supporting consensus meeting in many regions designed to provide recommendations regarding therapy. Initially, 14-day triple therapy was highly successful, but a rapid increase in clarithromycin resistance led to a fall in cure rates to 80% or less (Fig. **1**) such that triple therapy is now considered an outdated legacy therapy that should only be used in regions where clarithromycin resistance is low or in patients with proven susceptible organisms (*i.e.*, as a tailored therapy).

Choice of Therapy

When deciding on the treatment of infectious disease it is generally possible to extrapolate the results from one region to another provided the conditions are similar; *H. pylori* is no exception. If the regimens (specific drugs, formulations, routes of administration, does, dosing intervals, dosing in relation to meals, and treatment duration) are the same, they would be expected to yield similar if not identical results in any other region provided the pattern of resistance was similar between the two regions. On occasion one must consider additional variables that might result in differences in outcome such as differences in the prevalence of polymorphisms of enzymes involved in metabolism of the drugs. For example, the metabolism of PPIs such as omeprazole is influenced by polymorphisms in CYP2C19 and slow metabolizers tend to have better treatment success compared to rapid metabolizers [9]. The prevalence of slow metabolizers is relatively high in Asia whereas fast metabolizers are more common in Western countries. The effect is especially seen in the presence of clarithromycin resistance where slow metabolizers exhibit improved outcome with the dual amoxicillin-PPI component of triple therapy despite the presence of clarithromycin resistance. With this exception, if one takes into account the prevalence of antimicrobial resistance, regional differences in drug metabolizing enzymes can generally be ignored clinically.

Choice of therapy can be improved by knowledge of the local or regional patterns of drug resistance. In most regions the prevalence of antimicrobial resistance in *H. pylori* is not monitored and one must use indirect assessment to identify which antibiotics are likely to a problem. Widespread use of metronidazole, macrolides or fluoroquinolones practically ensures that the prevalence of resistance to these drugs will be high. The patient's history of prior antibiotic use is particularly important in identifying drugs where resistance is likely to be a problem. One of the best techniques to select regimens is to base the choices on what has proven to be effective locally (Fig. **1**) [10].

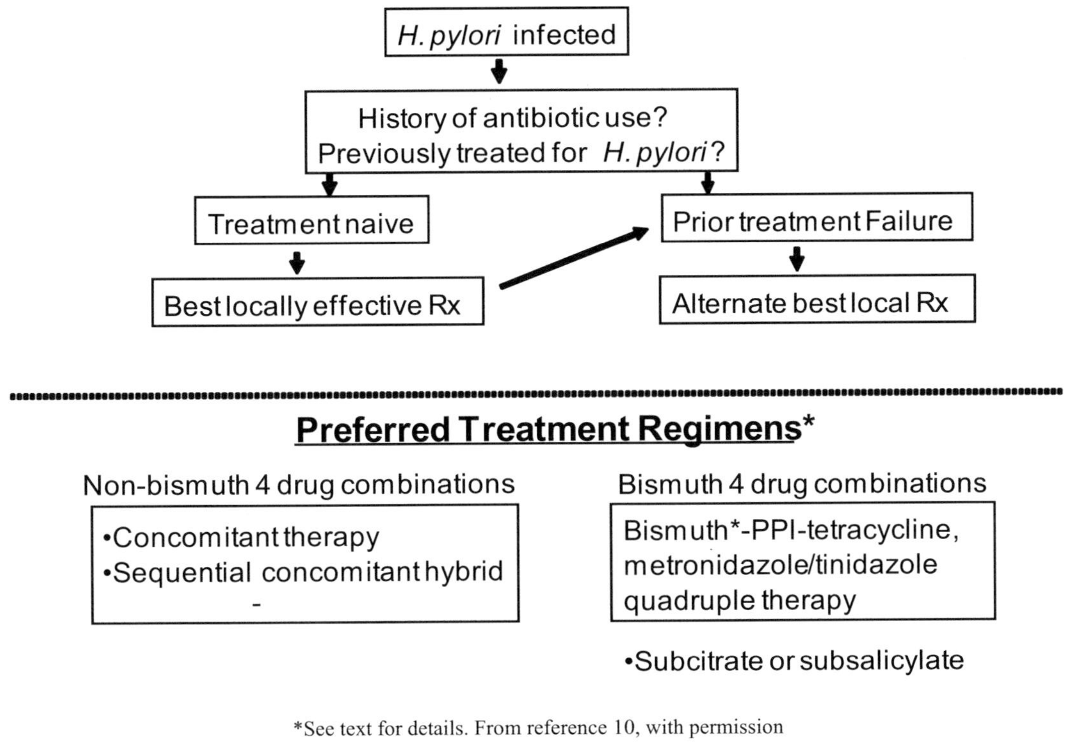

Figure 1: Suggested approach for empiric *H. pylori* therapy.

This information requires that post treatment testing for confirmation cure be done routinely, preferably with noninvasive tests. Monitoring the outcome of therapy provides clinicians with a reliable measure of the local effectiveness of particular therapies and also serves as an early warning of development of resistance[11,12].

Caveats Regarding Therapy: Drugs and Doses

The most commonly used antibiotics for the treatment of *H. pylori* infection are clarithromycin, amoxicillin, metronidazole, tinidazole, tetracycline and the fluoroquinolones (for example, levofloxacin, moxifloxacin and sitafloxacin) (Table **1**).

Table 1: Authors recommended doses of PPIs, bismuth compounds and antimicrobial agents commonly used in the *H. pylori* eradication regimens

Drug	Daily dose
Proton pump inhibitors	
Omeprazole	20 mg twice
Esomeprazole	40 mg once or 20 mg twice
Lansoprazole	30 mg once or twice
Rabeprazole	20 mg once or twice
Pantoprazole	40 mg once or twice four times
Bismuth compounds	
Bismuth subcitrate (BSC)	240 mg four times
Bismuth subsalicylate (BSS)	524 mg four times
Ranitidine bismuth citrate (RBC)	400 mg twice
Antimicrobial agents	
Amoxicillin	1,000 mg twice
Clarithromycin	500 mg twice
Metronidazole	500 mg twice or 500 mg four times
Tinidazole	500 mg twice
Tetracycline HCl	500 mg twice or four times
Rifabutine	150 mg twice
Levofloxacin	500 mg once
Moxifloxacin	400 mg once
Sitafloxacin	100 mg twice
Furazolidone	100 mg three times

Choice must always consider whether the patient is allergic to the drug as well as a drugs local availability. We recommend the following general rules [13]: 1) Do not use legacy triple therapy consisting of a PPI, clarithromycin and amoxicillin unless it has been proven to be highly effective locally (*e.g.*, eradication >90% in per-protocol analyses); 2) Use the higher of the commonly used doses of antibiotics (*e.g.,* 500 mg/dose of clarithromycin, metronidazole and tetracycline) unless it has been shown that lower doses reliably produce eradication rates of 90% or greater; 3) the duration of therapy should be 14 days unless a shorter duration has been shown locally to produce equally high treatment success; 4) following treatment failure (*i.e.*, for second line therapy) avoid reuse clarithromycin or fluoroquinolones as resistance had likely developed and cannot be overcome by increasing the dose or duration of therapy; and 5) avoid clarithromycin and fluoroquinolones in first line therapy if either has been used in the past even for a different indication.

First Line Therapies

First line therapies are those recommended for empiric use in areas where they are of proven effectiveness. Second-line therapy is given after the failure of one treatment attempt using first-line therapy. Therapy based on pretreatment susceptibility testing (*i.e.*, tailored to the infection) is always preferred but generally unavailable. When the pattern of antimicrobial resistance is unknown, clinicians should use an empiric regimen that is optimal in terms of efficacy, dose, duration, and dosing interval and proven to work well locally. In most countries we recommend using a four-drug combination as first line (*i.e.*, concomitant or bismuth-containing regimens) (Table **2**).

Table 2: Authors recommended regimens for *Helicobacter pylori* therapy

Treatment	**Drugs, Dosages and Duration**
Empiric Therapies	
Concomitant therapy	Amoxicillin (1 g), clarithromycin (500 mg), and tinidazole (500 mg) or metronidazole (500 mg) plus a PPI all given twice daily for 10–14 days
Sequential therapy (now considered obsolete)	Amoxicillin (1 g) plus a PPI twice daily for 5-7 days, followed by clarithromycin (500 mg) and tinidazole (500 mg) or metronidazole (500 mg) plus a PPI all twice daily for a further 5-7 days (total 10-14 days)
Sequential–concomitant hybrid therapy	Amoxicillin (1 g) plus a PPI twice daily for 7 days, followed by amoxicillin (1 g), clarithromycin (500 mg) and tinidazole (500 mg) or metronidazole (500 mg) for a further 7 days (total 14 days)
Bismuth quadruple therapy	Bismuth subsalicylate or bismuth subcitrate 2 tablets and tetracycline hydrochloride (500 mg) both four times daily with meals and at bedtime plus metronidazole (500 mg) or tinidazole (500 mg) three times daily with meals and a PPI twice daily preferably for 14 days.

Table 2: contd...

Tailored Therapy	
Triple therapy when *H. pylori* infection is known to be susceptible to clarithromycin	Amoxicillin (1 g) and either clarithromycin (500 mg), or tinidazole (500 mg) or metronidazole (500 mg) plus a PPI all given twice daily for 14 days
Fluroquinolone therapy when *H. pylori* is known to be susceptible to fluoroquinolones	Fluoroquinolone (*e.g.* levofloxacin 500 mg once daily), plus a PPI and amoxicillin 1 g twice daily for 14 days or Amoxicillin (1 g) plus a PPI twice daily for 5 days, followed by a fluoroquinolone (*e.g.* levofloxacin 500 mg once daily) and tinidazole (500 mg) or metronidazole (500 mg) plus a PPI all twice daily for a further 5 days (total 10 days)
Empiric Salvage Therapy	
Furazolidone quadruple therapy	Bismuth subsalicylate or bismuth subcitrate 2 tablets and tetracycline hydrochloride (500 mg) both four times daily with meals and at bedtime plus furazolidone 100 mg t.i.d., with means and PPI twice daily for 14 days
Rifabutin triple therapy	Rifabutin (150 mg daily), amoxicillin (1.5 g q.8.h., and a pantoprazole 80 mg (or an equivalent PPI) q.8.h. for 12 days
High dose PPI-amoxicillin dual therapy	PPI (*e.g.* omeprazole [40 mg] or lansoprazole [30 mg]) plus amoxicillin (500 mg) all four times daily at approximately 6 h intervals for 14 days (can used 8 hour interval at night)

Sequential – Concomitant – Hybrid Sequential Concomitant First Line Therapies

Sequential therapy is a two part 10-day regimen in which a PPI plus amoxicillin is given for 5 or preferably 7 days followed by a PPI plus clarithromycin and metronidazole (or tinidazole) for an additional 5 or preferably 7 days [14]. Sequential therapy is now considered obsolete as 14 day concomitant therapy will always be equal or most often superior. Concomitant therapy uses the same 4 drugs but they are all given simultaneously for the full duration of therapy. Concomitant therapy is also preferred as it is less complex as it does not require the patient to switch from a dual to a triple therapy at the half way point. Both sequential and concomitant therapies provide success rates of 90 to 94% in the presence of moderate levels of clarithromycin resistance (*e.g.* below 20%) sequential therapy is sensitive to metronidazole resistance. Both sequential and concomitant therapies are ineffective in the presence of dual clarthromycin and metronidazole resistance [15-18]. In countries where clarithromycin and metronidazole resistance are common, sequential therapy has proven to be ineffective (*e.g.*, 78% eradication with 10-day sequential therapy) and is not recommended [19, 20].

The choice of 10-day duration for sequential therapy was arbitrary and the average result is between 90 and 94% success in the face of moderate clarithromycin resistance. Extending the duration of sequential therapy to 14 days (7 days plus 7 days) instead improved the outcome [21]. However, hybrid sequential–concomitant therapy in which the duration was extended to 14 days and the amoxicillin was also given throughout provided 99% treatment success in per protocol suggesting that this combination may be the ideal use of these 4 drugs [22] except in populations with a high prevalance of clarithromycin and metronidazole resistance.

Bismuth-Containing 4 Drug Regimens First Line Therapies

As noted above bismuth triple therapy was the first successful regimen but evolved into bismuth quadruple therapy to overcome the problem of metronidazole resistance. Metronidazole is a prodrug that is activated by bacterial enzymes to become an antimicrobial. It differs from clarithromycin and fluoroquinolones in that there are a number of enzymes that can active the drug, the local concentration is very high such that resistance as assessed *in vitro* may not correlate with what is achieved *in vivo*. Clinical studies have shown that metronidazole resistance can be partially or even largely overcome by increasing the duration of therapy and administering 1,500 to 1,600 mg of metronidazole daily in divided doses. Bismuth quadruple therapy has often been given at inappropriately low doses or shorter durations especially when compared directly against standard clarithromycin-containing triple therapy where both regimens generally faired poorly with unacceptably low treatment success (equally bad results) [23,24]. In contrast, when given in full doses for 10-14 days treatment results have generally been excellent [11, 25-28]. Several studies have suggested that twice a day quadruple therapy (given at the noon and evening meals) may also be effective [29-31] and additional studies in populations with high prevalence metronidazole resistance are needed to confirm these results.

Approach After One Treatment Failure

Ideally, choice of antimicrobials would be based on the results of susceptibility testing. If that is not available, the preferred empiric approach for second-line therapy is to choose a therapy that contains antimicrobials that have not been used previously. As such if a clarithromycin-containing 4 drug therapy was used initially, the second line would be (if available) bismuth quadruple therapy and *vice versa*. This approach is consistent with the general rule that previously used antimicrobials to which resistance commonly occurs and cannot be overcome by increasing the dose/duration of therapy should not be reused (*e.g.*, macrolides and fluoroquinolones). Other options generally include a fluoroquinolone-containing sequential or triple therapy or rifabutin-containing triple therapy, or therapies tailored to the antimicrobial susceptibility pattern of the patient.

In general we do not recommend repeating the same regimen after one treatment failure. The one exception is bismuth quadruple therapy is often effective after one treatment failure. Sequential and concomitant treatments expose the patient to both clarithromycin and metronidazole (or tinidazole) so there is little to be gained from switching from one to the other or after failure of triple therapy and bismuth quadruple therapy.

Fluoroquinolone-Containing Therapies

Levofloxacin may be used as a substitute for clarithromycin in either a standard triple or sequential therapy. A large study comparing the antibiotics in either regimen shows a clear advantage to levofloxacin with no difference in compliance rates or adverse events in both standard triple and sequential combinations. A recent randomized, multicenter study involving 375 patients in an area of high prevalence (*i.e.,* 15-20%) of clarithromycin resistant *H. pylori* strains investigated the efficacy of a 10-day levofloxacin-containing sequential therapy which substituted levofloxacin (250 mg or 500 mg twice daily). The eradication rate of with 250 mg twice daily levofloxacin-containing sequential therapy by ITT analysis was 96% and superior to clarithromycin -containing sequential therapy (81%) in the same population [32]. However, the main disadvantage with use of levofloxacin-containing therapies is the rapid emergence of resistance to fluoroquinolones. Worldwide the prevalence of quinolone resistant *H. pylori* is rising rapidly in concert with the increased use of these agents of other indications [33].

Fluoroquinolone triple therapy is widely used as second line therapy. Early studies showed unequivocally that 7 and 10-day regimens of a PPI, amoxicillin and fluoroquinolone failed to reliably produce acceptable cure rates [34]. Recently, a study of 14-day fluoroquinolone triple therapy produced 95% cures compared to 78.9% with 7-day therapy suggesting that therapy should be at least for 14 days [35].

Rifabutin-Containing Therapy

A recent review of rifabutin-containing therapies (generally, a PPI, amoxicillin 1 gram and rifabutin 150 mg, all b.i.d.) shows average cure rates of below 80% (typically in the mid-70%'s)[36]. These are not very encouraging results and suggest that at the least, rifabutin triple therapy has not yet been optimized. One high dose regimen reported >95% success with a 12-day therapy consisting of 150 mg of rifabutin once daily (half dose), amoxicillin 1.5 g t.i.d. and pantoprazole 80 mg t.i.d. [37]. These results have not been confirmed but the regimen is worth considering (Table **2**). However, rifabutin is limited as a treatment option by a number of factors. Greater use of rifabutin in the treatment of *H. pylori* could potentially result in the development of more resistant strains of *Mycobacterium tuberculosis*. In addition, serious myelotoxicity and ocular adverse events have been reported with this treatment although they are uncommon and may be greatly reduced by not starting with full dose (*e.g.*, 300 mg or more) therapy [38,39].

Treatment After Multiple Treatment Failures with Different Antimicrobials – Salvage Therapy

Salvage therapy is a therapy given after multiple treatment failures with different regimens. Ideally, it should be chosen on the basis of the results of anti microbial susceptibility testing. One possibility is furazolidone quadruple therapy.

Furazolidone is a synthetic nitrofuran derivative, which has an antibacterial and antiprotozoal efficacy against many gram-negative enteric organisms. Furazolidone is available in many parts of the world but is largely unavailable in most Western countries. It is an old and often unfairly maligned drug that was widely used in animals but was withdrawn for that use because of its tendency to remain in the tissue and thus inadvertently expose humans [40,41]. It is also a monoamine oxidase inhibitor and thus interacts with many drugs and foods (*e.g.*, soy sauce, aged cheeses, *etc.*) leading to a relatively high rate of side effects. Like rifabutin, a general review of its use showed that overall high cure rates were often not obtained [40]. Nonetheless, in our experience, the furazolidone-containing bismuth quadruple therapy is highly effective and is recommended where available.

Personalized approaches include therapy based on susceptibility testing and carefully consideration of what drugs the patient has taken. Resistance to tetracycline, amoxicillin, rifabutin and furazolidone are rare. Resistance to bismuth probably does not occur. Increased doses of PPI generally improve treatment results as does extending the duration of therapy to 14 (or possibly more) days. In the absence of multiple drug allergies, it is generally possible for an experienced *H. pylori* therapist to come up with an effective regimen.

Use of Adjuvants and Probiotics

There is considerable interest in probiotics to enhance effectiveness of antimicrobial therapy for *H. pylori* by increasing tolerability, and reducing side effects and therefore improving compliance. Probiotics are microorganisms that help maintain normal gut flora and prevent colonization by pathogenic organisms *via* a number of mechanisms, including competitive inhibition of gut wall adhesion of pathogenic microorganisms and generalized immune system enhancement because of the ability of probiotics to bind to epithelial cells [42-44]. A randomized prospective study indicated adding 100 mg of bovine lactoferrin (bLf) and probiotics to the standard triple therapy for *H. pylori* infection improved eradication rate (72.5% to 88.6% by ITT analysis) [45]. In meta-analysis of 14 randomized trials (n = 1671), pooled *H. pylori* eradication rates were 83.6% (95% CI. 80.5–86.7%) and 74.8% (95% CI.71.1–78.5%) for patients with or without probiotics by ITT analysis, respectively [46].

Saccharomyces boulardii (*S. boulardii)* is another useful adjunct. In a cohort of patients in Korea who received *S. boulardii* for 4 weeks during and after a 1-week course of standard triple therapy, eradication rates were 10% better than for those who did not receive the supplement [47]. A meta-analysis recently published illustrated that supplementation with *S. boulardii* significantly increased the eradication rate and reduced the risk of overall *H. pylori* therapy-related adverse effects especially diarrhea [48]. Pronase and N-acetyl cysteine have been used to change the mucus layer and potentially expose the bacteria. In a single trial, pronase given as 18,000 tyrosine units of pronase twice daily for 2 weeks significantly increased the effectiveness of legacy triple therapy (*e.g.,* from 76.5 to 94%) [49]. The effect of other probiotics such as Lactobacillus acidophilus, *Bifidobacterium*-containing yoghurt is less well described, however, probiotics may produce a significant reduction of the incidence of eradication regimen-related side effects. Probiotics are not inexpensive and thus cost will need to be taken into consideration, especially if the benefits are minor.

ACKNOWLEDGEMENTS

Dr. Graham is supported in part by the Office of Research and Development Medical Research Service Department of Veterans Affairs, Public Health Service grant DK56338. which funds the Texas Medical Center Digestive Diseases Center, DK067366 and CA116845. The contents are solely the responsibility of the authors and do not necessarily represent the official views of the VA or NIH. Dr. Graham is a unpaid consultant for Novartis in relation to vaccine development for treatment or prevention of *H. pylori* infection. Dr. Graham is a also a paid consultant to RedHill Biopharma regarding novel *H. pylori* therapies and to Otsuka Pharmaceuticals Japan regarding diagnostic testing. Dr. Graham has received royalties from the Baylor College of Medicine for patents covering materials related to ^{13}C-urea breath test.

CONFLICT OF INTEREST

Dr. Shiotani has nothing to declare.

REFERENCES

[1] Lahner E, Annibale B, Delle FG. Systematic review: *Helicobacter pylori* infection and impaired drug absorption. Aliment Pharmacol Ther 2009;29:379-86.

[2] Malfertheiner P, Megraud F, O'Morain C, *et al.* Current concepts in the management of *Helicobacter pylori* infection: the Maastricht III Consensus Report. Gut 2007;56:772-781.

[3] Kandulski A, Selgrad M, Malfertheiner P. *Helicobacter pylori* infection: a clinical overview. Dig Liver Dis 2008;40:619-26.

[4] Fischbach LA, Goodman KJ, Feldman M, Aragaki C. Sources of variation of *Helicobacter pylori* treatment success in adults worldwide: a meta-analysis. Int J Epidemiol 2002;31:128-39

[5] Megraud F. *H. pylori* antibiotic resistance: prevalence, importance, and advances in testing. Gut 2004;53:1374-84.

[6] Zagari RM, Bianchi-Porro G, Fiocca R, Gasbarrini G, Roda E, Bazzoli F. Comparison of 1 and 2 weeks of omeprazole, amoxicillin and clarithromycin treatment for *Helicobacter pylori* eradication: the HYPER Study. Gut 2007;56:475-9.

[7] Borody TJ, Andrews P, Fracchia G, Brandl S, Shortis NP, Bae H. Omeprazole enhances efficacy of triple therapy in eradicating *Helicobacter pylori.* Gut 1995;37:477-81.

[8] de Boer WA. How to achieve a near 100% cure rate for *H. pylori* infection in peptic ulcer patients. A personal viewpoint. J Clin Gastroenterol 1996;22:313-6.

[9] Furuta T, Graham DY. Pharmacologic aspects of eradication therapy for *Helicobacter pylori* Infection. Gastroenterol Clin North Am 2010;39:465-80.

[10] Graham DY, Rimbara E. *Helicobacter pylori* therapy in the West. Japanese Journal of Helicobacter Research 2012;13:40-5.

[11] Rimbara E, Fischbach LA, Graham DY. Optimal therapy for *Helicobacter pylori* infections. Nat Rev Gastroenterol Hepatol 2011;8:79-88.

[12] Graham DY, Shiotani A. New concepts of resistance in the treatment of *Helicobacter pylori* infections. Nat Clin Pract Gastroenterol Hepatol 2008;5:321-31.

[13] Graham DY, Fischbach L. *Helicobacter pylori* treatment in the era of increasing antibiotic resistance. Gut, 2010; 9:143-1153.

[14] Zullo A, Rinaldi V, Winn S, *et al.* A new highly effective short-term therapy schedule for *Helicobacter pylori* eradication. Aliment Pharmacol Ther 2000;14:715-8.

[15] Essa AS, Kramer JR, Graham DY, Treiber G. Meta-analysis: four-drug, three-antibiotic, non-bismuth-containing "concomitant therapy" *vs.* triple therapy for *Helicobacter pylori* eradication. Helicobacter 2009;14:109-18.

[16] Gisbert JP, Calvet X, O'Connor A, Megraud F, O'Morain CA. Sequential therapy for *Helicobacter pylori* eradication: a critical review. J Clin Gastroenterol 2010;44:313-25.

[17] Gatta L, Vakil N, Leandro G, Di Mario F, Vaira D. Sequential therapy or triple therapy for *Helicobacter pylori* infection: systematic review and meta-analysis of randomized controlled trials in adults and children. Am J Gastroenterol 2009;104:3069-79.

[18] Jafri NS, Hornung CA, Howden CW. Meta-analysis: sequential therapy appears superior to standard therapy for *Helicobacter pylori* infection in patients naive to treatment. Ann Intern Med 2008;148:923-31.

[19] Nadir I, Yonem O, Ozin Y, Kilic ZM, Sezgin O. Comparison of two different treatment protocols in *Helicobacter pylori* eradication. South Med J 2011;104:102-5.

[20] Wu DC, Hsu PI, Wu JY,*et al.* Sequential and concomitant therapy with four drugs is equally effective for eradication of *H. pylori* infection. Clin Gastroenterol Hepatol 2010;8:36-41 e1.

[21] Liou JM, Chen CC, Chen MJ *et al.* Sequential *versus* triple therapy for the first-line treatment of *Helicobacter pylori*: a multicentre, open-label, randomised trial. Lancet 2013;381:205-213.

[22] Hsu PI, Wu DC, Wu JY, Graham DY. Modified sequential *Helicobacter pylori* therapy: proton pump inhibitor and amoxicillin for 14 days with clarithromycin and metronidazole added as a quadruple (hybrid) therapy for the final 7 days. Helicobacter 2011;16:139-45

[23] Luther J, Higgins PD, Schoenfeld PS, Moayyedi P, Vakil N, Chey WD. Empiric quadruple *vs.* triple therapy for primary treatment of *Helicobacter pylori* infection: Systematic review and meta-analysis of efficacy and tolerability. Am J Gastroenterol 2010;105:65-73.

[24] Graham DY, Dore MP. The QUADRATE study: a proposal for a change in the reporting of pharmaceutical supported trials. Gastroenterology 2003;125:639.

[25] Fischbach L, Evans EL. Meta-analysis: the effect of antibiotic resistance status on the efficacy of triple and quadruple first-line therapies for *Helicobacter pylori*. Aliment Pharmacol Ther 2007;26:343-57.

[26] Fischbach LA, van ZS, Dickason J. Meta-analysis: the efficacy, adverse events, and adherence related to first-line anti-*Helicobacter pylori* quadruple therapies. Aliment Pharmacol Ther 2004;20:1071-82.

[27] Laine L, Hunt R, El Zimaity H, Nguyen B, Osato M, Spenard J. Bismuth-based quadruple therapy using a single capsule of bismuth biskalcitrate, metronidazole, and tetracycline given with omeprazole *vs.* omeprazole, amoxicillin, and clarithromycin for eradication of *Helicobacter pylori* in duodenal ulcer patients: a prospective, randomized, multicenter, North American trial. Am J Gastroenterol 2003;98:562-7.

[28] Malfertheiner P, Bazzoli F, Delchier JC, *et al. Helicobacter pylori* eradication with a capsule containing bismuth subcitrate potassium, metronidazole, and tetracycline given with omeprazole *vs.* clarithromycin-based triple therapy: a randomised, open-label, non-inferiority, phase 3 trial. Lancet 2011;377:905-13.

[29] Dore MP, Marras L, Maragkoudakis E, *et al.* Salvage therapy after two or more prior *Helicobacter pylori* treatment failures: the super salvage regimen. Helicobacter 2003;8:307-9.

[30] Dore MP, Farina V, Cuccu M, Mameli L, Massarelli G, Graham DY. Twice-a-day bismuth-containing quadruple therapy for *Helicobacter pylori* eradication: a randomized trial of 10 and 14 days. Helicobacter 2011;16:295-300.

[31] Graham DY, Belson G, Abudayyeh S, Osato MS, Dore MP, El-Zimaity HM. Twice daily (mid-day and evening) quadruple therapy for *H. pylori* infection in the United States. Dig Liver Dis 2004;36:384-7.

[32] Romano M, Cuomo A, Gravina AG, *et al.* Empirical levofloxacin-containing *vs.* clarithromycin-containing sequential therapy for *Helicobacter pylori* eradication: a randomised trial. Gut 2010;59:1465-70.

[33] Glocker E, Stueger HP, Kist M. Quinolone resistance in *Helicobacter pylori* isolates in Germany. Antimicrob Agents Chemother 2007;51:346-9.

[34] Saad RJ, Schoenfeld P, Kim HM, Chey WD. Levofloxacin-based triple therapy *vs.* bismuth-based quadruple therapy for persistent *Helicobacter pylori* infection: a meta-analysis. Am J Gastroenterol 2006;101:488-96.

[35] Miehlke S, Krasz S, Schneider-Brachert W, *et al.* Randomized Trial on 14 *vs.* 7 days of Esomeprazole, Moxifloxacin, and Amoxicillin for Second-line or Rescue Treatment of *Helicobacter pylori* Infection. Helicobacter 2011;16:420-6.

[36] Gisbert JP, Calvet X. Review article: rifabutin in the treatment of refractory *Helicobacter pylori* infection. Aliment Pharmacol Ther 2012;35:209-21.

[37] Borody TJ, Pang G, Wettstein AR, *et al.* Efficacy and safety of rifabutin-containing 'rescue therapy' for resistant *Helicobacter pylori* infection. Aliment Pharmacol Ther 2006;23:481-8.

[38] Apseloff G. Severe neutropenia among healthy volunteers given rifabutin in clinical trials. Clin Pharmacol Ther 2003;74:591-2.

[39] Bhagat N, Read RW, Rao NA, Smith RE, Chong LP. Rifabutin-associated hypopyon uveitis in human immunodeficiency virus-negative immunocompetent individuals. Ophthalmology 2001;108:750-2.

[40] Zullo A, Ierardi E, Hassan C, De F, V. Furazolidone-based therapies for *Helicobacter pylori* infection: A pooled-data analysis. Saudi J Gastroenterol 2012;18:11-7.

[41] Graham DY, Lu H. Furazolidone in *Helicobacter pylori* therapy: Misunderstood and often unfairly maligned drug told in a story of French bread. Saudi J Gastroenterol 2012;18:1-2.

[42] Cremonini F, Di Caro S, Nista EC, *et al.* Meta-analysis: the effect of probiotic administration on antibiotic-associated diarrhoea. Aliment Pharmacol Ther 2002;16:1461-7.

[43] Kale-Pradhan PB, Jassal HK, Wilhelm SM. Role of *Lactobacillus* in the prevention of antibiotic-associated diarrhea: a meta-analysis. Pharmacotherapy 2010;30:119-26.

[44] McFarland LV. Meta-analysis of probiotics for the prevention of antibiotic associated diarrhea and the treatment of *Clostridium difficile* disease. Am J Gastroenterol 2006;101:812-22.

[45] de Bortoli N, Leonardi G, Ciancia E, *et al.* *Helicobacter pylori* eradication: a randomized prospective study of triple therapy *vs.* triple therapy plus lactoferrin and probiotics. Am J Gastroenterol 2007;102:951-6.

[46] Tong JL, Ran ZH, Shen J, Zhang CX, Xiao SD. Meta-analysis: the effect of supplementation with probiotics on eradication rates and adverse events during *Helicobacter pylori* eradication therapy. Aliment Pharmacol Ther 2007;25:155-68.

[47] Song MJ, Park DI, Park JH,*et al.* The effect of probiotics and mucoprotective agents on PPI-based triple therapy for eradication of *Helicobacter pylori*. Helicobacter 2010;15:206-13.

[48] Szajewska H, Horvath A, Piwowarczyk A. Meta-analysis: the effects of *Saccharomyces boulardii* supplementation on *Helicobacter pylori* eradication rates and side effects during treatment. Aliment Pharmacol Ther 2010;32:1069-79.

[49] Gotoh A, Akamatsu T, Shimizu T, *et al.* Additive effect of pronase on the efficacy of eradication therapy against *Helicobacter pylori*. Helicobacter 2002;7:183-91.

Send Orders for Reprints to reprints@benthamscience.net

Helicobacter Pylori: A Worldwide Perspective 2014, 2014, 276-279

CHAPTER 13

Helicobacter pylori Infection and Functional Dyspepsia: Epidemiology, Diagnosis and Current Treatment

Marko Duvnjak*, Ivan Lerotić, Neven Baršić and Vedran Tomašić

Department of Gastroenterology and Hepatology Sestre Milosrdnice University Hospital Center Zagreb, Croatia

Abstract: Dyspepsia comprises a group of symtpoms including epigastric pain, burning, postprandial fullness and early satiation. Its prevalence in general population ranges from 10 to 40%. Functional dyspepsia prevalence estimates are 5-12%. The relationship between *Helicobacter pylori* and functional dyspepsia is complicated. There are no differences between infected and uninfected patients in prevalence and severity of dyspepsia. The meta-analysis of the efficacy of eradication therapy in functional dyspepsia showed a small but significant benefit in curing dyspeptic symptoms after one year therapeutic gain in comparison with placebo was 8% and the number of patients needed to treat was 15. According to the Maastricht IV guidelines, eradication therapy is considered appropriate for patients that have a confirmed *Helicobacter pylori* infection and a diagnosis of functional dyspepsia (recommendation grade: A).

Keywords: Dyspepsia, functional dyspepsia, *H. pylori*, eradication treatment, endoscopy.

INTRODUCTION

Dyspepsia is defined as a group of symptoms that include epigastric pain, epigastric burning, postprandial fullness and early satiation. When there are no structural or organic causes that could explain these symptoms, dyspepsia is considered to be functional. The prevalence of dyspepsia in general population ranges from 10 to 40%, varying largely due to the heterogeneity of definitions used in the studies. When only functional dyspepsia is considered, prevalence estimates are 5-12% [1]. *Helicobacter pylori* (*H. pylori*) is considered to be one of

***Address correspondence to Marko Duvnjak:** Department of Gastroenterology and Hepatology Sestre Milosrdnice University Hospital Center, Zagreb, Croatia; Tel: +36-513-784-448; Fax: +38-513-787-448; E-mail: marko.duvjnak1@gmail.com

Buzás György Miklós (Ed.)

the most common worldwide infections. Estimations report that almost half of the world population is infected [2]. The infection, after it is acquired, can persist in the stomach with or without causing a gastroduodenal disease.

It is clearly associated with a broad variety of chronic gastrointestinal diseases such as chronic gastritis, peptic ulcer disease, gastric carcinoma, and MALT lymphoma – disorders that can all present with dyspeptic symptoms (structural dyspepsia). On the other hand, relationship between *H. pylori* infection and functional dyspepsia is complicated. Many studies have failed to demonstrate differences between *H. pylori* positive and *H. pylori* negative patients in dyspepsia prevalence, severity of dyspeptic symptoms or more specific findings like altered perception of gastric distension [3-5]. However, a meta-analysis of the efficacy of *H. pylori* eradication therapy in functional dyspepsia demonstrated that eradication of *H. pylori* provides a humble but statistically significant benefit in curing symptoms of dyspepsia after one year and can be cost-effective [6].

Therapeutic gain in comparison with placebo was 8% and the number of patients needed to treat was 15 (NNT 15, 95% CI 10-28). This is still better than any other treatment for functional dyspepsia and when effective, it can lead to a lasting improvement of symptoms. Currently, there are no prognostic models which could help identify which patients would benefit most from treatment. Still, there are additional reasons for eradication of *H. pylori* in patients that are diagnosed with functional dyspepsia that are related to the prevention of peptic ulcer disease and gastric malignancies. In summary, eradication therapy is considered appropriate for patients that have a confirmed *H. pylori* infection and a diagnosis of functional dyspepsia which is a grade A recommendation in Maastricht IV guidelines on *H. pylori* infection [7]. When approaching a patient with dyspepsia in clinical practice, usually the most important questions are when to test for *H. pylori* infection and when to perform the upper GI endoscopy. In populations with high *H. pylori* infection prevalence, detection and eradication of *H. pylori* in patients with dyspeptic symptoms are justified. There are two alternative approaches regarding the use of endoscopy. In younger patients (<45 years) with dyspeptic symptoms and no 'alarm' symptoms (dysphagia/odynophagia, gastrointestinal bleeding, iron deficiency anemia, involuntary weight loss, frequent vomiting, palpable abdominal mass, family history of gastric malignancies), 'test and treat' approach is recommended - testing for *H. pylori* infection with one of noninvasive methods (urea breath test, stool antigen testing, serology) and eradication in positive cases [7] This approach can significantly reduce (up to 60%) the number of unnecessary endoscopies, which avoids several problems related to the procedure - patient discomfort due to invasive nature of the procedure, procedure costs, unnecessary ambulatory patient visits, long waiting lists [8]. Patients above 45 years of age as well as patients that have so called alarm symptoms regardless of their age need to undergo upper GI endoscopy as a part of their dyspepsia work- up, primarily with the purpose of tumor detection ('scope and treat' approach) [7]. This approach has several advantages, including prompt and accurate diagnosis, consequent reduction of symptoms and abolishment of fear from malignant disease. This is demonstrated by the finding of marginally higher percentage of patients without symptoms after one year with this approach, compared to patients that underwent only noninvasive testing [9]. However, most studies have concluded that there were no significant differences between these two approaches regarding the percentage of patients that were without symptoms, had better quality of life and reduced primary care visits or reduced hospitalizations [8].

ACKNOWLEDGEMENT

None declared.

CONFLICT OF INTEREST

The author(s) confirm that this chapter content has no conflict of interest.

REFERENCES

[1] El-Serag HB, Talley NJ. Systemic review: the prevalence and clinical course of functional dyspepsia. Aliment Pharmacol Ther. 2004 Mar 15;19:643-54.

[2] Pounder RE, Ng D. The prevalence of *Helicobacter pylori* infection in different countries. Aliment Pharmacol Ther. 1995;9 Suppl 2:33-9.

[3] Tucci A, Corinaldesi R, Stanghellini V, Tosetti C, Di Febo G, Paparo GF, Varoli O, Paganelli GM, Labate AM, Masci C, *et al. Helicobacter pylori* infection and gastric function in patients with chronic idiopathic dyspepsia. Gastroenterology. 1992;103:768-74.

[4] Saslow SB, Thumshirn M, Camilleri M, Locke GR 3rd, Thomforde GM, Burton DD, Hanson RB. Influence of *H. pylori* infection on gastric motor and sensory function in asymptomatic volunteers. Dig Dis Sci. 1998;43:258-64.

[5] Mearin F, de Ribot X, Balboa A, Salas A, Varas MJ, Cucala M, Bartolomé R, Armengol JR, Malagelada JR. Does *Helicobacter pylori* infection increase gastric sensitivity in functional dyspepsia? Gut. 1995;37:47.

[6] Moayyedi P, Deeks J, Talley NJ, Delaney B, Forman D. An update of the Cochrane systematic review of *Helicobacter pylori* eradication therapy in nonulcer dyspepsia: resolving the discrepancy between systematic reviews. Am J Gastroenterol. 2003;98:2621-6.

[7] Malfertheiner P, Megraud F, O'Morain CA, *et al.* Management of *Helicobacter pylori* infection-the Maastricht IV/Florence Consensus Report. Gut 2012;61:646-664.

[8] Lassen AT, Pedersen FM, Bytzer P, *et al. Helicobacter pylori* test-and-eradicate *vs.* prompt endoscopy for management of dyspeptic patients: a randomised trial. Lancet. 2000;356(9228):455-60.

[9] Ford AC, Qume M, Moayyedi P, *et al. Helicobacter pylori* "test and treat" or endoscopy for managing dyspepsia: an individual patient data meta-analysis. Gastroenterology. 2005;128(7):1838-44.

Send Orders for Reprints to reprints@benthamscience.net

Helicobacter Pylori: A Worldwide Perspective 2014, 2014, 280-315

CHAPTER 14

The Contribution of Meta-Analyses to the Treatment of *Helicobacter pylori*

Javier P. Gisbert*

Department of Gastroenterology and Centro de Investigación Biomédica en Red de Enfermedades Hepáticas y Digestivas (CIBEREHD), Hospital Universitario de La Princesa, Instituto de Investigación Sanitaria Princesa (IP), Madrid, Spain

Abstract: After 30 years of experience in *Helicobacter pylori* treatment, however, the ideal regimen to treat this infection has still to be found. Systematic reviews and meta-analyses are essential to summarize evidence relating to efficacy and safety of health care interventions accurately and reliably. The aim of this chapter is to review published meta-analyses focused on *H. pylori* eradication treatments. Initially, dual therapies containing one antibiotic combined with bismuth compounds or proton pump inhibitors (PPIs) obtained sub-optimal cure rates. The most recommended therapies have been triple therapies containing a PPI and two antibiotics. PPI-based regimens are more effective than H_2-antagonists-based ones. Bismuth-containing quadruple therapy is roughly equivalent to triple therapy in terms of effectiveness, compliance and safety profile. The influence of the type of PPI, the dosage and the length of treatment have been discussed. Clarithromycin and metronidazole antibiotic resistance are the most relevant factors causing eradication failure. As a progressive decrease in the eradication rate after standard triple therapy has been reported, more recently, sequential and non-bismuth quadruple (concomitant) therapies have been recommended in settings where the efficacy of triple therapy is unacceptably low. The role of prebiotics and probiotics as adjunctive treatment for *H. pylori* infection has also been reviewed. Several rescue options have been proposed. Bismuth-based quadruple therapy is effective, but its complexity and the associated adverse effects affect compliance. PPI plus amoxicillin combined with levofloxacin or moxifloxacin is at least as effective, and better tolerated.

Keywords: *Helicobacter pylori*, meta-analysis, proton pump inhibitor, bismuth, ranitidine bismuth citrate, clarithromycin, amoxicillin, levofloxacin, treatment, therapy, omeprazole, lansoprazole, pantoprazole, rabeprazole, esomeprazole, sequential therapy, concomitant therapy, resistance.

***Address correspondence to Javier P. Gisbert:** Hospital Universitario de La Princesa Instituto de Investigation Sanitaria Princesa (IP), Department of Gastroenterology and Centro de Investigación Biomédica en Red De Enfermedades Hepáticas Digestivas, Madrid, Spain; Tel: +34-913093911; Fax: +31-914022299; E-mail: javier.p.gisbert@gmail.com

Buzás György Miklós (Ed.)

INTRODUCTION

Systematic reviews comprehensively examine the medical literature, seeking to identify and synthesize all relevant information to formulate the best approach to diagnosis or treatment [1]. A systematic review uses explicit, systematic methods that are selected with a view to minimizing bias, thus providing more reliable findings from which conclusions can be drawn and decisions made [2-3]. Systematic overviews of the medical literature that summarize scientific evidence (in contrast to unsystematic narrative reviews that mix together opinions and evidence) are becoming more prevalent, and are increasingly useful for clinicians trying to make optimal management decisions [4].

Meta-analyses are a special type of systematic review. They are statistical procedures that integrates the results of several independent studies considered to be "combinable" [5]. Meta-analyses use quantitative methods to analyze the literature and seek to answer a focused clinical question, using rigorous statistical analysis of pooled research studies [1]. Thus, meta-analysis provides a means of combining raw statistical data from all eligible primary studies addressing an identical question of interest to arrive at conclusions that are more precise and reliable than those presented in a single study [6]. Furthermore, well conducted meta-analyses allow a more objective appraisal of the evidence than traditional narrative reviews, provide a more precise estimate of a treatment effect, and may explain heterogeneity between the results of individual studies [5].

There are several reasons explaining why we need meta-analyses [6]: First, we are living in a time of information explosion. More than two million articles are published annually in more than 20,000 biomedical journals. As an example, if we look for the term "*H. pylori*" in PubMed (US National Library of Medicine, National Institutes of Health), we recover more than 32,000 references from published articles. Healthcare providers, consumers, researchers, and policy makers are inundated with unmanageable amounts of information, including evidence from healthcare research. It is unlikely that all will have the time, skills and resources to find, appraise and interpret this evidence and to incorporate it into healthcare decisions [2, 7]. Thus, most physicians are overwhelmed by this unmanageable volume of literature and prefer unbiased summaries of multiple original investigations [6]. Clinicians read meta-analyses to keep up to date with their field, and they are often used as a starting point for developing clinical practice guidelines [4, 8].

A second reason why we need meta-analyses is that single studies, even the most rigorously designed and conducted ones, rarely provide definitive answers to clinical questions. A third reason is that meta-analysis that uses a systematic and quantitative approach limits bias and helps improve the precision of estimates of study findings and the reliability of conclusions by increasing sample size and study power. Finally, because of the systematic approach, metaanálisis teases apart differences in studies that may lead to disparate findings, explores sources of heterogeneity and identifies study gaps and directions for future investigations [6].

Since it was first defined by Glass in 1976 [9] the number of meta-analysis-related publications has increased significantly in the last decades. As an example, between year 1981 and year 1986, only 21 references including the term meta-analysis in its heading were found in MEDLINE, whereas a decade later (period 1991-1996) this figure had increased up to 1,459 [10]. At present, a brief search on PubMed including the term "meta-analysis" yields more than 54,000 related citations. A final example: up to the year 2012, approximately 300 meta-analyses have been published on the topic of *H. pylori* infection, a relatively recently discovered micro-organism.

These figures strongly suggest that meta-analysis is increasingly recognized as a scientific method of investigation by the medical establishment as well as by editors of medical journals. Meta-analysis is an invaluable scientific research method that is widely used in many disciplines of science, including medicine [6]. And, in particular, meta-analysis has contributed to our understanding in the management of patients with *H. pylori* infection [11].

There are, however, several misconceptions and potential problems about meta-analysis [6, 12]: i) The belief that meta-analysis is about pooling studies is a typical and common one. The notion that "meta-analysis is the same as an ordinary review, only larger" is also not true. ii) Another common erroneous perception is that metaanálisis is a substitute for large good-quality individual experimental studies. It is important to understand that meta-analysis is not a hypothesis-testing experiment, but more a tool to identify where knowledge is currently lacking and a research directory for future investigations. It is supplementary to large randomized controlled clinical trials and is a cost-effective approach because it reduces the number of unnecessary primary studies [6]. iii) Finally, meta-analysis is no panacea for turning bad primary studies into good ones [6]. "Garbage in and garbage out"', is the most common mistake, in which good studies are mixed with bad ones in the meta-analysis [6]. In summary, it should not be forgotten that although meta-analysis has become increasingly accepted, it is a retrospective method of research and carries the potential disadvantages of such an approach [6].

OBJECTIVES AND METHODS

H. pylori infection is the main known cause of gastritis, gastroduodenal ulcer disease, and gastric cancer. After 30 years of experience in *H. pylori* treatment, however, the ideal regimen to treat this infection has yet to be found.

This chapter aims to review published meta-analyses focused on the treatments used in the eradication of *H. pylori* infection.

The bibliographical search was performed in the PubMed (Internet) database, including studies available until May 2012, looking for the following words: (*H. pylori* OR *Helicobacter pylori*) AND (meta-analysis OR metaanalysis) AND (treatment OR therapy). No language restriction was placed on the search strategy. Hand search of further relevant trials was performed on all reference lists of the selected trials from the electronic search. The abstracts from all selected articles in each of these were reviewed. All those meeting the inclusion criteria (that is, meta-analysis of randomized trials evaluating efficacy/tolerance of *H. pylori* eradication regimens) were recorded.

Only meta-analyses focused on the efficacy (or tolerance) of one or several treatments aimed at the eradication of *H. pylori*, were included. Therefore, those meta-analyses dealing with the role of *H. pylori* eradication on a particular disease related with *H. pylori* infection (for example, the efficacy of eradication treatment on functional dyspepsia, gastoesophageal reflux disease, gastric cancer, *etc.*), but not focusing on the efficacy/tolerance of the eradication regimen itself, were not included in the present review.

Dual Regimens

Aiming to systematically determine the best *H. pylori* eradication treatment, by meta-analysing pooled eradication rates, Chiba *et al.* identified in 1992 a total of 27 trials. Efficacies of single (19%), double (48%), and triple therapies (82%) were highly different statistically. Regarding bismuth-containing regimens, a combination with metronidazole offered better results than with amoxicillin (55% *vs.* 44%) [13].

The meta-analytical review published by Pipkin *et al.* in 1997 evaluated clarithromycin-containing dual therapies in *H. pylori* eradication. One hundred and four dual regimen arms evaluated in 75 trials were reviewed. Pooled eradication rate of Ranitidine bismuth citrate (RBC) plus clarithromycin was 85%, ranging from 70% to 96%,. The omeprazole plus clarithromycin treatment reported eradication rates ranging from 27% to 90%, with the pooled reported rate being 66% [14].

A two weeks course of either of these two dual regimens was approved by The Food and Drug Administration (FDA) of the USA to treat peptic ulcer [15]. However, at that time (1997) the European Maastricht Consensus Report only approved triple (PPI plus two of these antibiotics: metronidazole, amoxicillin and clarithromycin) and quadruple therapy (PPI, colloidal bismuth subcitrate, tetracycline and metronidazole) [16].

The pooled analysis of different therapeutic combinations performed by Unge in 1997, evaluating 101 randomized and 20 blind trials, showed an eradication rate ranging from 52% to 60% with dual therapy with omeprazole plus amoxicillin. PPI-based triple therapies were in this study the most effective and convenient regimens [17].

Proton Pump Inhibitor-Based Triple Therapies

The combination of PPI, clarithromycin and either amoxicillin or a nitroimidazole in triple therapies has been considered the most effective treatment of *H. pylori* infection. These are the most frequently recommended regimens world-wide due to their safety profile, simplicity and cost-effectiveness [18-19].

The different treatment strategies were meta-analysed in 1996, grouping them into 13 different classes [20]. Omeprazol-containing triple therapies achieved higher efficacy than the two classes of PPI-containing dual combinations analysed (with amoxicillin or clarithromycin), and than the triple regimens with H_2-receptor antagonists [20]. This benefitial effect has been confirmed including the abstracts from several international meetings between 1997 and 2002 in a more recent meta-analysis [21-22]. Thus, Buzás *et al.* [22] reviewed the randomised, controlled studies from European countries, including 102 studies comprising nearly 400 treatment arms and over 25.000 patients. The eradication rate of PPI-based first line triple therapies was 80.4%. On the contrary, PPI-based double combinations were efficient in only 47.1% (p=0.001 *vs.* triple regimens). Clarithromycin and amoxicillin or nitroimidazole combinations regimens achieved an eradication of 80% and 84%, respectively, while regimens with amoxicillin and nitroimidazole were less efficient (72%, p=0.006).

More recently, in 2006, this same author has updated this meta-analysis of European abstracts presented up to 2004 at the International Workshop on Helicobacter (by the European Helicobacter Study Group, United European Gastroenterology Week meetings and World Congresses of Gastroenterology [23]. The pooled eradication rates of PPI one week triple therapies was 81.4%. Again, PPI-based double combinations were less efficient than triple regimens (55%). Amoxicillin + nitroimidazole therapies eradicated the infection in only 73.5% (P<0.05 *vs.* clarithromycin-based regimens). These last meta-analyses emphasize the fact that high quality congress abstracts constitute a valuable pool of data which is suitable for meta-analytical workup.

Costs and outcomes of 8 antibiotic combinations with documented anti-*H.pylori* activity, *vs.* maintenance therapy with H_2-receptor antagonists, were evaluated in 1997[24]. Aggregate eradication rates were meta-analysed from nearly 20 studies including 6,416 patients. Health outcomes and annual costs were determined with a MonteCarlo simulation for a decision analytic model. The lowest costs and recurrence rates were achieved by 3 regimens: bismuth-based triple therapy (a combination of bismuth, metronidazole, and tetracycline) for 14 days, bismuth-based triple therapy with a PPI for 7 days, and a combination of clarithromycin, metronidazole, and a PPI for 7 days.

Two years later, trials with omeprazole combined with antibiotics (clarithromycin or nitroimidazoles, and amoxicillin) were evaluated with a meta-regression analysis [25]. One hundred and seventeen treatment arms from 74 trials involving 4,769 patients were included. Eradication rates of the dual regimens combining omeprazole with clarithromycin, and omeprazole with amoxicillin were 76%, and 65% respectively. However, triple regimens of omeprazole-amoxicillin-clarithromycin, omeprazole-amoxicillin-imidazole, and omeprazole-clarithromycin-imidazole achieved 82% 83% and 89% eradication rates respectively. The authors concluded that triple therapies were superior to dual therapies previously used.

Most recommend triple therapies combine PPI plus clarithromycin plus nitroimidazole or PPI plus clarithromycin plus amoxicillin. Whether these therapies are equivalent was meta-analysed in 2000[26]. Twenty-two trials comparing these regimens lasting one week were included. Pooled *H. pylori* eradication rates by intention-to-treat (ITT) were 81% in both combinations, which indicated that these therapies were similarly effective.

More recently, Rodgers *et al.* [27] reviewed all clinical trials containing Canadian data on the success rate of *H. pylori* treatment. Seventeen papers met the inclusion criteria. Both triple therapies consisting of a PPI + clarithromycin + amoxicillin/metronidazole performed relatively well, achieving a success rate of 84% and 82%, respectively. The cure rate of PPI-amoxicillin + metronidazole was 76%.

It is still unclear whether lower doses (250 mg. b.i.d.) of clarithromycin are sufficient to obtain eradication of the bacteria when 7-day PPI-containing triple regimens are prescribed. Several studies have obtained favourable results with this lower dose of clarithromycin when using this combination. The results from the aforementioned meta-analysis by Gisbert *et al.*, from trials using clarithromycin at low doses (250 mg b.i.d.) in both regimens (PPI, clarithromycin, and amoxicillin;

and PPI, clarithromycin, and nitroimidazole) showed higher eradication for the nitroimidazole-containing therapy (86%) than for the amoxicillin one (81%) [26]. Aiming to evaluate the importance of clarithromycin dose in PPI-containing therapies for the radication of the bacteria, another meta-analysis by Huang *et al.*, demonstrated that the PPI-clarithromycin-amoxicillin regimen achieved higher efficacy if clarithromycin was prescribed at 500 mg b.i.d. instead of 250 mg b.i.d. [28]. However, the authors concluded that, although in general low dose of clarithromycin should not be prescribed, in the PPI-clarithromycin-nitroimidazole regimen, efficacy was similar using both doses [28].

Some authors have evaluated whether adding azithromycin to first-line *H. pylori* eradication improved eradication and reduced side effects [29]. All randomized trials that compared azithromycin-containing with standard triple-therapy regimens for first-line treatment of *H. pylori* infection were included. Fourteen randomized trials (1,431 patients) were identified. Pooled *H. pylori* eradication rates were 72% and 70% for patients with or without azithromycin by ITT analysis, and the odds ratio (OR) was 1.17 (95% confidence interval (95% CI) = 0.64-2.14). The occurrence of side effects differed significantly and was 16% and 25% for treatment with or without azithromycin, respectively, and the summary OR was 0.58 (95% CI = 0.41-0.82). Furthermore, the azithromycin-containing group had a lower occurrence of diarrhoea, nausea and taste disturbance. Therefore, this review suggests that azithromycin-containing triple-therapy regimens could be equally effective in eradication of *H. pylori* compared with standard first-line triple-therapy regimens.

Finally, quinolones-based triple therapy has been suggested as an alternative first line therapy to clarithromycin-based triple therapy. Recently, some studies have evaluated levofloxacin and moxifloxacin, new fluoroquinolones, that may prove to be a valid alternative to more common antibiotics in rescue treatments [30]. However, the number of studies evaluating a combination of levofloxacin and amoxicillin (together with an antisecretor) as first-line regimen has been relatively small, and the number of patients included in each of the studies limited.

Zhang *et al.* [31] meta-analysed randomized studies evaluating the effectiveness and safety of PPI and levofloxacin-containing first-line triple therapy. Eleven randomized clinical trials including 1,926 cases were selected for analysis. As the first line treatment, PPI and levofloxacin-containing triple therapy was more effective than standard triple therapy (OR = 1.56; 95% CI = 1.25-1.94), and had lower side effect rate than standard triple therapy (OR = 0.57; 95% CI = 0.44-0.74).

Other authors [32] have systematically reviewed the efficacy and tolerance of moxifloxacin-based triple therapy, and have conducted a meta-analysis of studies comparing this regimen with clarithromycin-based triple therapy. Four randomized clinical trials totalling 772 patients were included. The meta-analysis showed that the mean eradication rate was 84% in the moxifloxacin-based triple therapy group and 74% in the clarithromycin-based triple therapy group (RR = 1.13; 95% CI = 1.01-1.27). There were no statistically significant differences in the overall side effects (RR = 0.61; 95% CI = 0.25, 1.48).

The authors of the aforementioned meta-analyses [31, 32] concluded that quinolone (levofloxacin- or moxifloxacin-containing triple therapy) should be advocated as first-line regimen in *H. pylori* eradication. However, the quick acquisition of resistance to quinolones may jeopardise its future efficacy and, consequently, it has been suggested to reserve quinolones for rescue treatment to avoid the increase of the resistance phenomenon [19].

Proton Pump Inhibitors *vs.* Histamine H_2-Receptor Antagonists

It may be considered whether the PPIs are superior to the histamine H_2-receptor antagonists. On one hand, while PPIs have intrinsic antibacterial activity against *H. pylori* and produces synergistic pharmacokinetic interactions with antibiotics; H_2-receptor antagonists do not offer these advantages [33]. On the other hand, the antisecretory capacity of PPIs is greater than that obtained with H_2-receptor antagonists at standard doses [33]. Therefore, that combining antibiotics with PPIs is more effective than with H_2-receptor antagonists may be proposed.

Year ago, no statistically significant difference was found between PPIs and H_2-receptor antagonists in a meta-analysis; [34]. However, the validity of its conclusion was considerably limited due to its publication in a German-Language journal as a "Letter to the Editor", and its serious limitations, such as suboptimal quality of methodology, small quantity and size (number of patients) of the included studies. For this reason, A recent updated meta-analysis evaluating the efficacy of both types of antisecretory drugs combined with antibiotics, has been carried out [35]. To this purpose, all randomized trials comparing PPIs and H_2-receptor antagonists, in combination with the same two antibiotics, were evaluated. Twenty studies were included and PPIs achieved higher ITT eradication rates (74%) than histamine H_2-receptor antagonists (69%; OR = 1.31; 95% CI = 1.09-1.58). This conclusion confirms the results from a previous meta-analysis, which evaluated 12 different therapies in terms of *H. pylori* eradication, and suggested that the combination of triple therapies with lansoprazole or omeprazole achieved higher eradication rates than with H_2-receptor antagonists [36]. Moreover, a recent meta-analysis including abstracts from several international meetings has confirmed these findings [22].

Lafutidine is a newly synthesized H_2-receptor antagonist and has been shown to exhibit antisecretory action. A meta-analysis investigated the efficacy of lafutidine-based triple therapy for *H. pylori* [37]. Three studies met the inclusion criteria, and overall it was demonstrated that *H. pylori* eradication rates were similar in the lafutidine group and the lansoprazole group (OR = 1.03; 95% CI = 0.64-1.66). Likewise, adverse events were similar in both groups.

Role of the Various Proton Pump Inhibitors in *H. pylori* Eradication Therapy

As mentioned, triple therapy containing a PPI and two antibiotics has been the first-line recommended treatment for *H. pylori* eradication, but until very recently it was unknown whether the efficacy of therapy may be different depending on the type of PPI used (omeprazole, lansoprazole, pantoprazole, rabeprazole, or esomeprazole). Therefore, several meta-analyses have consecutively aimed to compare the *H. pylori* eradication efficacy of the newer PPIs *vs.* omeprazole in combination with two antibiotics.

1) Lansoprazole

A first systematic review of literature evaluated all randomized studies published up to 1996, reporting the *H. pylori* eradication rate of lansoprazole combined with antibiotics or even as monotherapy [38]. This meta-analysis indicated that lansoprazole achieved high rates of *H. pylori* eradication, especially when combined with amoxicillin or clarithromycin, and nitroinidazoles. The reported rates were equivalent to those obtained with omeprazole.

2) Pantoprazole

Another meta-analysis including 12 studies compared the eradication rate of combinations of antibiotics with pantoprazole and other PPIs [39]. The pooled efficacies in *H. pylori* eradication were equivalent (the association's OR was 1) when prescribing pantoprazole and other PPIs (83% and 81% respectively).

3) Rabeprazole

Twelve randomized trials have been included in a recent meta-analysis evaluating rabeprazole-containing regimens [40]. The meta-analyss suggested that antibiotic treatments might achieve higher eradication rates in combination with rabeprazole (79%) than with other PPIs (77%). However, the OR for this association was 1.15 (95% CI = 0.93-1.42).

4) Esomeprazole

In 2004, esomeprazole-containing regimens were evaluated in a further meta-analysis [41]. Only 4 trials met the inclusion criteria in this case. Pooled eradication efficacies of antibiotics in combination with esomeprazole or omeprazole were 85%, and 82% respectively (OR = 1.19; 95% CI = 0.81-1.74). Subanalysing trials scoring as high quality, the homogeneity of results was increased, and the OR obtained for the association was closer to one (1.08). Two years later, another meta-analysis evaluated the rate *H. pylori* eradication in studies comparing antibiotic treatments containing esomeprazole and other PPIs [42]. After evaluating the 11 clinical trials (2,159 subjects) included, the pooled efficacy of combinations with esomeprazole (86%) was comparable to that achieved with other PPIs (81%) (OR = 1.38; 95% CI = 1.09-1.75). The subanalysis of high-quality trials (6 studies) increased homogeneity of results and the OR became closer to one (1.17).

Finally, Vergara *et al.* [43] compared the *H. pylori* eradication rate of each PPI as part of a triple regimen in a single meta-analysis. Eradication rates by ITT were similar for omeprazole and lansoprazole (74.7% *vs.* 76%), for omeprazole and rabeprazole (77.9% *vs.* 81.2%), for omeprazole and esomeprazole (87.7% *vs.* 89%), and also for lansoprazole and rabeprazole (81% *vs.* 85.7%).

As conclusion, the efficacies in *H. pylori* eradication of the different PPIs (omeprazole, lansoprazole, pantoprazole, rabeprazole, and esomeprazole) as part of a triple therapy are equivalent.

Dose of Proton Pump Inhibitors in Standard Triple Therapies

The standard regimens for *H. pylori* eradication are triple therapies prescribing antibiotics with a twice-daily dose of PPI. As some authors have suggested that once daily PPI is equivalent, Vallve *et al.* [44] meta-analysed 13 studies including 2,391 patients, comparing the eradication rate of both dosage schemes of PPI. Efficacy by ITT with twice-daily doses of PPI was higher (84% *vs.* 78%). However, this beneficial impact of the double doses of PPIs was limited to combination containing clarithromycin and amoxicillin in triple therapy, effect not found for the combinations including clarithromycin and metronidazole.

In addition, Padol *et al.* [45] recently showed that cure rates of triple therapy are less effective in extensive PPI metabolizers. Furthermore, direct evidence suggesting that high-dose PPI can improve the cure rates of *H. pylori* treatment comes from the recent meta-analysis of Villoria *et al.* [46], showing that high-dose PPIs increase cure rates by around 6-10% when compared with standard doses. A sub-analysis of these data showed that the maximal effect was observed in the studies comparing high doses of the more potent second generation PPIs, namely 40 mg esomeprazole, twice a day with a standard dose of a first line PPI also twice a day. The rationale for this finding is that the difference in the degree of gastric secretion between arms is much larger when using double doses of more potent PPIs. According to this last sub-analysis data, increasing the dose of PPI from, for example, 20 mg omeprazole b.i.d. to 40 mg of esomeprazole or rabeprazole b.i.d. may increase cure rates 8-12%.

In conclusion, high-dose PPI seems more effective than standard-dose for curing *H. pylori* infection in standard triple therapy.

Duration of Proton Pump Inhibitor-Based Triple Therapies

The duration that a PPI-containing triple therapy should be prescribed for is still unclear. On one hand, it has been evaluated whether short-term therapy (*e.g.*, for less than 7 day) is sufficient to eradicate *H. pylori* infection. Thus, Zhou *et al.* [47] performed a meta-analysis of the efficacy of short-term protocols, and reviewed the safety and adverse profiles of these eradication protocols. Mean ITT cure rates of 63% and 81% were achieved with short-term protocols and 7-day PPI-containing protocols, respectively. Thus, short-term therapy was inferior to 7-day triple regimen ($P<0.001$). In conclusion, although more economical, short-duration protocols are inferior to 7-day PPI-based triple protocols with regarding to eradication rate of *H. pylori*.

On the other hand, four meta-analyses have evaluated triple therapies lasting more than 7 days to assess whether the lengthening of treatment increased efficacy, achieving roughly similar results. All four consistently show that 14-day triple therapies increase cure rates when compared to 7 days. Ten-day therapies were also superior to 7-day therapies. The increases in cure rates were superior with 14 days than with 10 days of therapy in all meta-analyses.

Initially, Calvet *et al.* [48] performed a meta-analysis including 13 studies. They found that lengthening triple therapy from 7 to 14 days increased cure rates by 9%. Corresponding value for increasing from 7 to 10 days was 3%. Cure rates improvement was significant for 14-day therapies (OR = 0.62; 95% CI = 0.45-0.84) but not for the 10-day ones.

Ford *et al.* [49] found even superior increases in cure rates (relative risk reduction = 12%; 95% CI = 7-17%) when comparing 14-day to 7-day therapy.

Fuccio *et al.* [50] included 21 studies in a more recent study. Meta-analysis yielded relative risks (RRs) for eradication of 1.05 (95% CI = 1.01-1.10) for 7-day compared with 10-day triple therapy and 1.07 (CI, 1.02 to 1.12) for 7-day compared with 14-day therapy. Improvements on cure rates were 4% for 10-day therapy and 5% for 14-day therapy. When analyzing their data, the authors argue that increasing the length of treatment did not achieve clinically significant improvements in cure rates. This statement has, however, been challenged [51].

Finally, a recent meta-analysis presented at the *Digestive Disease Week* 2010 including 26 studies has yielded very similar results, with a RR of 0.79 (95% CI = 0.71-0.89) for 14-day therapy [52]. A similar benefit was seen with 10 days of treatment compared to 7 days (RR = 0.84; 95% CI = 0.73-0.96). Improvement of cure rates was around 6% for 14 days and 4% for 10 days of triple therapy.

As a conclusion, it should be emphasized that none of the aforementioned meta-analyses found significant differences regarding the rate of side effects with the different durations. Furthermore, except for some specific areas like some Scandinavian countries, cure rates with 7-day triple therapy are clearly unsatisfactory [53]. So, as safety seems similar and the increase in costs is small, it seems reasonable to recommend the length of treatment achieving maximal cure rates, even though the expected improvements will be moderate.

Duration of Proton Pump Inhibitor Therapy to Heal Peptic Ulcer

General agreement exists in that *H. pylori* eradication using a triple regimen combining a PPI and two antibiotics for 7 to 10 days is the gold standard of treatment. Nevertheless, while eradication of *H. pylori* is an appropriate end-point for clinical trials in patients with peptic ulcer disease, ulcer healing and relief of symptoms are the primary aims of treatment from the patient's perspective. The traditional strategy in peptic ulcer disease has been therefore to continue PPI monotherapy for a further 3 weeks after *H. pylori* eradication to ensure ulcer healing and symptom relief.

However, the optimal treatment of *H. pylori* is still a matter of debate. As mentioned, most ulcer patients have been traditionally treated with antisecretory drugs up to follow-up investigation 4 or more weeks after cessation of anti-*H. pylori* therapy, and it has been controversial whether eradication of *H. pylori* alone, without acid suppression, is sufficient to achieve the goal of both good efficacies in *H. pylori* eradication and peptic ulcer healing. This represents an important issue because there is a significant correlation between the complexity and duration of treatment, on one hand, and the cost of treatment and patient compliance, on the other.

In this context, Gisbert *et al.* [54] systematically reviewed the efficacy on ulcer healing of 1-week combination of a PPI plus two antibiotics and performed a meta-analysis of randomized clinical trials to evaluate whether 7 days of PPI-based triple therapy is sufficient to heal peptic ulcer (randomized clinical trials comparing the efficacy on ulcer healing of 7-day PPI-based triple therapy *vs.* this same regimen but prolonging the PPI for several more weeks were included in the meta-analysis). Twenty-four studies (including 2,342 patients) assessed ulcer healing with 1-week PPI. Mean healing rate was 86%, and 95% in *H. pylori*-eradicated patients. Six studies (862 patients), were included in the meta-analysis. Mean ulcer healing rate with a 7-day treatment was 91% *vs.* 92% when PPI was prolonged for 2-4 more weeks (OR = 1.11; 95% CI = 0.71-1.74). Therefore, the authors concluded that in patients with peptic ulcer and *H. pylori* infection, prolonging therapy with PPI after a triple therapy for 7 days with a PPI and two antibiotics is not necessary to induce ulcer healing.

Bismuth-Containing Quadruple Therapy

Owing to rising drug-resistant *H. pylori*, currently recommended PPI-based triple therapies are losing their efficacy, and regimens efficacious in the presence of drug resistance are needed [55-56]. Therefore, it seems reasonable to re-assess the efficacy and safety of first-line bismuth-containing quadruple therapies. Fischbach *et al.* [57] performed meta-regression models to identify factors explaining variation in the efficacy of first-line quadruple therapies from 145 treatment arms. The authors found that quadruple therapies combining a gastric acid inhibitor, bismuth, metronidazole and tetracycline were enhanced when omeprazole was included, and treatment duration lasted 10-14 days. On the other hand, treatment efficacy decreased as the prevalence of metronidazole resistance increased. However, the efficacy of quadruple therapy achieved over 85% eradication rate, even in areas with a high prevalence of metronidazole resistance, this quadruple regimen eradicated more than 85% of *H. pylori* infections when it contained a PPI and was given for 10-14 days. Furthermore, in the presence of clarithromycin resistance, this quadruple regimen eradicated 90-100% of *H. pylori* infections, while the most recommended triple regimen combining clarithromycin, amoxicillin and a PPI achieved lower than 50% eradication rate. These results support the recommendation of including bismuth-containing quadruple therapy among recommended first-line anti-*H. pylori* therapies [19].

The safety of bismuth used in *H. pylori* eradication therapy regimens has recently been assessed by Ford *et al.* [58] in a systematic review and meta-analysis. The authors identified 35 randomised controlled trials containing 4,763 patients. There were no serious adverse events occurring with bismuth therapy. Furthermore, there was no statistically significant difference detected in total adverse events with bismuth (RR = 1.01; 95% CI = 0.87-1.16), specific individual adverse events, with the exception of dark stools, or adverse events leading to withdrawal of therapy (RR = 0.86; 95% CI = 0.54-1.37). Therefore, it may be concluded that bismuth for the *H. pylori* eradication is safe and well-tolerated.

Finally, the adherence to, and safety of bismuth-containing quadruple therapy seem to be equivalent to currently recommended triple regimens, regardless of the higher complexity of quadruple regimen; and even despite results from a previous meta-analysis showing that in *H. pylori* eradication regimens; the higher the number of doses per day, the higher the rate of treatment discontinuation [59].

Proton Pump Inhibitor-Based Triple Therapy *vs.* Bismuth-Containing Quadruple Therapy

Gene *et al.* [60], in 2003 meta-analysed trials comparing triple *vs.* quadruple therapy as first-line therapy in *H. pylori* eradication, to evaluate if quadruple therapy could be considered as an alternative. The 4 trials included showed equivalent ITT efficacy for triple (78%) and quadruple therapy (81%). without statistically significant differences. Adherence and safety of both therapies were also equivalent.

In 2010 more studies have concluded comparable results, suggesting that quadruple therapies do not obtain higher eradication rates than triple therapies [61]. Thus, in the meta-analysis by Luther *et al.* [61], nine randomized clinical trials (including 1,679 patients) were selected. Bismuth quadruple therapy achieved eradication in 78% of patients, whereas clarithromycin triple therapy achieved an eradication rate of 77% (RR = 1; 95% CI = 0.936-1.073).

Therefore, it may be concluded that in first-line treatment for *H. pylori* eradication, triple and quadruple therapies offer similar results in terms of effectiveness, adherence to treatment and safety profile. From a different perspective, however, it may also be concluded that both therapies yielded suboptimal (<80%) eradication rates.

Proton Pump Inhibitors *vs.* Ranitidine Bismuth Citrate-Containing Regimens

RBC was developed as a novel compound that presented, on one hand, the antisecretory activity of ranitidine and, on the other, the mucosal protective and anti-*H. pylori* effects of certain other bismuth salts [62]. The appearance of RBC raised the question of whether this drug could compete with, or even overcome, PPI-based triple therapies.

In an initial meta-analysis, Gisbert *et al.* [63] compared the efficacy of PPI *vs.* RBC with two antibiotics for 1 week in *H. pylori* eradication, and concluded that both drugs had similar efficacy for *H. pylori* eradication when given with clarithromycin and amoxicillin for 1 week, but RBC seemed to have a higher efficacy than PPI when clarithromycin and a nitroimidazole were the co-prescribed antibiotics. More recently, these same authors have updated the meta-analysis [64]. Mean *H. pylori* eradication with 7-day RBC-clarithromycin-amoxicillin, RBC-clarithromycin-nitroimidazole, and RBC-amoxicillin-nitroimidazole was 83%, 86%, and 71%, respectively. Again, the meta-analysis presented equivalent efficacy for the combination of either RBC or PPI plus clarithromycin and amoxicillin (OR = 1.11; 95% CI = 0.88-1.40), and plus amoxicillin and metronidazole (OR = 0.92; 95%CI = 0.60-1.41). However, when clarithromycin and a nitroimidazole were the antibiotics used, higher eradication rates were found with RBC than with PPI (OR = 1.65; 95% CI = 1.15-2.37).

The explanation for better results obtained with RBC than with PPI (when given with clarithromycin and a nitroimidazole) is unknown, but several hypotheses may be suggested. Firstly, several studies have found a significant drop in efficacy with one-week PPI-based triple therapies with metronidazole when *H. pylori* strains are resistant to this antibiotic. On the contrary, the triple therapy with RBC plus antibiotics seems to achieve high eradication rates even in patients with metronidazole-resistant strains, perhaps due to a synergistic interaction of RBC with this antibiotic, even against *H. pylori*-resistant strains. On the other hand, *in vitro* and *in vivo* studies have demonstrated that RBC and clarithromycin given in combination have also a synergistic interaction [62].

Factors Influencing Efficacy of *H. pylori* Eradication Treatment (Mainly Standard Triple Therapy)

1) Antibiotic Resistance

Pre-treatment antibiotic resistance is the most important factor in non-response to initial treatment. To define the effect of pre-treatment *H. pylori* resistance to metronidazole or to clarithromycin on the success of antimicrobial therapy, Dore *et al.* [65] conducted a meta-analysis and identified 49 papers with 65 arms for metronidazole. Metronidazole resistance reduced effectiveness by an average of 38%. Susceptibility tests for clarithromycin were performed in 12 studies (501 patients), and resistance to this drug reduced effectiveness by an average of 55%. Another meta-analysis evaluated the influence of *in vitro* nitroimidazole resistance on the efficacy of nitroimidazole-containing anti-*H. pylori* regimens [66]. A total of 91 treatment arms, including 4,823 patients, were evaluated. Eradication rates were 90% in susceptible strains but <75% in resistant strains. The negative effect of metronidazole resistance has been confirmed in a more recent meta-analysis [67]. Finally, in 2007, Fischbach *et al.* [68] determined the effect of drug resistance on the efficacy of first-line treatment regimens for *H. pylori* and identified the most efficacious treatments in the presence of drug resistance. The authors analyzed data from 93 studies with 10,178 participants. For triple therapies, clarithromycin resistance had a greater effect on treatment efficacy than nitroimidazole resistance. Metronidazole resistance reduced efficacy by 26% in triple therapies containing a nitroimidazole, tetracycline and bismuth, while efficacy was reduced by only 14% when a gastric acid inhibitor was added to the regimen.

In conclusion, metronidazole and, mainly, clarithromycin pre-treatment resistant *H. pylori* are the main factors responsible for treatment failure with regimens using these compounds, emphasizing the fact that more effective treatments are needed for most populations of the world where drug resistance is common.

2) Smoking

Some studies have pointed to a link between *H. pylori* eradication failure with smoking. To investigate the effects of smoking on eradication outcome, a meta-analysis was recently performed [69]. Twenty-two published studies (including 5,538 patients), which provided information on eradication failure according to smoking status, were included in the analysis. The summary OR for eradication failure among smokers relative to non-smokers was 1.95 (95% CI = 1.55-2.45). It corresponded with the differences in eradication rates between smokers and non-smokers of about 8%.

3) CYP2C19 Genetic Polymorphisms

It has been suggested that PPI-related differences *H. pylori* eradication rates are partly because of CYP2C19 polymorphisms and there have been conflicting data in this area.

In 2006, Padol *et al.* [45] conducted a meta-analysis to investigate the evidence relating CYP2C19 to first-line *H. pylori* eradication rates. When all eradication rates, regardless of PPI used, were combined there was no significant difference between poor metabolizers (PM) and heterozygous extensive metabolizers (HetEMs) (OR = 1.35; 95% CI = 0.89-2.07); however, there was a significant difference between HetEM and homozygous extensive metabolizers (HomEMs) (OR = 1.90; 95% CI = 1.38-2.60). Additional subanalysis of individual PPIs revealed that dual and triple omeprazole therapies significantly favoured higher *H. pylori* eradication rates in PM over HomEMs (OR = 4.03; 95% CI = 1.97-8.28), and also over HetEMs (OR = 2.24; 95% CI =1.09-4.61). Dual and triple rabeprazole and triple lansoprazole therapies did not show significantly different *H. pylori* eradication rates between PM (OR = 1.04; 95% CI = 0.44-2.46) and HomEMs (OR = 1.80; 95% CI = 0.67-4.85).

More recently (in 2008), Zhao *et al.* [70] performed a similar meta-analysis to determine whether CYP2C19 polymorphism affect *H. pylori* eradication rates obtained with first-line PPI-based triple therapies. Eradication rates were significantly different between PM and HetEMs and between PM and HomEMs. Moreover, eradication rates were also significantly different between HetEMs and

HomEMs. Triple omeprazole and lansoprazole therapies achieved higher *H. pylori* eradication rates in PM than in HomEMs, and higher in HetEMs than those in HomEMs. Finally, rabeprazole therapies had no significant effect on *H. pylori* eradication rates depending on the CYP2C19 status.

In summary, the impact of CYP2C19 polymorphisms on *H. pylori* eradication rates appears clinically relevant in patients prescribed omeprazole as a component of their dual- or triple-drug therapy. The efficacy of lansoprazole-based first-line triple therapies at the standard doses may be also dependent on CYP2C19 genotype status. However, CYP2C19 polymorphisms appear not to affect the efficacy of the regimens including rabeprazole. It may be suggested, therefore, that choice of PPI and/or dose rather than CYP2C19 genotyping could be a more practical approach to assure the highest *H. pylori* eradication rates in clinical settings.

4) Virulence of H. pylori Strain (CagA)

Some, but not all studies have provided evidence that the CagA status of *H. pylori* strains is a predictive factor for the outcome of eradication therapy. Suzuki *et al.* [71] conducted a meta-analysis on the importance of CagA status for successful eradication of this infection. Fourteen studies (1,529 patients) were included of 325 articles identified in the search. The summary RR for eradication failure in CagA-negative relative to CagA-positive was 2.0 (95% CI = 1.6-2.4), corresponding with the summary risk difference for eradication success between the groups of 11% (95% CI = 3-19%). In conclusion, this meta-analysis confirmed the importance of the presence of CagA as a predictor for successful eradication of *H. pylori*.

5) Pre-Treatment with a PPI

There is much debate about the influence of pre-treatment with a PPI on *H. pylori* eradication. A recent meta-analysis, including 9 studies and a total of 773 patients, calculated pooled eradication rates of 81.3% for patients with pre-treatment and 81.2% for patients without pre-treatment [72]. Therefore, it may be concluded that pre-treatment with a PPI does not influence *H. pylori* eradication.

6) Underlying Disease (Peptic Ulcer vs. Non-Ulcer Disease)

Finally, it has been suggested that patients with peptic ulcer disease and with non-ulcer dyspepsia may respond differently to eradication treatment. To study risk factors for failure of *H. pylori* eradication treatment, individual data from 2,751 patients included in 11 multicentre clinical trials carried out in France and using a triple therapy, were gathered in a unique database [73]. There was a difference in failure rate between duodenal ulcer patients and non-ulcer dyspeptic patients, 22% and 34%, respectively, in accordance with a previous meta-analysis [25]. Therefore, this study concluded that ulcer and non-ulcer dyspeptic patients should be managed differently in medical practice and considered independently in eradication trials.

TIME TRENDS IN THE EFFECTIVENESS OF STANDARD TRIPLE THERAPY

A decrease in the *H. pylori* eradication rate after standard triple therapy has been suggested in recent years. Very recently, Gisbert *et al.* [74] assess the efficacy of standard triple therapy in the eradication of *H. pylori* through an epidemiological analysis of all published Spanish trials. Articles on *H. pylori* eradication published in peer-reviewed journals were identified. Studies that included a triple therapy consisting of any PPI with clarithromycin and amoxicillin for up to 14 days were selected. The pooled eradication rates by year from Spanish studies evaluating the efficacy of the standard triple regimen revealed a relatively constant rate over the years. Overall, the analysis of the 32 studies (4,727 patients) showed a mean *H. pylori* cure rate of 80% (95% CI = 77-82%) by ITT. From these results, it may be concluded that, although a decrease in the *H. pylori* eradication rate after triple therapy has been suggested in recent years, cure rates with this regimen did not change in Spain between 1997 and 2008. However, this by no means indicates that the efficacy of standard triple therapy in Spain is acceptable, as it was calculated to be around only 80%.

In this respect, it should be emphasized that although several therapeutic regimens have been eligible to cure *H. pylori* infection, none of the medication combinations have been able to cure the infection in more than 85% of the patients assessed by ITT in a published meta-analysis in 1999[75]. Thus, Laheij *et al.* reviewed as many as 132 different medication combinations to treat *H. pylori* infection, and cure rates of "only" 80-85% were achieved using combinations of a PPI with two antibiotics including clarithromycin, amoxicillin and metronidazole or tinidazole [75]. Therefore, it is evident that new strategies to improve first-line treatment are urgently needed.

SEQUENTIAL THERAPY

One recent therapeutic innovation, postulated as an alternative to standard triple therapy, is the so called "sequential" treatment. Strictly speaking, it is not a new approach, as it uses well-known drugs with approved indication for *H. pylori* eradication. However, the administration strategy is innovative. The sequential regimen is a simple dual therapy including a PPI plus amoxicillin 1 g (both twice daily) given for the first five days followed by a triple therapy including a PPI, clarithromycin 500 mg, and tinidazole (all twice daily) for the remaining five days. Therefore, it is a "five plus five" day therapy [76].

The first meta-analysis comparing the sequential therapy and the standard triple therapy was conducted by Jafri *et al.* [77] in 2008. The crude rates of *H. pylori* eradication in 10 randomized clinical trials involving 2,747 patients were 93% for sequential therapy and 77% for standard triple therapy (RR reduction = 71%; 95% CI = 64-77%; absolute RR = 16 percentage points; 95% CI = 14-19 percentage points). The median rates of adherence were 97.4% for sequential therapy and 96.8% for standard therapy. Sequential therapy appeared superior in pre-specified sensitivity (subgroup) analyses stratified by resistance to clarithromycin, imidazoles, or both. Finally, both treatments had similar side effect profiles.

A second meta-analysis evaluating the sequential therapy, conducted by Gatta *et al.* [78] in 2009, assess the efficacy of this regimen in adults and children. Ten randomized clinical trials enrolled 3,006 adult patients and the OR for eradication of *H. pylori* with sequential therapy compared with standard triple therapy was 2.99 (95% CI = 2.47-3.62), giving a number needed to treat (NNT) of 6. In patients with clarithromycin resistance, the OR for eradication with sequential therapy was 10.2 (95% CI = 3.01-34.6) compared with standard triple therapy. On the other hand, three studies enrolled 260 children, and the OR for eradication was

1.98 (95% CI = 0.96-4.07). As in the previous meta-analysis, there was no difference in the rate of side effects between both regimens.

A third meta-analysis, performed by Tong *et al.* [79], identified 11 randomized trials and, again, demonstrated clear superiority of the sequential therapy both over 7-day triple regimen (RR = 1.23; 95% CI = 1.19-1.27), and over 10-day triple regimen (RR = 1.16; 95% CI = 1.10-1.23). And, once more, adverse event rates were similar.

In summary, sequential therapy appears to be superior to standard triple therapy. Therefore, sequential therapy is a novel promising treatment approach that deserves consideration as a treatment strategy for *H. pylori* infection. However, further robust assessment across a much broader range of patients is required before sequential therapy could supplant existing treatment regimens and be generally recommended in clinical practice [76].

NON-BISMUTH QUADRUPLE (CONCOMITANT) THERAPY

A relevant question is whether it is necessary to provide the drugs sequentially or if the 4 constituent components of sequential therapy can be given concurrently [80]. In other words, does sequential administration represent an advantage or does it make therapy more complicated than necessary? In this regard, the triple combination of clarithromycin plus amoxicillin and a nitroimidazole with a PPI (but without bismuth) has previously been examined as a non-sequential regimen, which proved efficacious. The concept of a “non-bismuth quadruple regimen” or “concomitant” regimen (the term used hereafter) has recently resurfaced. Traditional standard triple therapy (PPI-clarithromycin-amoxicillin) can easily be converted to concomitant therapy by the addition of 500 mg of metronidazole or tinidazole twice daily [80].

Essa *et al.* [81] compared, in 2009,concomitant therapy with standard triple therapy for *H. pylori* infection. The authors identified nine studies (10 treatment arms) including five qualifying randomized clinical (576 subjects) comparing concomitant (duration 3 to 5 days) and triple therapy (duration 5 to 10 days). Pooled estimates of the five randomized clinical trials showed superiority of concomitant therapy over triple therapy (OR = 2.86; 95% CI = 1.73-4.73). Considering all 10 treatment arms, the ITT eradication rate with the concomitant therapy was 90% (95% CI = 86.8-92.1%).

More recently, in 2011, Gisbert *et al.* [80] critically reviewed evidence on the role of concomitant therapy in the treatment of *H. pylori* infection and updated previous meta-analysis. A meta-analysis of 15 studies (1,723 patients) revealed a mean *H. pylori* cure rate (ITT) of 90% for concomitant therapy. A tendency towards better results with longer treatments (7-10 days *vs.* 3-5 days) has been observed, so it seems reasonable to recommend the length of treatment by achieving maximal cure rates (10 days). Clarithromycin resistance may reduce the efficacy of concomitant therapy, although the decrease in eradication rates seems to be far lower than in standard triple therapy. These same authors have recently updated this last meta-analysis, including 19 studies (2,070 patients), and have confirmed a mean *H. pylori* cure rate (ITT) of 88% for concomitant therapy [82]. Moreover, the updated meta-analysis of the randomized clinical trials comparing the concomitant (481 patients) and the standard triple therapy (503 patients) showed that the former was more effective than the latter: 90% *vs.* 78% (ITT analysis) (OR = 2.36; 95% CI = 1.67-3.34).

In summary, non-bismuth quadruple "concomitant" therapy appears to be an effective, safe, and well-tolerated alternative to standard triple therapy and is less complex than sequential therapy. Therefore, this regimen appears well suited for use in settings where the efficacy of triple therapy is unacceptably low.

NITROFURAN (FURAZOLIDONE AND NITROFURANTOIN)-BASED REGIMENS

Buzás *et al.* [83] conducted a systematic review and meta-analysis of the effect of furazolidone- and nitrofurantoin-based regimens in the eradication of *H. pylori* infection. Primary triple regimens containing furazolidone were slightly less efficient than the standard primary combinations. Thus, the pooled eradication rate of primary PPI-based regimens containing furazolidone was 76%. The OR for standard triple therapies *vs.* furazolidone-based regimens was 2.34 (95% CI = 0.76-3.92). RBC plus furazolidone-based triple regimens were equally efficient.

Schedules including a H_2-antagonist plus furazolidone and another antibiotic achieved pooled eradication rates of 80% ($P < 0.05$). Bismuth-based triple therapies achieved 84% cure rate. Primary quadruple regimens containing furazolidone were superior to triple therapies. Second-line schedules containing furazolidone obtained eradication rates of 76%. Finally, third-line rescue therapies were efficient in 65% of the cases. Side-effects of the regimens containing furazolidone were more frequent than those of the standard therapies. Thus, the combined OR of side-effects for furazolidone-based *vs.* standard therapies was 0.74 (95% CI = 0.32-1.98). The duration of treatment, but not the furazolidone dose, influenced the treatment outcome.

Vitamins, Prebiotics and Probiotics

Problems with currently recommended *H. pylori* eradication therapies include unsatisfactory eradication rates and therapy-associated side effects. Measures to overcome these problems include the use of probiotics, which are live microbial food ingredients that are beneficial to health. The rationale for the use of probiotics as adjunctive treatment for *H. pylori* infection is based on the results of studies that have shown that some probiotics can inhibit or kill *H. pylori in vitro*.

Tong *et al.* [84] systematically evaluated whether adding probiotics to anti-*H. pylori* regimens could improve eradication rates and reduce side effects during anti-*H. pylori* treatment. The authors identified 14 randomized trials (including 1,671 patients). Pooled *H. pylori* eradication rates were 84% and 75% for patients with or without probiotics by ITT analysis, respectively (OR = 1.84; 95% CI = 1.34-2.54); the occurrence of total side effects were 25% and 38% for groups with or without probiotics (OR = 0.44; 95% CI = 0.30-0.66). These results suggest that supplementation with probiotics could be effective in increasing eradication rates of anti-*H. pylori* therapy, and could be considered helpful for patients with eradication failure. Furthermore, probiotics show a positive impact on *H. pylori* therapy-related side effects.

Recent evidence showed that Lactobacilli could exert an inhibitory effect on *H. pylori* both *in vitro* and *in vivo* models. Zou *et al.* [85] systematically evaluated whether adding *Lactobacilli* to *H. pylori* eradication regimens could improve eradication rates and reduce side effects during anti-*H. pylori* treatment. Eight randomized trials (including 1,372 patients) were identified. Pooled *H. pylori* eradication rates were 82% and 77% for patients with or without Lactobacilli by ITT analysis, respectively (OR = 1.78; 95% CI = 1.21-2.62). The occurrence of total side effects had no significant difference. However, Lactobacilli supplementation group had lower occurrence of diarrhoea, bloating and taste disturbance. The authors conclude that supplementation with Lactobacilli could be effective in increasing eradication rates of anti-*H. pylori* therapy for first-treated patients. Furthermore, Lactobacilli may have a positive impact on some *H. pylori* therapy-related side effects.

Sachdeva *et al.* [86] evaluated the effect of fermented milk-based probiotic preparations on *H. pylori* eradication. Ten randomized controlled trials were identified, including 963 patients. The pooled OR for eradication by ITT analysis in the treatment *vs.* control group was 1.91 (95% CI = 1.38-2.67). Therefore, the authors concluded that fermented milk-based probiotic preparations improve *H. pylori* eradication rates by approximately 10%, whereas the effect on adverse effects is heterogeneous.

Szajewska *et al.* [87] investigated the effects of *Saccharomyces boulardii* as supplementation to standard triple therapy on *H. pylori* eradication rates and therapy-associated side effects. Five randomized clinical trials involving a total of 1,307 participants were included. Compared with placebo or no intervention, *S. boulardii* given along with triple therapy significantly increased the eradication rate (RR = 1.13; 95% CI = 1.05-1.21) and reduced the risk of overall *H. pylori* therapy-related adverse effects (RR = 0.46; 95% CI = 0.3-0.7), particularly of diarrhoea (RR = 0.47; 95% CI = 0.32-0.69). Therefore, the authors concluded that in patients with *H. pylori* infection, there is evidence to recommend the use of *S. boulardii* along with standard triple therapy as an option for increasing the eradication rates and decreasing overall therapy-related side effects, particularly diarrhoea. More recently, McFarland *et al.* [88] confirmed these results in another meta-analysis, where it was demonstrated that *S. boulardii* reduced *H. pylori* treatment-related symptoms.

Recent evidence has shown that lactoferrin could exert an antimicrobial effect against *H. pylori* both *in vitro* and *in vivo* models. Sachdeva *et al.* [89] evaluated the effect of bovine lactoferrin supplementation in *H. pylori* eradication. Five eligible studies were identified, including 682 subjects. The pooled OR for eradication by ITT analysis was 2.22 (95% CI = 1.44-3.44). There was no significant difference in incidence of adverse effects. Similarly, Zou *et al.* [90] confirmed the beneficial effects of adding lactoferrin to *H. pylori* eradication regimens for the improvement of eradication rates. The authors identified nine randomized trials, including 1,343 patients. Pooled *H. pylori* eradication rates were 86% and 74% for patients with or without lactoferrin by ITT analysis, respectively (OR = 2.26; 95% CI = 1.70-3.00). Furthermore, in contrast with the aforementioned meta-analysis [89], the present one confirmed a lower occurrence of total side-effects in the group receiving lactoferrin (9% *vs.* 16%; OR = 0.15; 95% CI = 0.04-0.54). Therefore, supplementation with lactoferrin could be effective in increasing eradication rates of anti-*H. pylori* therapy. The positive impact on *H. pylori* therapy-related side-effects of lactoferrin, however, needs confirmation.

Vitamins C and E can act as potent antioxidants to reduce the damage caused by reactive oxygen species in gastric mucosa. Whether vitamin supplements for *H. pylori* eradication regimen could improve the rate of eradication remains uncertain. Therefore, Li *et al.* [91] performed a meta-analysis to evaluate the efficacy of vitamins C and E supplementation for the eradication of *H. pylori*. Six studies were included, although five had a low methodological quality. The result of the meta-analysis showed a non-significant difference in the eradication rate of *H. pylori* between the two groups. In conclusion, vitamins C and/or E supplements to the *H. pylori* eradication regimen could not improve the eradication rate.

Traditional Chinese Medicine

Lin *et al.* [92] evaluated the efficacy and safety of Traditional Chinese Medicine in the treatment of *H. pylori* infection. Sixteen trials were included. Clinical heterogeneity and substantial statistical heterogeneity existed among the trials, and therefore meta-analysis was not conducted. The average eradication rates following Traditional Chinese Medicine and triple therapy were 72% and 78%.

Therefore, available evidence is not convincing enough to show that Traditional Chinese Medicine has the same efficacy as triple therapy in *H. pylori* treatment.

H. pylori Eradication When First-Line Therapy Fails: Quinolone-Based Rescue Regimens

After failure of a combination of a PPI-based triple regimen, the use of the quadruple therapy (that is, PPI, bismuth, tetracycline and metronidazole) has been generally used as the optimal second-line therapy based on the relatively good results reported by several authors [93]. However, this regimen requires the administration of 4 drugs with a complex scheme, and is associated with a relatively high incidence of adverse effects. Furthermore, this quadruple regimen still fails to eradicate *H. pylori* in approximately 20 to 30% of the patients, and these cases constitute a therapeutic dilemma, as patients who are not cured with two consecutive treatments including clarithromycin and metronidazole will have at least single, and usually double, resistance [93].

Levofloxacin is a fluoroquinolone antibacterial agent with a broad spectrum of activity against Gram-positive and Gram-negative bacteria and atypical respiratory pathogens [94]. Recently, some studies have evaluated the efficacy of new fluoroquinolones, such as levofloxacin, that could prove to be a valid alternative to standard antibiotics not only as first-line therapies but, more interesting, as rescue-regimens [95]. The aim of a recent study was to conduct a meta-analysis of randomized clinical trials comparing the efficacy and tolerance of the quadruple therapy *vs.* levofloxacin-based triple regimens, for *H. pylori* eradication failures [96]. The meta-analysis demonstrated better results with levofloxacin than with the quadruple combination (81% *vs.* 70%; OR = 1.80; 95% CI = 0.94-3.46). This difference reached statistical significance and heterogeneity markedly decreased when a single outlier study was excluded or when only high-quality studies were considered. Furthermore, levofloxacin-regimen was associated with less adverse effects than the quadruple regimen. A similar meta-analysis simultaneously published achieved the same conclusion [97].

Finally, a third and more recent meta-analysis by Li *et al.* [98], including 13 randomized clinical trials, compared levofloxacin-based triple therapy *vs.* bismuth-based quadruple therapy. The eradication rates of the two regimens were shown to have no significant difference (OR = 1.43; 95% CI = 0.82-2.51). However, the eradication rates demonstrated superiority of the 10-day levofloxacin-based triple therapy over 7-day bismuth-based quadruple therapy (OR = 4.79; 95% CI = 2.95-7.79). And, again, levofloxacin-based triple therapy was demonstrated to be better tolerated than bismuth-based quadruple therapy with lower rates of side effects (OR = 0.41; 95% CI = 0.27-0.61), and lower rates of discontinuation of therapy due to adverse events (OR = 0.13; 95% CI = 0.06-0.33). Furthermore, this meta-analysis suggested that the eradication rates of the moxifloxacin-based triple therapy had a slight superiority to bismuth-based quadruple therapy, but there was no significant difference between them.

In 2011, Wu *et al.* [99] systematically reviewed the efficacy and tolerance of moxifloxacin-containing triple therapy in second-line *H. pylori* eradication, and conducted a meta-analysis of studies comparing this regimen with bismuth-containing quadruple therapy. Seven randomized clinical trials, including 787 patients, were assessed. The meta-analysis showed that the eradication rate in the moxifloxacin group was significantly higher than that in the quadruple therapy group (75 *vs.* 61%, OR = 1.89; 95% CI = 1.38-2.58); besides, the rates of side effects and discontinuing therapy because of side effects in the moxifloxacin group were significantly lower than those in the quadruple therapy group (OR = 0.27; 95% CI = 0.18-0.41; discontinuing therapy because of side effects: OR = 0.18; 95% CI = 0.08-0.40).

In summary, second-generation fluoroquinolone-based (especially 10-day levofloxacin-based) triple therapy can be suggested as the regimen of choice for rescue therapy in the eradication of persistent *H. pylori* infection. Moxifloxacin-containing triple regimen may also be an encouraging alternative to bismuth-containing quadruple therapy in the second-line treatment of *H. pylori* infection.

CONCLUSIONS

Helicobacter pylori infection is the main cause of gastritis, gastroduodenal ulcer disease, and gastric cancer. After 30 years of experience in *H. pylori* treatment, however, the ideal regimen to treat this infection has still to be found. Nowadays, apart from having to know well first-line eradication regimens, we must also be prepared to face treatment failures.

Systematic reviews and meta-analyses are essential to summarize evidence relating to efficacy and safety of health care interventions accurately and reliably. Meta-analyses use quantitative methods to analyze the literature and seek to answer a focused clinical question, using rigorous statistical analysis of pooled research studies. Well conducted meta-analyses allow a more objective appraisal of the evidence than traditional narrative reviews, provide a more precise estimate of a treatment effect, and may explain heterogeneity between the results of individual studies. Meta-analysis is an invaluable scientific research method that is widely used in many disciplines of science, including medicine.

In this chapter, we have reviewed published meta-analyses focused on *H. pylori* eradication treatments. Initially, dual therapy of either bismuth compounds or PPIs and one antibiotic obtained insufficient cure rates to be advisable. PPI-based triple therapies (combined with two antibiotics, among amoxicillin, nitroimidazole and clarithromycin) have been the most widely recommended. Bismuth-containing quadruple therapy is roughly equivalent to triple therapy in terms of effectiveness, compliance and side-effects profile. PPI-based regimens are superior to H_2-antagonists-based ones. The influence of the type of PPI, the dose and the duration of the treatment are discussed. Among the factors influencing the efficacy of therapy, resistance to clarithromycin and metronidazole are the most important risk factors for eradication failure. As a progressive decrease in the eradication rate after standard triple therapy has been suggested in recent years, more recently, the sequential therapy and the non-bismuth quadruple (concomitant) therapy have been recommended in settings where the efficacy of triple therapy is unacceptably low. The role of prebiotics and probiotics as adjunctive treatment for *H. pylori* infection is also reviewed. Several rescue therapies may be used. Bismuth-based quadruple therapy is effective, but the complexity of the regimen and the associated adverse effects limit the compliance. PPI-based triple with amoxicillin and levofloxacin or moxifloxacin is at least equally effective, and better tolerated.

In summary, it may be concluded that meta-analysis has contributed, in a relevant way, to our understanding in the management of patients with *H. pylori* infection.

ACKNOWLEDGEMENT

None Declared.

CONFLICT OF INTEREST

The author(s) confirm that this chapter content has no conflict of interest.

REFERENCES

[1] Siwek J, Gourlay ML, Slawson DC, Shaughnessy AF. How to write an evidence-based clinical review article. Am Fam Physician. 2002 Jan 15;65(2):251-8.
[2] Higgins JPT, Green S, (editors). Cochrane Handbook for Systematic Reviews of Interventions Version 5.1.0 [updated March 2011] The Cochrane Collaboration, 2011. Available from www.cochrane-handbook.org.
[3] Antman EM, Lau J, Kupelnick B, Mosteller F, Chalmers TC. A comparison of results of meta-analyses of randomized control trials and recommendations of clinical experts. Treatments for myocardial infarction. Jama. 1992 Jul 8;268(2):240-8.
[4] Oxman AD, Cook DJ, Guyatt GH. Users' guides to the medical literature. VI. How to use an overview. Evidence-Based Medicine Working Group. Jama. 1994 Nov 2;272(17):1367-71.
[5] Egger M, Smith GD, Phillips AN. Meta-analysis: principles and procedures. Bmj. 1997 Dec 6;315(7121):1533-7.
[6] Huang JQ, Hunt RH. Editorial: Uses and abuses of meta-analysis in gastroenterology. Chin J Dig Dis. 2002;3:39-42.
[7] Mulrow CD. Rationale for systematic reviews. Bmj. 1994 Sep 3;309(6954):597-9.
[8] Liberati A, Altman DG, Tetzlaff J, *et al.* The PRISMA statement for reporting systematic reviews and meta-analyses of studies that evaluate health care interventions: explanation and elaboration. Ann Intern Med. 2009 Aug 18;151(4):W65-94.
[9] Glass GV. Primary, secondary and meta-analysis of research. Educ Res. 1976;5:3-8.
[10] Gabriel-Sánchez R, Pladevall-Vila M. Evaluación de la evidencia en medicina: revisiones sistemáticas y metaanálisis. Medicine. 1998;7(104):4845-51.
[11] Gisbert JP, Pajares R, Pajares JM. Evolution of *Helicobacter pylori* therapy from a meta-analytical perspective. Helicobacter. 2007 Nov;12 Suppl 2:50-8.
[12] Petticrew M. Systematic reviews from astronomy to zoology: myths and misconceptions. Bmj. 2001 Jan 13;322(7278):98-101.
[13] Chiba N, Rao BV, Rademaker JW, Hunt RH. Meta-analysis of the efficacy of antibiotic therapy in eradicating *Helicobacter pylori*. Am J Gastroenterol. 1992 Dec;87(12):1716-27.
[14] Pipkin GA, Dixon JS, Williamson R, Wood JR. Clarithromycin dual therapy regimens for eradication of *Helicobacter pylori*: a review. Helicobacter. 1997 Dec;2(4):159-71.
[15] Hopkins RJ. Current FDA-approved treatments for *Helicobacter pylori* and the FDA approval process. Gastroenterology. 1997 Dec;113(6 Suppl):S126-30.
[16] Current European concepts in the management of *Helicobacter pylori* infection. The Maastricht Consensus Report. European *Helicobacter Pylori* Study Group. Gut. 1997 Jul;41(1):8-13.

[17] Unge P. What other regimens are under investigation to treat *Helicobacter pylori* infection? Gastroenterology. 1997 Dec;113(6 Suppl):S131-48.

[18] Malfertheiner P, Megraud F, O'Morain C, *et al.* Current concepts in the management of *Helicobacter pylori* infection: the Maastricht III Consensus Report. Gut. 2007 Jun;56(6):772-81.

[19] Malfertheiner P, Megraud F, O'Morain CA, *et al.* Management of *Helicobacter pylori* infection--the Maastricht IV/ Florence Consensus Report. Gut. 2012 May;61(5):646-64.

[20] Unge P. Review of *Helicobacter pylori* eradication regimens. Scand J Gastroenterol Suppl. 1996;215:74-81.

[21] Buzás GM. [Eradication of *Helicobacter pylori* infection in Hungary (1993-2002): a meta-analysis] Orv Hetil. 2003 Jun 1;144(22):1077-83.

[22] Buzás GM, Józan J. [Eradication of *Helicobacter pylori* infection in Europe: a meta-analysis based on congress abstracts, 1997-2002] Orv Hetil. 2004 Oct 3;145(40):2035-41.

[23] Buzás GM, Józan J. First-line eradication of *H. pylori* infection in Europe: a meta-analysis based on congress abstracts, 1997-2004. World J Gastroenterol. 2006 Sep 7;12(33):5311-9.

[24] Taylor JL, Zagari M, Murphy K, Freston JW. Pharmacoeconomic comparison of treatments for the eradication of *Helicobacter pylori*. Arch Intern Med. 1997 Jan 13;157(1):87-97.

[25] Schmid CH, Whiting G, Cory D, Ross SD, Chalmers TC. Omeprazole plus antibiotics in the eradication of *Helicobacter pylori* infection: a meta-regression analysis of randomized, controlled trials. Am J Ther. 1999 Jan;6(1):25-36.

[26] Gisbert JP, Gonzalez L, Calvet X, *et al.* Proton pump inhibitor, clarithromycin and either amoxycillin or nitroimidazole: a meta-analysis of eradication of *Helicobacter pylori*. Aliment Pharmacol Ther. 2000 Oct;14(10):1319-28.

[27] Rodgers C, van Zanten SV. A meta-analysis of the success rate of *Helicobacter pylori* therapy in Canada. Can J Gastroenterol. 2007 May;21(5):295-300.

[28] Huang J, Hunt RH. The importance of clarithromycin dose in the management of *Helicobacter pylori* infection: a meta-analysis of triple therapies with a proton pump inhibitor, clarithromycin and amoxycillin or metronidazole. Aliment Pharmacol Ther. 1999 Jun;13(6):719-29.

[29] Dong J, Yu XF, Zou J. Azithromycin-containing *vs.* standard triple therapy for *Helicobacter pylori* eradication: a meta-analysis. World J Gastroenterol. 2009 Dec 28;15(48):6102-10.

[30] Gisbert JP. Second-line rescue therapy of *helicobacter pylori* infection. Therap Adv Gastroenterol. 2009 Nov;2(6):331-56.

[31] Zhang ZF, Zhao G, Liu LN. [Effectiveness and safety of proton pump inhibitor and levofloxacin based first-line triple therapy in the eradication of *Helicobacter pylori*: a meta-analysis] Zhonghua Yi Xue Za Zhi. 2008 Oct 21;88(38):2722-5.

[32] Wenzhen Y, Kehu Y, Bin M, *et al.* Moxifloxacin-based triple therapy *vs.* clarithromycin-based triple therapy for first-line treatment of *Helicobacter pylori* infection: a meta-analysis of randomized controlled trials. Intern Med. 2009;48(24):2069-76.

[33] Gisbert JP. Potent gastric acid inhibition in *Helicobacter pylori* eradication. Drugs. 2005;65 Suppl 1:83-96.

[34] Holtmann G, Layer P, Goebell H. [Are proton pump inhibitors superior to H2 receptor antagonists within the scope of *H. pylori* eradication therapy? Meta analysis of current parallel group comparisons] Z Gastroenterol. 1996 May;34(5):267-72.

[35] Gisbert JP, Khorrami S, Calvet X, Gabriel R, Carballo F, Pajares JM. Meta-analysis: proton pump inhibitors *vs.* H2-receptor antagonists--their efficacy with antibiotics in *Helicobacter pylori* eradication. Aliment Pharmacol Ther. 2003 Oct 15;18(8):757-66.

[36] Dobrucali A, Canbakan B, Canbakan M, *et al.* [Meta-analysis of determining the pathogen eradicating efficacy of various therapeutic regimens in *Helicobacter pylori* infection] Wien Med Wochenschr. 1998;148(20):464-8.

[37] Ren Q, Ma B, Yang K, Yan X. Lafutidine-based triple therapy for *Helicobacter pylori* eradication. Hepatogastroenterology. 2010 Sep-Oct;57(102-103):1074-81.

[38] Bazzoli F, Pozzato P, Zagari M, *et al.* Efficacy of lansoprazole in eradicating *Helicobacter pylori*: a meta-analysis. Helicobacter. 1998 Sep;3(3):195-201.

[39] Gisbert JP, Khorrami S, Calvet X, Pajares JM. Pantoprazole based therapies in *Helicobacter pylori* eradication: a systematic review and meta-analysis. Eur J Gastroenterol Hepatol. 2004 Jan;16(1):89-99.

[40] Gisbert JP, Khorrami S, Calvet X, Pajares JM. Systematic review: Rabeprazole-based therapies in *Helicobacter pylori* eradication. Aliment Pharmacol Ther. 2003 Mar 15;17(6):751-64.

[41] Gisbert JP, Pajares JM. Esomeprazole-based therapy in *Helicobacter pylori* eradication: a meta-analysis. Dig Liver Dis. 2004 Apr;36(4):253-9.

[42] Wang X, Fang JY, Lu R, Sun DF. A meta-analysis: comparison of esomeprazole and other proton pump inhibitors in eradicating *Helicobacter pylori*. Digestion. 2006;73(2-3):178-86.

[43] Vergara M, Vallve M, Gisbert JP, Calvet X. Meta-analysis: comparative efficacy of different proton-pump inhibitors in triple therapy for *Helicobacter pylori* eradication. Aliment Pharmacol Ther. 2003 Sep 15;18(6):647-54.

[44] Vallve M, Vergara M, Gisbert JP, Calvet X. Single *vs.* double dose of a proton pump inhibitor in triple therapy for *Helicobacter pylori* eradication: a meta-analysis. Aliment Pharmacol Ther. 2002 Jun;16(6):1149-56.

[45] Padol S, Yuan Y, Thabane M, Padol IT, Hunt RH. The effect of CYP2C19 polymorphisms on *H. pylori* eradication rate in dual and triple first-line PPI therapies: a meta-analysis. Am J Gastroenterol. 2006 Jul;101(7):1467-75.

[46] Villoria A, Garcia P, Calvet X, Gisbert JP, Vergara M. Meta-analysis: high-dose proton pump inhibitors *vs.* standard dose in triple therapy for *Helicobacter pylori* eradication. Aliment Pharmacol Ther. 2008 Oct 1;28(7):868-77.

[47] Zhou N, Chen WX, Zhang W, Li L, Jin X, Li YM. Is short-term therapy really sufficient to eradicate *Helicobacter pylori* infection? J Zhejiang Univ Sci B. 2010 Sep;11(9):690-701.

[48] Calvet X, Garcia N, Lopez T, Gisbert JP, Gene E, Roque M. A meta-analysis of short *vs.* long therapy with a proton pump inhibitor, clarithromycin and either metronidazole or amoxycillin for treating *Helicobacter pylori* infection. Aliment Pharmacol Ther. 2000 May;14(5):603-9.

[49] Ford A, Moayyedi P. How can the current strategies for *Helicobacter pylori* eradication therapy be improved? Can J Gastroenterol. 2003 Jun;17 Suppl B:36B-40B.

[50] Fuccio L, Minardi ME, Zagari RM, Grilli D, Magrini N, Bazzoli F. Meta-analysis: duration of first-line proton-pump inhibitor based triple therapy for *Helicobacter pylori* eradication. Ann Intern Med. 2007 Oct 16;147(8):553-62.

[51] Calvet X, Villoria A, Vergara M. Could increasing the duration of triple therapy be a clinically useful strategy? Ann Intern Med. 2008 Apr 15;148(8):624; author reply -5.

[52] Flores HB, Salvana A, Ang ELR, *et al.* Duration of Proton-Pump Inhibitor-Based Triple Therapy for *Helicobacter pylori* Eradication: a Meta-Analysis. Gastroenterology. 2010;138:M1138.

[53] Graham DY, Fischbach L. *Helicobacter pylori* treatment in the era of increasing antibiotic resistance. Gut. 2010 Aug;59(8):1143-53.

[54] Gisbert JP, Pajares JM. Systematic review and meta-analysis: is 1-week proton pump inhibitor-based triple therapy sufficient to heal peptic ulcer? Aliment Pharmacol Ther. 2005 Apr 1;21(7):795-804.

[55] Megraud F. *H. pylori* antibiotic resistance: prevalence, importance, and advances in testing. Gut. 2004 Sep;53(9):1374-84.

[56] Megraud F, Doermann HP. Clinical relevance of resistant strains of *Helicobacter pylori*: a review of current data. Gut. 1998 Jul;43 Suppl 1:S61-5.

[57] Fischbach LA, van Zanten S, Dickason J. Meta-analysis: the efficacy, adverse events, and adherence related to first-line anti-*Helicobacter pylori* quadruple therapies. Aliment Pharmacol Ther. 2004 Nov 15;20(10):1071-82.

[58] Ford AC, Malfertheiner P, Giguere M, Santana J, Khan M, Moayyedi P. Adverse events with bismuth salts for *Helicobacter pylori* eradication: systematic review and meta-analysis. World J Gastroenterol. 2008 Dec 28;14(48):7361-70.

[59] Buring SM, Winner LH, Hatton RC, Doering PL. Discontinuation rates of *Helicobacter pylori* treatment regimens: a meta-analysis. Pharmacotherapy. 1999 Mar;19(3):324-32.

[60] Gene E, Calvet X, Azagra R, Gisbert JP. Triple *vs.* quadruple therapy for treating *Helicobacter pylori* infection: a meta-analysis. Aliment Pharmacol Ther. 2003 May 1;17(9):1137-43.

[61] Luther J, Higgins PD, Schoenfeld PS, Moayyedi P, Vakil N, Chey WD. Empiric quadruple *vs.* triple therapy for primary treatment of *Helicobacter pylori* infection: Systematic review and meta-analysis of efficacy and tolerability. Am J Gastroenterol. 2010 Jan;105(1):65-73.

[62] Gisbert JP, Pajares JM, Valle J. Ranitidine bismuth citrate therapy regimens for treatment of *Helicobacter pylori* infection: a review. Helicobacter. 1999 Mar;4(1):58-66.

[63] Gisbert JP, Gonzalez L, Calvet X, Roque M, Gabriel R, Pajares JM. *Helicobacter pylori* eradication: proton pump inhibitor *vs.* ranitidine bismuth citrate plus two antibiotics for 1 week-a meta-analysis of efficacy. Aliment Pharmacol Ther. 2000 Sep;14(9):1141-50.

[64] Gisbert JP, Gonzalez L, Calvet X. Systematic review and meta-analysis: proton pump inhibitor *vs.* ranitidine bismuth citrate plus two antibiotics in *Helicobacter pylori* eradication. Helicobacter. 2005 Jun;10(3):157-71.

[65] Dore MP, Leandro G, Realdi G, Sepulveda AR, Graham DY. Effect of pretreatment antibiotic resistance to metronidazole and clarithromycin on outcome of *Helicobacter pylori* therapy: a meta-analytical approach. Dig Dis Sci. 2000 Jan;45(1):68-76.

[66] van der Wouden EJ, Thijs JC, van Zwet AA, Sluiter WJ, Kleibeuker JH. The influence of *in vitro* nitroimidazole resistance on the efficacy of nitroimidazole-containing anti-*Helicobacter pylori* regimens: a meta-analysis. Am J Gastroenterol. 1999 Jul;94(7):1751-9.

[67] Fischbach LA, Goodman KJ, Feldman M, Aragaki C. Sources of variation of *Helicobacter pylori* treatment success in adults worldwide: a meta-analysis. Int J Epidemiol. 2002 Feb;31(1):128-39.

[68] Fischbach L, Evans EL. Meta-analysis: the effect of antibiotic resistance status on the efficacy of triple and quadruple first-line therapies for *Helicobacter pylori*. Aliment Pharmacol Ther. 2007 Aug 1;26(3):343-57.

[69] Suzuki T, Matsuo K, Ito H, *et al.* Smoking increases the treatment failure for *Helicobacter pylori* eradication. Am J Med. 2006 Mar;119(3):217-24.

[70] Zhao F, Wang J, Yang Y, *et al.* Effect of CYP2C19 genetic polymorphisms on the efficacy of proton pump inhibitor-based triple therapy for *Helicobacter pylori* eradication: a meta-analysis. Helicobacter. 2008 Dec;13(6):532-41.

[71] Suzuki T, Matsuo K, Sawaki A, *et al.* Systematic review and meta-analysis: importance of CagA status for successful eradication of *Helicobacter pylori* infection. Aliment Pharmacol Ther. 2006 Jul 15;24(2):273-80.

[72] Janssen MJ, Laheij RJ, de Boer WA, Jansen JB. Meta-analysis: the influence of pre-treatment with a proton pump inhibitor on *Helicobacter pylori* eradication. Aliment Pharmacol Ther. 2005 Feb 15;21(4):341-5.

[73] Broutet N, Tchamgoue S, Pereira E, Lamouliatte H, Salamon R, Megraud F. Risk factors for failure of *Helicobacter pylori* therapy--results of an individual data analysis of 2751 patients. Aliment Pharmacol Ther. 2003 Jan;17(1):99-109.

[74] Gisbert JP, Calvet X. Review article: the effectiveness of standard triple therapy for *Helicobacter pylori* has not changed over the last decade, but it is not good enough. Aliment Pharmacol Ther. 2011 Dec;34(11-12):1255-68.

[75] Laheij RJ, Rossum LG, Jansen JB, Straatman H, Verbeek AL. Evaluation of treatment regimens to cure *Helicobacter pylori* infection--a meta-analysis. Aliment Pharmacol Ther. 1999 Jul;13(7):857-64.

[76] Gisbert JP, Calvet X, O'Connor A, Megraud F, O'Morain CA. Sequential therapy for *Helicobacter pylori* eradication: a critical review. J Clin Gastroenterol. 2010 May-Jun;44(5):313-25.

[77] Jafri NS, Hornung CA, Howden CW. Meta-analysis: sequential therapy appears superior to standard therapy for *Helicobacter pylori* infection in patients naive to treatment. Ann Intern Med. 2008 Jun 17;148(12):923-31.

[78] Gatta L, Vakil N, Leandro G, Di Mario F, Vaira D. Sequential therapy or triple therapy for *Helicobacter pylori* infection: systematic review and meta-analysis of randomized controlled trials in adults and children. Am J Gastroenterol. 2009 Dec;104(12):3069-79; quiz 1080.

[79] Tong JL, Ran ZH, Shen J, Xiao SD. Sequential therapy *vs.* standard triple therapies for *Helicobacter pylori* infection: a meta-analysis. J Clin Pharm Ther. 2009 Feb;34(1):41-53.

[80] Gisbert JP, Calvet X. Review article: non-bismuth quadruple (concomitant) therapy for eradication of Helicobater *pylori*. Aliment Pharmacol Ther. 2011 Sep;34(6):604-17.

[81] Essa AS, Kramer JR, Graham DY, Treiber G. Meta-analysis: four-drug, three-antibiotic, non-bismuth-containing "concomitant therapy" *vs.* triple therapy for *Helicobacter pylori* eradication. Helicobacter. 2009 Apr;14(2):109-18.

[82] Gisbert JP, Calvet X. Update on non-bismuth quadruple (concomitant) therapy for eradication of *Helicobacter pylori*. Clin Exp Gastroenterol. 2012;5:23-34.

[83] Buzás GM, Józan J. Nitrofuran-based regimens for the eradication of *Helicobacter pylori* infection. J Gastroenterol Hepatol. 2007 Oct;22(10):1571-81.

[84] Tong JL, Ran ZH, Shen J, Zhang CX, Xiao SD. Meta-analysis: the effect of supplementation with probiotics on eradication rates and adverse events during *Helicobacter pylori* eradication therapy. Aliment Pharmacol Ther. 2007 Jan 15;25(2):155-68.

[85] Zou J, Dong J, Yu X. Meta-analysis: Lactobacillus containing quadruple therapy *vs.* standard triple first-line therapy for *Helicobacter pylori* eradication. Helicobacter. 2009 Oct;14(5):97-107.

[86] Sachdeva A, Nagpal J. Effect of fermented milk-based probiotic preparations on *Helicobacter pylori* eradication: a systematic review and meta-analysis of randomized-controlled trials. Eur J Gastroenterol Hepatol. 2009 Jan;21(1):45-53.

[87] Szajewska H, Horvath A, Piwowarczyk A. Meta-analysis: the effects of Saccharomyces boulardii supplementation on *Helicobacter pylori* eradication rates and side effects during treatment. Aliment Pharmacol Ther. 2010 Nov;32(9):1069-79.

[88] McFarland LV. Systematic review and meta-analysis of Saccharomyces boulardii in adult patients. World J Gastroenterol. 2010 May 14;16(18):2202-22.

[89] Sachdeva A, Nagpal J. Meta-analysis: efficacy of bovine lactoferrin in *Helicobacter pylori* eradication. Aliment Pharmacol Ther. 2009 Apr 1;29(7):720-30.

[90] Zou J, Dong J, Yu XF. Meta-analysis: the effect of supplementation with lactoferrin on eradication rates and adverse events during *Helicobacter pylori* eradication therapy. Helicobacter. 2009 Apr;14(2):119-27.

[91] Li G, Li L, Yu C, Chen L. Effect of vitamins C and E supplementation on *Helicobacter pylori* eradication: a meta-analysis. Br J Nutr. 2011 Dec;106(11):1632-7.

[92] Lin J, Huang WW. A systematic review of treating *Helicobacter pylori* infection with Traditional Chinese Medicine. World J Gastroenterol. 2009 Oct 7;15(37):4715-9.

[93] Gisbert JP, Pajares JM. Review article: *Helicobacter pylori* "rescue" regimen when proton pump inhibitor-based triple therapies fail. Aliment Pharmacol Ther. 2002 Jun;16(6):1047-57.

[94] Croom KF, Goa KL. Levofloxacin: a review of its use in the treatment of bacterial infections in the United States. Drugs. 2003;63(24):2769-802.

[95] Gisbert JP, Pajares JM. *Helicobacter pylori* "rescue" therapy after failure of two eradication treatments. Helicobacter. 2005 Oct;10(5):363-72.

[96] Gisbert JP, Morena F. Systematic review and meta-analysis: levofloxacin-based rescue regimens after *Helicobacter pylori* treatment failure. Aliment Pharmacol Ther. 2006 Jan 1;23(1):35-44.

[97] Saad RJ, Schoenfeld P, Kim HM, Chey WD. Levofloxacin-based triple therapy *vs.* bismuth-based quadruple therapy for persistent *Helicobacter pylori* infection: a meta-analysis. Am J Gastroenterol. 2006 Mar;101(3):488-96.

[98] Li Y, Huang X, Yao L, Shi R, Zhang G. Advantages of Moxifloxacin and Levofloxacin-based triple therapy for second-line treatments of persistent *Helicobacter pylori* infection: a meta analysis. Wien Klin Wochenschr. 2010 Jul;122(13-14):413-22.

[99] Wu C, Chen X, Liu J, Li MY, Zhang ZQ, Wang ZQ. Moxifloxacin-containing triple therapy *vs.* bismuth-containing quadruple therapy for second-line treatment of *Helicobacter pylori* infection: a meta-analysis. Helicobacter. 2011 Apr;16(2):131-8.

Send Orders for Reprints to reprints@benthamscience.net

CHAPTER 15

From Chronic Gastritis to Gastric Cancer: The Role of *Helicobacter pylori*

Krisztina Hagymási, László Herszényi* and Zsolt Tulassay

2nd Department of Medicine, Semmelweis University, Budapest, Hungary

Abstract: *Helicobacter pylori* (*H. pylori*) infects more than half of the world's human population, but only 1 to 3% of infected persons develop gastric adenocarcinoma. *H. pylori* is a definite or class I carcinogen in humans. The mechanisms of *H. pylori*-associated gastric carcinogenesis are still poorly defined. The clinical outcome of the infection is determined by host genetic predisposition (IL-1*β*, TNF*a*, IL-10), bacterial virulence factors (*VacA, CagA*), as well as environmental factors (salt intake, smoking). Eliminating *H. pylori* from a large part of the population may be unfeasible economically, and the long-term consequences are still unpredictable; this is why identifying high-risk individuals is very important.

Keywords: Adhesins, gastric cancer, *Helicobacter pylori,* helminths infection, interleukins, outer membrane proteins, peptidoglycans, polymorphisms, salt intake, smoking, tumor necrosis factor-ά, virulence factors.

Gastric cancer is the fourth or fifth most common cancer worldwide, the second leading cause of cancer-related death [1-3]. Almost 1 million cases are diagnosed each year [1], causing approximately 700,000 deaths on an annual basis [4]. Although the incidence rate is declining, its prognosis remains poor. The five-year survival rate is low (10-20%) [5]. Despite a major decline in incidence and mortality, gastric cancer remains a severe public health burden worldwide, especially in developing countries [3].

Environmental factors play a major role in the carcinogenesis, but immunological, genetic and immunogenetic factors are also thought to contribute to the etiopathogenesis of gastric carcinoma [5]. The main risk factors are *Helicobacter pylori* infection, chronic gastritis, pernicious anaemia, intestinal metaplasia,

***Address correspondence to László Herszényi:** Semmelweis University 2nd Medical Clinic; Tel: +36-1-266-0926; Fax: +36-1-266-0816; E-mail: herlasz@yahoo.com familial adenomatous polyposis or gastric polyps. Blood group A, previous gastric resection, a salt-rich diet, preserved pickles and foods, low intake of fruits and vegetables, alcohol consumption, smoking, familial history of stomach cancer, exposure to coal mines and the processing of rubber, and nickel can elevate the risk of gastric neoplasms developing [4, 6].

The Gram-negative, micro-aerophilic, spiral-shaped bacterial pathogen, *H. pylori* is considered to be the most common etiological factor of infection-related cancers. 16.1% of the worldwide cancers are considered to be associated with infectious diseases. The ratio was higher in less developed countries (22.9%) than in more developed countries (7.4%), and varies from 3.3% in Australia and New Zealand to 32.7% in sub-Saharan Africa [7]. *H. pylori* infection represents.

5.5% of the global cancer burden [1], followed by human papilloma viruses, hepatitis B and C viruses, Epstein-Barr virus, human immunodeficiency virus and human herpesvirus-8 [2, 7]. *H. pylori* is a definite or class I carcinogen in humans, as concluded by the WHO in 1994 [2]. At the moment, gastric cancer is generally considered the end result of a chronic process, beginning with *H. pylori*-associated chronic gastritis, and followed by atrophy, metaplasia and dysplasia [8].

H. pylori infects more than half of the world's human population [2]. Colonisation causes no symptoms. Approximately 10% of infected individuals develop peptic ulcer disease, 1 to 3% develop gastric adenocarcinoma, and <0.1% develop mucosa-associated lymphoid tissue (MALT) lymphoma [9].

Some colonised individuals may develop corpus gastritis, associated with gastric hypochlorhydria, gastric atrophy, gastric ulcers and an increased risk of gastric cancer. However, others may develop antral-predominant gastritis, associated with gastric hyperchlorhydria and an increased risk of duodenal ulcers [10, 11].

Gastric cancer develops in 2.9 percent of the infected and none of the uninfected patients [12]. *H. pylori* infection is responsible for about 75% of all noncardia gastric cancers and 63.4% of all stomach cancers worldwide [2]. Statistically the prevalence of infection is significantly higher in specimens from patients with the intestinal type (89.2%) than in specimens from patients with the diffuse type (31.8%) of gastric cancer [13].

Eradication of *H. pylori* infection decreases the risk of gastric cancer in infected individuals, as well as the presence of premalignant lesions [14-16]. Endoscopic abnormalities are common in gastric ulcer patients and persist after proton-pump inhibitor-based triple therapy for *H. pylori* eradication. Follow-up endoscopy and histology may be necessary, even in patients with apparently non-malignant gastric ulcer, to improve the detection rate of gastric malignancy in populations with a high prevalence of gastric cancer [17].

H. pylori plays a role in the development and progression of gastric mucosa associated lymphoid tissue (MALT) lymphoma [18]. Eradicating the bacterium ensues with the treatment of localised stage I gastric MALT lymphoma with *H. pylori* infection [18].

Connection Between *H. pylori* and Gastric Cancer

Colonisation of the bacteria is differs in different parts of the stomach. Data shows that *H. pylori* infection plays a crucial role in noncardia gastric carcinogenesis, but its association with cardia cancer is still ambiguous. *H. pylori* infection increases the risk of noncardia gastric cancer by six-fold over non-infected individuals [4].

The carcinogenic effect of *H. pylori* can be modified by dietary and environmental factors. *H. pylori* infection is more frequent in less developed Asian countries (India, Bangladesh, Pakistan, Thailand) in comparison to more developed Asian countries (Japan, China). However the frequency of gastric cancer is paradoxically very low in less developed regions compared to that in Japan and China ("Asian enigma"). The rice and more salty fish consumption, alcohol consumption, as well as smoking are responsible for the higher frequency of gastric cancer in the developed Asian countries [19]. Several other large populations with a high infection prevalence reveal a very low rate of gastric cancer. The so-called "African enigma" remains unexplained as well, but it does verify that not all *H. pylori* infected patients have increased risk of gastric cancer [13, 20].

Virulence Factors of *H. pylori*

Bacterial virulence factors play an important role in the progression and outcome of *H. pylori* infection [21].

The *cag* pathogenicity island (*cag* PAI) contains 27-31 genes and encodes the CagA protein [1]. The *cag* PAI is not expressed in all strains. In western countries, 60% of the isolated strains are *cag* PAI positive, while almost all of the East Asian strains isolated are *cag* PAI-positive [2].

cag PAI (*cag*+) amplifies the risk for severe gastritis, atrophic gastritis, and distal gastric cancer in comparison with *cag*-deficient mutant. At least 18 *cag* genes encode components of a bacterial secretion apparatus type IV, which exports bacterial protein across the bacterial membrane and into host gastric epithelial cells [1].

Reactive oxygen species and oxidative damage play a role in the inflammation-to-carcinoma sequence of *H. pylori* infection. *H. pylori* strains bearing the *cag* pathogenicity island induced higher levels of intracellular oxygen metabolites than isogenic *cag* PAI-deficient mutants [22].

CagA

Cytotoxin-associated gene A product (*CagA*) is a well-known virulence factor of *H. pylori*. When it translocated into the host cell by the type IV secretion system it is phosphorylated at the glutamate-proline-isoleucine-tyrosine-alanine (EPIYA) motifs by members of the Abl and Src kinases, which results in morhological changes of the cell: elongation and scattering, development of so-called "hummingbird phenotype". Four EPIYA motifs (-A,-B, -C, -D) are distinguished by different amino acid sequence surrounding the motif. EPIYA-A, -B sites are less phosphorylated than EPIYA-C. EPIYA-C is typically found only in strains from western countries (Europe, North America, Australia), and is and an indicator of the gastric cancer risk. EPIYA-D containing strains induce greater interleukin-8 release from gastric epithelial cells. EPIYA-D is found in East Asian strains [1].

Phosphorylated *CagA* activates an eukaryotic tyrosine phosphatase (SHP-2), resulting in sustained activation of extracellular signal-regulated kinases 1 and 2 (ERK ½), Crk adaptor, C-terminal Src kinase. East Asian A-B-D type *CagA* binds more strongly to SHP-2 than Western type A-B-C type CagA [1]. The activation of ERK, focal adhesion kinase (FAK), a defect in cell retraction, and the inhibition of the catalytic activity of c-Src, result in tyrosine dephosphorylation of the actin binding proteins cortractin, ezrin, vinculin, leading to cell elongation [1, 2].

Nonphosphorylated *CagA* also exerts effects within the cell. The main effects and targets of nonphosphorylated *CagA*: adhesion protein E-cadherin, cadherin-associated protein β-catenin, hepatocyte growth factor receptor c-Met, phospholipase C gamma (PLC-γ), adaptor protein Grb2, the kinase partitioning-defective 1b/microtubule affinity-regulating kinase 2 (PAR1b/MARK2), epithelial tight junction scaffolding protein zonula occludens 1 (ZO-1) and the transmembrane protein junctional adhesion molecule A (JAM-A), which lead to pro-inflammatory and mitogenic responses, disruption of cell-cell junctions, and loss of cell polarity that may be important in the development of gastric carcinoma [1, 2].

CagA is an oncogenic protein, its expression leads to gastric epithelial cell proliferation and carcinoma, based on transgenic mice studies. However the details are not fully understood, because only a small part of individuals colonised by *Cag+ H. pylori* will develop gastric cancer [1].

Activity of *CagA* on tumor suppressor pathways has also been investigated. Data show that *CagA* is able to modulate the apoptotic signal that *H. pylori* itself induces, but the exact mechanism has yet to be elucidated. The initial host response upregulates p53 expression, followed by a *CagA* action that induces p53 degradation. *CagA* can interact with the tumor suppressor apoptosis-stimulating protein of p53-2 (ASPP2). DNA damage or oncogenic stimuli activate the binding of ASPP2 to the tumor suppressor p53, inducing apoptosis. *CagA* inhibits the apoptotic processes by the proteosomal degradation of p53 [10].

There are 2 types of clinical *H. pylori* isolates: cagA gene-positive strains and cagA gene-negative strains. There are geographical differences in the presence of *cagA*. In western countries, however, it has been reported that individuals infected with cagA-positive strains are at a higher risk of peptic ulcer and/or gastric cancer than those infected with cagA-negative strains [23].

Almost all cagA-positive strains are classified as the vacA s1 strain (either m1 or m2), whereas almost all cagA-negative strains are classified as the vacA s2/m2 strain (see below) [23]. Specific *vacA* genotypes of *H. pylori* strains are associated with a level of *in vitro* cytotoxin activity as well as clinical consequences [24].

Peptidoglycans

The cag secretion system translocates the bacterial peptidoglycans into the host cells. Peptidoglycans (α4β1 integrin) interact with the nucleotide-binding oligomerization domain 1 (Nod1) molecule which leads the activation of nucear factor kB (NF-κB) pro-inflammatory responses: secretion of (interleukin- (IL-) 8, β-defensin-2 [1, 25]. *H. pylori* enhances phosphoinositide 3-kinase (PI3K) - Akt signaling in a Src and epidermal growth factor receptor- (EGFR-) dependent manner, which was also mediated by a functional cag secretion system, and peptidoglycan. The activation of PI3K-AKT signaling will result in decreased apoptosis and increased cell migration. NOD1 binding to its ligand can activate the interferon(IFN)-stimulated gene factor 3 (ISGF3) signaling a pathway resulting in I IFN production that is usually associated with protection against viral infection and possibly other mucosal infections [26].

VacA Toxin

The another bacterial virulence factor is the vacuolating cytotoxin gene *vacA* present in all strains. *vacA* encodes the cytotoxin *VacA* that induces the vacuolation of the cells and multiple cellular activities as well. *VacA* induces the disruption of the gastric epithelial barrier function, late endosomal compartments, decreases the mitochondrial transmembrane potential, the release of cytochrome c from mitochondria, activates caspase-8, -9, modulates the inflammatory response, and induces apoptosis *in vitro*. The suppressed T-cell activation and proliferation prolong the *H. pylori* infection [1, 27].

The binding of the *VacA* to receptor-type protein tyrosine phosphatase (RPTPβ) regulates cell proliferation, differentiation and adhesion. Wild type RPTPβ $^{+/+}$ mice develop gastric ulcer and atrophy in comparison with RTPTβ $^{-/-}$ mice [28].

Variations of the *vacA* gene structure (in the signal /s: s1, s2/, in the middle regions /m: m1, m2/) trigger differences in vacuolating activities. s region variants affect the vacuolating activity of *VacA*, whereas m region polymorphisms determine the cell specificity of vacuolation [2]. *vacA* s1/m1 strains can induce greater vacuolation (than do s1/m2, and s2/m2 strains). s1/m1 allel is associated with peptic ulcer disease and gastric cancer in Westen countries, but has no pathogenic role in East Asian countries [1, 2].

The intermediate (i) region also plays a role in the vacuolating activity of *H. pylori*. All s1/m1 strains were classified as i1 (vacuolating) type, and all s2/m2 strains were classified as i2 (non-vacuolating) type, while s1/m2 alleles could be i1 or i2 [2]. Colonisation with *vacA* i1 strains was associated with gastric cancer in Iranian patients [29], but the connection between *vacA* i subtypes and gastric cancer was missed in East Asian and Southeast Asian population [30]. i1 genotype appeared to be a better predictor of carcinoma-associated *H. pylori* strains than s or m genotype [2]. It is suggested that i region typing may be useful for identifying of all pathogenic forms of *vacA* and for cancer prevention [18]. In a recent study, a novel intermediate variant (i3) was identified [23].

The fourth pathogenic region is a region d, a 69-81 bp-region between the m and the i region. d1 strains without the deletion of d region are predictors of histological inflammation and atrophy and generate a higher risk of peptic ulceration and gastric cancer compared with the presence of the *vacA* s-, m-, and i-region genotypes in Western countries [31].

The variants of the s and the m regions seem to be good markers of clinical outcomes. However, the roles of the i and d regions should be further investigated [23].

CagA and *VacA* can downregulate each effect and activity, enabling the bacteria can to avoid the induction of excess cellular damage and maintaining the long-term colonisation of the gastric niche [1].

Adhesins and Outer Membrane Proteins (OMPs)

4% of the *H. pylori* genome encodes OMPs (*BabA, BabB, SabA, OipA*) which has been associated with gastroduodenal diseases, and may increase the risk of gastric cancer. Bacterial OMPs have multiple functions as adhesins, porins, or in complement resistance and immune regulation [32].

The best described *H. pylori* OMP is the blood group antigen binding adhesin *BabA* encoded by *babA2* gene, which is thought to mediate host/bacterial interactions and has been linked to microbial pathogenicity, as well as the sustained colonisation of the *H. pylori* targeting human Lewis(b) surface epitopes [32, 33]. The *babA2* gene is associated with duodenal ulcers and gastric cancer. However the results are conflicting in connection with the biomarker role of *babA2* depending on the geographic origin of the *H. pylori* strains [1]. In conjuction with *cagA* and *vacA* s1 alleles ("triple-positive strains") it is associated with a greater risk of severe diseases: duodenal ulcers and gastric adenocarcinoma in Western population [2, 33].

Sialic acid-binding adhesin (*SabA*) is also a *H. pylori* adhesin. It binds to the carbohydrate structure of the sialyl-Lewis^x antigen expressed on the gastric epithelium. *SabA* positive status was associated with gastric cancer, intestinal metaplasia, and corpus atrophy, and negatively associated with duodenal ulcer neutrophil infiltration [27]. *SabA* can mediate the binding of *H. pylori* to neutrophils, and erythrocytes, but the pathophysiological importance of these findings is uncertain [2].

Outer inflammatory protein (*OipA*) is an inflammatory-related outer membrane protein, its expression is linked to increased IL-1, -8, -17 and tumornecrosis factor- (TNF-) α production *in vitro* [1]. However its precise function is still unclear. It is suggested that *OipA* induces inflammation and actin dynamics through the phosphorylation of multiple signaling pathways that usually interact with cag PAI (CagA)-related pathways [23]. The upregulation of matrix metalloproteinase 1 (MMP-1), the inhibition of glycogen synthase kinase 3β (GSK-3β), the accumulation of β-catenin in the nucleus and the transcriptional activation of genes that influence carcinogenesis play a role in *H. pylori* carcinogenesis [1].

OipA positive status was significantly associated with high *H pylori* density, severe neutrophil infiltration and the presence of duodenal ulcer and gastric cancer [27]. Only the *OipA*-positive status was an independent determining predictor of gastric cancer in a multiple logistic regression analysis, however clinical isolates that contain the cag PAI typically have an oipA "on" status [23].

The duodenal ulcer promoting gene (*dupA*) is another novel virulence marker of *H. pylori*. It induces the production of IL-8, -12 [23]. Data are controversial. It seems that *DupA* may enhance duodenal ulceration and /or decrease gastric cancer development in some, but not all, populations [1, 2, 23].

H. pylori is a flagellated bacteria. Motility is essential for gastric colonisation and may contribute to pathogenesis [1]. Variants of gene-encoding flagellar proteins (*flaA*) may affect the motility and colonisation of the *H. pylori*. Less motile strains are less carcinogenic [1].

The oipA gene is located approximately 100 kbp from the cag PAI on the *H. pylori* chromosome. oipA status is also linked to the vacA s region type, and the presence of the babA gene. These links between the virulence factors may show that they possibly interact with one another [23].

Other Factors

H. pylori has a genome of approximately 1.600 genes, so there may be other novel virulence factors [23].

A recent study provides new insight into potential mechanisms of *H. pylori*-induced gastric carcinogenesis. Annexin family members (*AnxA1* and *AnxA4*) are involved in an epithelial cell membrane repair response induced by *H. pylori*-generated *VacA* and *CagA*-independent plasma membrane disruption. Plasma membrane disruption and *AnxA4* can promote cell proliferation [34].

TNF-α-inducing protein (*Tipα*) is an unique carcinogenic factor of *H. pylori* and has no similarity to any other virulence factors of *H. pylori*. *Tipα* protein specifically binds to cell-surface nucleolin and then enters the gastric cancer cells, where TNF-α and chemokine gene expressions are induced by NF-κB activation in a *cag* PAI independent manner [35].

Regulatory T cells (Treg) suppress the activity of most other lymphoid cells as well as dendritic cells through cell-to-cell contact mechanisms which are not fully defined. Antigen-specific Treg accumulate in gastric tissue during both *H. pylori*-induced gastritis and peptic ulcer disease. The local Treg response protects the gastric mucosa from exaggerated inflammation and tissue damage, and decrease the risk of peptic ulcer disease. However Treg activity leads to increased bacterial density through the reduction of the inflammatory response, resulting in chronic infection and in some patients in the development of atrophic gastritis and gastric cancer progression [36].

H. pylori can induce the activation of several proteolytic enzymes, which may have an important role in gastric mucosal inflammation, gastric cancer progression and the development of distant metastasis [37].

New mechanisms of gastric cancer development with *H. pylori* provide a new targeted preventive strategy in the future [34, 35] (Table **1**).

Table 1: *H. pylori* virulence factors and role in gastric carcinogenesis

Virulence Factor	Abbreviation	Effect
Cytotoxin-associated gene A product	CagA	Disruption of cell-cell junctions, loss of polarity, cell elongation Pro-inflammatory response Mitogenic response
Peptidoglycans		Pro-inflammory responses Decreased apoptosis Increased cell migration
Vacuolating cytotoxin	VacA	Cell vacuolation, cell differentiation, adhesion
Blood group antigen binding adhesin	BabA	Modulation of host/bacterial interaction Maintaining bacterial colonization
Sialic acid-binding adhesin	SabA	Mediation of binding of *H. pylori* to neutrophils and erythrocytes
Outer inflammatory protein	OipA	Pro-inflammatory response Signaling pathways
Duodenal ulcer promoting gene product	DupA	Pro-inflammatory response
Flagellar proteins	FlaA	Motility, colonisation
Others		
Annexin family member 4	AnxA4	Plasma membrane disruption
TNF-α inducing protein	Tipα	Pro-inflammatory response

Host Factors

Most persons colonised with diseases-associated *H. pylori* strains remain asymptomatic, while some develop gastroduodenal disease, which underlines the possible role of host factors [1, 20].

Genetic variants of the inflammation- (IL-10, IL-17, IL-RN, TNF-α) [38, 39] and non-inflammation-related genes (mucin carrier gene 1, 6, MUC1, MUC6; DNA methyltransferase 3B, DNMT3B; SMAD4, and serpin peptidase inhibitor, clade E, member 1, SERPINE1) modify the risk of developing gastric cancer. Several genes have been newly associated with gastric carcinogenesis, both through oncogenic activation (synthase kinase3β, GSK3β; transmembrane protein CD133; desmocollin-2, DSC2; P-Cadherin, member of the cadherin superfamily, CDH17; CD168, CD44, metalloproteinases MMP7 and MMP11, and a subset of miRNAs) and through tumour suppressor gene inactivation mechanisms (trefoil factor 1, TFF1; pancreatic duodenal homebox 1, PDX1; BCL2L10; XRCC; endogenous retrovirus-related gene, psi TPTE-HERV; HAI-2, GRIK2, and RUNX3) [38].

Most of the host factors are restricted either to histological type (intestinal *vs.* diffuse), ethnical background (particularly Caucasian *vs.* Asian) and tumour localization (non-cardia *vs.* cardia cancer) [40].

IL-1

The pro-inflammatory molecule IL-1β is increased within the gastric mucosa of *H. pylori* infected persons. Polymorphism of the IL-1β gene cluster can alter, increase or decrease the IL-β production [1]. Persons with high-expression IL-1β polymorphisms (C–T or T–C transitions, at positions −511, −31, and +3954 bp from the transcriptional start site) have an increased risk of hypochorhydria, gastric atrophy, and distal gastric adenocarcinoma in comparison with low-expression polymorphisms [41, 42].

High-expression IL-1β genotype appears to increase the risk of noncardia gastric cancer, while it has no effect on cancers associated with high acid exposure such as esophageal adenocarcinomas and some cardia cancers [42].

The importance of the background prevalence of gastric cancer in the population was highlighted. Positive associations were easier to demonstrate in low-incidence regions compared with high-incidence regions. Some reports, particularly from Asian countries, failed to find an association between IL-1 markers and gastric cancer risk [42].

The combined effects of pro-inflammatory IL-1 genotypes and *H. pylori* bacterial virulence factors (*cagA* positive, *VacA s1* and *VacA m1*), report that for each combination of bacterial and host genotype the odds of having a gastric carcinoma were greatest in those with both bacterial and host high-risk genotypes [42].

TNF-a

Polymorphisms (308 G > A) of the pro-inflammatory cytokine gene TNF-α which increase the expression of the cytokine have been associated with an increased risk of chronic atrophic gastritis and distal cancer [42, 43]. It is suggested that macrophage-derived TNF-alpha promotes Wnt/beta-catenin signalling through inhibition of GSK3beta, which may contribute to tumour development in the gastric mucosa [44].

IL-10

Polymorphisms (promoter polymorphisms at positions −592, −819 and −1082) that reduce the production of the anti-inflammatory cytokine (IL-10) can enhance the risk of distal gastric cancer [45]. A relative deficiency of IL-10 may result in a T helper-1-driven hyper-inflammatory response to *H. pylori* with greater damage to the gastric mucosa [42].

Pro-inflammatory IL-1β, TNF-α and IL-10 genotypes were each associated with the progressively increased risk. Three high-risk polymorphisms elevate the risk of cancer 27-fold over the baseline [1, 45].

Others

IL-8 is a potent chemoattractant for neutrophils and lymphocytes. It also has effects on cell proliferation, migration and tumour angiogenesis [42]. High-expression polymorphisms of IL-8 do not increase the risk of inflammation and premalignant lesion in every population [42].

Polymorphisms of IL-4 and IL-6 were not associated with upper gastrointestinal cancers (gastric cardia, noncardia adenocarcinoma, esophageal squamous cell carcinoma, adenocarcinoma) [45].

Functional polymorphisms of toll like receptor 4 (TLR4) increase the risk of severe inflammation and subsequent development of hypochlorhydria and gastric atrophy, and cancer in white population *via* the deficiency in production of antiinflammatory cytokine IL-10 [42].

Localisation of nucleolin on the cell surface may be a limiting factor that is induced in the very early stage of carcinogenesis. Cells with nucleolin on cell surface become more sensitive to Tipα, associated with tumour promoting activity. Cell surface nucleolin is one of the key determinants in a host factor for developing of gastric cancer based on *H. pylori* infection. Ligands (*e.g.* lactoferin), which bind to nucleolin and inhibiting the interaction between Tipα and nucleolin, resulting in inhibition of the *H. pylori* infection have anticancer activity, and could potentially be used for preventing and treating gastric cancer in humans [35].

The renin-angiotensin system (RAS) plays an important role not only in homeostasis but also in carcinogenesis. *H. pylori* infection gradually increases the RAS expression in the gastric mucosa after the infection with respect to the severity of inflammatory cell infiltration. It follows from this that RAS genotypic variation may affect the component expression levels (*e.g.* angiotensin I converting enzyme, chymase and angiotensinogen), and thereby the risk of gastric cancer. RAS inhibitors may provide tools for specifically preventing this disease [36].

There is interaction between host and bacterial virulence factors. *H. pylori* genotype and host genetic polymorphisms together determine the clinical consequences of *H. pylori* infection. The odds of having gastric carcinoma were greatest in those with both bacterial and host high-risk genotypes: *vacAs1/IL-1B-511*T* carrier OR = 87, (95% CI = 11 to 679) (Table **2**) [47].

Table 2: Host factors in gastric carcinogenesis

	Effect
IL-1β	Pro-inflammatory response
TNF-α	Pro-inflammatory response
IL-10	Anti-inflammatory response
Other possible factors	
IL-8	Pro-inflammatory response
TLR4	Pro-inflammatory response
Nucleolin	Pro-inflammatory response
RAS	Pro-inflammatory response, angiogenesis, cell proliferation

Environmental Factors

Beyond bacterial characteristics and host genetic features, environmental factors can affect the risk of gastric carcinogenesis in *H. pylori* infected individuals as well.

Salt

High dietary salt intake unequivocally increases the risk of gastric cancer supported by epidemiological and experimental studies [6]. The pathogenetic role of salt intake was confirmed. The property of salt intake that entails an increased gastric cancer risk is not fully clear. Salt can cause stomach cancer by directly damaging gastric mucosa, improving temporary epithelial proliferation and the incidence of endogenous mutations. Hypergastrinemia induced by the bacteria leads to eventual parietal cell loss and progression to gastric cancer [48]. Direct damages of the gastric mucosa and upregulated production of cytokines are mentioned as well. Damages of the mucosa potentiates exposure to carcinogens such as N-nitroso compounds as well [48].

H. pylori and salt exert synergistic effects on the development of premalignant lesions or gastric cancer. High dietary salt intake may potentiate the colonisation of *H. pylori* through the increase of surface mucous cell mucin and the decrease of gland mucous cell mucin [48]. Salt-induced hypergastrinemia can synergise with *H. pylori* infection and result in parietal cell loss and progression to gastric cancer [48]. High salt concentration can modulate *H. pylori* gene expression, especially virulence factors. Up-regulation of *H. pylori cagA* expression in response to high salt concentration may be a factor contributing to the development of gastric adenocarcinoma [49].

Helminth Infection

Coinfection with helminths (Ascaris lumbricoides) and Toxoplasma gondii can alter the outcome of *H. pylori* infection, reducing the severity of *H. pylori*-induced gastritis. Reduced Th1 response with higher levels of Th2 cytokines partially explain decreased gastric cancer risk in *H. pylori*-induced atrophy [50].

Dietary Antioxidants

Modulating dietary patterns can reduce the risk of gastric cancer. Further studies are needed to evaluate the possible protective effects of dietary antioxidants against gastric cancer among *H. pylori*-infected patients [1].

Fruit and vegetables are rich sources of carotenoids, vitamin C, folate, and phytochemicals, which may play a preventive role in the carcinogenesis process [51]. Modulating xenobiotic-metabolising enzymes, in particular phase II enzymes, and antioxidant activity contribute to this putative preventive mechanism [51].

The beneficial effects of fruit and vegetable intake, dietary antioxidants, vitamin C and β-carotene supplementation must be studied in the future, because the protective effect of dietary supplementation and no significant interaction between *H. pylori* infection and vitamin C treatment [52] was also reported [1]. Vitamin C might protect against *H. pylori* associated gastric carcinogenesis by enhancing mucosal immune responses, neutralising reactive oxygen species, reducing the formation of gastric N-nitroso compounds, inhibiting the growth of cancer cells and directly affecting *H. pylori* growth and virulence. However, vitamin C can significantly enhance *H. pylori* induced apoptosis in gastric cancer cells, indicating it is possible that vitamin C increases *H. pylori* induced DNA damage [53].

Smoking

Smoking is an established risk factor for gastric cancer. Relatively few studies have investigated which step of smoking has effects in *H. pylori* related gastric carcinogenesis [54]. A recent study demonstrated that smoking habits and *H. pylori i*nfection mean an 11-fold higher risk of gastric cancer. The increased risk of gastric carcinogenesis observed for smokers in comparison with control subjects with gastric atrophy would be explained by the effect of swallowed carcinogenic substances (nitrosamine, other nitrosocompounds), greater concentrations of smoking-related DNA adducts in gastric mucosa of the smokers, lower levels of free radical scavengers (ascorbic acid, β-carotene), as well as by the increased mRNA expression of chemokines in gastric mucosa [55]. Positive association is possible, but no statistically significant association was reported [1].

CONCLUSIONS

The mechanisms of *H. pylori*-associated gastric carcinogenesis are still poorly defined, further recognition may provide possibilities to develop effective strategies for gastric cancer prevention and treatment [2].

The clinical outcome of *H. pylori* infection is determined by host genetic predisposition, bacterial strain factors as well as environmental factors [2]. Bacterial virulence factors (*VacA, CagA*) modulate the immune response involved in the initiation of the carcinogenesis in the stomach. Host genetic factors (IL-1*b*, TNF*a*, IL-10) regulate the inflammatory response and the aggravation of mucosal damage. The environmental factors, salt intake and smoking of tobacco are well-known harmful etiological factors. The ingestion of fruit and vegetables has some protective effect [56].

H. pylori screening and treatment is a recommended gastric cancer risk reduction strategy in high-risk populations. In populations at low risk of gastric cancer, *H. pylori* screening is not recommended [57]. Eliminating *H. pylori* from a large part of the population may be unfeasible economically, and the long-term consequences are still unpredictable: this is why identification of high-risk individuals is very important (Table **3**) [18].

Table 3: Open-unresolved questions

Exact mechanism of *H. pylori* carcinogenesis.
Role of *H. pylori* in the development of cardia cancer.
Exact-novel virulence factors. Interactions of the virulence factors.
Exact-novel host factors. Intercations of the host factors.
Exact-novel environmental factors. Exact role of vegetables and dietary antioxidants.
Interactions of bacterial-host-environmental factors.
Identification and screening of high-risk individuals.
Development effective strategies for gastric cancer prevention and treatment.

ACKNOWLEDGEMENT

None Declared.

CONFLICT OF INTEREST

The author(s) confirm that this chapter content has no conflict of interest.

REFERENCES

[1] Wroblevski LE, Peek RM, Wilson KT., *Helicobacter pylori* and gastric cancer: Factors that modulate disease risk, Clin Microbiol Rev 2010; 23:713-39.

[2] Wen, S & Moss, SF. *Helicobacter pylori* virulence factors in gastric carcinogenesis. Cancer Letters 2009; 282; 1, 1-8.

[3] Herszényi L, Tulassay Z. Epidemiology of gastrointestinal and liver tumors. Eur Review Med Pharmacol Sci 2010; 14: 249-58.

[4] Venkateshwari A, Krishnaveni D, Venugo, S & Shashikumar, P & Vidyasagar, A & Jyothy, A. *Helicobacter pylori* infection in relation to gastric cancer progression. Indian J Cancer 2011; 48: 94-8.

[5] Khan FA,Shukla AN. Pathogenesis and treatment of gastric carcinoma: an up-date with brief review. J Cancer Res Therap 2006; 2: 196-99.

[6] Nagini S. Carcinoma of the stomach: A review of epidemiology, pathogenesis, molecular genetics and chemoprevention. World J Gastrointest Oncol 2010; 4: 156-69.

[7] de Martel C, Ferlay J,Franceschi S,Vignat J, Bray F, Forman D, Plummer M. Global burden of cancers attributable to infections in 2008: a review and synthetic analysis. Lancet Oncol 2012;13: 607-15.

[8] Juhász M,Herszényi L, Tulassay Z, Malfertheiner P, Ebert MP. *Helicobacter pylori* and molecular mechanisms of gastric carcinogenesis: targets for prevetion and therapy. Expert Review of Anticancer Therapy, 2004; 4: 97-103.

[9] Peek RM, Crabtree JE. *Helicobacter pylori* infection and gastric neoplasia. J Pathol *Pathology* 2008; 2: 233-48.

[10] Ruggiero P. *Helicobacter pylori* infection: what's new. Curr Opin Infect Dis 25;3: 337-44.

[11] Malfertheiner P. The intriguing relationship of *Helicobacter pylori* infection and acid secretion in peptic ulcer disease and gastric cancer. Dig Dis 2011;29: 459-64.

[12] Uemura, N & Okamoto, S & Yamamoto, S & Matsumura, N & Yamaguchi, S & Yamakido M,Taniyama K, Sasaki N, Schlemper RJ.*Helicobacter pylori* infection and the development of gastric cancer. N Eng J Med 2001; 345: 784-89.

[13] Pandey R, Misra V, Misra SP, Dwivedi M, Kumar A,Tiwari BK. *Helicobacter pylori* and gastric cancer. Asian Pacific Journal of Cancer Prevention 2011; 11: 583-88.

[14] Wong BC, Lam SK, Wong WM, Chen JS, Zheng TT, Feng RE, Lai KC, Hu WH, Yuen ST, Leung SY, Fong DY, Ho J, Ching CK, Chen JS, China Gastric Cancer Study Group *Helicobacter pylori* eradication to prevent gastric cancer in a high-risk region of China: a randomized controlled trial. J Am Med Ass 2004; 291: 187-94.

[15] Mera R, Fontham ET,Bravo LE,Bravo JC, Piazuelo MB, Camargo MC,Correa P. Long term follow up of patients treated for *Helicobacter pylori* infection. *Gut* 2005; 54: 1536-40.

[16] Farinati F, Cardin R, Della Libera G, Herszenyi L, Marafin C, Molari A, Plebani M, Rugge M, Naccarato R. The role of anti-oxidants in the chemoprevention of gastric cancer. Eur J Cancer Prev 1994; 3: Suppl 2, 93-97.

[17] Tulassay Z, Stolte M, Engstrand L, Butruk E, Malfertheiner P, Dítê P, Tchernev V, Wong BC, Gottlow M, Eklund S, Wrangstadh M, Herszényi L, Nagy P and the HELIX Study Investigators. Twelve-month endoscopic and histological analysis following proton-pump inhibitor-based triple therapy in *Helicobacter pylori*-positive patients with gastric ulcers. Scand J Gastroenterol 2010; 45: 1048-58.

[18] Ferreira AC, Isomoto H, Moriyama M, Fujioka T, Machado JC, Yamaoka Y. Helicobacter and gastric malignancies Helicobacter 2008; 13: Suppl.1, 28-34.

[19] Singh K, Ghoshal UC.Causal role of *Helicobacter pylori* infection in gastric cancer: an Asian enigma. World J Gastroenterol 2006;12: 1346-51.

[20] Suzuki R, Shiota S, Yamaoka Y. Molecular epidemiology, population genetics, and pathogenic role of *Helicobacter pylori*. Infection, Genetics and Evolution 2012; 12: 203-13.

[21] Molnar B, Galamb O, Sipos F, Leiszter K, Tulassay Z. (2010), Molecular pathogenesis of *Helicobacter pylori* infection: the role of bacterial virulence factors. Dig Dis 2010; 28: 604-08.

[22] Ding SZ, Minohara Y, Fan XJ, Wang J, Reyes VE, Patel J, Dirden-Kramer B, Boldogh I, Ernst PB, Crowe SE. *Helicobacter pylori* infection induces oxidative stress and programmed cell death in human gastric epithelial cells. Infection and Immunity 2007; 75: 4030-39.

[23] Yamaoka Y. Pathogenesis of *Helicobacter pylori*-Related Gastroduodenal Diseases from Molecular Epidemiological Studies. Gastroenterological Research and Practice 2012: 2012,371503.

[24] Atherton JC, Cao P, Peek RM, Tummuru MK, Blaser MJ, Cover TL. (1995), 'Mosaicism in vacuolating cytotoxin alleles of *Helicobacter pylori*. Association of specific vacA types with cytotoxin production and peptic ulceration. J Biol Chem 1995; 270: 17771-17777.

[25] Backert S, Naumann M. What a disorder: proinflammatory signaling pathways induced by *Helicobacter pylori*. Trends in Microbiology, 2010; 18: 479-86.

[26] Watanabe T, Asano N, Fichtner-Feigl S, Gorelick PL, Tsuji Y, Matsumoto Y, Chiba T, Fuss IJ, Kitani A, Strober W. NOD1 contributes to mouse host defense against *Helicobacter pylori via* induction of type I IFN and activation of the ISGF3 signaling pathway. J Clin Invest 2010; 120: 1645-62.

[27] Yamaoka Y, Ojo O, Fujimoto S, Odenbreit S, Haas R, Gutierrez O, El-Zimaity HM, Reddy, R, Arnqvist A, Graham DY. *Helicobacter pylori* outer membrane proteins and gastroduodenal disease. Gut*,* 2006; 55: 775-81.

[28] Fujikawa A, Shirasaka D, Yamamoto S, Ota H, Yahiro K, Fukada M, Shintani T, Wada A, Aoyama N, Hirayama T, Fukamachi H, Noda M. Mice deficient in protein tyrosine phosphatase receptor type Z are resistant to gastric ulcer induction by VacA of *Helicobacter pylori*. Nature Genetics 2003; 33: 375-81.

[29] Rhead JL, Letley DP, Mohammadi M, Hussein N, Mohagheghi MA, Eshagh Hosseini M, Atherton JC. A new *Helicobacter pylori* vacuolating cytotoxin determinant, the intermediate region, is associated with gastric cancer. Gastroenterology 2007; 133: 926-36.

[30] Ogiwara H, Graham DY, Yamaoka Y. vacA i-Region Subtyping. Gastroenterology, 2008; 134: 1267.

[31] Ogiwara H, Sugimoto M, Ohno T, Vilaichone RK, Mahachai V,Graham, DY, Yamaoka Y. Role of deletion located between the intermediate and middle regions of the *Helicobacter pylori* vacA gene in cases of gastroduodenal diseases. J Clin Microbiol 2009; 47: 3493-3500.

[32] Dossumbekova, A & Prinz, C & Gerhard, M & Brenner, L & Backert, S & Kusters, JG & Schmid RM, Rad R. *Helicobacter pylori* outer membrane proteins and gastric inflammation. Gut 2006:55: 1360-61.

[33] Gerhard M, Lehn N, Neumayer N, Borén T, Rad R, Schepp W, Miehlke S, Classen M, Prinz C. Clinical relevance of the *Helicobacter pylori* gene for blood-group antigen-binding adhesin. Proc Natl Acad Sci 1999; 96: 12778-83.

[34] Lin LL, Huang HC, Ogihara S, Wang JT, Wu MC, McNeil PL, Chen CN, Juan HF. *Helicobacter pylori* Disrupts Host Cell Membranes, Initiating a Repair Response and Cell Proliferation. Int J Molec Sci 2012;13: 10176-92.

[35] Suganuma M, Watanabe T, Yamaguchi K, Takahashi A, Fujiki H. Human gastric cancer development with TNF-α-inducing protein secreted from *Helicobacter pylori*. Cancer Letters 2012; 322: 133-38.

[36] Raghavan S, Quiding-Järbrink M. Immune modulation by regulatory T cells in *Helicobacter pylori*-associated diseases. Endocrine, Metabolic & Immune Disorders - Drug Targets. 2012; 12: 71-85.

[37] Plebani M, Herszènyi L, Cardin R, Roveroni G, Carraro P, Paoli MD, Rugge M, Grigioni, WF, Nitti D, Naccarato R. Cysteine and serine proteases in gastric cancer. Cancer 1995;76: 367-75.

[38] Resende C, Thiel A, Machado JC, Ristimäki A. Gastric cancer: basic aspects. Helicobacter 2011;16: Suppl 1, 38-44.

[39] Persson, C & Canedo, P & Machado, JC & El-Omar, EM & Forman, D. Polymorphisms in inflammatory response genes and their association with gastric cancer: A HUGE systematic review and meta-analyses. Am J Epidemiol 2011; 173: 259-70.

[40] Wex T, Bornschein J, Malfertheiner P. Host polymorphisms of immune regulatory genes as risk factors for gastric cancer. Minerva Gastroenterologica e Dietologica 2009; 55: 395-408.

[41] Hwang IR, Kodama T, Kikuchi S, Sakai K, Peterson LE, Graham DY, Yamaoka Y. Effect of interleukin 1 polymorphisms on gastric mucosal interleukin 1beta production in *Helicobacter pylori* infection.Gastroenterology. 2002; 123: 1793-1803.

[42] Shanks AM, El-Omar EM. *Helicobacter pylori* infection, host genetics and gastric cancer. J Dig Dis 2009; 10: 157-64.

[43] Machado JC, Figueiredo C, Canedo P, Pharoah P, Carvalho R, Nabais S, Castro Alves C, Campos ML, Van Doorn LJ, Caldas C, Seruca R, Carneiro F, Sobrinho-Simões M. A proinflammatory genetic profile increases the risk for chronic atrophic gastritis and gastric carcinoma. Gastroenterology, 2003; 125: 364-71.

[44] Oguma K, Oshima H, Aoki M, Uchio R, Naka K, Nakamura S, Hirao A, Saya H, Taketo MM, Oshima M. Activated macrophages promote Wnt signalling through tumour necrosis factor-alpha in gastric tumour cells. EMBO Journal 2005; 27: 1671-81.

[45] El-Omar EM, Rabkin CS, Gammon MD, Vaughan TL, Risch HA, Schoenberg JB, Stanford JL, Mayne ST, Goedert J, Blot WJ, Fraumeni JF, Chow WH. Increased risk of noncardia gastric cancer associated with proinflammatory cytokine gene polymorphisms. Gastroenterology 2003;124: 1193-1201.

[46] Sugimoto M, Yamaoka Y, Shirai N, Furuta T. Role of renin-angiotensin system in gastric oncogenesis. J Gastroenterol Hepatol 2012; 17: 442-51.

[47] Figueiredo, C & Machado, JC & Pharoah, P & Seruca, R & Sousa, S & Carvalho, R & Capelinha AF, Quint W, Caldas C, van Doorn LJ, Carneiro F, Sobrinho-Simões M. *Helicobacter pylori* and interleukin 1 genotyping: an opportunity to identify high-risk individuals for gastric carcinoma. J Natl Cancer Inst 2002; 9: 1680-87.

[48] Wang XQ, Terry PD, Yan H. Review of salt consumption and stomach cancer risk: epidemiological and biological evidence. World J Gastroenterol 2009; 15: 2204-13.

[49] Loh JT,Torres VJ, Cover TL. Regulation of *Helicobacter pylori* cagA expression in response to salt. Cancer Research 2005; 67: 4709-15.

[50] Ek C, Whary MT, Ihrig M, Bravo LE, Correa P,Fox JG. Serologic evidence that ascaris and toxoplasma infections impact inflammatory responses to *Helicobacter pylori* in Colombians. Helicobacter 2012; 17: 107-15.

[51] Tsugane S, Sasazuki, S, Diet and the risk of gastric cancer: review of epidemiological evidence. Gastric Cancer 2007; 10: 75-83.

[52] Ma JL, Zhang L, Brown LM, Li JY, Shen L, Pan KF, Liu WD,Hu Y, Han ZX, Crystal-Mansour S, Pee D, Blot WJ, Fraumeni JF,You WC, Gail MH. Fifteen-year effects of *Helicobacter pylori*, garlic, and vitamin treatments on gastric cancer incidence and mortality. Journal of the National Cancer Institute 2012;104: 488-92.

[53] Zhang ZW, Farthing MJ. The roles of vitamin C in *Helicobacter pylori* associated gastric carcinogenesis. Chinese Journal of Digestive Diseases 2005; 6: 53-8.

[54] Hishida A, Matsuo K, Goto Y,Naito M, Wakai K, Tajima K, Hamajima N. Smoking behavior and risk of *helicobacter pylori* infection, gastric atrophy and gastric cancer in Japanese. Asian Pacific Journal of Cancer Prevention 2010; 1: 313-17.

[55] Shikata K, Doi Y, Yonemoto K, Arima H, Ninomiya T, Kubo M, Tanzaki Y, Matsumoto, T,Iida M, Kiyohara Y. Population-based prospective study of the combined influence of cigarette smoking and *Helicobacter pylori* infection on gastric cancer incidence: the Hisayama Study'. Am J Epidemiol 2008; 168: 1409-15.

[56] Bornschein J, Malfertheiner P. Gastric carcinogenesis. Langenbeck's Arch Surg 2011; 396: 729-42.

[57] Fock KM,Talley N, Moayyedi P, Hunt R, Azuma T, Sugano K, Xiao SD,Lam SK, Goh KL,Chiba T, Uemura N, Kim JG, Kim N, Ang,TL, Mahachai V, Mitchell H, Rani AA, Liou JM, Vilaichone RK, Sollano J. Asia-Pacific Gastric Cancer Consensus Conference, Asia-Pacific consensus guidelines on gastric cancer prevention. J Gastroenterol Hepatol 2008; 23: 351-65.

Send Orders for Reprints to reprints@benthamscience.net

Helicobacter Pylori: A Worldwide Perspective 2014, 2014, 336-395

CHAPTER 16

Extradigestive Manifestations of *Helicobacter pylori* Infection: What is Proven and Unproven in 2014?

Natale Figura*, Giulia Fiorilli, Francesco Langone, Leonardo Vaglio, Elena Moretti

Department of Internal Medicine, Endocrino-Metabolic Sciences and Biochemistry and Department of Biomedical Sciences, Applied Biology Section, University of Siena, Siena, Italy

Abstract: It has long been known that chronic bacterial infections have an impact upon the overall organism. *H. pylori* infection is no exception to the rule. Indeed, the infection is acquired early in life and induces an intense/moderate local and systemic inflammatory status that lasts for the entire patients' life. During this time, different organs and systems of infected individuals are exposed to injures exerted by the inflammation and immune responses to the infection, as well as to autoimmune reactions triggered by mechanisms of antigenic mimicry between human tissue cells and *H. pylori*. The *CagA-positive* bacterial genotype is mostly involved in extradigestive manifestations of such an infection, due to the increased inflammatory potential of this organism. The organs and systems that most of all may suffer from the detrimental consequences of *H. pylori* infection are the cardiovascular (ischaemic heart diseases), haematological (purpura, urticaria *etc.*), central nervous (Parkinson's and Alzheimer's diseases) and endocrine systems (autoimmune thyroid disorders). There is an increasing evidence, however, that no district of the human body is sheltered from the harmful effects of *H. pylori* infection. In conclusion, *H. pylori* infection may have deleterious consequences on organs and systems different from the gastroduodenal tract. To better understand the pathogenic mechanisms of extradigestive disorders associated with *H. pylori* infection, is essential to determine the CagA status of the infecting organisms.

Keywords: *H. pylori* infection, CagA, extradigestive diseases, ischaemic heart disease, idiopathic arrhythmia, migraine, Raynaud's disease, autoimmune thyroid disease, diabetes mellitus, osteoporosis, iron deficiency anemia, Schönlein-Henoch purpura, MALT lymphoma, rosacea, chronic urticaria, glaucoma, Parkinson's disease, Alzheimer's disease, systemic sclerosis, Sjögren's syndrome, reproductive disorders.

*Address correspondence to Natale Figura: Associate Professor of Gastroenterology, University of Siena, Italy; Tel: + 39 0577585463; Fax: + 39 0566233446; E-mail: figura@unisi.it

Buzás György Miklós (Ed.)

INTRODUCTION

Helicobacter pylori is a successful primary pathogen: this microorganism colonizes the gastroduodenal tract of more than half of the world population and arouses a solid inflammatory and immune response that lasts for the entire patients' life, if the infection is not adequately treated. *H. pylori* infection is the main cause of chronic gastritis, the *condicio sine qua non* for the development of gastroduodenal ulceration and the principal contributory cause of stomach's neoplastic diseases.

Starting in the early nineties, epidemiological surveys have indicated that the possible pathological consequences of *H. pylori* infection may not be restricted to the gastroduodenal tract. It was suggested that *H. pylori* infection may be correlated with a wide range of extra-digestive diseases, whose signs and symptoms are overlooked most of the time. Such diseases may affect heart, vessels, skin, and various systems, such as the endocrine, respiratory, haemopoietic, immune and central nervous systems. The most common extra-digestive diseases associated with *H. pylori* infection are reported in Table **1**.

Table 1: Most common extradigestive diseases associated with *H. pylori* infection

System, Region, Organ	Suggested Association	Degree of Association
Cardiovascular or vascular system	Atherosclerosis (coronary heart disease, strock, aneurysm), migraine, Raynaud's disease, idiopathic arrhythmia	Strong
Endocrine system	Autoimmune thyroid disorders, resistance to insulin/diabetes, post-prandial hypoglicemia	Both positive/indifferent
Haemopoietic system	Iron deficiency anemia, idiopathic thrombocytopenic purpura, extra-gastric MALT lymphoma	Strong
Immune system	Food allergy	Both positive/negative
Skin	Rosacea, primitive chronic urticaria, pruritus cutaneus, Sweet syndrome, angioedema, alopecia areata, prurigo nodularis, lichen planus	Moderate
Respiratory system	Chronic otitis media with effusion	Moderate
Eye	Glaucoma, blefaritis	Moderata/strong
Central nervous system	Parkinson's and Alzheimer's disease, hepatic encephalopathy	Strong/moderate

System, Region, Organ	Suggested Association	Degree of Association
Periferal nervous system	Guillain-Barrè syndrome	Mild
Reumatologic diseases	Systemic sclerosis, Sjögren syndrome, Behçet disease	Moderate/strong
Reproductive system	Male and female reproductive disoerders	Moderate
Miscellanea	Sudden infant death syndrome, *hyperemesis gravidarum*, halitosis, growth delay, IgA nephropathy	Mild/moderate

CARDIOVASCULAR AND VASCULAR SYSTEM

Cardiovascular Organic Diseases

Ischaemic Heart Disease

The existence of an association between infectious agents and atherosclerosis was initially proposed by Osler in 1908 [1]. The hypothesis that infectious diseases may be associated with cardiovascular disorders was demonstrated when coxsackievirus B4 was found to be involved in the development of coronary arteritis. Later on, cytomegalovirus, *herpes simplex* virus, *Chlamydia pneumoniae* and recently *H. pylori* have been reputed to contribute to the atherogenesis and clinical implications of atherosclerosis, such as ischemic heart disease, stroke and aneurysm.

Since 1994, several researchers have investigated the existence of an association between *H. pylori* infection and atherosclerosis. This association, theoretically plausible, still remains controversial from a practical point of view. Epidemiological and animal studies, as well as some trials aimed at eradicating *H. pylori* infection, gave conflicting results, possibly due to differences in the study design, subjects enrolled and diagnostic tools used to demonstrate the infection [2-4]. Surprisingly, studies investigating the specific mechanisms of molecular mimicry triggered by *H. pylori* strongly support such an association [5, 6]. These studies showed an immune cross reactivity between CagA and the artery wall [5] and an increased mean level of systemic antibodies to heat-shock protein 60 (hsp60) in patients with coronary heart disease respect to controls [7], suggesting that the immune reaction to the bacterial hsp could cross react with hsp of the eukaryotic cells.

In spite of a remarkable number of studies on *H. pylori*-related atherosclerosis, the real mechanisms involved in these phenomena are still controversial; many pathogenic hypotheses were therefore postulated [8]; some of them are typical of this condition, such as the ability of *H. pylori* to induce an atherogenic modified lipid profile, the establishment of a hypercoagulable state, changes regarding homocysteine levels, the induction of endothelial dysfunction, an increase of vasoconstrictor factors, the stimulation of platelet aggregation, the direct effect of *H. pylori* on the progression and instability of atherosclerotic plaques *etc.* Other phenomena are shared with various conditions, including the systemic increase of inflammatory markers and mediators, the molecular mimicry, the oxidative modifications that contribute to atherogenesis *etc.* [8]. A recent metanalysis demonstrated in humans that some strains of *H. pylori* are capable of binding the von Willebrand factor and interacting with glycoprotein Ib to induce platelet aggregation [9]. In the long run, such mechanism, together with other factors of increased atherosclerotic risk, may concur to damaging the arteries, including the coronary vessels.

In animal models, such infection promotes the formation of platelet aggregates through a marked increase in the flux of rolling leukocytes and the appearance of platelet and leukocyte-platelet aggregates in gastric venules. This aggregate formation was abrogated by antibodies against specific adhesion molecules (L-selectin and P-selectin) [9]. As in many other extra-digestive manifestations of *H. pylori* infection, the most important pathogenetic factor is the presence of the so-called pathogenicity island (PAI) *cag* in the bacterial genome [10]. *cag* PAI is harboured by 50%-90% of *H. pylori* isolates and contains genes involved in virulence. One of the 31 *cag* genes, called *cagA*, encodes for the oncoprotein CagA (cytotoxin associated gene A), a major virulent factor that also induces massive inflammatory and immune responses consisting in an overproduction of various pro-inflammatory cytokines, such as interleukin-1 (IL-1), IL-8 *etc.*, which, over a long period of time, may contribute to damaging the vessels.

In 2002, our group observed an increased prevalence of infection by *H. pylori* expressing CagA in patients with ischaemic heart disease respect to controls and hypothesized that the reason that could account for the contradictory results present in the scientific literature may include the variable circulation in different areas of *H. pylori* strains endowed with a greater inflammatory potential, *i.e.* the CagA-positive [11]. Our study confirmed the findings of Pasceri *et al.* [12] who first hypothesized a pathogenic role of infection by *H. pylori* strains expressing CagA in the development of ischaemic heart disorders. We also observed more severe electrocardiographic ischaemic alterations in infected cardiac patients seropositive for CagA [11]. It is therefore important to consider the CagA status of patients and subjects in studies aimed at investigating the possible association between *H. pylori* infection and development or worsening of cardiovascular diseases. The majority of publications that do not explore the CagA status do not reach unequivocal results, at least from a statistical point of view. In this respect, some researchers published a metanalysis that included 26 studies considering the CagA status, determined serologically, in the development of atherosclerotic disease [13]. Data revealed that chronic infection by *H. pylori* virulent strains (*i.e.* those expressing CagA) increased the risk of ischemic strokes and coronary heart diseases, yielding pooled ORs of 2.68 (95% CI: 2.20, 3.27) and 2.11 (95% CI: 1.70, 2.62), respectively. In another study, the following parameters were investigated in patients infected by CagA-positive and –negative *H. pylori* strains: levels of high sensitivity C-reactive protein, total cholesterol, low-density protein (LDL), oxidized LDL and apolipoprotein B [14]. Interestingly, the systemic concentrations of all these markers were significantly increased in CagA-positive patients; in addition, patients with serum antibodies to CagA showed a more severe coronary atherosclerosis [14].

In 2012, in a population-based cohort study, Schöttker *et al.* examined 9953 old adults and found that neither CagA-negative nor CagA-positive *H. pylori* infections were associated with an increased risk of myocardial infarction, stroke or all-cause mortality. Intriguingly, infection with CagA-positive *H. pylori* strains was inversely associated with cardiovascular mortality suggesting that CagA-positive *H. pylori* infection could be a protective factor towards fatal cardiovascular events [15]. A recent Iranian work, in which more than 400 patients were tested for classic ischaemic heart disease risk factors and *H. pylori* infection, reported that seropositivity for *H. pylori* was significantly associated with the risk of short-term adverse outcomes, but results failed to show any association between *H. pylori* seropositivity and long-term unfavourable outcomes [16].

Aneurysm

Only a few works are published investigating the correlation between aneurysm and *H. pylori* infection and the majority of them have not found any association. This can be due to differences in the research methods: for example, some researchers, using PCR or immunohistochemical techniques, failed to demonstrate the direct presence of this pathogen in aortic atherosclerotic lesions [17-19]. Others found an interesting association between complicated aortic aneurysm and *H. pylori* IgG positivity [20, 21]. A closer association was also detected with infection by strains secreting the particular VacA (the vacuolating cytotoxin) subtype s1/m1 (which is endowed with an increased cytotoxic power), suggesting that infection by strains expressing CagA and VacA s1/m1 may have a more important role than infection by strains expressing CagA alone in the development of aneurysms, rupture of abdominal aortic aneurysm and acute aortic dissection.

Functional Vascular Diseases

Idiopathic Arrhythmia

The putative association between cardiac idiopathic arrhythmias and *H. pylori* infection is a new object of study. The first publication that substantiated this hypothesis was performed in 2005 [22]. The authors found, in a group of patients with atrial fibrillation (AF), that *H. pylori* seropositivity levels and C-reactive protein (CRP) systemic concentrations were significantly increased, respect to the control group; these values were further augmented in patients with persistent AF *vs.* paroxysmal AF. The following pathogenic mechanism has been proposed: some patients with *H. pylori* infection have autoantibodies to the H+/K+-ATPase of the gastric parietal cells that can determine corpus atrophy. The existence of a linear homology between the gastric proton pump and Na+/K+-ATPase of the cardiac cells (which is inhibited by cardiac glycosides such as digoxin), suggests that autoantibodies to H+/K+-ATPase may also react with Na+/K+-ATPase, thus determining atrial damage. In fact, the cardiac and the gastric ATPases share a similar 35 kDa domain, necessary to exert their catalytic activity. The role of these pumps is to maintain an ionic homeostasis by hydrolyzing ATP; a loss of this balance may therefore trigger AF by determining an abnormal automaticity or causing delay after depolarization, thus inducing rapid premature atrial contractions [22]. Other researchers showed that atrial dimension and CRP levels (independent predictors of AF) were significantly increased in the CagA seropositive subgroup respect to the control group [23].

Some investigators underlined that young *H. pylori* seropositive patients (<50 years) have a greater relative risk of AF compared to seronegative patients [24]. In comparison, older patients seropositive for *H. pylori* have only a slight increased risk of AF. An additional pathogenic mechanism was hypothesized in a recent study, in which it was demonstrated that elevated levels of tumour necrosis factor-α (TNF-α), IL-6 and CRP were associated with AF, while concentrations of transforming growth factor-β1 (TGF-β1) was significantly reduced in AF patients [25]. In addition, AF was associated with elevated systemic levels of antibodies to VacA, compared to the control group. TGF-β1 may act as an anti-atherogenic factor by suppressing the Th1 pathogenic immune responses. Therefore, the elevation of TNF-α, coupled with suppressed TGF-β1, may increase the risk of AF [25].

H. pylori is not only an inflammatory agent but also an immune regulator. Considering the role of TGF-β1 in modulating Th1/Th2 balance, *H. pylori* might be involved in the mechanism underlying AF pathogenesis mediated by suppressed TGF-β1 and elevated Th1 responses. VacA-induced Th1 suppression could possibly abrogate Treg (T regulatory) cell function, which determines a loss of balance between Th1 and Th2 cells. On the other hand, a study by Platonov *et al.* who explored a role of *C. pneumoniae* and *H. pylori* infections in patients with idiopathic permanent AF, did not show any significant serologic correlation in the pathogenesis of such disorder [26].

In conclusion, these data show a general association of *H. pylori* infection with AF in patients with multiple cardiovascular risk factors, but conclusions are questionable.

Migraine

Since the late nineties, *H. pylori* infection has been associated with a largely diffuse functional vascular disorder, primary headache and migraine. One of the first studies based on this hypothesis was accomplished by Gasbarrini *et al.* in 1998. The infection was found in almost 40% of the participants and the prevalence of migraine without aura was significantly greater in infected patients that subsequently underwent eradication therapy: the intensity, duration and frequency of migraine attacks were significantly reduced in all patients in whom the infection was eradicated. The authors concluded that eradication reduces the vasoactive substances produced along the infection, substances that are the pathogenic factors underlying this painful phenomenon [27]. Another study by the same working group found that infection by CagA-positive *H. pylori* was strongly associated with migraine with aura [28]. The proposed pathogenic mechanism consisted in an increased inflammatory gastric mucosa response to strains endowed with a greater inflammatory potential (those expressing CagA), consisting in an enhanced release of cytokines (in particular IL-1, IL-6, IL-8, interferon-γ [IFN-γ]) and others molecules possessing proinflammatory, vasospastic and proalgogen properties [29]. These peptides may act as triggers of vasospasm in peculiar cerebral arterial districts, probably implicated in the aura phenomenon. In agreement with these publications, some researchers recommended that *H. pylori* infection should be investigated in all migrainous patients and concluded that eradication of the infection may be helpful for the treatment of the disease, since 84.6% of patients treated with eradication therapy referred benefits, *vs.* 75% of patients treated with the classic protocols [30, 31]. Other authors highlighted the role of *H. pylori* infection as probable independent environmental risk factor for migraine without aura, especially in patients that are not genetically or hormonally susceptible to migraine [32, 33]. In opposition, an Italian group suggested that chronic *H. pylori* infection is not more frequent in patients with migraine than in controls and that the infection does not modify the clinical features of the disease [34]. Some researchers claim that *H. pylori* infection does not modify the plasma oxidative status and the systemic NO bioavailability of migraineurs, concluding that results do not support any specific correlation between *H. pylori* infection and migraine [35]. Similar results were obtained in another study, but the blood samples examined for the levels of nitric oxide had been taken from patients with migraine during the headache-free period, instead of during the episodes of headache [30].

Raynaud's Disease

Raynaud's phenomenon (Rp), described for the first time by the French physician Maurice Raynaud (1834-1881) in 1861, is a vasospastic disorder mainly involving distal limbs. This disease is characterized by vasospasm after exposure to some motivating factors, like cold or emotional status, with classical paleness of distal finger's skin. Secondary Raynaud's syndrome is associated with many rheumatologic diseases (the most important example is the systemic sclerosis), whereas the primary Raynaud's syndrome (pRp) is idiopathic.

It was observed that *H. pylori* infection is correlated with many vascular diseases. Some studies have ascertained an increased prevalence of *H. pylori* infection in patients with Rp [36]. In other surveys, this correlation was denied; a low prevalence of infection was even observed in Rp patients [37, 38]. However, it seems that the eradication treatment produces benefits: symptoms completely disappeared in 17% of 36 pRp patients and were significantly reduced in 72% of them after cure of the infection. According to the authors, this effect may be due to a reduction of vasoactive mediators linked to *H. pylori* infection [39].

ENDOCRINE SYSTEM

Autoimmune Thyroid Disease

H. pylori infection might be involved in the onset of autoimmune thyroid disease (AITD), but currently there are some controversies. Our group in 1996 and de Luis *et al.* in 1998 underlined that the prevalence of *H. pylori* infection was markedly increased in patients with AITD compared with that observed in controls; in addition, a positive linear regression was found between levels of microsomal autoantibodies and those of anti-*H. pylori* IgG in patients with AITD [40, 41] This suggests that *H. pylori* antigens might be involved in the development of AITD, possibly through the production of immune cross reactive antibodies.

In late nineties, some researchers found that monoclonal antibodies to an *H. pylori* strain expressing CagA reacted with human tissues, including thyroid follicular cells [42]. Another group sequenced the chromosome of an *H. pylori* strain possessing the *cag* PAI and showed that the microorganism carries a gene encoding for an endogenous peroxidase [43]. These observations prompted us [44] to perform a study, whose results showed that the overall prevalence of infection by CagA-positive *H. pylori* was significantly greater in patients with autoimmune thyroid disease than in controls and hypothesized that mechanisms of antigenic mimicry could sustain the association between *H. pylori* and AITD. Some authors, in a small case-control study, have observed a reduction of thyroid autoantibodies (anti-thyroid peroxidase, -TPO, and anti-thyroglobulin,-TG) after eradication of *H. pylori* infection *vs.* no reduction in patient that did not undergo eradication treatment [45].

A possible mechanism to explain how an infection in the stomach can produce pathological effects upon distant organs may consist in the induction of an autoimmune reaction through mechanisms of antigenic mimicry [46, 47]. The bacterial components involved in this cross-reaction have partly been identified as antigens of the Lewis blood groups, present both on *H. pylori* lipopolysaccharide and on host gastric epithelium. Lewis antigens are expressed at high concentration in the gastric mucosa and in extragastric sites, even though at lower concentrations. In normal conditions, the thyroid gland expresses few antigens of the Lewis group, whereas their expression increases in the presence of inflammatory processes or neoplasms [48]. Anti-*H. pylori* monoclonal antibodies cross reacting with Lewis X and Lewis Y antigens were tested on normal thyroid tissue. No reactivity was observed with thyrocytes, whereas a strong reactivity was observed with the oxyphil cells of the Hashimoto's thyroiditis and epithelial neoplasms, whether benign or malignant. It may therefore be argued that the thyroid gland is a target of a cross-reaction in the human immune response to *H. pylori* infection. Gastric mucosa infected by *H. pylori* and thyroid tissue in AITD are both characterized by the presence of mucosal-associated lymphoid tissue (MALT). MALT lymphoid cells have a strong tendency to recirculate to MALT due to their specific receptors. A chronic immune response induced by *H. pylori* continues to activate cross-reactive B and T lymphocytes, whose migration to the thyroid gland is further facilitated by the homing tendency of these cells to MALT.

Larizza *et al.* investigated in a pediatric setting the possibility that a susceptible immunogenetic profile could influence the development of AITD in subjects with

H. pylori infection. A significant interaction between HLA-DRB1*0301 and *H. pylori* infection was present in AITD patients and not in controls, suggesting that the co-presence of these two factors might favor AITD development; they concluded that the target of *H. pylori*-elicited immune inflammatory response might be the thyroid gland in subjects with a peculiar immunogenic profile, so that the consequence of this particular setting may be the development of AITD [49]. Recent data showed an increased prevalence of *H. pylori* infection in patients with Graves' disease (GD) with an overall high prevalence of infection by strains expressing CagA compared to the control group, suggesting a possible role of this bacterium in the onset and/or the maintenance of the disease. Subsequently, the same group [50, 51] determined the prevalence of *H. pylori* infection in AITD, especially in Hashimoto's thyroiditis (HT) and observed a positive correlation with GD alone (independently of the CagA status) and not also with HT. To explain the different results regarding *H. pylori* prevalence in GD and HT, these researchers singled out different autoimmune mechanisms: cellular response and Th1 profile for HT; humoral response and Th2 profile for GD.

The seroprevalence of *H. pylori* infection in patients with type 1 diabetes mellitus and AITD was significantly higher than in healthy controls [52]; in addition, anti-*H. pylori* IgG and IgA titers were positively and significantly correlated with anti-TPO and -TG titers in patients with type 1 diabetes mellitus [52]. The conclusion of this group was that *H. pylori* infection could be considered as an environmental trigger for the development of AITD in these patients.

Recently, some investigators compared the seroprevalence of *H. pylori* infection in patients affected by HT or GD with that observed in healthy individuals and found that the rates of infection were similar in the two groups, but there was a significant association between AITD (both HT and GD) and infection by strains expressing CagA; in addition, anti-CagA antibody levels correlated with titres of thyroid autoantibodies [53].

In contrast to previous observations, a small Italian pilot study noticed a similar prevalence of *H. pylori* infection (independently of the CagA status) in patients with HT and controls, indicating that an association between *H. pylori* infection and AITD was unlikely [52]. Similar results were obtained on patients who underwent gastroscopy for dyspeptic symptoms: *H. pylori* positivity, prevalence of anti-TPO and anti-TG autoantibodies and thyroid hormonal levels in dyspeptic patients were not different from those in controls. A weakness of this study, however, consisted in the patients' selection; in fact, only persons with dyspeptic symptoms were enrolled, ignoring the fact that up to 80% of *H. pylori* infected individuals are asymptomatic [55]. For a comprehensive overview of this subject, the publication by Papamichael *et al.* can be consulted [56].

ENDOCRINO-METABOLIC SYSTEM

Diabetes Mellitus

Despite the finding that *H. pylori* infection may also be related to the development of diabetes mellitus (DM) is relatively recent, there is a fierce contentious on this matter [56]. There are discordant data on the prevalence of *H. pylori* infection in type 1 and type 2 DM, the presence of gastro-intestinal symptoms or disorders (*e.g.* delayed gastric emptying, dyspepsia, esophagitis, peptic ulcer, chronic gastritis and upper gastrointestinal symptoms) and DM complications. One point on which all studies seem to converge is that the success of eradication regimens of *H. pylori* infection is significantly lower in diabetics than in non-diabetics, whereas re-infection rates seem to be greater, especially in patients with type 2 DM compared to the general population [57-61]. This may be due to alterations in the gastric microvasculature, which could lead to diminished absorption of antibiotics. Alternatively, the frequent antibiotic use in diabetics may result in the selection of *H. pylori* resistant strains. The difference in the eradication rate observed between adults and children affected by diabetes could be due to the fact that the latter have no history of repeated infectious diseases and antibiotic treatments, with negligible selection of antibiotic-resistant *H. pylori* strains [62]. The clinical consequences of *H. pylori* infection in terms of metabolic control, however, seem to be negligible [63]. No correlation between *H. pylori* infection and glycemic status in both type 1 and 2 DM patients was found in different surveys [64;65]. No association was found between infection by several pathogens and DM status [66]. Similar results were obtained also in a very recent Nigerian study [67].

Another issue concerns insulin resistance. In a study on the possible association between *H. pylori* infection and insulin resistance on 1107 patients, it was found that *H. pylori* infection significantly and independently contributed to promoting insulin resistance [68]. Results of another study, conducted on 130 type 2 DM patients, showed that *H. pylori* infection had a significant effect on the daily blood glucose levels and blood glucose fluctuation in those who were infected [69]. *H. pylori* infection was also associated with increased fasting serum insulin levels [70]. Finally, in a study on the effect of *H. pylori* on pancreatic beta-cell function in 288 Chinese subjects, it was found that anti-*H. pylori* antibody titer, as well as adiponectin levels and white cell blood count, were shown to be independent predictors for hyperglycemia and reduced insulin sensitivity [71]; in addition, such study contributes to explain the reason why this Chinese population have a high occurrence of type 2 DM, in spite of their relatively low adiposity [72]. Data of a systematic review, summarizing the epidemiologic evidence concerning the association between *H. pylori* infection and insulin resistance quantitative indexes, suggest the existence of a potential association between *H. pylori* infection and insulin resistance, even though there is a significant heterogeneity in studies regarding the methods to detect the *H. pylori* infection and the study populations [73]. A recent review, focused on the possible association between metabolic syndrome and *H. pylori* infection, gave controversial results with emphasis on the possible linkage between them [74].

Finally, in a recent study, Chen and Blaser found that *H. pylori* seropositivity and especially the CagA-positive status, were associated with increased HbA1c (glycosylated hemoglobin) levels, also after the exclusion of individuals with a history of diabetes and control for potential confounders [75].

Postprandial Hypoglycemia

In the literature there is only a few articles on this topic. In a study on 12 patients with postprandial symptomatic hypoglycemia and *H. pylori* infection, it was found that serum insulin responses decreased, whereas the plasma glucose levels increased significantly following a mixed meal in patients successfully treated [76]. The number and the clinical severity score of postprandial hypoglycemia attacks that occurred in a one-month period and the area under the curve for symptom scores decreased significantly. These findings suggest that *H. pylori* gastritis may contribute to the development of postprandial symptomatic hypoglycemia. The increased insulin secretion may be due to an imbalance between gastrin and somatostatin production in gastrointestinal tract: *H. pylori*-induced gastritis stimulates gastrin secretion and down-regulates D-cell production of somatostatin, concurrently causing an exaggerated acute insulin release following meals; consequently, reduced postprandial levels of plasma glucose occur. Soon after, other investigators concluded that this infection has a significant effect on the daily blood glucose levels and blood glucose fluctuation in patients with type 2 DM [66]. Finally, a case of an old *H. pylori* infected man with hypoglycemia and severe insulin-resistance induced by anti-insulin receptor antibodies was published; his condition improved only after bacterial eradication, supporting a causal involvement of this pathogen in insulin resistance syndrome [77].

Osteoporosis

There is only a few publications regarding the possible association between osteoporosis and *H. pylori* infection. The first study was made by our group in 2005, 240 men were examined in a whole: 80 osteoporotic patients and 160 controls. Both the *H. pylori* infectious and the CagA status were investigated. The following parameters were considered: bone mineral density (BMD) (by dual x-ray absorptiometry), urinary cross-laps - a marker of bone resorption - and systemic levels of estradiol. The prevalence of CagA-positive *H. pylori* infection was increased in osteoporotic patients; in infected patients with anti-CagA antibodies the levels of estradiol were significantly lower and levels of urinary cross laps were significantly increased compared to those measured in CagA-negative infected patients [78, 79]. As regards BMD, the results of our study and those of another publication did not show any correlation with *H. pylori* infection or CagA status. Taken together these data are not conclusive, but we can suppose that the presence of the *cag* pathogenicity island in the infecting isolates could be a risk factor for the development of osteoporosis [80, 81].

HAEMOPOIETIC SYSTEM

Iron Deficiency Anemia (IDA)

Anemia, defined as a hemoglobin concentration below established cut-off levels (normally, 12 g/dL), affects about two billion people in the world (WHO source) and approximately 50% of all anemia cases are diagnosed as iron deficiency anemia (IDA) [48, 290]. IDA remains one of the most common nutritional deficiencies of mankind and can be induced by a variety of causes, as an inadequate iron intake, chronic blood loss, malabsorption, hemolysis, chronic diseases, or a combination of these disorders [84, 85, 86].

It is reported that *H. pylori* infection is observed in over 50% of people in the world with peaks of 70%-90% in some countries. Since IDA affects billions people in the world, the obvious conclusion is that when two diseases have such a high prevalence in the population, the possibility that they are associated is very high.

If gastroenterological evaluation fails to disclose a reasonable cause of IDA, especially if anemia is refractory to oral iron treatment, screenings for celiac disease, autoimmune gastritis and *H. pylori* infection are recommended. Recent studies indicate that 20%-27% of patients with unexplained IDA have autoimmune gastritis, about 50% have evidence of active *H. pylori* infection and 4%-6% have celiac disease.

The mechanisms that may cause IDA in patients infected by *H. pylori* range from occult bleeding for erosive gastritis to an inadequate absorption of dietary iron. *H. pylori* induces chronic pangastritis with resultant achlorhydria and decreases ascorbic acid secretion in the gastric mucosa. This may lead to a diminished iron absorption, which can justify anemia for 20% of patients without gastrointestinal bleeding. Since *H. pylori* infected individuals have elevated levels of circulating antibodies to H+, K+-ATPase of the gastric parietal cells, it is reasonable to assume that this bacterium can cause autoimmune atrophic gastritis *via* an autoimmune response [87].

Although some studies have reached inconclusive or negative results [88, 89, 90], the great majority of them conclude for an association. A meta-analysis published in 2010 evaluated the association between *H. pylori* infection and IDA and examined the effect of *H. pylori* eradication upon serum hemoglobin and ferritin levels. The aim of that study was in particular to evaluate the randomized controlled trials (RCTs) on the association between *H. pylori* and IDA. Fifteen observational studies and five RCTs were identified and used for calculation. Meta-analysis on observational studies indicates an association. In RCTs, eradication of *H. pylori* can improve hemoglobin and serum ferritin levels but not significantly [91]. Another meta-analysis suggests that treatment of *H. pylori* infection could be effective in improving anemia and iron status in IDA patients, particularly in those with moderate or severe anemia [92].

A recent study showed a high occurrence of *H. pylori* infection in pregnant women with IDA. Eradication treatment resulted in a better response to iron oral supplementation [93].

Schönlein-Henoch Purpura

Schönlein-Henoch purpura (SHP) is a systemic vasculitis characterized by palpable purpura (the appearance of red or purple discolorations on the skin), colicky abdominal pain, gastrointestinal hemorrhage, arthralgia and renal involvement. The pathogenesis is unclear, but a great variety of conditions, including bacterial and viral infections, may be responsible for the onset. Only a few authors have described an association between SHP and *H. pylori* infection, mostly by case report. One of the first publications concerns an *H. pylori* infected woman with SHP, in whom clinical manifestations of vasculitis disappeared after successful *H. pylori* eradication treatment [94]. SHP signs and symptoms recurred ten months later alongside with re-infection; the same therapy was effective in curing both the infection and SHP. Similarly, other researchers treated successfully a patient with SHP and duodenal ulcer by eradicating *H. pylori* [95]. According to some physicians, it could be useful to examine for *H. pylori* infection all patients with gastrointestinal manifestations of SHP, such as bleeding and important epigastric pain, since in this case the patient had complained severe gastrointestinal symptoms associated with vasculitis [96]. Others conducted a research on 11 consecutive adults patients presenting with SHP; they found that IgG antibodies against *H. pylori* were mostly present in acute SHP, while IgA antibodies possibly sustained gastrointestinal symptoms underlying the chronic phase of the disease and supporting the hypothesis that *H. pylori* infection might be associated with the development and progression of SHP. It should also be considered the possibility that the association of *H. pylori* infection with SHP may be underestimated, as endoscopic examination is not systematically performed in patients with this disease [97].

In children, the prevalence of *H. pylori* infection in SHP patients with gastro-intestinal manifestations was as high as 58.3% and the prevalence of infection in patients with gastro-intestinal manifestations who relapsed was 81.3%; the rates of infection in SHP patients without gastro-intestinal manifestations and healthy children were significantly lower: 28.1% and 6.7%, respectively [98].

In conclusion, should gastric *H. pylori* infection play an important role in the onset of SHP, its eradication would be a definitive remedy, either in terms of improved prognosis and of protection against recurrences and renal complications (renal failure and end stage renal disease), which are more difficult to treat. Additional studies with a greater number of cases are needed in order to verify whether the association of *H. pylori* infection with SHP is causal or occasional and to evaluate the usefulness of *H. pylori* eradication therapy in this condition.

Extra-Gastric MALT Lymphoma

The stomach is the most common site of MALT lymphoma, but this neoplasia may also occur in lungs, thyroid gland, salivary glands and other organs, such as intestine. Approximately two-thirds of MALT lymphoma affecting the stomach are caused by *H. pylori* infection and it has been shown that eradication of the organism can lead to regression of lymphoma.

A new entity in the field of infection-associated lymphoma is the ocular adnexal lymphoma, which is often associated with *Chlamydia psittaci* ocular infection. Successful antimicrobial treatment against chlamydia was associated with remission of such malignancy.

Primary thyroid lymphoma seems to be involved in *H. pylori* infection, too. In the literature, only one case is described, which concerned a 69-year-old man presented with right neck tumour. Primary thyroid MALT lymphoma occurring in Hashimoto's thyroiditis was diagnosed. He also had gastric cancer and *H. pylori* infection. After subtotal gastrectomy, thyroid lymphoma became smaller spontaneously, but transiently. Then, the patient was treated with *H. pylori* eradication therapy, resulting in the complete disappearance of lymphoma. Although *H. pylori* organisms were not detected in the lymphoma tissue by PCR, it is reasonable to believe that the infection was implicated in the pathogenesis of such neoplasia.

Conversely, one study suggested that patients with an autoimmune disease might not be optimal candidates for *H. pylori* eradication, even in case of an early stage gastric MALT lymphoma, since very few patients responded to the eradication therapy [99]. The development of primary cutaneous B-cell lymphomas, as with gastric lymphoma, is regarded as being dependent on the acquisition of B-cell lymphoid tissue. There are cases in literature that have demonstrated that skin lesions progressively regressed after repeated eradication therapy. This suggested that a close relation exists between primary cutaneous MALT-type lymphoma and *H. pylori* colonization of the stomach [100].

H. pylori infection has been involved in MALT of the urinary bladder, too. The literature reports a case of an *H. pylori* positive woman in whom, after eradication therapy, the lymphoma disappeared; in addition, the patient did not have any tumor recurrence for the past 25 months [101].

Nishimura *et al.* described a case of salivary gland MALT lymphoma associated with localized *H. pylori* infection: no recurrence of the tumor after radiotherapy, surgery and bacterial eradication was noticed. The authors sustain that *H. pylori* infection plays a key role as an additional antigenic stimulus in the development of salivary gland MALT lymphoma [102].

Another interesting case concerns a woman with parotid MALT lymphoma and concomitant *H. pylori* infection. Although *H. pylori* was not detected in the recurrent parotid lymphoma, antibiotic therapy determined both the eradication of infection and the disappearance of recurrent lymphoma [103].

IMMUNE SYSTEM

Food Allergy

Food allergy manifestations can be observed in 6% of children and in 1%-2% of adults in the world, with a growing prevalence especially in occidental countries.

Clinical manifestations of food allergy can involve the gastrointestinal tract, the respiratory system and the skin; only in rare occasions, an anaphylactic shock can develop. It is also possible that some factors could influence the clinical presentation of food allergy and bacterial infections could be one of these factors.

H. pylori infection has a controversial role in this context. In 1999, we studied the possible interactions between *H. pylori* and food allergy, examining 38 patients with history of food allergy and determining the levels of IgE to alimentary antigens; 53 controls living in the same area were also examined. The prevalence of *H. pylori* infection between the two groups was similar, but the prevalence of anti-CagA seropositivity in patients with food allergy was increased compared to controls (62.5% *vs.* 28 %). In addition, the mean IgE titer to the most common food allergens in patients infected by CagA-positive *H. pylori* strains was greater than in patients infected by CagA-negative strains [104]. We hypothesized that the enhanced mucosal damage commonly found in gastric mucosa of patients infected by virulent strains could intensify the gastric epithelial permeability and decrease the selectivity of the allergen passage, with consequent augmented IgE response in atopic individuals [104]. In another study, the possible correlation between *H. pylori* infection and food allergy in chronic gastritis was examined and it was observed that a long-term exposure to food allergens may increase the intensity of gastritis in patients with *H. pylori* infection [105].

The stimulation of pro-inflammatory cytokines by *H. pylori* could have a role in the development of alimentary allergy, as it was observed that the concentration of mucosal cytokines in children with food allergy and *H. pylori* infection (especially IL-2, IL-8 and TNF-α) was increased compared to controls [106].

Opposite results were obtained in a recent study, which suggested a protective role of *H. pylori* in food allergy: the urinary excretion of N-tele-methylhistamine and serum levels of eosinophilic cation protein (ECP, a basic protein located in the eosinophils, which is released during their degranulation) and mast cell tryptase were measured in *H. pylori* infected and non-infected patients; concentrations of allergy mediators (*i.e.*, ECP) were lower in the first group of patients [107].

SKIN DISEASES

Pruritus Cutaneous

Some researchers found that the great majority (88%) of *H. pylori* infected patients with this symptoms, who were unresponsive to conventional therapy, improved after eradication [108]. Others observed that more than half of a large group of Japanese patients affected by intractable skin diseases were *H. pylori* positive. After eradication of infection, symptoms improved in most patients [109].

An interesting study was conducted in 2002 in order to understand the pathogenic relationship between *H. pylori* infection and skin disease. The authors examined the serum level of IgG antibodies against *H. pylori* and performed gastroscopic examinations in Japanese patients with chronic skin diseases. Considered the high prevalence of infection in those patients, they hypothesized that persistent *H. pylori* infection may contribute to the development of disease and that the infection may worsen the disease and lead to an intractable and chronic form [109].

Rosacea

Rosacea is a chronic dermatitis involving central areas of face. The main signs are constituted by erythema, teleangectasias and acneiform eruptions. Rosacea is an idiopathic syndrome; nevertheless, many researchers have been investigating the possible role of infective agents, such as *Staphylococcus aureus, C. pneumoniae* and *H. pylori*. An increased prevalence of *H. pylori* infection in patients with rosacea has recently been reported. The anti-*H. pylori* mean antibody titer was augmented in 29 patients with rosacea, compared to controls [92]. Other investigators detected an improvement of rosacea symptoms after *H. pylori* eradication, suggesting that investigation on *H. pylori* infectious status and antibiotic treatment of those who are infected can be helpful in a large percentage of patients [110, 111]. Anyhow, not all the researchers believe in this association: some authors, for instance, did not find a greater frequency of gastric disease and *H. pylori* infection in patients with rosacea at different stages [112].

As far as the putative pathogenic mechanism is concerned, in an immunoproteomic study, we found an IgE antibody-mediated reactivity against catalase produced by *H. pylori* (Kata protein) in a serum sample from a patient with rosacea. Kata is an antioxidant enzyme required for a complete protection against superoxide radicals. Since one of the causes of rosacea could consist in a reduced catalase activity of patients' cells (which implies an insufficient anti-oxidant response), we hypothesized that *H. pylori* infection may induce an antibacterial catalase immune response that may cross react with the host catalase, making inadequate the human antioxidative defense [113].

Sweet's Syndrome

Sweet's syndrome, also known as acute febrile neutrophilic dermatosis, is an idiopathic syndrome characterized by painful papulonodular lesions localized on the whole body, most frequently on face, neck and upper and lower limbs. The etiology of Sweet's syndrome is still unknown, but it seems to be associated with tumors, inflammatory diseases, vaccinations and infections. The infective involvement in this syndrome and in particular the putative contribution of *H. pylori* infection, are described in a case report of a 42-years-old patient. The authors assert that *H. pylori* could trigger a hypersensitivity response, considering the abnormal immunologic reaction behind this syndrome [114].

Chronic Urticaria

Chronic urticaria (CU) is a common condition characterized by the persistence of urticaria symptoms over six weeks. It is difficult to determine a starting factor for CU (in the 70%-90% of patients the cause is unclear) even though many infectious agents have been investigated, including *H. pylori*. For example, in a study in which 184 patients with urticaria (idiopathic or allergic) were examined, *H. pylori* infection was found more frequently in patients with idiopathic CU, compared to those with allergic urticaria. Moreover, *H. pylori* eradication reduced the frequency of CU exacerbations [4]. Others found a similar correlation between different clinical variants of CU and *H. pylori* infection, which, also in this study, was detected most frequently in patients with idiopathic CU than in patients with allergic CU. In these cases the eradication therapy lead to an improvement of symptoms in patients with idiopathic CU, while in the allergic urticaria group there was no evidence of improvement [115].

In another survey, in which 82 patients with CU and 17 patients with *prurigo chronica multiformis* were examined, a remission of symptoms, especially in the second group, was detected after antibiotic treatment and it was suggested that the eradication treatment of infection can be helpful in the intractable cases [116]. An improvement of CU symptoms after bacteriological cure was also found in a more recent study [117].

Molecular mimicry and the consequent production of autoantibodies can be the pathway through which *H. pylori* may contribute to CU exacerbation: in fact, it was recently observed that 30%-50% of CU cases could be provoked by an autoimmune process [118]. Our group found an increased seropositivity for anti-heat-shock protein 60 in patients with idiopathic CU [119]. Since this chaperonin is highly conserved in the evolutive pathway, we hypothesized that the infection could modulate CU pathogenesis by stimulating the production of cross reactive antibodies. Another mechanism proposed is the increased gastric vascular permeability during *H. pylori* infection, that could derive from a prolonged exposure to host allergic antigens [118].

The disagreement existing on this topic is accentuated by a review of ten studies performed in 2010, nine of which showing no benefit after successful *H. pylori* treatment [120]. A German review, however, reached opposite conclusions, as the authors observed that a statistically significant number of CU patients received benefits from the eradication therapy [121, 122].

In conclusion, we believe that this association can be defined weak or controversial.

Angioedema

Angioedema is a quick swelling of skin, mucosal or submucosal tissues, frequently associated with allergic manifestations or C1-inibitor protein deficiency (hereditary angioedema autosomal dominant or acquired C1-esterase inhibitor deficiency). Some researchers described the possible role of *H. pylori* infection in C1-esterase inhibitor (C1-INH) acquired deficiency, a condition often associated with lymphoproliferative diseases, malignancy, immune disordes, and infections. A complete resolution of symptoms and the normalization of C1-INH serum level were achieved after *H. pylori* eradication [123]. Others suggested that *H. pylori* can act as a triggering factor in autoimmune angioedema with autoantibodies against C1-INH [124].

The eradication of *H. pylori* infection may be also an improvement factor in hereditary angioedema. In fact, a high prevalence of such infection was found in patients with this pathology, especially in those with a history of recurrent episodes of abdominal pain (hereditary angioedema is frequently associated with upper respiratory obstruction with dyspnea and abdominal pain). The eradication therapy reduced drastically the frequency of edematous episodes, suggesting that a screening for *H. pylori* should be carried out in these patients [125].

Alopecia Areata

Alopecia areata is a form of immune-mediated hair loss. The possible contribution of *H. pylori* infection in this disease was recently investigated. The prevalence of the infection (18 out of 31 patients were infected), however, was not significantly different from that in controls [126, 127]. On the contrary, others described the complete reverse of hair loss in a patients infected by *H. pylori* after eradication therapy [128]. Larger case-control studies, however, do not confirm this relationship [126, 127].

Prurigo Nodularis

In 1909, Hyde described a rare and untreatable idiopathic eruption - characterized by numerous persistent nodules mainly affecting the extensor surface of arms and legs of women - that he called prurigo nodularis (PN) [129]. Some authors studied 42 cases of Hyde's prurigo nodularis and an evidence for *H. pylori* infection was found in 40 out of the 42 patients examined. Eradication of *H. pylori* was confirmed in 39/40 cases and in these patients pruritus decreased markedly [130].

Lichen Planus

Lichen planus (LP) is a mucocutaneous inflammatory disease of unknown origin. Skin and oral mucosa are the most frequently involved areas. Other mucous membranes (including genitalia, esophagus and conjunctiva) and skin appendages (*e.g.*, scalp hair and nails) can also be affected. One or several areas can be involved, concomitantly or sequentially [131]. Etiology and pathogenesis of LP are not fully understood, but infections and stress are suspected to be the most common triggering factors. Most studies did not demonstrate an evidence of a causal association between *H. pylori* infection and LP [132, 133, 134].

Also recent surveys have not been able to effectively prove a link between infection by *H. pylori* and LP [135]. Only a recent study on oral lichen planus, found that the concomitant presence of erosive lichen planus, *H. pylori* DNA in erosive lesions and *H. pylori* organisms in gastric mucosa may imply a possible pathogenic connection between such species and this disorder [136]

RESPIRATORY SYSTEM

Chronic Otitis Media with Effusion

Recently, it was suggested that tonsil and adenoid tissues may act as a reservoir for *H. pylori* [137]. A connection between chronic tubotympanal disorders and gastroesophageal reflux is well recognized, but the mechanism underlying this relationship is unclear. Some authors investigated the possible presence of *H. pylori* in adenoid tissue and middle ear effusion samples from patients with chronic otitis media with effusion (OME) and compared the results with the data obtained with children who had adenoid hypertrophy without OME. They showed that *H. pylori* was present in middle ear of children with chronic OME and suggested that *H. pylori* has conceivably a role in the pathogenesis of such disease. In addition, they demonstrated *H. pylori* presence in only one out of 38 adenoid specimens, concluding that adenoid tissue does not act as a reservoir for *H. pylori* [138, 139].

Some studies, despite they confirmed the presence of *H. pylori* in the nasopharynx and middle ear, do not support a role for this bacterium in the pathogenesis of OME, or even deny that *H. pylori* can colonize the nasopharynx of children with middle ear disease, whether dyspeptic or not, concluding that there is no apparent role for this bacterium in middle ear pathology [140].

Numerous other respiratory disorders have tentatively been associated with *H. pylori* infection, including laryngeal carcinoma, vocal folds' lesions, lung carcinoma, nasal polyps and chronic obstructive pulmonary disease, but at present, there is no definite proof of a causal relationship between *H. pylori* infection and respiratory diseases. The primary evidence comes from case-control studies, which, however, concern relatively small numbers of patients. We have therefore decided not to treat them.

EYE

Glaucoma

Glaucoma (primary chronic open angle, POAG) is a progressive optic neuropathy mainly due to an augmented intraocular pressure. Glaucoma is the second most common cause of blindness in the world: it is estimated that 60 million people are affected by glaucoma and 8.4 million are bilaterally blind [141]. Glaucoma is a multifactorial disease, but the most important risk factor is an increased intraocular pressure. Other determinants, however, may damage the neural tissue in glaucomatous optic neuropathy, including an endothelium-dependent vascular disregulation, blood hyperviscosity and the action of cytokines.

Over the last decade, various researchers have examined the existence of a possible link between *H. pylori* infection and glaucoma. Some studies have supported such association and the underlying pathogenic mechanisms include the induction of inflammatory responses, as well as apoptotic processes that may lead to glaucomatous neuropathy.

Some researchers observed that *H. pylori* infection is more frequent among patients with glaucoma than in the general population. When compared with the control group, glaucoma patients have less often a normal endoscopic appearance of the gastric mucosa and more often an antral gastritis or peptic ulcer disease [142, 143].

In another study, the authors reported increased anti-*H. pylori* IgG levels in aqueous humor of glaucoma patients and the titer correlated with the degree of vertical cupping, possibly reflecting the severity of glaucomatous damage [144]. In an extension of this study the same authors demonstrated that *H. pylori* eradication may positively influence glaucoma parameters (intraocular pressure and visual field) [145].

Also an Indian study [146], in which the levels of anti-*H. pylori* IgG in aqueous humor and serum of patients with primary open glaucoma (POAG), exfoliation syndrome (pseudoexfoliation glaucoma, PXFG) and normotensive cataract patients were investigated, it was demonstrated that anti-*H. pylori* antibody levels in sera of individuals with POAG were significantly increased compared to those in PXFG and control groups. Thus, also the Indian physicians supported the hypothesis that anti-*H. pylori* antibodies may have a role in the development of POAG.

The role of *H. pylori* infection on the pathophysiology of glaucoma may depend on the release of various proinflammatory and vasoactive substances and by the influence on infection upon the apoptotic process [I47]. The mechanisms involved are numerous:

1. Promotion of platelet and platelet–leukocyte aggregation.

2. Releasing of large amounts of proinflammatory and vasoactive substances, such as cytokines ([IL-1, IL-6, IL-8, IL-10, IL-12, TNF-α, interferon-γ), eicosanoids (leukotrienes, prostaglandins), and acute phase proteins (fibrinogen, C-reactive protein). In particular, increased endothelin-1 (a potent constrictor of arterioles and venules), nitric oxide, and nitric oxide synthase levels are associated with *H. pylori* infection. Endothelin-1–induced vasoconstriction of the anterior optic nerve vessels and nitric oxide modulation of vascular tone in the ophthalmic artery may produce glaucomatous damage.

3. Stimulation of mononuclear cells to produce a tissue factor-like procoagulant that converts fibrinogen into fibrin.

4. Existence of an antigenic mimicry between endothelial and bacterial antigens.

5. Production of reactive oxygen metabolites such as lipid peroxides.

6. Influence upon the apoptotic process.

H. pylori, through the release of inflammatory mediators (such TNF-α), may induce a breakdown of the blood-brain barrier (BBB) and blood-ocular barrier; this could explain the pathogenesis of some neuropathies such as glaucoma. In addition, antibodies to *H. pylori* might also diffuse into the aqueous circulation through the destruction of BBB. In fact, when serum-specific antibodies pass into the brain, they are able to kill the cells of the retina [142-143]. Not all researches, however, agree on the existence of such association [148].

Some authors suggest that *H. pylori* infection may be associated with an increased risk of normal tension glaucoma (NTG) as a secondary aggravating factor because of the coexistence of other main causes [25]. Mechanisms involved in the pathogenesis of NTG include an altered ocular blood flow, an autoimmune reaction, vasoactive substances, alterations of platelet functions and molecular mimicry. These factors seem to be more related to *H. pylori* infection than POAG, in which a high intra-ocular pressure is recognized as a major pathogenic factor.

In any case, there are also studies that are skeptical of such an association [149, 150].

Blepharitis

Blepharitis is an ocular condition characterized by chronic inflammation of the eyelid. Even if some cases resolve spontaneously in 2-4 weeks, generally it is a long-standing inflammation with different degrees of severity. In the past, the potential eye involvement along *H. pylori* infection had been evaluated by the same researchers that had investigated the link between *H. pylori* and glaucoma [149, 144], chronic ocular inflammation [151] and individuals affected by central serous chorioretinopathy [152]. In 2006, some authors confirmed the existence of an association between *H. pylori* infection and blepharitis, even though causal associations were disclaimed. The most important result was that the bacteriological eradication improved ocular cytology results.

The infection may induce lid inflammatory changes by several mechanisms, including the production of NO and gastrin, which are potent vasodilators that may play a role in producing flushing reactions on face and neck. Eyelids and conjunctiva are certainly involved in vasodilation and this effect may constitute the starting point of a chronic inflammation. Also the chronic release of large amounts of inflammatory mediators caused by *H. pylori* infection or, more likely, cross-mimicry mechanisms between bacterial and eukaryotic cell antigens, could affect organs distant from the gastroduodenal tract. At last, *H. pylori* has been found in the mouth, but it is not known whether the oral cavity acts as a permanent reservoir for this bacterium. However, from the oral cavity, it may reach the anterior surface of the eye, causing or worsening blepharitis, at least on the basis of cytological criteria [153]. The most important datum from this study is that blepharitis improved in approximately 50% of patients after eradication treatment of *H. pylori* infection.

CENTRAL NERVOUS SYSTEM

Parkinson's Disease

The first researcher who clearly hypothesized the existence of an etiologic correlation between Parkinson's disease (PD) and *H. pylori* infection was Altschuler in 1996 [154]. However, it should be acknowledged that James Parkinson himself, almost two centuries ago (1817), conjectured that there might be a causative relationship between gastrointestinal problems and PD. In 1965, in a study on 200 PD patients and 200 age- and sex-matched controls, Strang noted a statistically augmented prevalence of peptic ulcer (diagnosed by X-ray or surgery) in PD patients compared to controls. Interestingly, ulcers typically preceded PD diagnosis by 10 up to 20 years [38]. Among the first authors, Charlettand (one of Strang's colleagues), in 1999, observed a greater prevalence of seropositivity for *H. pylori* and brady/hypokinesia, rigidity and abnormal posture in siblings of PD patients, compared to controls. Subsequently, they affirmed that *H. pylori* infection, through immunosuppression and predisposing to autoimmunity, could be considered as a model to study the pathogenesis of parkinsonism and parkinsonian-like aspects of ageing. They also claimed that the eradication of a putative trigger of the disease had the potential of changing the approach to the parkinsonism, just as the eradication of *H. pylori* infection sorted out for peptic ulcer [155]. Furthermore, these researchers found that the cure of the infection in late parkinsonism with cachexia - a stage usually considered intractable - can result in an U-turn. The eradication treatment, however, may not provide a definite solution. Persistence of antibodies against CagA increases the predicted probability of being labelled as having parkinsonism [156]. A successive study, despite it showed a clinical improvement and a reduced deterioration of brady/hypokinesia, had to register a worsening of rigidity after a successful eradication therapy [157]. In 2008, the same authors proposed a two stage pathogenesis for the potential association of *H. pylori* infection and small intestinal bacterial overgrowth (SIBO) in PD: in stage 1, *H. pylori* evokes autoimmunity against mitochondria and this mechanism underlies brady/hypokinesia predominant parkinsonism. In stage 2, acquisition of SIBO causes further mitochondrial dysfunctions, resulting in a rigidity-predominant picture. They hypothesize that peripheral infection would increase traffic and signaling into brain through afferent nerve stimulation. *Substantia nigra* is considered particularly vulnerable to everyday insults, such as products of dopamine oxidation. Nigral glial activation would increase stress and recruit immune cells locally [158].

An original pathogenetic mechanism to explain the association between PD and *H. pylori* infection was provided by Schulz *et al.* [159]: amyotrophic lateral sclerosis-parkinsonism dementia complex (ALS-PDC) - a neurological disorder characterized by features of parkinsonism and for which no consistent genetic explanation has been found - is linked to the consumption of cycad (*Cycas micronesica*). Recent experiments in their laboratory have identified several sterol glycosides in cycads, which have neurotoxic properties *in vitro* and that are possibly linked to the development of neurodegenerative diseases *in vivo*. Specifically, mice fed on cycads displayed behavioural symptoms of parkinsonism such as reduced gait length and neuropathological signs, such as those deriving from loss of striatal dopaminergic terminals and upregulation of the dopamine D2 receptor. These cycad-derived sterol glycosides are structurally similar to cholesterol glycosides that account for a significant part of the lipid profile of *H. pylori*. They formally hypothesized that cholesterol glycosides arising from *H. pylori* infection may act as neurotoxins, promoting the degeneration of the dopaminergic neurons affected in parkinsonism, similarly to the mechanism that presumably links cycad consumption to ALS-PDC [159].

Pierantozzi *et al.* reported in 2001 that the area under the curve of L-dopa plasma concentration, following the administration of a single dose of 250 mg L-dopa, was augmented after *H. pylori* eradication in six PD patients with high antibody titers to *H. pylori*. This finding suggested that infection-activated gastric alterations may be responsible, at least in part, for the reported erratic efficacy of oral L-dopa therapy in some patients with advanced PD; they therefore recommended *H. pylori* eradication in all PD patients under L-dopa therapy [160]. Subsequently, they noted that motor fluctuations were related with pharmacokinetic modifications and that *H. pylori* eradication was followed by a significant improvement of clinical disability and a prolonged "on-time" duration, whereas gastritis/duodenitis scores significantly decreased in line with an improved L-dopa pharmacokinetic: they therefore attributed the impaired L-dopa absorption to an active gastro-duodenitis induced by *H. pylori* infection [160, 161]. A similar pharmacokinetic effect was described by other investigators: L-dopa "onset" time was longer and the "on-time" duration was shorter in *H. pylori* infected respect to non-infected patients; *H. pylori* eradication improved the effects of L-dopa treatment [162]. In a systematic review, the authors proposed that a plausible mechanism of impaired drug absorption may consist in a decreased acid secretion in patients with *H. pylori* related chronic gastritis. They found that the absorption of orally administered L-dopa (as well as L-thyroxine and delavirdine) improved after successful *H. pylori* eradication therapy (an increase of 21%-54% for L-dopa in Parkinson's disease and of 150% for delavirdine in HIV-positive patients) [163].

Some investigators suggested a potential interaction of L-dopa with *H. pylori* adhesins, confirming the clinical alterations found in pharmacokinetics of L dopa given to by *H. pylori*-positive patients with PD. The evaluation of time- and concentration-dependent incubation experiments indicated a significant decrease in L-dopa concentrations when exposed to *H. pylori*. *H. pylori* organisms, pre-incubated with different L-dopa concentrations, showed a significantly reduced adhesion to gastric epithelial cells. These results demonstrate a direct interaction of L-dopa with the outer membrane proteins of *H. pylori* responsible for the adhesion to gastric epithelial cells. As a result of this interaction, the unbound L-dopa concentration in bacterial suspension was strongly reduced [164]. Lyte hypothesized that the direct utilization of L-dopa by *H. pylori* was targeted to maintain its ecological niche within the gastrointestinal tract; sequestration of L-dopa by *H. pylori* for its growth requirement would consequently decrease the amount of the drug available for the treatment of Parkinson's disease-related pathology [165]. A recent systematic review on the prevalence of *H. pylori* infection in PD patients and clinical and pharmacokinetic improvement after *H. pylori* eradication therapy, concluded that the prevalence of *H. pylori* infection in PD patients reported in collected studies ranged from 37% to 59%, which is similar to that observed in the general population [166]. There is currently lack of evidence on the effects of screening and treating the infection in patients with PD and there is therefore limited evidence to suggest that *H. pylori* eradication improves the absorption of levodopa and motor symptoms. Other researchers, in a population study, found that prescriptions of *H. pylori*-eradication drugs and proton pump inhibitors, five or more years prior to the diagnosis of PD, were associated with a 45% and 23% increase in PD risk, respectively [167]. Hospitalization and outpatient visits for gastritis and peptic ulcers, however, were not associated with PD. Consequently, they suggested that chronic *H. pylori* infections and/or gastritis may contribute to PD or that these PD-related pathologies may precede motor symptoms.

In summary, the reasons of biological plausibility that may account for the association between *H. pylori* infection and PD are:

- Autoimmunity and chronic inflammation.
- The presence of cholesterol glycosides that act as dopaminergic neurotoxin.
- Impaired absorption of L-dopa due to active gastro-duodenitis induced by the infection.
- Mucosal damage and reduced absorption of levodopa due to hypochlorhydria.
- Direct interaction of L-dopa with outer membrane proteins of bacterium.
- Direct utilization of L-dopa by *H. pylori* to increase growth and persistence in the stomach.

Alzheimer's Disease

Alzheimer's disease (AD) is a progressive neurodegenerative disease of the central nervous system, which mainly affects old people and is characterized by dementia. Recent data and experimental studies support the role of inflammation and chronic bacterial infections, including *H. pylori* infection, in the development of such disorder [168, 169]. *H. pylori* can potentially influence AD pathogenesis through different pro-apoptotic pathways, such as oxidative stress, overexpression of the nitrate system and molecular mimicry of host structures. The release of pro-inflammatory cytokines (TNF-α, and vascular endothelial growth factor [VEGF]) may modulate the vascular permeability and promote a blood-brain barrier injury. TNF-α, TNF-β, IFN-γ, IL-1 and IL-2 also promote nerve leukocyte and macrophages activation and direct myelotoxic effects [168]. Furthermore, *H. pylori* chronic gastritis induces vitamin B_{12} and folic acid malabsorption, resulting in a reduced 5-metil-tetraidrofolate methylation with consequent omocistein accumulation. Omocistein can trigger a mechanism of endothelium damage, resulting in a thrombophilic state and contributing to the AD development [169].

Another pathogenic mechanism that may contribute to AD development consists in platelet activation and aggregation. Platelets are the source of the major constituents of Abeta plaques, whose formation is considered the most important event in the etiology of AD. Abeta plaques may damage vessels and increase the permeability of blood-brain barrier. In addition, platelets aggregation and brain vasoconstriction could promote or predispose to thrombotic and ischemic events. Reactive oxygen species and circulating lipid peroxides could be also involved in plaque development [170].

Due the possible existence of cross-mimicry phenomena between endothelial cells and *H. pylori* antigens, we aligned some endothelial cell proteins with *H. pylori* epitopes and found numerous partial homologies. In Fig. **1** for instance, we reported the alignment between BMP-binding endothelial regulator protein and *H. pylori*, which shows an identity of 21% (with 39/97 positive amino acids and only one gaps) with a bacterial product, glutamate-1-semialdehyde aminotransferase, an enzyme that participates in porphyrin metabolism).

(taxid:85963).

```
Query 54 GEVLQIPFITDNPCIMCVCLNKEVTCKREKCPVLSRDCALAIKQRGACCERCKGCTHEGR 113
G V Q ++ NP +C L+ KR+K + +R ALA++ + +
Sbjct 290 GGVYQAGTLSGNPLAVCAGLSALYKIKRDKT-LYTRLNALAVRLTQGLQKSAQNYNIALE 348
Query 114 TYNSSFKWQTPAEPCVLRQCQEGVVTESEVRCVVHCK 150
T N + +R + + +++E+ H K
Sbjct 349 TLNMGSMFGFFFNENAVRDFDDALKSDTEMFAKFHQK
```

Figure 1: Alignment of BMP-binding endothelial regulator protein with glutamate-1-semialdehyde aminotransferase of *H. pylori* J99.

In conclusion, the bases of biological plausibility of such association are solid and also prevalence studies conclude in favour of an association: Kounturas *et al.* proved an increased prevalence of *H. pylori* infection in 30 patients with AD (88%), respect to controls (46.7%) ($P < 0.001$) [169]; in a recent study, a more severe dementia was observed in patients with *H. pylori* infection, which may support the existence of such an association [171].

Hepatic Encephalopathy

H. pylori infection is an important factor of increased blood ammonia concentration and hepatic encephalopathy (HE) in cirrhotic patients. HE is a frequent complication of liver cirrhosis. Ammonia retention in cirrhotics depends on an intricately balanced enzyme and transport systems, involving liver, large and small bowel, muscles and kidneys [172]. Although the pathogenesis is unclear, ammonia is certainly one of the key factors involved.

Several studies have confirmed a correlation between HE and *H. pylori* infection [173]. *H. pylori* infection can increase serum ammonia concentrations in patients with liver dysfunction [174]. Eradication of *H. pylori* in cirrhotic patients may prevent HE. Other researchers concluded that, although in their opinion the amount of ammonia produced by *H. pylori* is too small to contribute to hepatic encephalopathy, eradication of *H. pylori* might reduce the systemic levels of ammonia and improve HE [175]. Finally, a recent study reported a significant association between *H. pylori* infection and HE in patients with liver cirrhosis; the eradication treatment resulted in a reduction of the blood ammonia levels and an improvement of HE [176].

Although *H. pylori* produces ammonia in the stomach, several studies have shown that both the basal ammonia levels and HE prevalence did not significantly differ in cirrhotics, with or without infection. Moreover, some prospective studies have documented that both ammonia blood levels and mental status in cirrhotics with HE are not significantly affected by *H. pylori* eradication. Even if a small subgroup of cirrhotics with high bacterial density and severe hepatic impairment seems to benefit from bacterial eradication, some data indicate that ammonia production in the stomach by *H. pylori* urease appears to be inadequate to clinically affect ammonia levels in the majority of cirrhotic patients [172].

Several studies, however, did not demonstrate the existence of a correlation [177-181].

PERIPHERAL NERVOUS SYSTEM

Guillain-Barrè Syndrome

Guillain-Barrè syndrome (GBS) is a multifactorial disease, characterized by an acute demyelinating inflammatory polyradiculoneuropathy. GBS is the most common cause of spastic paralysis with areflexia. The causative role of infections and immune response in the development of GBS is supported by the observation that 60%-70% of the patients report a history of recent vaccination, or respiratory and gastro-enteric infections.

H. pylori infection could play an important role in GBS pathogenesis. An increased prevalence of *H. pylori* infection was observed in patients with GBS and elevated anti-*H. pylori* antibody titers were found in patients with advanced GBS [182, 183]. In one of our study, the frequency of anti-*H. pylori* serum IgG in GBS patients was similar to that found in a large cohort of sex- age- and social class-matched healthy Italian subjects (NF personal observation). To assess the influence of antibodies on the duration of hospitalization and clinical score at discharge, a survival analysis was performed and patients with anti-GM1 antibodies (the pathogenetic basis of such disorder consists in the development of anti-ganglioside GM1 antibodies) along with anti-*H. pylori*, -cytomegalovirus and -*Campylobacter jejuni* antibodies were analyzed. Patients with anti-GM1 and -*H. pylori* antibodies had significantly longer hospitalization to reach low clinical score at discharge than those with anti-GM1 antibodies alone (P= 0.004), which suggests that *H. pylori* infection may contribute to exacerbate the disease (NF personal observation).

In the late nineties, specific IgG antibodies to the VacA cytotoxin were detected in cerebrospinal fluid of 13 patients with GBS, who, in addition, showed a significant demyelination of peripheral nerves [184]. These data suggest the existence of an antigenic mimicry mechanism at the basis of such association: the targets of cross-reacting antibodies are probably the surface components of gangliosides of peripheral nerves or the Schwann abaxonal cells. However, the exact target of anti-VacA antibodies is still unknown [183, 184]. The molecular mimicry is not the only way through which *H. pylori* can contribute to the pathogenesis of GBS. The release of inflammatory mediators (TNF-α, IFN-γ, VEGF) may induce leucocyte transmigration, macrophages proliferation and activation and mast cells degranulation, with direct nerve damage and blood-brain barrier impairment [184].

REUMATOLOGIC DISEASES

Systemic Sclerosis

Systemic sclerosis (SSc) is a chronic and progressive autoimmune disorder, characterized by loss of epidermic elasticity. SSc could appear as a localized form - defined by single or multiple plaques of skin hardening (*morphea*) or linear lesions - or as a systemic form that goes along with C.R.E.S.T. syndrome (**C**alcinosis, **R**aynaud, **E**sophageal motility disorders, **S**clerodactyly and **T**elangiectasia), limited or diffuse skin thickening and overlap syndromes.

It was observed that infections could be implicated in SSc. Radic *et al.* studied the possible influence of various infective agents in SSc, in particular parvovirus B19, cytomegalovirus and *H. pylori* [185]. The pathogenetic pathway behind the possible association between *H. pylori* and SSc is an autoimmune response. An improvement of SSc symptoms after antibiotic therapy was achieved in some studies [186]. Certain researchers have observed a high prevalence of *H. pylori* infection in patients with SSc [187]. Others investigated the frequency of *H. pylori* infection in 12 patients with SSc by ^{13}C-urea breath test and found a positive result in five patients (41.6%) [188]. In a larger survey, 124 patients were examined serologically and 55.6% of them were infected: a positive correlation between infection and esophageal hypomotility was also found [189]. In another study, 23 SSc patients, out of 35 patients (65.7%) examined by serum antibody detection and urease breath test, were infected [190]. Furthermore, it was observed an improvement of SSc-associated Raynaud's phenomenon after *H. pylori* eradication [191, 192].

Many pathogenetic hypotheses can be postulated to explain the correlation between *H. pylori* and SSc development. *H. pylori* infection stimulates the release of pro-inflammatory products, leading to the development of antigen-antibody complexes and the production of cross-reacting antibodies. Molecular mimicry could be an important step in the endothelial damage (which is the first manifestation of SSc), the associated microangiopathy and Raynaud's phenomenon. Underlining the importance of autoimmunity, some researchers detected a high prevalence of *H. pylori* infection in SSc patients (78%) and showed the production of antibodies against a 60-kDa protein belonging to the family of heat-shock proteins (in particular, human hsp60 and mycobacterial hsp65) in those who were infected [193]. It is also possible, however, that the high prevalence of *H. pylori* infection in these patients could be promoted by the upper gastro-intestinal motility disorders existing in SSc [194].

Sjögren's Syndrome

Sjögren's syndrome (SS), also known as "sicca syndrome", is an autoimmune disorder characterized by xerostomia and keratoconjunctivitis sicca, associated with other organ dysfunctions, such kidneys, lungs, liver, pancreas, blood vessels, stomach and peripheral nervous system. Our group first hypothesized an association of SS with *H. pylori* infection [195]: the treatment of three infected patients with eradication therapy was followed by a decrease in the severity of the symptoms and an improvement of the Shirmer's test results in all patients [195]. A significantly increased prevalence of *H. pylori* infection was thereafter found in Sjögren's patients [196, 197]; however, the *H. pylori* positive status had no influence on the serum levels of autoantibody [197]. Other investigators underlined the high prevalence of *H. pylori* infection in patients with primary SS

(80.6%) respect to patients with secondary SS and patients with various connective diseases not suffering from sicca syndrome: 71% and 60.9 %, respectively. In addition, serum antibodies titers to *H. pylori* were correlated with other clinical indexes, like age, disease duration and C-reactive protein levels. The authors conclude recommending an *H. pylori* evaluation in older patients, in particular those with a long history of SS (more than 3 years) [198]. As far as the role of the infection in the pathogenesis of SS is concerned, in late nineties, a probable role of the bacterial hsp60 was supposed, since infected SS patients also had anti-hsp60 antibodies [199].

Finally, in an Italian study, the authors focused on the role of *H. pylori* infection in SS-associated gastritis: the prevalence in the case group and controls was similar and the lymphocytic infiltration and atrophy of gastric mucosa persisting after eradication of infection was considered as the expression of an endogenous, even though unknown, condition [200].

Behçet Disease

Behçet disease (BD), first described by Hulusi Behçet in 1937, is a multisystemic, chronic, relapsing vasculitis of unknown origin that affects nearly all organs and systems. The involvement of the gastrointestinal system is called entero-Behçet disease. The most frequent extraoral sites of gastrointestinal involvement are the ileocecal tract and colon. Compared with the other parts of the digestive system, the gastric mucosa is involved less frequently. Endoscopic findings consist of aphthous ulcers, esophagitis, fistulae and stricture in esophagus, aphthous ulcers and erosions in the stomach, aphthous ulcers, erosions and bulbitis in the duodenum. The most frequent gastric lesions of BD are aphthous ulcers. Symptoms consist of abdominal colicky pain, nausea, vomiting, diarrhea, with or without blood in stools, and constipation. The hepatic complication known as Budd-Chiari syndrome is relatively common [201].

More than one mechanism seems to be operative in the pathogenesis of BD, including genetic and environmental factors, such as infections, causing different manifestations of the syndrome. Basic researches on both viruses and bacteria suggest that microorganisms could play a role, possibly through heat-shock proteins and T-cell hypersensitivity.

The role of microorganisms, including *H. pylori*, in the pathogenesis of BD has long been investigated; however, none of these infectious agents have been proved to cause BD. Also *H. pylori* infection has been involved in the pathogenesis of the disease. Although there is no information supporting the role of a single microorganism as the specific cause, a problem with disregulation in innate immunity, with an altered response to more than one infectious agent, is a generally accepted theory. An infectious agent could operate through molecular mimicry. This mimicked interaction or false signaling could attract the inflammatory cells into the field of action, and this may in turn result in vasculitis. Subsequently, the disease could be perpetuated by an abnormal immune response to an autoantigen in the absence of ongoing infection.

Some researchers reported that endoscopic findings, eradication rates and prevalence of *H. pylori* infection were similar in patients with BD and control group [201]. Subsequently, it was reported a case of an *H. pylori* infected young woman with recurrent aphtous ulcers (RAU) and dyspeptic symptoms. After eradication treatment, her dyspeptic symptoms decreased, but new oral aphtous ulcers developed; the frequency of RAU diminished proportionally in the first two weeks of the follow up period. After a few weeks, however, RAU relapsed. According to other investigators, there could be a potential relationship between RAU and *H. pylori* infection eradication therapy for *H. pylori*. After the eradication treatment, the periods between recurrences of RAS in patients recovered from infection were significantly longer compared with those before treatment. Another important observation was that the clinical status of patients who became negative after eradication therapy was comparable with that of patients who were *H. pylori* negative from the beginning of the study [202]. These findings were confirmed by other researchers who concluded that the anti-*H. pylori* antibiotic therapy in patients with BD can reduce the development of new oral aphthous ulcers and the frequency of recurrent attacks for a limited period of time [203].

REPRODUCTIVE DISORDERS

Male and Female Reduced Fertility

Reproductive disorders are a very interesting topic to study because, in many cases, the causes of infertility are unclear. During the last decade more and more clues have been acquired on the possible negative influence of *H. pylori* infection on the reproductive sphere.

Our group first found that the infection is significantly more common in both men and women with reproductive problems; in addition, infected individuals have specific antibodies in semen, follicular fluid and vaginal secretions, which cross react *in vitro* with sperm, suggesting the existence of autoimmune phenomena. A partial linear homology was observed between human tubulin, the main constituent of sperm flagellum, and some *H. pylori* proteins (flagellin, CagA and VacA). We therefore concluded that such an antigenic mimicry may stimulate cross-reactive antibodies [204]. At this purpose, an immune reaction was observed between anti-*H. pylori* antibodies and the centriolar region and flagellum (structures rich in tubulin) of human sperm.

Furthermore, *H. pylori* was proposed as a risk factor for alterations of sperm quality in a group of idiopathic infertile men; infected men, especially those with serum antibodies to CagA, showed increased systemic levels of TNF-α - a proinflammatory cytokine that may cause sperm damage - reduced sperm motility *in vitro* and a greater number of necrotic and apoptotic sperm in their ejaculates [205]. The effects of this infection on the reproductive sphere is not limited to sperm alterations; we found in fact that the infection may influence the semen concentration of some hormones as demonstrated for ghrelin, an hormone endowed with anti-inflammatory properties and involved in reproduction [206].

As far as the female reproductive sphere is concerned, in a retrospective study including 204 patients with idiopathic infertility tested for anti- *H. pylori* antibodies, Kurotsuchi *et al.* reported that the infection was twice as much more frequent in women in whom no known cause of infertility was found, compared to women with recognized determinants of reduced fertility; thus, they concluded that *H. pylori* infection may increase the risk of infertility [207]. Soon after, some investigators described the existence of an association between polycystic ovary syndrome (PCOS), one of the most common endocrinopathies causing infertility, and *H. pylori* seropositivity (PCOS 40%; *vs.* 20% of controls, $P= 0.007$) [208]. Recently, anti-*H. pylori* antibodies have been detected in the cervical mucus of *H. pylori* infected women with unexplained infertility [209] and such antibodies interfered *in vitro* with sperm progression. The most recent paper on this topic suggests that women infected by CagA-positive *H. pylori* strains have an increased risk of early pregnancy loss after intracytoplasmic sperm injection [210], probably owing to an increased release of inflammatory cytokines. Even mice infected by *H. pylori* showed an increased number of embryo resorptions and lower fetal weights compared to non-infected controls [211]. The proposed mechanism of action is interesting: under particular physiopathological conditions of active tissue and vascular formation, such as pregnancy, the local Th1 response, induced by *H. pylori* infection, could alter the systemic Th1/Th2 cytokine balance [211].

There are therefore indications that *H. pylori* infection should be listed among the putative causes of reduced fertility in males and females and could decrease the probability of pregnancy.

A question arises as to whether it is possible that, in developing countries, where practically everyone is infected, the birth rate is progressively increasing.

In European and American countries, *H. pylori* causes a predominant and prolonged Th1-type response, which is unable to eliminate the organism, damages the gastric mucosa and increases the systemic inflammatory status. As an additional possible consequence, high levels of proinflammatory cytokines in the blood stream may injure extra-digestive organs, including the reproductive apparatus [212, 213]. In developing countries, the endemic helminthiasis and other parasitic infestation change the Th-cell immune response from a predominantly Th1-type to a Th2-type, which is considered protective and is characterized by the release of the non-inflammatory cytokines IL-4, IL-5, IL-6 and IL-10 [214]. The results of a study performed in Colombian children, for instance, suggest that intestinal helminthiasis promotes Th2-polarizing responses to *H. pylori* and reduces the mucosal damage caused by the inflammation; the decreased inflammatory status is reputed to prevent the progression of gastritis to gastric atrophy, dysplasia, and cancer [215]. Studies performed in animals, experimentally infected by *H. pylori* and parasites, have confirmed the observations made in humans; in particular the production of anti-inflammatory cytokines triggered by parasitic infestation could protect the gastric mucosa [216,

217]. The protection may have systemic effects: the release of anti-inflammatory cytokines due to the Th2 response may counteract the adverse effects of inflammation and possibly spare the involvement of extra-digestive organs and fluids, such as the ejaculate.

Are these enough clues to propose that individuals with reproductive disorders have to be routinely examined for *H. pylori* infection and anti-CagA serum antibodies?

MISCELLANEA

Sudden Infant Death Syndrome

Sudden infant death syndrome (SIDS) is marked by the sudden death of an infant that cannot be explained after a complete case investigation, including a scene examination, forensic autopsy and review of the clinical history. Sudden unexpected infant death (SUID) is a term used to describe any sudden and unexpected death, whether explained or unexplained (including SIDS), that occurs during infancy. After case investigation, SUIDs can be attributed to suffocation, asphyxia, entrapment, infections, ingestions, metabolic diseases, arrhythmia-associated cardiac channelopathies, and traumas (accidental or non-accidental) [218].

In the past, it was proposed a link between *H. pylori* infection and SIDS. Pattison and Marshall, in 1997, proposed for the first time this association. They proposed that, once *H. pylori* has infected the newborn and microaspiration of vomiting and gastroesophageal reflux have reached the alveoli, the hydrolysis of plasma urea would produce ammonia, which would cause respiratory arrest because it is toxic. In addition, gastric inflammation caused by *H. pylori* increases IL-1 cytokine synthesis with production of fever, activation of the immune system and deep sleep [219]. Other investigators examined gastric, tracheal, and pulmonary tissue looking for evidence of *H. pylori* in SIDS victims and control, reporting a highly significant association between *H. pylori ureC* and *cagA* genes in the stomach, trachea, and lung in cases of SIDS when compared to controls [220].

Other authors found elevated IL-6 levels in cerebrospinal fluid, that represent signs of central immune stimulation, in *H. pylori* seropositive SIDS victims compared with seronegative victims ($P = 0.045$). The detection of *H. pylori* antigen in stool is associated with SIDS and deaths due to infections. They concluded that *H. pylori* infection may be involved in SIDS, during the first five months after birth, as a trigger pathogen [221].

Conversely, recent studies do not related *H. pylori* infection with SIDS. In 2000, 25 pairs of gastric and tracheal tissue specimens obtained from autopsies of 25 children with previous diagnoses of SIDS, were analyzed for *H. pylori* DNA by nested PCR. Six different tissue specimens (four samples from the stomach and two from trachea) were positive, but in no case *H. pylori* DNA was detected in both tissues. This study concluded that *H. pylori* infection is most likely not associated with SIDS. There are other surveys that deny a role of *H. pylori* infection in the development of SIDS [222].

Hyperemesis Gravidarium

Hyperemesis gravidarium (HG) is a condition characterized by frequent and intense episodes of vomit and nausea during pregnancy. *H. pylori* infection was considered an aggravating factor in several studies. Two systematic reviews concluded that studies performed until 2007 were unconvincing because they did not support any evidence, the number of patients was very little and results were considerably heterogeneous [223, 224]. In a Greek study, no connection between *H. pylori* infection and HG was observed [225]. The authors, using a multi-variable questionnaire and serum IgG tests for *H. pylori* status, did not support a direct correlation with number of vomit episodes per day, age and history of gastrointestinal symptoms, but there was a link only with the number of deliveries (65% of *H. pylori* infection prevalence in multigravida) [225].

The prevalence of *H. pylori* infection in 105 cases of HG and 58 controls was recently investigated and an association was found, especially in African women. The conclusion was that this infection is a potential risk factor of HG [226]. Then, the same group presented a systematic review and a meta-analysis of case-control studies, underlining once more that the exposure to *H. pylori* is associated with an increased risk of HG; nonetheless, heterogeneity between different studies subsisted [227]. More recently, the role of *H. pylori* in HG was evaluated in 80 patients and it was observed that the employment of a non-teratogenic treatment of infection in positive subjects reduced the frequency of vomiting and the severity of HG symptoms, suggesting that this treatment can be advisable in intractable cases [228].

Halitosis

About 90% of halitosis cases originate within the oral cavity. Bacterial formation of the odorous volatile sulfur compounds (VSCs) hydrogen sulfide (H_2S) and methyl mercaptan (MM, CH3SH) within the oral cavity, especially in the tongue coating, is the main cause of oral malodour. An estimated 5%–10% has non-oral causes and the smell is mostly due to the presence of dimethyl sulfide produced in the intestine; then, the gas dissolves in the blood stream and is therefore exhaled in the environment [229].

Several studies have detected *H. pylori* in the oral cavity, particularly in patients with gingivitis and chronic periodontitis, concluding that the oral cavity may act as a reservoir for transmission of *H. pylori* [119, 230]. In the past some authors demonstrated that *H. pylori* was able to produce the VSCs H_2S and MM, suggesting that *H. pylori* can contribute to the development of halitosis. Several reports have examined this relationship, but results are controversial. The problem of these studies is that the authors use the method of self-reported subjective halitosis, which is unreliable.

In a recent research [229], the possible correlation between *H. pylori* infection and halitosis has been evaluated using an objective method like gas chromatography to detect VSCs, responsible for halitosis. The result was that halitosis nearly always originates within the oral cavity, very rarely within the stomach. In addition, no statistical difference was obtained between measurements performed in infected and uninfected individuals [229].

Growth Delay

H. pylori infection is a common problem in pediatric practice. *H. pylori* is generally acquired early in life and socioeconomic conditions are considered as the most important risk factors for acquisition of the infection.

Like other chronic diseases, *H. pylori* infection might impair growth. Three studies have already shown a difference in height between infected and non-infected children. The first study, in which *H. pylori* infection was detected mostly in poor children in developing world, revealed that short stature was related to a low nutrient intake rather than to *H. pylori* infection itself [231]. A subsequent study from Europe showed that over half of children investigated for short stature were infected with *H. pylori* [232, 233]. However, no controls were considered. A Scottish study found that *H. pylori* infection was associated with growth delay only in girls around puberty [234, 235]. Common to all these studies, however, is a lack of information about the socioeconomic conditions which may affect height, as shown by the positive correlation between increasing height observed over the past centuries and improved living conditions in industrially developed societies. The exact mechanism of this association has not been completely elucidated, but the gradual disappearance of chronic infections is a plausible explanation. A large cross-sectional population-based study (3315 children, five to seven year old) [236] concluded that *H. pylori* infection is associated with growth delay, growth retardation, or both in affected children.

Finally, a recent and interesting study [237] demonstrated that children who were always negative, or who had cleared the infection, grew significantly faster than those who remained positive after adjusting for other covariates. This study suggests that the growth of school-age children benefits from being treated for *H. pylori* infection.

The effect of *H. pylori* infection on growth retard seems to be more evident in older children with a long lasting infection than in younger children with a recently acquired infection, because, once acquired in early childhood, *H. pylori* infection takes several years before starting to affect growth. The mechanisms through which *H. pylori* infection might lead to short stature are largely unknown. The hypothesis are:

1) The infection could cause dyspeptic symptoms;

2) The infection could result in a low energy intake and malnutrition;

3) long standing infections induce low grade chronic gastric inflammation and the release of cytokines, which in turn would affect growth [238, 239];

4) *H. pylori* infection may be associated with a poor socioeconomic background, malnutrition, and exposure to other chronic diseases which could independently affect growth. In childhood itself, *H. pylori* is known to cause gastritis, and may cause recurrent abdominal pain [63].

In any case, most studies agree on the fact that infected children have weight loss and short stature [232-235, 240].

The hypotheses that *H. pylori* infection acquired in childhood is associated with short stature and poor socioeconomic conditions have at least two implications. First, *H. pylori* infection could be one of the environmental causes of growth delay. The decline in the incidence of *H. pylori* infection related to general improvements of socioeconomic conditions could be responsible, at least in part, for the trend toward increased height growth observed during the last century in developed countries. Second, therapeutic intervention against *H. pylori* infection in children could be recommended not only to prevent ulcer disease or gastric cancer but also to avoid interference with growth [241].

IgA Nephropathy

IgA nephropathy (IgAN) is the most common form of idiopathic glomerulonephritis leading to chronic kidney disease in developed country. Regarding the pathogenesis, current data implicate an important genetic factor, especially in promoting the overproduction of an aberrant form of IgA1. The first step of immunochemical aberrancy of IgAN is characterized by the undergalactosylation of glycans in the hinge region of IgA1. The next stage of renal injury development requires the formation of glycan-specific IgG and IgA antibodies that recognize the undergalactosylated IgA1 molecule. These antibodies often react with antigens of extrinsic microorganisms and might be produced for recurrent mucosal infections.

H. pylori has been reported to be present in coccoid forms in the palatine tonsillar crypts of IgAN patients. In a recent study that involved 55 patients, 43 patients (78.2%) had tonsillar *H. pylori*, and 15 patients (27.3%) were infected by *H. pylori* in the gastroduodenal tract. All patients with gastric *H. pylori* also had these bacteria in their tonsils ($p < 0.01$). CagA was observed in 38 (88.4%) of 43 patients with tonsillar *H. pylori*. Tonsillar *H. pylori* could not be cultured in any conditions. All patients with IgA nephropathy had tonsillar *H. pylori* ($p < 0.01$) [137]. This may indicate that tonsillar *H. pylori* is one of the antigens causative of IgAN.

Even if the indication of tonsillectomy in IgAN is controversial, tonsillectomy is associated with a favorable renal outcome of the disease in terms of clinical remission and delayed renal deterioration, even in non-steroid-treated patients. Such observation is a strong point in favour of a role of this bacterium in the development of IgAN.

CONCLUSIONS

Some investigators are skeptical that *H. pylori* infection could contribute to the development of extradigestive diseases. These bacteria colonize the stomach, an organ large 800 cm^2 *ca.*, in most cases since the first years of life. Through the activity of vacuolating toxin, mucinase and other enzymes, such bacterial species demolishes the mucus layer and wrecks the epithelium. Bacterial components and products attract and activate immunocytes infiltrating the gastric mucosa and circulating in the blood stream. Immunocytes, vasoactive substances and cellular mediators, such as cytokines, which are washed away from the stomach by the blood stream, can be transported in any district of the human body and promote or worsen inflammatory responses in organs distant from the digestive tracts. Those organs and apparatus already compromised by other concomitant inflammatory diseases could be the most affected sites. In such a way, *H. pylori*-triggered inflammation could also bring out sub-clinical disorders of other systems, which therefore become manifest. These events take place every day, starting from the infancy, and last for the entire patients' life. For all such considerations, it is plausible that this infection may have systemic effects.

H. pylori infection is *per se* a condition in which autoimmunity is exalted; in addition, many helicobacter antigens possess structural homologies with different human tissue cells. It is therefore reasonable that certain extradigestive disorders associated with *H. pylori* infection are based on phenomena of cross mimicry. As far as the majority of the above-reported disorders is concerned, most studies have been given conflicting results; less frequently, sporadic studies have demonstrated a significant association. The lack of consistent results makes it hard to assert that *H. pylori* is definitely associated with any of these disorders, although two conditions—iron deficiency anaemia and idiopathic thrombocytopenic purpura — have the highest claim.

The list of disorders linked to *H. pylori* infection grows every day. For instance, while the present manuscript was in preparation, a possible connection between autoimmune bullous disease and *H. pylori* infection has been hypothesized (Sagi L *et al.* Autoimmun Rev 2011;10:527-35). Furthermore, the pathogenetic mechanisms of extradigestive *H. pylori*-associated diseases become clearer every day. For example some researchers, studying (with the aid of an experimental animal model) the mechanisms of brain damage putatively induced by *H. pylori* infection in patients with Alzheimer's disease, found that *H. pylori* directly induces tau hyperphosphorylation (tau is an important component of neuronal cytoskeleton; the protein stabilizes microtubules, maintains cell shape and axonal transport mechanisms) and cognitive impairment, likely through the release of toxins that could be sensed by the neuron (Wang X. Alzheimer's & Dementia 2012;8 Supplement:468-9).

To conclude, it is not unreasonable to conjecture that the reduced incidence of such infection - with its negative repercussions upon different organs and systems - may contribute to prolongation of life expectancy in the Western world.

ACKNOWLEDGEMENT

None Declared.

CONFLICT OF INTEREST

The author(s) confirm that this chapter content has no conflict of interest.

REFERENCES

[1] Osler W. Diseases of the arteries. In: Osler W, McCrae T (eds). Modern Medicine: Its Theory and Practice in Original Contributions by Americans and Foreign Authors (vol. 4). Lea & Febiger, 1908, Philadelphia, PA, USA:pp 426–47.

[2] Cammarota G, Pasceri V, Gasbarrini A *et al. H. pylori* is an etiological factor for ischaemic heart disease: the case against. Dig Liver Dis 2000;32:65–8.

[3] Gasbarrini G, Pretolani S, Bonvicini F *et al.* Population based study of *Helicobacter pylori* infection in a European country: the San Marino Study. Relations with gastrointestinal diseases. Gut 1995;36:838–44.

[4] Yamaoka Y, Graham D Y. CagA status and gastric cancer unreliable serological tests produce unreliable data. Gastroenterology 1999;117:745

[5] Franceschi F, Leo D, Fini L, *et al. Helicobacter pylori* infection and ischaemic heart disease: an overview of the general literature. Dig Liver Dis 2005;37:301-8.

[6] Gennari L, Figura N, Merlotti D *et al. Helicobacter pylori* CagA-positive strains negatively affect bone health: a population based study. J Bone Miner Res 2010;25 (Suppl.1):MO0365.

[7] C Lenzi, A Palazzuoli, N Giordano *et al. Helicobacter pylori* infection and systemic antibodies to CagA and heat-shock protein 60 in patients with coronary heart disease and controls. World J Gastroenterol 2006;12:7815-20.

[8] Manolakis A, Kapsoritakis AN, Potamianos SP. A review of the postulated mechanisms concerning the association of *Helicobacter pylori* with ischemic heart disease. *Helicobacter* 2007;12:287-97.

[9] Fagoonee S, De Angelis C, Elia C, *et al.* Potential link between *Helicobacter pylori* and ischemic heart disease: does the bacterium elicit thrombosis? Minerva Med 2010;101:121–5.

[10] Censini S, Lange C, Xiang Z *et al. cag*, a pathogenicity island of *Helicobacter pylori*, encodes type I-specific and disease-associated virulence factors. Proc Natl Acad Sci U S A 1996;93:14648-53.

[11] Figura N, Palazzuoli A, Faglia S *et al.* Infection by CagA-positive *Helicobacter pylori* strains in patients with ischaemic heart disease: prevalence and association with exercise-induced electrocardiographic abnormalities. Dig Dis Sci 2002,47.831-6.

[12] Ojetti V, Pitocco D *et al.* Efficacy of different *Helicobacter pylori* eradication regimens in patients affected by insulin-dependent diabetes mellitus. Scand J Gastroenterol 2000;35:260-3

[13] Zimmermann MB, Hurrell RF. Nutritional iron deficiency. Lancet 2007;370:511-20

[14] Altschuler EL. Association of *Helicobacter pylori* infection and Parkinson's disease already proposed. Acta Neurol Scand 1999;100:122.

[15] Schöttker B, Adamu MA, Weck MN *et al. Helicobacter pylori* infection, chronic atrophic gastritis and major cardiovascular events: a population-based cohort study. Atherosclerosis 2012;220:569-74.

[16] Eeskandarian R, Ghorbani R, Shiyasi M *et al.* Prognostic role of *Helicobacter pylori* infection in acute coronary syndrome: a prospective cohort study. Cardiovasc J Afr 2012;23:131-5.

[17] Blasi F, Denti F, Erba M, *et al.* Detection of *Chlamydia pneumoniae* but not *Helicobacter pylori* in atherosclerotic plaques of aortic aneurysms. J Clin Microbiol 1996;34:2766-9.

[18] Falkensammer B, Duftner C, Seiler R, *et al.* Innsbruck Abdominal Aortic Aneurysm Trial-Group. Lack of microbial DNA in tissue specimens of patients with abdominal aortic aneurysms and positive *Chlamydiales* serology. Eur J Clin Microbiol Infect Dis 2007;26:141-5.

[19] Koullias GJ, Korkolis DP, Hatzaras IS *et al.* Immunohistochemical testing for *Helicobacter pylori* infection in ascending aortic aneurysms and penetrating aortic ulcers. Am J Cardiol 2004;93:122-3.

[20] Mannacio VA, De Amicis V, Di Tommaso L *et al.* The association of acute aortic dissection with *Helicobacter pylori* virulence specific serotypes: Distinct diversity of systemic antibodies to CagA and VacA genotypes. Surgery 2011;149:240-6.

[21] Zullo A, Hassan C, Morini S. Hepatic encephalopathy and *Helicobacter pylori*: a critical reappraisal. J Clin Gastroenterol 2003;37:164-8.

[22] Montenero AS, Mollichelli N, Zumbo F *et al. Helicobacter pylori* and atrial fibrillation: a possible pathogenic link. Heart 2005;91:960-1.

[23] Badran HM, Mahfouz ME. Cytotoxin-associated gene-A bearing strains of *Helicobacter pylori* and atrial fibrillation due to ischemic origin: is there a link? Eur J Cardiovasc Prev Rehabil 2007;14:518-20.

[24] Bunch TJ, Day JD, Anderson JL *et al.* Frequency of *Helicobacter pylori* seropositivity and C-reactive protein increase in atrial fibrillation in patients undergoing coronary angiography. Am J Cardiol 2008;101:848-51.

[25] Ki MR, Shin DG, Park JS *et al.* Frequency of vacuolating cytotoxin A (VacA)-positive *Helicobacter pylori* seropositivity and TGF-ß1 decrease in atrial fibrillation. Int J Cardiol 2010;145:345-6.

[26] Platonov P, Ekesbo R, Hansson A *et al.* Permanent atrial fibrillation in patients without structural heart disease is not associated with signs of infection by *Chlamydia pneumoniae* and *Helicobacter pylori.* Acta Cardiol 2008;63:479-84.

[27] Gasbarrini A, De Luca A, Fiore G *et al.* Beneficial effects of *Helicobacter pylori* eradication on migraine. Hepatogastroenterology 1998;45:765-70.

[28] Gasbarrini A, Gabrielli M, Fiore G *et al.* Association between *Helicobacter pylori* cytotoxic type I CagA-positive strains and migraine with aura. Cephalalgia 2000;20:561-5.

[29] Bodger K, Crabtree JE. *Helicobacter pylori* and gastric inflammation. Br Med Bull 1998;54:139-50.

[30] Tunca A, Ardiçoglu Y, Kargili A *et al.* Migraine, *Helicobacter pylori,* and oxidative stress. *Helicobacter* 2007;12:59-62.

[31] Tunca A, Türkay C, Tekin O *et al.* Is *Helicobacter pylori* infection a risk factor for migraine? A case-control study. Acta Neurol Belg 2004;104:161-4.

[32] Yilmaz MD, Aktepe O, Cetinkol Y *et al.* Does *Helicobacter pylori* have role in development of otitis media with effusion? Int J Pediatr Otorhinolaryngol 2005;69:745-9.

[33] Hosseinzadeh M, Khosravi A, Saki K *et al.* Evaluation of *Helicobacter pylori* infection in patients with common migraine headache. Arch Med Sci 2011;7:844-9.

[34] Pinessi L, Savi L, Pellicano R *et al.* Chronic *Helicobacter pylori* infection and migraine: a case-control study. Headache 2000;40:836-9.

[35] Ciancarelli I, Di Massimo C, Tozzi-Ciancarelli MG *et al. Helicobacter pylori* infection and migraine. Cephalalgia 2002;22:222-5.

[36] Gasbarrini A, Serricchio M, Tondi P *et al.* Raynaud's phenomenon and *Helicobacter pylori* infection. Int J Angiol 1998;7:307-9.

[37] Hervé F, Cailleux N, Benhamou Y *et al.* *Helicobacter pylori* prevalence in Raynaud's disease. Rev Med Interne 2006;27:736-41.

[38] Strang R R. The association of gastro-duodenal ulceration and Parkinson's disease. Med J Austr 1965, 52: 842-3

[39] Gasbarrini A, Serricchio M, Tondi P *et al.* Association of *Helicobacter pylori* infection with primary Raynaud phenomenon. Lancet 1996;348:966-7.

[40] Figura N, Guarino E, Gragnoli A *et al.* *H. pylori* (HP) infection and thyroid diseases. Gut 1996;39 suppl 2:A93.

[41] de Luis DA, Varela C, de La Calle H. *Helicobacter pylori* infection is markedly increased in patients with autoimmune atrophic thyroiditis. J Clin Gastroenterol 1998;26:259-63.

[42] Ko GH, Park HB, Shin MK *et al.* Monoclonal antibodies against *Helicobacter pylori* cross-react with human tissue. *Helicobacter* 1997;2:210-5.

[43] Tomb J-F, White O, Kerlavage AR *et al.* The complete genome sequence of the gastric pathogen *Helicobacter pylori.* Nature 1997;388: 539-47

[44] Figura N, Di Cairano G, Lorè F *et al.* The infection by *Helicobacter pylori* strains expressing CagA is highly prevalent in women with autoimmune thyroid disorders. J Physiol Pharmacol 1999;50:817-26.

[45] Bertalot G, Montresor G, Tampieri M *et al.* Decrease in thyroid autoantibodies after eradication of *Helicobacter pylori* infection. Clin Endocrinol (Oxf) 2004;61:650-2.

[46] Negrini R, Savio A, Appelmelk BJ. Autoantibodies to gastric mucosa in *Helicobacter pylori* infection. *Helicobacter* 1997;2 Suppl 1:S13-6.

[47] Negrini R, Savio A, Poiesi C *et al.* Antigenic mimicry between *Helicobacter pylori* and gastric mucosa in the pathogenesis of body atrophic gastritis. Gastroenterology 1996;111:655–65.

[48] Gonzalez-Campora R, Garcia-Santana JA, Jorda' i Heras MM *et al.* Blood group antigens in differentiated thyroid neoplasms. Arch Pathol Lab Med 1998;12:957– 65.

[49] Larizza D, Calcaterra V, Martinetti M *et al.* *Helicobacter pylori* infection and autoimmune thyroid disease in young patients: the disadvantage of carrying the human leukocyte antigen-DRB1*0301 allele. J Clin Endocrinol Metab 2006;91:176-9.

[50] Bassi V, Marino G, Iengo A *et al.* Autoimmune thyroid diseases and *Helicobacter pylori*: The correlation is present only in Graves's disease. World J Gastroenterol 2012;18:1093-7.

[51] Bassi V, Santinelli C, Iengo A *et al.* Identification of a correlation between *Helicobacter pylori* infection and Graves' disease. *Helicobacter* 2010;15:558-62.

[52] El-Eshmawy MM, El-Hawary AK, Abdel Gawad SS *et al.* *Helicobacter pylori* infection might be responsible for the interconnection between type 1 diabetes and autoimmune thyroiditis. Diabetol Metab Syndr 2011;3:28.

[53] Soveid M, Hosseini Asl K, Omrani GR. Infection by CagA-positive strains of *Helicobacter pylori* is associated with autoimmune thyroid disease in Iranian patients. Iran J Immunol 2012;9:48-52.

[54] Franceschi F, Satta MA, Mentella MC *et al.* *Helicobacter pylori* infection in patients with Hashimoto's thyroiditis. *Helicobacter* 2004;9:369.

[55] Tomasi PA, Dore MP, Fanciulli G *et al.* Is there anything to the reported association between *Helicobacter pylori* infection and autoimmune thyroiditis? Dig Dis Sci 2005;50:385-8

[56] Papamichael KX, Papaioannou G, Karga H *et al.* *Helicobacter pylori* infection and endocrine disorders: is there a link? World J Gastroenterol 2009;15:2701-7.

[57] Gasbarrini A, Ojetti V, Pitocco D, *et al. Helicobacter pylori* infection in patients affected by insulin-dependent diabetes mellitus. Eur J Gastroenterol Hepatol 1998;10:469-72.

[58] Gasbarrini A, Ojetti V, Pitocco D *et al.* Efficacy of different *Helicobacter pylori* eradication regimens in patients affected by insulin-dependent diabetes mellitus. Scand J Gastroenterol 2000;35:260-3.

[59] Ojetti V, Pitocco D, Bartolozzi F *et al.* High rate of *Helicobacter pylori* re-infection in patients affected by type 1 diabetes. Diabetes Care 2002;25:1485.

[60] Ojetti V, Pitocco D, Ghirlanda G *et al.* Role of *Helicobacter pylori* infection in insulin-dependent diabetes mellitus. Minerva Med 2001;92:137-44.

[61] Sargyn M, Uygur-Bayramicli O, Sargyn H *et al.* Type 2 diabetes mellitus affects eradication rate of *Helicobacter pylori*. World J Gastroenterol 2003 May;9(5):1126-8.

[62] Ojetti V, Pellicano R, Fagoonee S *et al. Helicobacter pylori* infection and diabetes. Minerva Med 2010;101:115-9.

[63] Sullivan PB. *Helicobacter pylori* infection in children. Baillieres Clin Gastroenterol. 1995;9:519-28.

[64] Ciortescu I, Sfarti C, Stan M *et al.* Prevalence of *Helicobacter pylori* infection in patients with diabetes mellitus. Rev Med Chir Soc Med Nat Iasi 2009;113:1048–55.

[65] Krause I, Anaya JM, Fraser A *et al.* Anti-infectious antibodies and autoimmune-associated autoantibodies in patients with type I diabetes mellitus and their close family members. Ann N Y Acad Sci 2009;1173:633–9.

[66] Lutsey PL, Pankow JS, Bertoni AG *et al.* Serological evidence of infections and Type 2 diabetes: the Multi- Ethnic Study of Atherosclerosis. Diabet Med 2009;26:149–52.

[67] Oluyemi A, Anomneze E, Smith S *et al.* Prevalence of a marker of active *Helicobacter pylori* infection among patients with type 2 diabetes mellitus in Lagos, Nigeria. BMC Res Notes 2012;5:284.

[68] Gunji T, Matsuhashi N, Sato H *et al. Helicobacter pylori* infection significantly increases insulin resistance in the asymptomatic Japanese population. *Helicobacter* 2009;14:144–50.

[69] Wang SZ, Shi YN, Zhao J *et al.* Effects of *Helicobacter pylori* on blood glucose fluctuation in type 2 diabetic patients. Zhonghua Yi Xue Za Zhi 2009;89:958–61.

[70] Eshraghian A, Hashemi SA, Hamidian Jahromi A *et al. Helicobacter pylori* infection as a risk factor for insulin resistance. Dig Dis Sci 2009;54:1966–70.

[71] So WY, Tong PC, Ko GT *et al.* Low plasma adiponectin level, white blood cell count and *Helicobacter pylori* titre independently predict abnormal pancreatic beta-cell function. Diabetes Res Clin Pract 2009;86:89–95.

[72] Figura N, Franceschi F, Santucci A *et al.* Extragastric manifestations of *Helicobacter pylori* infection. *Helicobacter* 2010;15 Suppl 1:60-8.

[73] Polyzos SA, Kountouras J, Zavos C *et al.* The association between *Helicobacter pylori* infection and insulin resistance: a systematic review. *Helicobacter* 2011;16:79-88.

[74] Albaker WI. *Helicobacter pylori* infection and its relationship to metabolic syndrome: is it a myth or fact? Saudi J Gastroenterol 2011;17:165-9.

[75] Chen Y, Blaser MJ. Association Between Gastric *Helicobacter pylori* colonization and glycated hemoglobin levels. J Infect Dis 2012, 205:1195-202.

[76] Açbay O, Celik AF, Kadioglu P *et al. Helicobacter pylori* -induced gastritis may contribute to occurrence of postprandial symptomatic hypoglycemia. Dig Dis Sci 1999;44:1837-42.

[77] Imai J, Yamada T, Saito T *et al.* Eradication of insulin resistance. Lancet 2009;374:264.

[78] Figura N, Gennari L, Merlotti D *et al.* *H. pylori* (HP) infection and osteoporosis: a population based study. *Helicobacter* 2010;15:316.
[79] Figura N, Gennari L, Merlotti D *et al.* Prevalence of *Helicobacter pylori* infection in male patients with osteoporosis and controls. Dig Dis Sci 2005;50:847-52.
[80] Kakehasi AM, Mendes CM, Coelho LG *et al.* The presence of *Helicobacter pylori* in postmenopausal women is not a factor to the decrease of bone mineral density. Arq Gastroenterol 2007;44:266-70.
[81] Kakehasi AM, Rodrigues CB, Carvalho AV *et al.* Chronic gastritis and bone mineral density in women. Dig Dis Sci 2009;54:819-24.
[82] Clark SF. Iron deficiency anemia: diagnosis and management. Curr Opin Gastroenterol 2009;25:122-8.
[83] Ojetti V, Migneco A, Silveri NG, Ghirlanda G, Gasbarrini G, Gasbarrini A. The role of *H. pylori* infection in diabetes. Curr Diabetes Rev 2005;1:343-7.
[84] Gasche C, Lomer MC, Cavill I *et al.* Iron, anaemia and inflammatory bowel diseases. Gut 2004;53:1190-7.
[85] Weiss G, Goodnough LT. Anemia of chronic disease. N Engl J Med 2005;352:1011-23.
[86] World Health Organization, United Nations University, The United Nations Children's Fund. Iron deficiency anaemia. Assessment, prevention and control:A guide for programme managers. Available from: URL: http://whqlibdoc.who. int/hq/2001/WHO_NHD_01.3.pdf, accessed 2001.
[87] Rad R, Schmid RM, Prinz C. *Helicobacter pylori*, iron deficiency, and gastric autoimmunity. Blood 2006;107:4969-70.
[88] Bini EJ. *Helicobacter pylori* and iron deficiency anemia: guilty as charged? Am J Med 2001;111:495-7.
[89] DuBois S, Kearney DJ. Iron-deficiency anemia and *Helicobacter pylori* infection: a review of the evidence. Am J Gastroenterol 2005;100:453-9.
[90] Malfertheiner P, Megraud F, O'Morain C *et al.* Current concepts in the management of *Helicobacter pylori* infection: the Maastricht III Consensus Report. Gut 2007;56:772-81.
[91] Qu XH, Huang XL, Xiong P *et al.* Does *Helicobacter pylori* infection play a role in iron deficiency anemia? A meta-analysis. World J Gastroenterol 2010;16:886-96.
[92] Zandi S, Shamsadini S, Zahedi MJ *et al.* *Helicobacter pylori* and rosacea. East Mediterr Health J 2003;9, 167-71.
[93] Malik R, Guleria K, Kaur I *et al.* Effect of *Helicobacter pylori* eradication therapy in iron deficiency anaemia of pregnancy - a pilot study. Indian J Med Res 2011;134:224-31.
[94] Reinauer S, Megahed M, Goerz G *et al.* Schönlein-Henoch purpura associated with gastric *Helicobacter pylori* infection. J Am Acad Dermatol 1995;33:876-9.
[95] Cecchi R, Torelli E. Schönlein-Henoch purpura in association with duodenal ulcer and gastric *Helicobacter pylori* infection. J Dermatol 1998;25:482-4.
[96] Mozrzymas R, d'Amore ES, Montini G *et al.* Schönlein-Henoch vasculitis and chronic *Helicobacter pylori* associated gastritis and duodenal ulcer: a case report. Pediatr Med Chir 1997;19:467-8.
[97] Novák J, Szekanecz Z, Sebesi J *et al.* Elevated levels of anti-*Helicobacter pylori* antibodies in Henoch-Schönlein purpura. Autoimmunity 2003;36:307-11.
[98] Wang BH, Zhou LQ, Zuo YH. Relationship between *Helicobacter pylori* infection and Henoch-Schonlein purpura with gastrointestinal involvement in children. Zhongguo Dang Dai Er Ke Za Zhi 2007;9:367-9.

[99] Raderer M, Osterreicher C, Machold K *et al.* Impaired response of gastric MALT-lymphoma to *Helicobacter pylori* eradication in patients with autoimmune disease. Ann Oncology 2001;12:937-9.

[100] Mandekou- Lefaki I, Delli FS, Kountouras J *et al.* Primary cutaneous MALT-type lymphoma and *Helicobacter pylori*: a possible relationship. J Eur Acad Dermatol Venereol 2006;20:606-8.

[101] Ojetti V, Pellicano R, Fagoonee S *et al. Helicobacter pylori* infection and diabetes. Minerva Med 2010;101:115-9.

[102] Nishimura M, Miyajima S, Okada N. Salivary gland MALT lymphoma associated with *Helicobacter pylori* infection in a patient with Sjögren's Syndrome. J Dermatol 2000;27:450-2.

[103] Iwai H, Nakamichi N, Nakae K *et al.* Parotid mucosa-associated lymphoid tissue lymphoma regression after *Helicobacter pylori* eradication. Laryngoscope 2009;119:1491-4.

[104] Figura N, Perrone A, Gennari C *et al.* Food allergy and *Helicobacter pylori* infection. Ital J Gastroenterol Hepatol 1999;31:186-91.

[105] Bartuzi Z, Korenkiewicz J, Romański B. Correlation between *Helicobacter pylori* infection and food allergy in chronic gastritis. Med Sci Monit 2000;6:530-8.

[106] Maciorkowska E, Panasiuk A, Kaczmarsk M. Concentrations of gastric mucosal cytokines in children with food allergy and *Helicobacter pylori* infection. World J Gastroenterol 2005;11:6751-6.

[107] Konturek PC, Rienecker H, Hahn EG *et al. Helicobacter pylori* as a protective factor against food allergy. Med Sci Monit 2008;14:452-8.

[108] Kandyil R, Satya NS, Swerlick RA. Chronic pruritus associated with *Helicobacter pylori*. J Cutan Med Surg 2002;6:103-8.

[109] Sakurane M, Shiotani A, Furukawa F. Therapeutic effects of antibacterial treatment for intractable skin diseases in *Helicobacter pylori* -positive Japanese patients. J Dermatol. 2002;29:23-7.

[110] Joon Mo K, Seok Hwan K, Park KH *et al.* Investigation of the association between *Helicobacter pylori* infection and normal tension glaucoma. Invest Ophthalmol Vis Sci 2011;52:665-8.

[111] Utaş S, Ozbakir O, Turasan A *et al. Helicobacter pylori* eradication treatment reduces the severity of rosacea. J Am Acad Dermatol 1999;40:433-5.

[112] Bonamigo RR, Leite CS, Wagner M *et al.* Rosacea and *Helicobacter pylori*: interference of systemic antibiotic in the study of possible association. J Eur Acad Dermatol Venereol 2000;14:424-5.

[113] Mini R, Figura N, D'ambrosio C *et al. Helicobacter pylori* immunoproteomes in case reports of rosacea and chronic urticarial. Proteomics 2004;5:777–87.

[114] Kürkçüoğlu N, Aksoy F. Sweet's syndrome associated with *Helicobacter pylori* infection. J Am Acad Dermatol 1997;37:123-4.

[115] Sebekina OV, Trubitsyna IE, Masharova AA *et al.* Clinical variants of chronic urticaria associated with *Helicobacter pylori*. Eksp Klin Gastroenterol 2011;(5):20-5.

[116] Akashi R, Ishiguro N, Shimizu S *et al.* Clinical study of the relationship between *Helicobacter pylori* and chronic urticaria and prurigo chronica multiformis: effectiveness of eradication therapy for *Helicobacter pylori*. J Dermatol 2011;38:761-6.

[117] Ben Mahmoud L, Ghozzi H, Hakim A *et al.* *Helicobacter pylori* associated with chronic urticaria. J Infect Dev Ctries 2011;5:596-8.

[118] Heidt PJ, Vossen JM. Experimental and clinical gnotobiotics: influence of the microflora on graft-*vs.*-host disease after allogeneic bone marrow transplantation. J Med 1992;23:161–73.

[119] Cherubini Di Simplicio F, Giannace R, Menchini M *et al.* Skin disorders and *Helicobacter pylori* infection: a negative association. J Physiol Pharmacol 1999;50 (suppl 2):5.

[120] Shakouri A, Compalati, Lang DM E *et al.* Effectiveness of *Helicobacter pylori* eradication in chronic urticaria: evidence-based analysis using the Grading of Recommendations Assessment, Development, and Evaluation system. Curr Opin Allergy Clin Immunol 2010;10:362-9.

[121] Wedi B, Kapp A. *Helicobacter pylori* infection and skin diseases. J Physiol Pharmacol 1999;50:753-6.

[122] Wedi B, Raap U, Wieczorek D *et al.* Infections and chronic spontaneous urticaria. A review. Hautarzt 2010;61:758-64.

[123] Farkas H, Gyeney L, Majthényi P *et al.* Angioedema due to acquired C1-esterase inhibitor deficiency in a patient with *Helicobacter pylori* infection. Z Gastroenterol 1999;37:513-8.

[124] Mukeba D, Chandrikakumari K, Giot JB *et al.* Autoimmune angioneurotic edema in a patient with *Helicobacter pylori* infection. *Helicobacter* 2009;14:9-11.

[125] Farkas H, Füst G, Fekete B *et al.* Eradication of *Helicobacter pylori* and improvement of hereditary angioneurotic oedema. Lancet 2001;338:1695-6.

[126] Abdel-Hafez HZ, Mahran AM, Hofny ER *et al.* Is *Helicobacter pylori* infection associated with alopecia areata? J Cosmet Dermatol 2009;8:52-5.

[127] Abdel-Hafez HZ, Mahran AM, Hofny ER *et al.* Alopecia areata is not associated with *Helicobacter pylori.* Indian J Dermatol 2009;54:17–9.

[128] Campuzano-Maya G. Cure of alopecia areata after eradication of *Helicobacter pylori*: A new association? World J Gastroenterol 2011;17:3165–70.

[129] Accioly-Filho LW, Nogueira A, Ramos-e-Silva M. Prurigo nodularis of Hyde: an update. J Eur Acad Dermatol Venereol 2000;14:75-82.

[130] Neri S, Ierna D, D'Amico RA *et al.* *Helicobacter pylori* and prurigo nodularis. Hepatogastroenterology 1999;46: 2269-72.

[131] Le Cleach L, Chosidow O. Clinical practice. Lichen planus. N Engl J Med 2012;366:723-32.

[132] Dauden E, Cabrera MM, Onate MJ *et al.* *Helicobacter pylori* CagA seropositivity is not strongly associated with lichen planus. J Am Acad Dermatol 2003;49:1199.

[133] Dauden E, Vazquez-Carrasco MA, Penas PF *et al.* Association of *Helicobacter pylori* infection with psoriasis and lichen planus: prevalence and effect of eradication therapy. Arch Dermatol 2000;136:1275-6.

[134] Vainio E, Huovinen S, Liutu M *et al.* Peptic ulcer and *Helicobacter pylori* in patients with lichen planus. Acta Derm Venereol 2000;80: 427-9.

[135] Izol B, Karabulut AA, Biyikoglu I *et al.* Investigation of upper gastrointestinal tract involvement and *H. pylori* presence in lichen planus: a case-controlled study with endoscopic and histopathological findings. Int J Dermatol 2010;49:1121-6.

[136] Attia EA, Abdel Fattah NS, Abdella HM. Upper gastrointestinal findings and detection of *Helicobacter pylori* in patients with oral lichen planus. Clin Exp Dermatol 2010;35:355-60.

[137] Kusano K, Inokuchi A, Fujimoto K *et al.* Coccoid *Helicobacter pylori* exists in the palatine tonsils of patients with IgA nephropathy. J Gastroenterol 2010;45:406-12.

[138] Yilmaz T, Ceylan M, Akyön Y *et al. Helicobacter pylori*: a possible association with otitis media with effusion. Otolaryngol Head Neck Surg 2006;134:772-7.

[139] Yuan W, Li Yumin, Yang Kehu *et al.* Iron deficiency anemia in *Helicobacter pylori* infection: meta-analysis of randomized controlled trials. Scand J Gastroenterol 2010;45:665-76.

[140] Fancy T, Mathers PH, Ramadan HH. Otitis media with effusion: a possible role for *Helicobacter pylori*? Otolaryngol Head Neck Surg 2009;140:256-8.

[141] Quigley HA, Glaucoma. Lancet 2011;377:1367-77.

[142] Kountouras J, Mylopoulos N, Boura P *et al.* Relationship between *Helicobacter pylori* infection and glaucoma. Ophthalmology 2001;108:599-604.

[143] Kountouras J, Mylopoulos N, Chatzopoulos D *et al.* Eradication of *Helicobacter pylori* may be beneficial in the management of chronic open-angle glaucoma. Arch Intern Med 2002;162:1237-44.

[144] Kountouras J, Zavos C, Deretzi G *et al.* Neuroprotection in glaucoma: is there a future role of *Helicobacter pylori* eradication? Exp Eye Res 2011;92:436–8.

[145] Kountouras J, Zavos C. Further data on the association between *Helicobacter pylori* infection and primary open-angle glaucoma. Clin Ophthalmol 2012;6:243–5.

[146] Deshpande N, Lalitha P, Krishna das SR, *Helicobacter pylori* IgG antibodies in aqueous humor and serum of subject with primary open glaucoma and pseudo-exfoliation glaucoma in a South Indian population. J Glaucoma 2008;17:605-10.

[147] Izzotti A, Saccà SC, Bagnis A *et al.* Glaucoma and *Helicobacter pylori* infection: correlations and controversies. Br J Ophtalmol 2009;93:1420-7.

[148] Zullo A, Ridola L, Hassan C, *et al.* Glaucoma and *Helicobacter pylori*: eyes wide shut? Dig Liver Dis 2012;44:627-8.

[149] Galloway PH, Warner SJ, Morshed MG *et al. Helicobacter pylori* infection and the risk for open-angle glaucoma. Ophtalmology 2003;110:922-5.

[150] Tzolaki F, Gogaki E, Sakkias F *et al. Helicobacter pylori* infection and primary open-angle glaucoma: is there a connection? Clin Ophtalmol 2012;6:45-7.

[151] Franceschi F, Gasbarrini A, Fontana L. Role of *Helicobacter pylori* infection in ophthalmology. Ophthalmology 1998;105:1351–2.

[152] Giusti C. Association of *Helicobacter pylori* with central serous chorioretinopathy: hypotheses regarding pathogenesis. Med Hypotheses 2004;63:524–7.

[153] Saccà, Pascotto A, Venturino GM *et al.* Prevalence and treatment of *Helicobacter pylori* in patients with blepharitis. Invest Ophtalmol Vis Sci 2006;47:501-8.

[154] Altschuler E. Gastric *Helicobacter pylori* infection as a cause of idiopathic Parkinson disease and non-arteric anterior optic ischemic neuropathy. Med Hypotheses 1996;47:413-4.

[155] Dobbs SM, Dobbs RJ, Weller C *et al.* Link between *Helicobacter pylori* infection and idiopathic parkinsonism. Med Hypotheses. 2000;55:93-8.

[156] Weller C, Oxlade N, Dobbs SM *et al.* Role of inflammation in gastrointestinal tract in aetiology and pathogenesis of idiopathic parkinsonism. FEMS Immunol Med Microbiol 2005;44:129-35.

[157] Dobbs SM, Dobbs RJ, Weller C *et al.* Differential effect of *Helicobacter pylori* eradication on time-trends in brady/hypokinesia and rigidity in idiopathic parkinsonism. *Helicobacter* 2010;15:279-94.

[158] Dobbs RJ, Dobbs SM, Weller C *et al. Helicobacter* hypothesis for idiopathic parkinsonism: before and beyond. *Helicobacter* 2008;13:309-22.

[159] Schulz JD, Hawkes EL, Shaw CA. Cycad toxins, *Helicobacter pylori* and parkinsonism: cholesterol glucosides as the common denomenator. Med Hypotheses 2006;66:1222-6.

[160] Pierantozzi M, Pietroiusti A, Brusa L *et al. Helicobacter pylori* eradication and l-dopa absorption in patients with PD and motor fluctuations. Neurology 2006;66:1824-9.

[161] Pierantozzi M, Pietroiusti A, Sancesario G *et al.* Reduced L-dopa absorption and increased clinical fluctuations in *Helicobacter pylori* -infected Parkinson's disease patients. Neurol Sci 2001;22:89-91.

[162] Lee WY, Yoon WT, Shin HY *et al. Helicobacter pylori* infection and motor fluctuations in patients with Parkinson's disease. Mov Disord 2008;23:1696-700.

[163] Lahner E, Annibale B, Delle Fave G. Systematic review: *Helicobacter pylori* infection and impaired drug absorption. Aliment Pharmacol Ther 2009;29:379-86.

[164] Loddenkötter B, Becker K, Hohoff C *et al.* Real-time quantitative PCR assay for the detection of *Helicobacter pylori*: no association with sudden infant death syndrome. Int J Legal Med 2005;119:202-6.

[165] Lyte M. Microbial endocrinology as a basis for improved L-DOPA bioavailability in Parkinson's patients treated for *Helicobacter pylori*. Med Hypotheses 2010;74:895-7.

[166] Rees K, Stowe R, Patel S *et al. Helicobacter pylori* eradication for Parkinson's disease. Cochrane Database Syst Rev 2011;(11):CD008453.

[167] Nielsen HH, Qiu J, Friis S. Treatment for *Helicobacter pylori* infection and risk of parkinson's disease in Denmark. Eur J Neurol 2012;19:864-9.

[168] Balin BJ, Appelt DM. Role of infection in Alzheimer's disease. J Am Osteopath Assoc 2001;12 Suppl Pt 1:S1-S6.

[169] Kountouras J, Tsolaki M, Gavalas E *et al.* Relationship between *Helicobacter pylori* infection and Alzheimer disease. Neurology 2006;66:938-40.

[170] Kountouras J, Gavalas E, Zavos C *et al.* Alzheimer's disease and *Helicobacter pylori* infection: Defective immune regulation and apoptosis as proposed common links. Med Hypotheses 2007, 68:378-8.

[171] Raubeaud-Baudron C, Krolak-Salmon P, Quadrio I *et al.* Impact of chronic *Helicobacter pylori* infection on Alzheimer's disease: preliminary results. Neurobiol Aging 2012;33:11-9.

[172] Zullo A, Hassan C, Morini S. Hepatic encephalopathy and *Helicobacter pylori*: a critical reappraisal. J Clin gastroenterol 2003;37:164-8.

[173] Dasani BM, Sigal SH, Lieber CS. Analysis of risk factors for chronic hepatic encephalopathy: the role of *Helicobacter pylori* infection. Am J Gastroenterol 1998;93:726-31.

[174] Si J, Cao Q, Gao M *et al.* Changes in serum ammonia concentration in cirrhotic patients with *Helicobacter pylori* infection. Med J (Engl) 2000;113:1080-1.

[175] Duseja A, Sachdev A, Dhiman RK *et al. Helicobacter pylori* and hepatic encephalopathy. Indian J Gastroenterol 2003;22(Suppl 2):S31-2.

[176] Abdel-Hady H, Zaki A, Badra G *et al. Helicobacter pylori* infection in hepatic encephalopathy: Relationship to plasma endotoxins and blood ammonia. Hepatol Res 2007;37:1026-33.

[177] Calvet X, Nogueras C, Roqué M *et al. Helicobacter pylori* is not a risk factor for hepatic encephalopathy. Dig Liver Dis 2001;33:414-9.

[178] Huber M, Rössle M, Siegerstetter V *et al.* *Helicobacter pylori* infection does not correlate with plasma ammonia concentration and hepatic encephalopathy in patients with cirrhosis. Hepatogastroenterology 2001;48:541-4.

[179] Kini D, Aggarwal R, Saraswat VA *et al.* Role of *Helicobacter pylori* infection in hyperammonemia and subclinical hepatic encephalopathy in cirrhosis of liver. Indian J Gastroenterol 2001;20:237-40.

[180] Săndulache L, Stanciu C. Prevalence of *Helicobacter pylori* in liver cirrhosis complicated with hepatic encephalopathy. Rev Med Chir Soc Med Nat Iasi 2009;113:1056-60.

[181] Vásconez C, Elizalde JI, Llach J *et al.* *Helicobacter pylori,* hyperammonemia and subclinical portosystemic encephalopathy: effects of eradication. J Hepatol 1999;30:260-4.

[182] Ghabaee M, Ghanbarian D, Brujeni GN *et al.* Could *Helicobacter pylori* play an important role in axonal type of Guillain-Barré syndrome pathogenesis? Clin Neurol Neurosurg. 2010;112:193-8

[183] Kountouras J, Deretzi G, Zavos C *et al.* *Helicobacter pylori* infection may trigger Guillain-Barré syndrome, Fisher syndrome and Bickerstaff brainstem encephalitis. J Neurol Sci 2011;305:167-8.

[184] Chiba S, Sugiyama T, Matsumoto H *et al.* Antibodies against *Helicobacter pylori* were detected in the cerebrospinal fluid obtained from patients with Guillain-Barré syndrome. Ann Neurol 1998;44:686-8.

[185] Radić M, Kaliterna DM, Radić J. *Helicobacter pylori* infection and systemic sclerosis-is there a link? Joint Bone Spine 2011;78:337-40.

[186] Hernando-Harder A, Booken N, Goerdt S *et al.* *Helicobacter pylori* infection and dermatologic diseases. Eur J Dermatol 2009;19:431-44.

[187] Danes S, Zoli A, Cremonini F *et al.* High prevalence of *Helicobacter pylori* type I virulent strains in patients with systemic sclerosis. J Rheumatol 2000;27:1568-9.

[188] Reinauer S, Goerz G, Ruzicka T *et al.* *Helicobacter pylori* in patients with systemic sclerosis: detection with the 13C-urea breath test and eradication. Acta Derm Venereol 1994;74:361-3.

[189] Yazawa N, Fujimoto M, Kikuchi K *et al.* High seroprevalence of *Helicobacter pylori* infection in patients with systemic sclerosis: association with esophageal involvement. J Rheumatol 1998;25:650-3.

[190] Farina G, Rosato E, Francia C *et al.* High incidence of *Helicobacter pylori* infection in patients with systemic sclerosis: association with Sicca Syndrome. Int J Immunopathol Pharmacol 2001;14:81-5.

[191] Gasbarrini A, Massari I, Sericchio M *et al.* *Helicobacter pylori* eradication ameliorates primary Raynaud's phenomenon. Dig Dis Sci 1998;43:1641-5.

[192] Wipff J, Allanore Y, Soussi F *et al.* Prevalence of Barrett's esophagus in systemic sclerosis. Arthritis Rheum 2005;52:2882–8.

[193] Kalabay L, Fekete B, Czirják L. *Helicobacter pylori* infection in connective tissue disorders is associated with high levels of antibodies to mycobacterial hsp65 but not to human hsp60. *Helicobacter* 2002;7:250-6.

[194] Radić M, Kaliterna DM, Radić J. *Helicobacter pylori* infection and systemic sclerosis-is there a link? Joint Bone Spine 2011;78:337-40.

[195] Figura N, Giordano N, Burroni D *et al.* Sjögren syndrome and *Helicobacter pylori* infection. Eur J Gastroenterol Hepatol 1994;6:321-2.

[196] Aragona P, Magazzu G, Macchia G *et al.* Presence of antibodies against *Helicobacter pylori* and its heat-shock protein 60 in the serum of patients with Sjögren's syndrome. J. Rheumatol 1999;26:1306-11.

[197] Theander E, Nilsson I, Manthorpe R *et al.* Seroprevalence of *Helicobacter pylori* in primary Sjögren's syndrome. Clin Exp Rheumatol 2001;19:633-8.

[198] El Miedany YM, Baddour M, Ahmed I *et al.* Sjogren's syndrome: concomitant *H. pylori* infection and possible correlation with clinical parameters. Joint Bone Spine 2005;72:135-41.

[199] Anand P S, Nandakumar K, Shenoy K T. Are dental plaque, poor oral hygiene, and periodontal disease associated with *Helicobacter pylori* infection? J Periodontol 2006;77:692-8.

[200] Sorrentino D, Faller G, DeVita S *et al. Helicobacter pylori* associated antigastric autoantibodies: role in Sjögren's syndrome gastritis. *Helicobacter* 2004;9:46-53.

[201] Ersoy O, Ersoy R, Yayar O. *et al. Helicobacter pylori* infection in patients with Behçet's disease. World J Gastroenterol 2007;13:2983–5.

[202] Albanidou-Farmaki E, Giannoulis L, Markopoulos A *et al.* Outcome following treatment for *Helicobacter pylori* in patients with recurrent aphthous stomatitis. Oral Dis 2005;1:22–6.

[203] Aksoz MK, Unsal B, Zeren I *et al.* The upper gastrointestinal endoscopic and rectosigmoidoscopic windings in Behcet's disease. Turk J Gastroenterol 1995;6:172–4.

[204] Figura N, Piomboni P, Ponzetto A *et al. H. pylori* infection and infertility. Eur J Gastroenterol Hepatol 2002;14:663-9.

[205] Collodel G, Moretti E, Campagna MS *et al.* Infection by CagA-positive *Helicobacter pylori* strains may contribute to alter the sperm quality of men with fertility disorders and increase the systemic levels of TNF-α. Dig Dis Sci 2010;55:94-100.

[206] Moretti E, Collodel G, Campagna MS *et al.* Influence of *Helicobacter pylori* infection on levels of ghrelin and obestatin in human semen. J Androl 2011 dec 15. [epub ahead of print], PMID: 22174388.

[207] Kurotsuchi, S, Hisao Ando H, Iwase A *et al.* The plausibility of *Helicobacter pylori*-related infertility in Japan. Fertil Steril 2008;90:866-8.

[208] Yavasoglu I, Kucuk M. Anti-*Helicobacter pylori* antibodies and polycystic ovary syndrome. Eur J Obstet Gynecol Reprod Biol 2012;163:243.

[209] Ambrosini G, Andrisani A, Fiore C *et al.* Anti-*Helicobacter pylori* antibodies in cervical mucus: a new cause of infertility. Eur J Obstet Gynecol 2011;155:157-60.

[210] Hajishafiha M, Ghasemi-Rad M, Memari A *et al.* Effect of *H. pylori* infection on pregnancy rates and early pregnancy loss after intracytoplasmic sperm injection. Int J Womens Health 2011;3:329-35.

[211] Qu XH, Huang XL, Xiong P *et al.* Does *Helicobacter pylori* infection play a role in iron deficiency anemia? A meta-analysis. World J Gastroenterol 2010;16:886-96.

[212] Bamford KB, Fan X, Crowe SE *et al.* Lymphocytes in the human gastric mucosa during *Helicobacter.pylori* have a T helper cell 1 phenotype. Gastroenterology 1998;114:482–92.

[213] D'Elios M M, Andersen L P, Del Prete G. Inflammation and host response. Curr Opin Gastroenterol 1998;14:15–9.

[214] Gordon D. Solving the African enigma: parasites may have their place. Gastroenterology 2000;119: 611.

[215] Weller C, Oxlade N, Dobbs SM *et al.* Role of inflammation in gastrointestinal tract in aetiology and pathogenesis of idiopathic parkinsonism. FEMS Immunol Med Microbiol. 2005;44:129-35.

[216] Fox JG, Wang TC, Nagler-Anderson C. The African enigma: the parasite's perspective. Gut 2001;49:156–7.

[217] Mitchell HM, Ally R, Wadee A *et al.* Major differences in the IgG subclass response to *Helicobacter pylori* in the first and third worlds. Scand J Gastroenterol 2002;37:517-22.

[218] Task Force on Sudden Infant Death Syndrome, Moon RY. SIDS and other sleep-related infant deaths: expansion of recommendations for a safe infant sleeping environment. Pediatrics. 2011;128:e1341-67.

[219] Pattison CP, Marshall BJ. Proposed link between *Helicobacter pylori* and sudden infant death syndrome. Medical Hypothesis 1997;49:365-9.

[220] Kerr JR, Al-Khattaf A, Barson AJ *et al.* An association between sudden infant death syndrome (SIDS) and *Helicobacter pylori* infection. Arch Dis Child 2000;83:429-34.

[221] Stray-Pedersen, A Vege A, Rognum T. *Helicobacter pylori* antigen in stool is associated with SIDS and sudden infant deaths due to infectious disease. Pediatr Res 2008;64:405-10.

[222] Ho GY, Windsor HM, Snowball B *et al. Helicobacter pylori* is not the cause of sudden infant death syndrome. Am J Gastroenterol 2001;96:3288-94.

[223] Golberg D, Szilagyi A, Graves L. Hyperemesis gravidarum and *Helicobacter pylori* infection: a systematic review. Obstet Gynecol 2007;110:695-703.

[224] Rosenstock SJ, Jørgensen T, Andersen LP *et al.* Association of *Helicobacter pylori* infection with lifestyle, chronic disease, body-indices, and age at menarche in Danish adults. Scand J Public Health 2000;28:32-40.

[225] Hatziveis K, Tourlakis D, Hountis P *et al.* Relationship between *Helicobacter pylori* seropositivity and hyperemesis gravidarum with the use of questionnaire. Minerva Ginecol 2007;59:579-83.

[226] Sandven I, Abdelnoor M, Wethe M *et al. Helicobacter pylori* infection and Hyperemesis gravidarum. An institution-based case-control study. Eur J Epidemiol 2008, 23:491-8.

[227] Sandven I, Abdelnoor M, Nesheim BI *et al. Helicobacter pylori* infection and hyperemesis gravidarum: a systematic review and meta-analysis of case-control studies. Acta Obstet Gynecol Scand 2009;88:1190-200.

[228] Mansour GM, Nashaat EH. Role of *Helicobacter pylori* in the pathogenesis of hyperemesis gravidarum. Arch Gynecol Obstet 2011;284:843-7.

[229] Tangerman A, Winkel E G. Extra-oral halitosis: an overview. J Breath Res. 2010;4:017003.

[230] Souto R, Colombo A P. Detection of *Helicobacter pylori* by polymerase chain reaction in the subgingival biofilm and saliva of non-dyspeptic periodontal patients. J Periodontol 2008;79:97-103.

[231] Klein PD, Graham DY, Gaillour A *et al.* Water source as risk factor for *Helicobacter pylori* infection in Peruvian children. Lancet 1991;337:1503–6.

[232] Raymond J, Bergeret M, Benhamou PH *et al.* A 2-year study of *Helicobacter pylori* in children. J Clin Microbiol 1994;32:461-3.

[233] Raymond J, Bergeret M, Kalach N. *Helicobacter pylori* infection in children. Presse Med 2008;37(3 Pt 2):513-8.

[234] Patel P, Mendall MA, Khulusi S *et al. Helicobacter pylori* infection in childhood: risk factors and effect on growth. Br Med J 1994;309:1119–23.

[235] Patel P, Mendall MA, Khulusi S *et al. Helicobacter pylori* infection in childhood: risk factors and effect on growth. Br Med J 1994;309:1119-23.

[236] Richter T, Richter T, List S *et al.* Five- to 7-year-old children with *Helicobacter pylori* infection are smaller than *Helicobacter*-negative children: a cross sectional population-based study of 3,315 children. J Pediatr Gastroenterol Nutr 2001;33:472-5.

[237] Mera RM, Bravo LE, Goodman KJ *et al.* Long-term effects of clearing *Helicobacter pylori* on growth in school-age children. Pediatr Infect Dis J 2012;31:263-6.

[238] Crabtree JE, Peichl P, Wyatt J *et al.* Gastric interleukin-8 and IgA IL-8 autoantibodies in *Helicobacter pylori* infection. Scand J Immunol 1993;37:65–70.

[239] Murch SH, Lamkin VA, Savage MO *et al.* Serum concentrations of tumour necrosis factor alpha in childhood chronic inflammatory disease. Gut 1991;32:913–7.

[240] Mendall MA, Pajares-Garcia J. Epidemiology and transmission of *Helicobacter pylori.* Curr Opin Gastroenterol 1995;11(suppl 1):1-4.

[241] Perri F, Pastore M, Leandro G *et al. Helicobacter pylori* infection and growth delay in older children. Arch Dis Child 1997;77:46–9.

[242] Shiotani A, Okada K, Yanaoka K, *et al.* Beneficial effect of *Helicobacter pylori* eradication in dermatologic diseases. *Helicobacter* 2001, 6: 60-5.

Send Orders for Reprints to reprints@benthamscience.net

Helicobacter Pylori: A Worldwide Perspective 2014, 2014, 396-410

CHAPTER 17

Helicobacter pylori Infection Up-date in Pediatric Population

Aron Cseh*, **Hedvig Bodanszky and Gabor Veres**

I[st] Department of Pediatrics, Semmelweis University, Budapest, Hungary

Abstract: *Helicobacter pylori* (*H. pylori*) infection is the main cause of ulcerous conditions affecting half of the world population. Previously the symptoms described only in adults but recently the studies focusing on chronic childhood gastrointestinal diseases. Besides the chronic inflammation resulting in gastritis and peptic ulcers, the *H. pylori* thought to be the root of some malignancies, like adenocarcinomas and lymphomas of gastrointestinal system. As long as the presence of *H. pylori* in stomach can be observed lifelong without treatment, the serious complications of the infection need to be prevented even in childhood. However, the presenting signs and symptoms are not clearly described in pediatric population and also the screening is not resolved; recent recommendations are well defined the therapeutic strategy in children.

Keywords: *Helicobacter pylori,* pediatrics, epidemiology, peptic ulcer disease, pathomechanism, extraintestinal manifestations

INTRODUCTION

Helicobacter pylori (*H. pylori*) is a spiral-shaped Gram-negative bacterium that causes one of the most common infection worldwide. It colonizes the stomach every second adults, with higher prevalence's in developing countries [1]. This infection is responsible for peptic ulcer disease as demonstrated by Marshall and Warren, who was awarded with Nobel Prize in 2005 for their discovery [2].

According to the latest theories, the chronic inflammation caused by *H. pylori* has a central role in the pathogenesis of adenocarcinoma of the stomach, B-cell lymphoma and mucosa-associated lymphoid tissue lymphoma even in children associated with epigenetic alterations [3].

While the symptoms of *H. pylori* infection are remarkable in most cases only in

***Address correspondence to Aron Cseh:** University Semmelweis 1st Department of Pediatrics, Budapes, Hungary; Tel: +36-1-334-3186; Fax: +36-1-301 38212; E-mail: cseharon@gmail.com adulthood, the infection is thought to be acquired in childhood, as early before 10 years of age. In childhood the symptoms, diagnostic possibilities, complications and therapeutic regimens largely differed from that in adults.

Epidemiology

In developing countries two thirds of children are infected by the age of two, while in developed countries even at the age of ten the rate of *H. pylori* infection is only around 10% [4]. In developing countries by the age of 15-20 some 90% of the population becomes infected. In developed countries only 20% of under-40's and 50% of over-60's carry the pathogen. The socioeconomics status of families and their hygiene conditions are decisive factors in the occurrence of the infection.

Several factors including differences in immunoglobulin prevalence's, estrogen receptors and antibiotic exposure may solved the phenomenon of male predominance in *H. pylori* infection [5-7]. However, it is present only in adult population [5].

The risk of infection is affected by some factors such as ethnic origin, jobs and therefore exposure for infection. Indeed, health workers are overrepresented compared to the population average, particularly those administering endoscopy. Transmission of infection is usually *via* the faecal-oral route, but as living bacteria have been detected, besides faeces, also in saliva and dental plaque, the oral-oral route may also be assumed. Cross-infection is more common inside families than among single persons. Infection between parents and children is 18-20%, with mother-child infection being more common.

The prevalence of *H. pylori* infection is constantly decreased in the last decade, but recent studies demonstrated a stable state in developed countries [8]. In addition, in developed countries the reinfection is still a major problem and in developing country the spontaneous clearance is less prevalent in *H. pylori* infection [9]. The reinfection rate of *H. pylori* in children after one to nine years of successful eradication was 18%, indicating a higher rate in children compared to adults [10].

Pathomechanism

H. pylori is a member of Helicobacter spp., among these species most of the members are microaerophile, but *H. pylori* is able to grow equally under microaerobic or aerobic conditions at high bacterial density [11]. The urease enzyme producing capability of *H. pylori* is not only of diagnostic importance, but that of pathogenic attribution. The setting of microenvironment pH is also important as the biofilm forming ability of *H. pylori* for pathogenic reasons [12]. In addition, the susceptibility of hosts is also play a role according to the latest proteomics and immunological studies; however the results are still controversial. The importance of some virulence markers (cagA, vacAs1, iceA) was also demonstrated in adult patients followed by studies in childhood populations [13,14]. The comparative genomics assays demonstrated the strong impact of these genes on severity of *H. pylori* infection along with increased inflammatory status of gastric mucosa and also esophageal lesions in children. The carrying of these genes in host organism is responsible for proinflammatory cytokine production combined with increased regulatory T cells prevalence's and therefore suppressive predominance [15].

The routes of early life *H. pylori* infections have not been well identified; however the protective role of maternal milk is already demonstrated. According to a meta-analysis, breast-feeding decreases the risk of *H. pylori* infections [16]. This effect is even stronger in developing countries, underlying the hypotheses that - due to higher prevalence of infections - mothers living in low-income countries have elevated titer of *H. pylori* IgA antigen. Nevertheless, the transmission of *H. pylori* infection by infected mother was also demonstrated in children [17,18]. The *H. pylori* seropositivity was highest when both parent are seropositive, and also even higher in only seropositive mother, then in only seropositive father compared with uninfected parents (16.0%, 14.9%, 9.9% and 3.5%, respectively) [19,20]. Moreover, the risk of children *H. pylori* infection was higher in symptomatic mother's and also when soothers were used. Along with others, these data suggest that through direct contact the infected mothers are the main source of *H. pylori* infection in their children.

Transplacental transmission of *H. pylori* infection during pregnancy was also investigated in experimental models, but no connection was demonstrated [21]. However, one study conducted in neonates and very young children demonstrated an unexpectedly high *H. pylori* antigen detection rate [22]. It is suggested that some transient colonization presents after birth and therefore in vaginal births the antigen prevalence's is higher than that of cesarean section (59% and 10%, respectively).

Signs and Symptoms

The complications of *H. pylori* infection can be divided into local and systemic ones [23]. Local problems are gastritis, dyspepsia, ulcers and gastric cancer. In addition, malignancies can be also the consequences of systemic changes in infection, but systemic manifestations of the infection can be also detected such as anemia, growth retardation and neurological disabilities [24].

In childhood there is no typical clinical manifestation. At the beginning of the infection usually epigastric pains, loss of appetite and weight loss are experienced. Diverse forms of abdominal pain are common symptoms in childhood population and it is suggested that *H. pylori* infection can be stay in the background of chronic complaints. However, a meta-analysis found no association between recurrent abdominal pain (RAP) or epigastric pain and *H. pylori* infection [25]. They only described a partial connection between children with unspecified abdominal pain and acute infection, but it can not be demonstrated widely and therefore recommended for screening purposes.

Intestinal Symptoms

Abdominal complaints such as pain, cramps and nausea are very common in pediatric population. One of the most common gastrointestinal symptoms, RAP is non-specific and occurs in 10-15% of school-age children. A multidimensional measure consisting four scales (pain intensity scale, symptoms scale, disability scale, and satisfaction scale) found no association between RAP and *H. pylori* infection [26]. Between 5 and 10 years of age, the prevalence of *H. pylori* in symptomatic children decreased, while in children without symptoms increased (20% to 7% *vs.* 11% to 40%, respectively). Early acquisition of *H. pylori* may cause chronic abdominal symptoms, however it is still not clear whether infections without ulcerative conditions can cause abdominal symptoms in childhood population or not [27]. Therefore recent studies indicated that testing for *H. pylori* should only be performed when alarming symptoms are present or organic disease is suspected [27,28].

Extraintestinal Manifestations

H. pylori infection is associated with hematological and neurological symptoms, such as anemia, immune thrombocytopenic purpura and short stature, neurological disabilities, and migraine [29]. Recently it is also raised that autoimmune hepatitis is associated with *H. pylori* infection, but it can not be demonstrated in children [30].

One of the most common complications of *H. pylori* infection is iron deficiency anemia [31]. One explanation for this symptom is blood loss due to bleeding, while an other more sophisticated is the changes of iron absorption in this disease. However, the exact pathomechanism is not fully understood, the hypothesis that anemia leads to neurodevelopmental disabilities in childhood is widely accepted [32]. In addition, idiopathic thrombocytopenic purpura characterized by low platelet count is a remarkable complication of *H. pylori* infection, which can be improved with the antimicrobial therapy [33]. It is hypothesized that the chronic immunological stimulus caused by *H. pylori* is responsible for the autoimmune thrombocytopenia; however the exact pathomechanism is still unknown. Several studies reported amelioration of low platelet count after triple therapy in adults, but theses results are not fully strengthened in children.

The *H. pylori* infection was also implicated in other conditions including upper respiratory tract infections, periodontal disease and also food allergy. However the causal relationship between these status and the colonization with the pathogen is still in debate. However recent studies demonstrated that in adenoidal tissues and middle ear fluids taken from children with otitis with effusion there is a significantly increased colonization of *H. pylori* compared with controls [34]. In order to clarify these results, more studies are needed for definitive conclusions.

Along with neurodevelopmental disabilities, growth retardation can be also a complication of *H. pylori* infection [23]. Several studies have been published about the connection between growth retardation and *H. pylori* infection in pediatric population [35]. One study concluded that short stature was associated with *H. pylori* infection only in older children (8-14 years) compared with children without infection in a low-income community [36]. Others found no positive correlation between the eradication of *H. pylori* and improvements in any of the growth outcomes (height, weight, and body mass index) investigated in children (7-11 years) infected with *H. pylori* [37]. As already demonstrated, the plasma levels of hunger-stimulating ghrelin are in inverse association with the presence of *H. pylori* infection which may lead to the alterations of the appetite and dyspeptic symptoms observed in infected patients [38, 39].

The levels of serum ferritin and vitamin B_{12} are lower, while that of serum folate and zinc are comparable in children with *H. pylori* infection and controls [40]. It has been previously demonstrated that the infected status with *H. pylori* was associated with a decrease in gastric juice ascorbic acid concentration, and this effect was more pronounced inpatients with the *cagA*-positive strain. In addition, pangastritis was found more common in patients whose *H. pylori* infection was accompanied by anemia than whose not [41]. Previously mentioned study also suggested that in some cases headache but not of abdominal pain or dyspepsia is the only symptom in children affected by *H. pylori* infection [8]. The remission of primary gastric lymphoma is elongated in immuncompromised pediatric patients and the treatment of *H. pylori* infection alone contributed to the recovery of patient's lymphoma during the follow-up [42].

Recently some data published about the possible beneficial effects of *H. pylori* infections. It was hypothesized that *H. pylori* can be protective against gastroesophageal reflux disease (GERD) and allergies. The most of these data are from epidemiological studies and some contradictions are also present in the results, therefore no conclusions can be made [1]. However *H. pylori* infection recently describe as a protective factor for asthma and allergic disorders, the pathomechanism and the concrete connection between these diseases is not known.

Diagnosis

H. pylori tests are divide into invasive and non-invasive ones. Invasive diagnostic methods using gastric tissue samples to detect *H. pylori* with culture, histopathology, polimerase chain reaction (PCR) and rapid urease test. Non-invasive tests are for detection of *H. pylori* antigen in stool and antibodies in serum, urine and oral samples. In addition, urea breath test (UBT) is based on the urease enzyme activity of *H. pylori* and therefore have high sensitivity and specificity for ongoing infection [43].

An UBT can serve to establish the diagnosis and provide basic information. The stool antigen test is specific, reliable (90%) and suitable for routine examination. It is recommended for use with children who are not infected. The stool test is relatively simple and can be used when nothing else is available. It is a very important tool particularly in the developing countries. In North America and Europe a consensus has been reached about establishing a diagnosis of *H. pylori* according to which endoscopy is indispensable while other forms of examination such as the urease test, stool culture *etc.* can only be used to verify the effectiveness of treatment. However, as summarized in a review, endoscopy and histopathology remained the only method that can detect undoubtedly the presence of *H. pylori* in pediatric population [43]. The surest way is endoscopy but in several developing countries where infection in on a wider scale it is not available, and also the invasiveness is limiting the routine use.

The diagnostic modalities for *H. pylori* infection especially in children less than 6 years of age are uncertain, therefore further investigation needed to establish the optimal protocol [44,45]. A comprehensive analysis planed to validate the invasive and non-invasive tests to detect *H. pylori* with setting up a gold standard from histology, culture, and rapid urease tests comparing [46]. The sensitivity and specificity was highest in case of UBT and stool enzyme-linked immunosorbent assay (ELISA) kit (UBT, 98% and 89%, ELISA, 94% and 81%, respectively), while that of was lower with serologic tests (50%). Along with these results, others demonstrated also higher sensitivity and specificity in patients less than 5 years of age with *H. pylori* infection (UBT, 93.3% and 95.5%, stool antigen, 93.3% and 98.7%, respectively) [47]. In line with this, a new meta-analysis concluded that UBT have high specificity and sensitivity (95.9% and 95.7%, respectively) in pediatric population, even more in children older than 6 year of age [44]. However, as recently described, stool-antigen tests are independent from age and has similar accuracy compared with UBT kits [48]. ELISA monoclonal antibodies have the highest sensitivity and specificity, in comparison with that of polyclonal antibodies and one-step monoclonal tests (97% and 97%, 92% and 93%, 88% and 93%, respectively). In addition, lower-dose (1 mg/kg of bodyweight, maximum 25 mg) of urea for the test is also effective to the determination of *H. pylori* infection in children [49]. However it should be noted that result of UBT does not estimate the severity of histological and results should be interpreted qualitatively in children with *H. pylori* infection.

When compared the UBT to histological results and rapid urease test the sensitivity and specificity of UBT is 83% and 91%, respectively [50]. The accuracy of *H. pylori* rapid test from serum, including the sensitivity, specificity, positive predictive value and negative predictive values were 75.7%, 95.0% 94.6% and 77.0% respectively [51]. The sensitivity and specificity of monoclonal antibody-based enzyme immunoassay were 95% and 90%, respectively [52].

In contrast, a test kit that measures *H. pylori* serum antibodies and pepsinogens I an II and gastrin 17 was insensitive (47%-73%) to recommend *H. pylori* screening, even when pepsinogens and gastrin included in the analysis [53]. A urine test for detection *H. pylori* IgG antibodies was also not sensitive (34%-66%) indicating limited diagnostic role in *H. pylori* infections [54].

Treatment

H. pylori infection is established early as less than 10 years of life and without antibiotic treatment generally persist lifelong [55]. Its eradication is the definitive treatment to prevent gastritis and peptic ulcer. In addition to diseases caused by the inflammation, malignant transformation is also plausible. Several studies demonstrated that *H. pylori* infections are implicated in the development of adenocarcinoma of the stomach and low-grade B cell lymphoma of gastric mucosa-associated lymphoid tissue.

The European Society for Paediatric Gastroenterology, Hepatology and Nutrition (ESPGHAN) and North American Society of Pediatric Gastroenterology, Hepatology and Nutrition (NASPGHAN) recommended triple therapy including amoxicillin, imidazole and proton pump inhibitor (PPI), or amoxicillin, clarithromycin and PPI, or amoxicillin, imidazole and bismuth salts [56]. However, the triple therapy is the first choice treatment for *H. pylori* infection in children, sequential therapy is also recommended. The sequential 10-day therapy typically consists from amoxicillin and PPI given for the first 5 days, followed by a triple therapy for another 5 days. A recent meta-analysis described that the effect of this is two-step therapy comparable with that of triple therapy [57]. The most commonly used antibiotic combinations in the treatment of *H. pylori* infections are containing PPIs. The PPIs have favorable role in facilitating the antimicrobial effects of antibiotics through the adjustment of gastric pH. Using individualized doses of PPIs, these drugs are safe and effective choices in the therapy of *H. pylori* infection in childhood [55]. According to one of the first meta-analyses which assessed the effectiveness of *H. pylori* treatments it can be concluded that further evaluation of new randomized placebo-controlled trials are needed, especially in population of developing areas [58]. In countries with high clarithromycin resistance rate, culture and susceptibility testing are needed to the optimal therapeutic choice [56]. However, the above mentioned sequential therapy thought to be useful in low clarithromycin resistance areas, but in this case it can be more effective than regular therapy. Recently a new diagnostic method was developed to the PCR detection of clarithromycin resistance with high sensitivity and specificity (83.3% and 100%, respectively) from stool samples [59].

The increasing number of antibiotic resistant strain of *H. pylori* affected pediatric population emerged the evaluation of new protocols and registers [60]. Therefore a new online register was established by the European Society for Pediatric

Gastroenterology Hepatology and Nutrition to collect data on treatment (Pediatric European Register for Treatment of *Helicobacter pylori*, PERTH) [61].

The treatment protocols recommended for adults maybe not suitable for children, as suggested by recent reports. Triple therapies containing bismuth salts were more effective than PPI-containing ones (77% *vs.* 64%, respectively) [62]. Also the eradication rate of *H. pylori* was higher in pediatric patients with ulcer than without (79.7% and 63.9%, respectively), but the two-week therapy was not superior to one-week therapy.

In addition, the efficacy of eradication was higher in case of triple therapy (omeprazole, clarithromycin and amoxicillin for 10 days) than quadruple therapy (omeprazole, amoxicillin, metronidazole and bismuth citrate for 10 days) in childhood patient population (92-75.5% *vs.* 84-68.8%, respectively) [63]. Indeed, triple therapy (esomeprazole, amoxicillin and clarithromycin/metronidazole) was highly effective for eradication of *H. pylori* in symptomatic children with moderate resistance to clarythromycin and to medronidazole (9% and 16%, respectively) [64]. In patients with *H. pylori* gastritis the triple therapy (omeprazole, amoxicillin and clarithromycin) offered higher eradication rate than dual therapy (amoxicillin and clarithromycin) (69% *vs.* 15%, respectively) [65]. However, a reduced triple therapy that lasts for one week instead of two, showed moderate results in *H. pylori* treatment (73.7%, 84,8%, respectively) [66].

Recent studies focused on the importance of probiotic therapy as possible immunmodulatory supplements. Indeed, it is already demonstrated from basic research that probiotics have impact on antigen presenting functions of innate immunity. The evaluation of probiotic effects as an adjuvant to the standard triple therapy and the correct selection of possible beneficial probiotic strain is the most important questions. It is already demonstrated that *Lactobacillus reuteri* reduced the antibiotic-associated side-effects of eradication therapy [67], while *Bifidobacterium animalis* and *Lactobacillus casei* did not showed similar results [68].

The major limiting factors of *H. pylori* treatments are bacterial resistance and low compliance for drug intake [69]. The resistance to clarithromycin among pediatric population was observed in 20% before therapy and 42% in treatment failure, and to metronidazole it was 23% and 35%, respectively. Interestingly, resistance was higher in boys and in subpopulation of children under 6 years of age, while almost no resistance was observed to amoxicillin [70]. On one hand it is suggested that the antibiotics given for upper respiratory diseases can be sometimes curative also for the *H. pylori* infection, but on other hand the abuse of antibiotics thought to be the major risk factor for the development of primary resistance.

CONCLUSIONS

As far as we can observed from the literature, the prevalence of *H. pylori* infection decreased in recent years worldwide. In addition, in 2011 a new therapeutic guideline was developed for the treatment of *H. pylori* infection in children population [56]. These are favorable tendencies in the story of *H. pylori*, however, our knowledge about the correct pathomechanism of the disease and of the complications developing in chronic state of the infection is still incomplete.

ACKNOWLEDGEMENTS

Declared None.

CONFLICT OF INTEREST

The author(s) confirm that this chapter content has no conflict of interest.

REFERENCES

[1] Homan M, Hojsak I, Kolaček S. *Helicobacter pylori* in pediatrics. Helicobacter. 2012; 17: 43-8.

[2] Talley NJ, Richter J. Nobel Prize in Medicine awarded to a Gastroenterologist in 2005. Am J Gastroenterol 2006; 101: 211.

[3] Moya DA, Crissinger KD. *Helicobacter pylori* persistence in children: distinguishing inadequate treatment, resistant organisms, and reinfection. Curr Gastroenterol Rep. 2012; 14: 236-42.

[4] Veres G, Pehlivanoglu E. *Helicobacter pylori* infection in pediatrics. Helicobacter. 2007; 12: 38-44.

[5] de Martel C, Parsonnet J. *Helicobacter pylori* infection and gender: a meta-analysis of population-based prevalence surveys. *Dig Dis Sci* 2006; 51: 2292-301.

[6] Nalbandian G, Kovats S. Understanding sex biases in immunity: Effects of estrogen on the differentiation and function of antigen-presenting cells. *Immunol Res* 2005; 31: 91-106.

[7] Morell V. Zeroing in on how hormones affect the immune system. *Science* 1995; 269: 773-775.

[8] Ozen A, Ertem D, Pehlivanoglu E. Natural history and symptomatology of *Helicobacter pylori* in childhood and factors determining the epidemiology of infection. *J Pediatr Gastroenterol Nutr* 2006; 42: 398-404.

[9] Jacobson K. The changing prevalence of *Helicobacter pylori* infection in Canadian children: should screening be performed in high-risk children? *Can J Gastroenterol* 2005; 19: 412-4.

[10] Halitim F, Vincent P, Michaud L, Kalach N, Guimber D, Boman F, Turck D, Gottard F. High rate of *Helicobacter pylori* reinfection in children and adolescents. *Helicobacter* 2006; 11: 168-72.

[11] Bury-Mone S, Kaakoush NO, Asencio C, Megraud F, Thibonnier M, De Reuse H, Mendz GL. Is *Helicobacter pylori* a true microaerophile? *Helicobacter*. 2006; 11: 296-303.

[12] Coticchia JM, Sugawa C, Tran VR, Gurrola J, Kowalski E, Carron MA. Presence and density of *Helicobacter pylori* biofilms in human gastric mucosa in patients with peptic ulcer disease. *J Gastrointest Surg* 2006; 10: 883-9.

[13] Shiota S, Watada M, Matsunari O, Iwatani S, Suzuki R, Yamaoka Y. *Helicobacter pylori* iceA, clinical outcomes, and correlation with cagA: a meta-analysis. PLoS ONE 2012;7:e30354

[14] Freire de Melo F, Rocha AM, Rocha GA, Pedroso SH, de Assis Batista S, Fonseca de Castro LP, *et al.* A regulatory instead of an IL-17 T response predominates in *Helicobacter pylori*-associated gastritis in children. Microbes Infect 2012;14:341–7.

[15] Oleastro M, Monterio L, Lehours P, Megraud F, Menard A. Identification of markers for *Helicobacter pylori* strains isolated from children with peptic ulcer disease by suppressive subtractive hybridization. *Infect Immun* 2006; 74: 4064-74.

[16] Chak E, Rutherford GW, Steinmaus C. The role of breast-feeding in the prevention of *Helicobacter pylori* infection: a systematic review. Clin Infect Dis. 2009; 48: 430-7.

[17] Rothenbacher D, Winkler M, Gonser T, Ader G, Brenner H. Role of infected parents in transmission of *Helicobacter pylori* to their children. *Pediatr Infect Dis* J 2002; 21: 674-9.

[18] Konno M, Fujii N, Yokota S. Five-year follow-up study of mother-to-child transmission of *Helicobacter pylori* infection detected by a random amplified polymorphic DNA fingerprinting method. *J Clin Microbiol* 2005; 43: 2246-50.

[19] Ito LS, Oba-Shinjo SM, Shinjo SK, Uno M, Marie SK, Hamajima N. Community-based familial study of *Helicobacter pylori* infection among healthy Japanese Brazilians. *Gastric Cancer* 2006; 9: 2008-16.

[20] Weyermann M, Adler G, Brenner H, Rothenbacher D. The mother as source of *Helicobacter pylori* infection. *Epidemiology* 2006; 17: 332-4.

[21] Lee JU, Jung K, Kim O. Absence of vertical transmission of *Helicobacter pylori* in an experimental murine model. *J Vet Sci* 2006; 7: 225-8.

[22] Stray-Pedersen A, Gaustad P, Stray-Pedersen B, Rognum TO. Detection rate of *Helicobacter pylori* stool antigen in newborn infants and small children. *J Perinat Med* 2007; 35: 155-8.

[23] Pacifico L, Anania C, Osborn JF, Ferraro F, Chiesa C. Consequences of *Helicobacter pylori* infection in children. World J Gastroenterol. 2010; 16: 5181-94.

[24] Kindermann A, Lopes AI. *Helicobacter pylori* infection in pediatrics. Helicobacter. 2009; 14: 52-7.

[25] Spee LA, Madderom MB, Pijpers M, van Leeuwen Y, Berger MY. Association between *Helicobacter pylori* and gastrointestinal symptoms in children. Pediatrics. 2010; 125: e651-69.

[26] Malaty HM, Abudayyeh S, Graham DY, Gilger MA, Rabeneck L, O'Malley K. A prospective study for the association of *Helicobacter pylori* infection to a multidimensional measure for recurrent abdominal pain in children. *Helicobacter* 2006; 11: 250-7.

[27] Tam YH, Chan KW, To KF, Cheung ST, Mou JW, Pang KK, Wong YS, Sihoe JD, Lee KH. Impact of pediatric Rome III criteria of functional dyspepsia on the diagnostic yield of upper endoscopy and predictors for a positive endoscopic finding. J Pediatr Gastroenterol Nutr. 2011;52:387–91.

[28] Buonavolonta R, Miele E, Russo D, Vecchione R, Staiano A. *Helicobacter pylori* chronic gastritis in children: to eradicate or not to eradicate? J Pediatr 2011;159:50–6.

[29] Sýkora J, Rowland M. *Helicobacter pylori* in pediatrics. Helicobacter. 2011; 16: 59-64.

[30] Dzierzanowska-Fangrat K, Nilsson I. Wozniak M, Jozwiak P, Rozynek E, Woynarowski M. Socha J, Ljungh A, Wadstrom T. Lack of an association between *Helicobacter* infection and autoimmune hepatitis in children. *Pol J Microbiol* 2006; 55: 157-9.

[31] Mourad-Baars P, Hussey S, Jones NL. *Helicobacter pylori* infection and childhood. Helicobacter. 2010; 15: 53-9.

[32] Lee A. Early influences and childhood development. Does helicobacter play a role? Helicobacter. 2007; 12: 69-74.

[33] Lionetti E, Indrio F, Pavone L, Borrelli G, Cavallo L, Francavilla R. Role of probiotics in pediatric patients with *Helicobacter pylori* infection: a comprehensive review of the literature. Helicobacter. 2010; 15: 79-87.

[34] Yilmaz T, Ceylan M, Akyion Y, Ozcakyr O, Gursel B. *Helicobacter pylori*: a possible association with otitis media with effusion. *Otolaryngol Head Neck Surg* 2006; 134: 772-7.

[35] Windle HJ, Kelleher D, Crabtree JE. Childhood *Helicobacter pylori* infection and growth impairment in developing countries. A vicious cycle? *Pediatric* 2007; 119: e754-9.

[36] Fialho AM, Brage AB, Queiroz DM, Rodrigues MN, Herbster ID, Braga LL. The association between *Helicobacter pylori* infection and height in children from an urban community in north-east Brazil. *Ann Trop Paediatr* 2007; 27: 55-61.

[37] Chimonas MA, Baggett HC, Parkinson AJ, Muth PT, Dunaway E, Gessner BD. Asymptomatic *Helicobacter pylori* infection and iron deficiency are not associated with decreased growth among Alaska Native children aged 7-11 years. *Helicobacter* 2006; 11: 159-67.

[38] Konturek PC, Czesnikiewicz-Guzik M. Bielanski W., Konturek SJ. Involvement of *Helicobacter pylori* infection in neuro-hormonal control of food intake. *J Physiol Pharmacol* 2006; 57 Suppl 5: 67-81.

[39] Plonka M, Konturek PC, Bielanski W, Pawlik T, Brozowski T, Konturek SJ. Relationship between ghrelin and *Helicobacter pylori* infection in Polish adult shepherds and their children. *Aliment Pharmacol Ther* 2006; 24 suppl 4: 160-8.

[40] Akcam M, Ozdem S, Yilmaz A, Gultekin M, Artan R. Serum ferritin, vitamin B[12] folate, and zinc levels in children infected with *Helicobacter pylori*. Dig Dis Sci 2007; 52: 405-10.

[41] Baysoy G, Ertem D, Ademoglu E, Kotiloglu E, Keskin S, Pehlivanoglu E. Gastric histopathology, iron status and iron deficiency anemia in children with *Helicobacter pylori* infection. *J Pediatr Gastroenterol Nutr* 2004; 38: 146-51.

[42] Ohno Y, Kosaka T, Muraoka I, Kanematsu T, Tsuru A, Kinoshita E, Moriuchi H. Remission of primary low-grade gastric lymphomas of the mucosa-associated lymphoid tissue type in immunocompromised pediatric patients. *World J Gastoenterol* 2006; 12: 2625-8.

[43] Guarner J, Kalach N, Elitsur Y, Koletzko S. *Helicobacter pylori* diagnostic tests in children: review of the literature from 1999 to 2009. Eur J Pediatr. 2010; 169: 15-25.

[44] Leal YA, Flores LL, Fuentes-Panana EM, Cedillo-Rivera R, Torres J. 13C-urea breath test for the diagnosis of *Helicobacter pylori* infection in children: a systematic review and meta-analysis. Helicobacter 2011; 16: 327–37.

[45] Megraud F; European Paediatric Task Force on *Helicobacter pylori*. Comparison of non-invasive tests to detect *Helicobacter pylori* infection in children and adolescents: results of a multicenter European study. *J Pediatr* 2005;146:198-203

[46] Frenck RW Jr, Fathy HM, Sherif M, Mohran Z, El Mohammedy H, Francis W, Rockabrand D, Mounir BI, Rozmajzl P, Frierson HF. Sensitivity and specificity of various test for the diagnosis of *Helicobacter pylori* in Egyptian children. *Pediatrics* 2006; 118: e1195-202.

[47] Dondi E, Rapa A, Boldorini R, Fonio P. Zanetta S, Oderda G. High accuracy of noninvasive tests to diagnose *Helicobacter pylori* infection in very young children. *J Pediatr* 2006; 149: 817-21.

[48] Leal YA, Cedillo-Rivera R, Simon JA, Velazquez JR, Flores LL, Torres J. Utility of stool sample-based tests for the diagnosis of *Helicobacter pylori* infection in children. J Pediatr Gastroenterol Nutr. 2011;52:718–28.

[49] Yang YJ, Sheu BS, Lee SC. Wu JJ. More economic 25 mg 13C-urea breath test can be effective in detecting primary *Helicobacter pylori* infection in children. *J Gastroenterol Hepatol* 2007; 22: 335-9.

[50] Jolley CD, Wagner DA. Comparison of the 13C-urea blood test to histology and rapid urease testing in the diagnosis of *Helicobacter pylori* infection in children. *J Pediatr Gastroenterol Nutr* 2007; 44: 68-70.

[51] Pelerito A, Oleastro M. Lopes AI, Ramalho P, Cabral J, Monteriro L. Evaluation of rapid test Assure *Helicobacter pylori* for diagnosis of *H. pylori* in pediatric population. *J Microbiol Methods* 2006; 66: 331-5.

[52] Kolho KL, Klemola T, Koivusalo A, Rautelin H. Stool antigen tests for the detection of *Helicobacter pylori* in children. *Diagn Microbiol Infect Dis* 2006; 55: 269-73.

[53] Koivusalo AI, Pakarinen MP, Kolho KL. Is GastroPanel serum assay useful in the diagnosis of *Helicobacter pylori* infection and associated gastritis in children? *Diagn Microbiol Infect Dis* 2007; 57: 35-8.

[54] Muhsen K, Athamma A, Athamma M, Spungin-Bialik A, Cohen D. Evaluation of urine-based enzyme-linked immunosorbent assay test for the detection of *Helicobacter pylori* infection among 3- to 5-year-old Israeli Arab healthy children. *J Pediatr Gasroenterol Nutr* 2006; 43: 398-401.

[55] Chiesa C, Anania C, Pacifico L, Olivero G, Osborn JF. *Helicobacter pylori* therapy in children: a focus on proton pump inhibitors. Chemotherapy. 2011; 57: 85-93.

[56] Kolctzko S, Jones NL, Goodman KJ, Gold B, Rowland M, Cadranel S, Chong S, Colletti RB, Casswall T, Elitsur Y, Guarner J, Kalach N, Madrazo A, Megraud F, Oderda G; H *pylori* Working Groups of ESPGHAN and NASPGHAN. Evidence-based guidelines from ESPGHAN and NASPGHAN for *Helicobacter pylori* infection in children. J Pediatr Gastroenterol Nutr. 2011; 53: 230-43.

[57] Horvath A, Dziechciarz P, Szajewska H. Meta-analysis: sequential therapy for *Helicobacter pylori* eradication in children. Aliment Pharmacol Ther. 2012; 36: 534-41.

[58] Khurana R, Fischach L, Chiba N, VAN Zanten SV, Sherman PM, George BA, Goodman KJ, Gold BD. Meta-analysis: *Helicobacter pylori* eradication treatment efficacy in children. *Aliment Pharmacol Ther* 2007; 25: 523-36.

[59] Scaletsky IC, Aranda KR, Garcia GT, Goncalves ME, Cardoso SR, Iriya K, *et al.* Application of real-time PCR stool assay for *Helicobacter pylori* detection and clarithromycin susceptibility testing in Brazilian children. Helicobacter 2011;16:311–5.

[60] Bourke B, Ceponis P, Chiba N, Czinn S, Ferraro R, Fischbach L, Gold B, Hyunh H, Jacobson K, Jones NL, Koletzko S, Lebel S, Moayyedi P, Ridell R, Sherman P, van Zanten S, Beck I, Best L,

Boland M, Bursey F, Chaun H, Cooper G, Craig B, Creuzenet C, Critch J, Govender K, Hasall E, Kaplan A, Keelan M, Noad G, Robertson M, Smith L, Stein M, Taylor D, Walters T, Persaud R, Whitaker S, Woodland R; Canadian *Helicobacter* Study Group, Canadian *Helidobacter* Study Group Consensus Conference: Update on the approach to *Helicobacter pylori* infection in children and adolescents-an evidence-based evaluation. *Can J Gastroenterol* 2005; 19: 399-408.

[61] Oderda G, Shcherbakov P, Bontems P, Urruzuno P, Romano C, Gottrand F, Gomez MJ, Ravelli a, Gandullia P, Roma E, Candranel S, De Giacomo C, Canani RB, Rutigliano v, Pehlivanoglu E, Kalach N, roggero P, Celinska-Cedro D, Drumm B, Casswall T, Ashorn M, Arvenitakis SN; European Pediatric Task Force on *Helicobacter pylori*. Results from the pediatric European register for treatment of *Helicobacter pylori* [PERTH]. Helicobacter 2007; 12: 150-6.

[62] Tam YH, Yeung CK, Lee KH. Seven-day is more effective than 4-day ranitidine bismuth citrate-based triple therapy in eradication of *Helicobacter pylori* in children: a prospective randomized study. *Aliment Pharmacol Ther* 2006; 24: 81-6.

[63] Bahremand S, Nematollahi LR, Fourutan H, Tirgari F, Nouripour S, Mir E, Aghakhani S. Evaluation of triple and quadruple *Helicobacter pylori* eradication therapies in Iranian children: randomized clinical trial. *Eur J Gastroenterol Hepatol* 2006; 18: 511-4.

[64] Arenz T, Antos D, Russmann H, Alberer M, Buderus S, Kappler M, Koletzko S. Esomeprazole-based 1-week triple therapy directed by susceptibility testing for eradication of *Helicobacter pylori* infection in children. *J Pediatr Gastroenterol Nutr* 2006; 43: 180-4.

[65] Cadranel S, Bontemps P, Van Biervliet S, Alliet P, Lauvau D, Vandenhoven G, Vandenplass Y. Improvement of the eradication rate of *Helicobacter pylori* gastritis in children is by adjuction of omeprazole to a dual antibiotherapy. *Acta Paediatr* 2007; 96: 82-6.

[66] Kawakami E, Machado RS, Ogata K, Langner M, Fukushima E, Carelli AP, Bonucci VC, Patricio FR. Furazolidone-based triple therapy for *H. pylori* gastritis in children. *World J Gasrtroenterol* 2006; 12: 5544-9.

[67] Lionetti E, Miniello VL, Castellaneta SP, Magista AM, de Canio A, Maurogiovanni G, Ierardi E, Cavallo L, Francavilla R. *Lactobacillus reuteri* therapy to reduce side-effects during anti-*Helicobacter pylori* treatment in children: a randomized placebo controlled trial. *Aliment Pharmacol Ther* 2006; 24: 1461-8.

[68] Goldman CG, Barrado DA, Balcarce N, Rue EC, Oshiro M, Calcagno ML, Janjetic M, Fuda J, Weill R, Salgueiro MJ, Valencia ME, Zubillaga MB, Boccio JR, Effect of a probiotic food as an adjuvant to triple therapy for eradication of *Helicobacter pylori* infection in children. *Nutrition* 2006; 22: 984-8.

[69] Horvitz G, Gold BD. Gastroduodenal diseases of childhood. *Curr Opin Gastroenterol* 2006; 22: 632-40.

[70] Koletzko S, Richy F, Bonems P, Crone J, Kalach N, Monteiro ML, Gottrand F, Celinska-Cedro D, Roma-Giannikou E, Orderda G, Kolacek S, Urruzuno P, Martizen-Gomez MJ, Casswall T, Ashorn M, Bodanszky H, Megraud F. Prospective multicentre study on antibiotic resistance of *Helicobacter pylori* strains obtained from children living in Europe. *Gut* 2006; 55: 1711-6.

Send Orders for Reprints to reprints@benthamscience.net
Helicobacter Pylori: A Worldwide Perspective 2014, 2014, 411-428

CHAPTER 18

Antibiotic Resistance of *Helicobacter pylori*: Worldwide Prevalence, Mechanisms and Impact on Therapy

Vincenzo de Francesco*

University of Foggia, Department of Medical Sciences, Section of Gastroenterology, Foggia, Italy

Abstract: *H. pylori* antibiotic resistance is the main factor affecting the efficacy of the current *H. pylori* eradicating therapies. Epidemiological aspects and different resistance mechanisms (point mutations, redox intracellular potential, pump efflux systems, membrane permeability) to clarithromycin, metronidazole, quinolones, amoxicillin and tetracycline, are accurately detailed on the **basis** of the most recent data available from the literature. In addition, the impact of resistance toward each antibiotic on efficacy of current therapies is thoroughly described.

Keywords: *Helicobacter pylori*, epidemiology, therapy, eradication, antibiotic, resistance, clarithromycin, metronidazole, amoxicillin, levofloxacin, tetracycline, rifabutin, quinolones, point mutation, efflux pump.

EPIDEMIOLOGY

H. pylori treatment still remains a challenge for physicians since no current first-line therapies is able to cure the infection in all treated patients. Although different factors may simultaneously act in reducing therapeutic efficacy in the same patient, bacterial antibiotic resistance plays the more relevant role [1]. Clarithromycin, metronidazole, amoxicillin, levofloxacin, and tetracycline are the antibiotics included in current therapeutic regimens for *H. pylori* infection. However, prevalence of both primary clarithromycin and metronidazole resistance has increased substantially in recent years, with a parallel reduction of efficacy of standard therapies [2]. Indeed, two meta-analyses demonstrated a risk of treatment failure of 55% and of 37% in presence of clarithromycin and metronidazole resistant strains, respectively, following standard therapies [3, 4]. Similarly, the

***Address correspondence to Vincenzo de Francesco:** University of Foggia, Department of Medical Sciences, Section of Gastroenterology, Foggia, Italy; Tel: +39-0881-650220; Fax: +39-0881-733776; E-mail: vdefrancesco@alice.it resistance toward quinolones, restrictively used in the past decades in second line therapies, is increasing in developed countries because of their more extensive use [5]. On the contrary, a very highly variable - but generally low- worldwide resistance rate against either amoxicillin or tetracycline has been observed.

On this basis, the surveillance of antibiotic resistance appears to be relevant in order to address local and national therapeutic strategies. Indeed, a tailored therapy based on prevalence of primary antibiotic resistance may be potentially chosen by improving the knowledge of both epidemiological and microbiological aspects of antibiotic resistance.

Primary Clarithromycin Resistance

Since clarithromycin is one of the most powerful antibiotic currently available for *H. pylori* infection [6,7], the knowledge of actual prevalence of resistance towards this drug is of pivotal relevance for clinical practice.

A recent systematic review, including 31 studies, with 11697 patients enrolled from 1993 to 2009, reveals an increasing trend for clarithromycin resistance from Europe (11.1%), to Asia (18.9%), and America (29.3%) [8]. Among the European countries, the highest resistance was reported in Spain (49.2%) [9], whilst the lowest in Sweden (1.5%) [10] and in The Netherlands (0.8%) [11].

Besides differences between continental areas, a significant increase in the resistance rate was worldwide observed over long period. In an Italian study, recruiting patients in two different periods (1989-90 and 2004-2005), clarithromycin resistance increased from 10.2% to 21.3%. The increase was even more evident in females and in patients with non-ulcer dyspepsia [12], confirming previous observations [13]. The higher resistance in females has been related to a cross resistance between clarithromycin and clindamycin which is largely used in bacterial vaginitis [14]. In contrast, the resistance rate did not increase with patient age [8, 13]. In Portugal, resistance values of > 30% were constantly observed over a 10 year period (2000-2009) [15].

In Asian countries, a high clarithromycin resistance rate was detected in Japan (40.7%) [16] whilst such a resistance was not detected in Malaysia (0.0%) [17].

The resistant rates significantly increase from 2000 to 2009 in Shanghai.(8.6% to 20.7%) [18].

In North America, a very high resistance rate (>30%) was observed in Alaska between 1999-2003 and between 2000-2008 [19, 20].

Both consumption in general population and duration of marketing are considered the main factors involved in different clarithromycin resistance rates reported in diverse geographic areas. In detail, each additional course of clarithromycin for different diseases has been associated with a 50% increase in the risk of *H. pylori* primary resistance [14, 21-23].

Several epidemiological studies clarified that point mutations in the peptidyltransferase region encoded in domain V of the *H. pylori* 23S ribosomal RNA are responsible of resistance. These researchers found that three mutate genotypes, *i.e.* A2143G, A2142G, A2142C, are detectable in more than 90% of resistant bacterial strains in Western countries [24, 25] whilst other point mutations, such as A2115G, G2141A, T2117C, and T2182C, T2289C, G224A, C2245T, C2611A, have been inconstantly detected in presence of clarithromycin resistance [26].

Primary Metronidazole Resistance

Metronidalole is widely used for *H. pylori* eradication. A decreasing trend for primary metronidazole resistance has been observed from Africa (92.4%) to America (44.1%), Asia (37.1%) and to Europe (17.0%) [8].

Among European **countries,** the lowest metronidazole resistance was observed in Sweden (14.4%) and The Netherlands (14.4%) [10,11], the highest being detected in Spain (45.1%) [27].

In Asia, metronidazole resistance rate was very high in Malaysia (75.5%) [17] and low in Japan (14.7%) [16]. In Africa, highest rates of resistance were observed in Cameroon, (93.2%) and in Senegal (90.%) [28, 29].

Several evidences underline the relevance of the consumption of metronidazole as a risk factor of resistance. Indeed each additional course of metronidazole was associated with a 60% increase in the risk of primary resistance in *H. pylori* strains [14]. In the last decade a clear preference in the management of the *H. pylori* infection for amoxicillin-clarithromycin-based first line therapies has determined a significant restriction of metronidazole use and a decrease of resistance in diverse developed countries. In contrast, persistent large application of metronidazole-based treatments to cure parasitic and gynaecologic infections could explain higher resistance rates in developing countries and in female patients, respectively [23].

Primary Amoxicillin Resistance

In European countries, a very low amoxicillin resistance rate has been constantly reported with values ranging from 0 in Sweden [10] and in Poland [30] to 1.4% in Spain [27]. Discordant data were reported in two African studies. Indeed, amoxicillin resistance was absent in Senegal [29] whilst it appears astonishingly high in Cameroon (85.6%) [28]. In Asian countries, resistance rates ranging from 8.8% in Korea, to 36.1% in Taiwan have been detected [31, 32]. A single study found a 2.2% amoxicillin resistance prevalence in Alaska [19]. Methodological differences in epidemiological studies can explain high variability of resistance rates in extra-European countries. Gender and previous consumption of amoxicillin did not seem to favour resistance onset [8, 14].

Primary Levofloxacin Resistance

Higher prevalence of quinolones resistance was reported in Europe (24.1%) as compared to Asia (11.6%) and Africa where it is virtually absent. The constant increase of resistance in different European countries is most likely related to wide use of levofloxacin in general population, whilst such an expensive drug in not used in developing countries [3, 5, 23]. In Asia, different values between countries were detected, the resistance rate being 14.9% in Japan [33] and 2.6% in Hong Kong [34].

Female gender, age (from 40 to 64 years) and number of previous treatments for other diseases were significantly correlated with a higher risk of primary resistance of *H. pylori* strains to levofloxacine [14].

Primary Tetracycline Resistance

Overall resistance rates did not significantly differ among Europe (2.1%), Asia (2.4%), and America (2.7%), while significantly higher values were found in Africa (43.9%).

Tetracycline resistance occurs similarly in male and female [8]. The previous use of tetracycline for other diseases was not significantly associated with resistance in *H. pylori* [5].

Primary Rifabutin Resistance

In the last seven years rifabutin resistance was tested in only three studies, the resistance rates being1.4% in Germany [5], 6.6% in England [35] and 0.24% in Japan [36]. Previous rifampin treatment for pulmonary tuberculosis is recognized as the main risk factor for rifabutin resistance.

Primary Multiple Antibiotic Resistance

Multiple-drug resistance has been worldwide reported, the rate being 8.3% in Asia, 15% in America and 8.9% in Europe [8]. Among European countries, the lowest value in Sweden (0.6%) [10] and the highest value in Germany (15.1%) [37] was observed. In Belgium, a detailed study has shown a significant increasing trend, with a multidrug-resistance rising from 22.2% to 39.8% for metronidazole-clarithromycin dual resistance, from 13.6% to 20.5% for levofloxacin-clarithromycin dual resistance, from 6.3% to 13% for clarithromycin-levofloxacin-metronidazole triple resistance, going from 2003 to 2009 [23].

MECHANISMS OF RESISTANCE

Clarithromycin

The bacteriostatic activity of clarithromycin depends on its capacity to inhibit the protein synthesis by binding to the 50S bacterial ribosomal subunit. Clarithromycin remains an available, powerful antibiotic against *H. pylori*, with very low minimal inhibitor concentrations (MICs) in comparison to the other currently used compounds [26].

Point mutations in the peptidyltransferase region encoded in domain V of 23S rRNA of the 50S bacterial ribosomal subunit are mainly responsible for clarithromycin resistance. These mutations are able to inhibit the binding between clarithromycin and the ribosomal subunit, thus preventing the inhibition of protein synthesis. The transition adenine to guanine in 2143 and 2142 positions of rRNA, and the substitution of adenine with cytosine in 2142 position are more frequent point mutation in resistant strains from developed countries [6, 38, 39]. In detail, the mutation at position 2143 seems to be associated with different resistance levels rather than with a behavior on/off, with MIC values widely ranging from 0.016 to 256 mg/L. Conversely, the mutations at position 2142 are associated with lower MIC values, close to 64 mg/L [6, 40-43].

Another relevant mechanism for clarithromycin resistance depend on the Efflux Pump Systems. These complex systems are able to excrete and to reduce intracellular concentrations of several compounds and drugs reducing their effect on bacterial metabolism. Among the five conserved families of drug efflux system the Resistance-Nodulation-cell Division (RND family) is responsible of the intrinsic clarithromycin resistance in different bacterial species [44].

Of note, this efflux pump system may either induce clarithromycin resistance *de novo* by reducing its intracellular concentration, or reinforce resistance in the presence of bacterial point mutations. Based on these findings, it has been hypothesized that the administration of specific Efflux Pumps Inhibitors (EPI) could improve the efficacy of the clarithromycin-based therapies by increasing antibiotic intracellular entrapment. In addition, there is evidence for a significant interaction between the RND efflux pump system and Proton Pump Inhibitors (PPIs) due to structural PPI-analogies with EPI drugs. Besides the profound gastric acid inhibition, PPIs may inhibit the activity of bacterial efflux pumps similarly to EPI drugs. Of note, MIC values of clarithromycin, as well as of metronidazole, amoxicillin, and furazolidone, has been found to be 4-fold and 3-fold lower in *H. pylori* multi-resistant strains by using rabeprazole and pantoprazole, respectively, whilst no significant effect was observed with omeprazole, esomeprazole and lansoprazole [45].

Metronidazole

Metronidazole is an inactive pro-drug and its activation requires a reaction of reduction of nitro-groups to anionic radicals, nitroso-derivates and hydroxylamines which are able to damage the DNA-helicoidal. The reaction of reduction is strongly affected by the intracellular redox potential of components of electron transport chain which needs to be effectively negative. In detail, electrons are produced by the Pyruvate Oxido Reductase complex (POR) and are transferred to either ferrodoxin or flavodoxin which, in turn, reduce other molecules as metronidazole. This process is particularly active in anaerobe or microaereophilic species, which are highly susceptible to metronidazole [26, 46].

Metronidazole resistance depends on the capacity to maintain the antibiotic in an inactive, not reduced form by the interruption of electron transport chain and/or by the loss of intracellular negative redox potential. In experimental conditions the essential role of the intracellular potential in the activation of metronidazole is sustained by finding that the pre-exposure to anaerobic conditions is associated with restoration of metronidazole susceptibility in resistant strains.

Different mutational events that inactivate the *rdxA* gene, encoding for an oxygen insensitive NADPH nitro-reductase, are identified as the main mechanism which confers *H. pylori* resistance under real microaerophilic/anaerobe conditions in. In susceptible strains, NADPH nitro-reductase reduces several compounds, including metronidazole, by two electrons transfer and generating toxic nitro-derivates for DNA. In resistant strains, this enzyme is inactive and the drug can not be reduced into the active form. Rare cases of metronidazole resistant strains in the absence of *rdxA* mutations have been attributed to mutations involving genes outside of the *rdxA* which can, in turn, down-modulate its expression [47, 48]. The inactivation of other reductases, encoded by genes such *frxA* (for NADPH flavin oxidoreductase) and *frxB* (for ferrodoxin-like enzymes) seem reinforce bacterial resistance exclusively in the presence of *rdxA* gene mutations [49, 50].

Besides inactive reductases, active transport systems, named Outer membrane Efflux Proteins (OEP), are recognized as a relevant factor of resistance by interacting with several intracellular translocases and reducing intracellular metronidazole concentrations. Indeed, the inactivation of 2 OEPs (HP0605 and HP0971) in a double-knockout mutant strain significantly increased susceptibility to metronidazole [51].

Finally, *Fur* regulatory genes which controls transcription of least dozens genes in response to iron availability, acidity and oxidative stress were involved in *H. pylori* metronidazole resistance occurrence. *Fur* gene mutations affect susceptibility to metronidazole by altering the expression "at cascade" of some genes that control cellular redox potential or by eliminating toxic **active** metronidazole compounds [52].

Amoxicillin

Amoxicillin is a β-lactam antibiotic constantly included in *H. pylori* therapies because of a very low occurrence of resistance [53]. The resistance of *H. pylori* strains towards amoxicillin is quite complex. Besides a stable amoxicillin resistant strains – with a MIC of 8 mg/L – data would indicate the possibility of an instable resistance. Indeed, the resistance may be lost upon freezing the culture at -80 °C [54]. Such unusual condition has been defined as 'amoxicillin tolerance' rather than resistance.

Amoxicillin acts by interfering with the synthesis of the peptidoglycans of the bacterial wall by mean a glycosyl transferase-acyl transpeptidase activity that block transporters named Penicillin Binding Proteins (PBP). These enzymes are involved in the synthesis of the peptidoglycan layer of the bacterial wall by a glycosyl transferase-acyl transpeptidase activity. PBP1, PBP2, PBP3 are reported as high molecular weight PBPs iso-enzymes whilst PBP4 is reported as low molecular weight iso-enzyme. The β-lactam binding to PBPs motifs is able to make a bactericidal effect by the interruption and destruction of the peptidoglycan layer, as well as inducing an osmotic shock.

Multiple point mutations in *pbp1* gene are well-known as the major mechanism of amoxicillin resistance, leading to a loss of affinity between amoxicillin and PBP-transpeptidase [55, 56].

In detail the substitution of Asn_{562} aminoacid with a Tyr residue in proximity to KTG motif of PBP1 is able to confer high resistance to all strains *"in vitro"* and is considered the main mutation conferring resistance. Other substitutions in PBP1, inconstantly associated to Asn_{562}-Tyr, seem contribute to increase MIC values of the resistant strains similarly to point mutations in PBP2, in PBP3 and PBP4 [55-

57]. Surprisingly, production of β-lactamase – *i.e.* the main mechanism of penicillin resistance in other bacteria – has been consistently found to be inactive in *H. pylori* [55, 56].

Interestingly, *H. pylori* resistant strains obtained by transformation *in vitro* from susceptible naive strains, exhibit MIC values 5-10 fold lower than naïve resistant strains [56], suggesting that different mechanisms probably interact in conferring the high levels observed in natural antibiotic resistance.

The variable fluidity of outer bacterial membrane seems contribute to not specific resistance by limiting the intracellular diffusion of several small lipophilic molecules. In detail "porin" narrow channels, encoded in *H. pylori* by *hopB* and *hopC* genes, regulate the penetration of small solutes and of several drugs. Point mutations in *hopB* and deletion in *hopC* genes can reduce amoxicillin penetration sustaining conferring variable resistance levels or reinforcing the amoxicillin resistance in presence of *pbp* point mutations [58]. In addition, significant alterations of permeability are likely associated to expression of genes involved in import/export/binding of metals [59].

On the other hand, the efflux pump systems seem play a marginal role in amoxicillin resistance because of a very low hydrophobicity of this drug, which is a necessary requisite for substrates of multidrug efflux pumps [60].

Fluoroquonolones

Fluroquinolones exert a dose-dependent bactericide effect by binding the subunit A of DNA gyrase (topoisomerase II), an essential enzyme for the maintenance of DNA helicoidal structure. In susceptible strains, levofloxacin stops DNA and, at high doses, even RNA synthesis. Surprisingly, when the dose is further increased, quinolones become bacteriostatic agents.

H. pylori resistance toward quinolones involves the *gyrA* gene in a specific genomic region, named Quinolones Resistance-Determining Region (QRDR). Point mutations of this gene preclude binding between the antibiotic and the enzyme, conferring antibiotic bacterial resistance [26, 61]. Mutations in both 91 (Asp91Gly, Asn, Ala, or Tyr) and 87 (Asn87Lys) position have been observed in the 100% of levofloxacin resistant isolates [62]. A new mutation consisting in the substitution of Asn with Tyr in position 87 of *gyrA* has been also identified. Other rare mutations in *gyrA* gene (Asp86Asn in position 86; Ala88Valin in 88 position) or in *gyrB* gene seem contribute to resistance exclusively in presence of 87 and 91 *gyrA* positions.

More recently the complete sequencing of the genome of two strains – *i.e.,* the 26695 and the J99 demonstrated that an aminoacidic polymorphism in the codon 87 of *gyrA* genes is significantly involved in *H. pylori* quinolones resistance [61].

Tetracycline

Tetracycline acts as bacteriostatic against either Gram positive or Gram negative species by inhibiting codon-anticodon link at level of 30S ribosomal subunit and blocking the attachment of aminoacyl-tRNA to the acceptor site. Tetracycline-ribosome interaction occurs at level of 2–6 possible sites at high affinity and at level of multiple likely hundreds sites at low affinity. Point mutations involving 30S ribosomal subunit are considered mostly responsible in resistance occurrence by reducing antibiotic-ribosome affinity [63].

Simultaneous triple point mutations from 965 to 967 position in the loop of helix 31of 30S ribosomal subunit, the essential part of primary acceptor site (site P), is recognized as the major mechanism of tetracycline resistance. The levels of resistance are proportional to the number of changes in the AGA 965-967 triplet. Single and double point mutations are associate with low and intermediate MIC values, whilst loss of affinity of 52% and high resistance levels are observed in the presence of a complete triple substitution from AGA to TTC [64, 65]. Mutations in Tet-4 site, in proximity of primary P site, can act as secondary mechanism of resistance. In particular, a deletion of G942 in Tet-4 site is observed in all resistant strains. Since the affinity of tetracycline for naive Tet-4 site is significantly lower than those for primary P site, the loss of affinity due to a deletion of G492 can play a subsidiary role for resistance [66].

Besides point mutations at ribosomal level, other accessory mechanisms appeared involved in resistance onset.

Indeed, further reduction of affinity between antibiotic and the ribosomal site may be acquired by chemical modifications of tetracycline by a bacterial oxidoreductase NADP-dependent [63]. In addition, the soluble protein Tet(O) is able to remove the antibiotic from ribosome preventing the arrest of protein synthesis and the bacteriostatic effect [67]. A decreased membrane permeability and a reduced intracellular accumulation of tetracycline have been observed in tetracycline resistant strains which are also cross-resistant to amoxicillin. Finally, the possible role of a specific tetracycline efflux pumps systems has been investigated with discordant evidences [66, 68].

Rifabutin

Rifabutin shows good *in vitro* activity against *H. pylori*, with the lowest minimal inhibitor concentrations (MICs) in comparison to the other molecules (69). Rifabutin exerts bactericide activity inhibiting the β-subunit of *H. pylori* DNA-dependent RNA polymerase, encoded by the *rpoB* gene. Recently the resistance to rifabutin has been related to amino acid exchanges in codons 524–545 or in codon 585 of the *rpoB* gene by reducing antibiotic affinity for RNA polymerase binding site [69].

IMPACT ON THERAPY SUCCESS

Undeniably antibiotic resistance is the main factor affecting efficacy of current treatment for *H. pylori* infection. Current European guidelines on *H. pylori* management suggest that first-line therapy should be tailored according to both clarithromycin and metronidazole resistance in each specific country since these antibiotics remain key drugs for current therapies [53]. There is evidence that primary clarithromycin resistance reduces by 55% and metronidazole resistance by 38% the efficacy of standard triple therapies [3].

Different PCR-based techniques for assessment the involvement of resistant mutate strains allowed new evidences.

The occurrence of point mutations in peptidyltransferase region may be considered a spontaneous process and the identification of novel *H. pylori* resistant genotypes shows a increasing trend. Highly variable MIC values are associated to different point mutations. Variable concordance in assessment of clarithromycin resistance between traditional culture-dependent methods and biomolecular techniques may be found, the κ values ranging from 70% to 100% [70, 71]. Discordance is attributed to higher sensitivity of PCR-based techniques in assessing even minimal traces of resistant strains in heteroresistant status (mixture of resistant and susceptible strains) [58]. The high sensitivity of the biomolecular methods does not seem to meaningfully affect therapeutic outcome. Genotypic resistance affects eradication rates only when it reaches phenotypic expression in the culture. This requisite occurs when a specific point mutations, namely A2143G, is involved in the clarithromycin resistance.

The lower impact of metronidazole as compared clarithromycin resistance on therapeutic out come may depend on the observation that metronidazole resistance could be overcome, at least partially, by an efficacious inhibition of gastric acid secretion or by increasing the dose/duration of treatment. In two studies the eradication rate increased from 76% to 91% and from 43% to 76% when a PPI is added [72, 73] and using 800 mg instead of 400 mg when the dosage passes from 400 mg to 800 mg (54% *vs.* 75%) [74]. In contrast, drug administration twice or three times daily did not overcome metronidazole resistance [75]. Similarly to clarithromycin, metronidazole exerts acceptable bactericide activity *in vivo* also in strains which are resistant in culture. This effect might also be explained by microenvironmental conditions within the gastric mucosa (such as oxygen tension and redox potential) which are known to influence the antibiotic activation in reduced form [46]. On the basis of this discordance, metronidazole-based therapies are still considered by current guidelines [53].

The effect of primary quinolone resistance on the efficacy of levofloxacin-containing first-line therapy has been poorly investigated. Following a first-line therapy failure, a levofloxacin-amoxicillin triple therapy achieved a 75.5% eradication rate in levofloxacin susceptible strains and in 33.3%-55.5% in resistant strains [76, 77]. Similarly, by using moxifloxacin as first line therapy, the eradication rates were 98% and 66% in susceptible and resistant strains, respectively. Resistance to tetracycline remained very low, suggesting that this agent can be still included in the management of *H. pylori* infection [14]. In contrast remarkable concerns regard the use of rifabutin. In fact high treatment costs, relevance of associated adverse side-effects (mainly myelotoxicity) and concrete risks to increase *M. tuberculosis* resistance in population with high prevalence of tuberculosis induce to use this antibiotic with extreme caution and exclusively in refractory *H. pylori* infection [69].

ACKNOWLEDGEMENTS

Dr. Borelli Grazia Maria, biologist doctor, for microbiological assistance and for the linguistic assistance in English.

CONFLICT OF INTEREST

The author(s) confirm that this chapter content has no conflict of interest.

REFERENCES

[1] Vakil N, Megraud F. Eradication therapy for *Helicobacter pylori.* Gastroenterology 2007; 133: 985–1001.

[2] Graham DY, Fischbach L. *Helicobacter pylori* treatment in the era of increasing antibiotic resistance.Gut 2010; 59: 1143-53.

[3] Dore, M. P., G. Leandro, G. Realdi, A. R. Sepulveda, and D. Y. Graham. Effect of pretreatment antibiotic resistance to metronidazole and clarithromycin on outcome of *Helicobacter pylori* therapy: a meta-analytical approach. Dig Dis Sci 2000; 45:68–7.

[4] Van der Wouden, E. J., J. C. Thijs, A. A. Van Zwet, W. J. Sluiter, and J. H. Kleibeuker. The influence of *in vitro* nitroimidazole resistance on the efficacy of nitroimidazole-containing anti-*Helicobacter pylori* regimens: a meta-analysis. Am J Gastroenterol 1999; 94:1751–59.

[5] Glocker, E., Stueger, H.P. and Kist, M. Quinolone resistance in *Helicobacter pylori* isolates in Germany. Antimicrob Agents Chemother 2007; 51: 346-49.

[6] Mégraud F, Lehours P. *Helicobacter pylori* detection and antimicrobial susceptibility testing. Clin Microbiol Rev. 2007; 20: 280-322.

[7] Elviss NC, Owen RJ, Breathnach A, Palmer C, Shetty N. *Helicobacter pylori* antibiotic-resistance patterns and risk factors in adult dyspeptic patients from ethnically diverse populations in central and south London during 2000. J Med Microbiol. 2005; 54: 567-74.

[8] De Francesco V, Giorgio F, Hassan C, *et al.* Worldwide *H. pylori* antibiotic resistance: a systematic review. J Gastrointestin Liver Dis. 2010; 19: 409-14.

[9] Agudo S, Alarcón T, Cibrelus L, Urruzuno P, Martínez M, López-Brea M. High percentage of clarithromycin and metronidazole resistance in *Helicobacter pylori* clinical isolates obtained from Spanish children. Rev Esp Quimioter 2009; 22: 88–92.

[10] Storskrubb T, Aro P, Ronkainen J, *et al.* Antimicrobial susceptibility of *Helicobacter pylori* strains in a random adult Swedish population. Helicobacter 2006; 11: 224–30.

[11] Janssen MJ, Hendrikse L, de Boer SY, *et al. Helicobacter pylori* antibiotic resistance in a Dutch region: trends over time. Neth J Med 2006; 64: 191–95.

[12] De Francesco V, Margiotta M, Zullo A, *et al.* Prevalence of primary clarithromycin resistance in *Helicobacter pylori* strains over a 15 year period in Italy. J Antimicrob Chemother. 2007; 59: 783-5.

[13] Kist M, Glocker E, Wolf B, *et al.* Resi-Net-A nationwide German sentinel study on the development and risk factors of antimicrobial resistance in *Helicobacter pylori.* Helicobacter 2003; 8: 465.

[14] McNulty CA, Lasseter G, Shaw I, *et al.* Is *Helicobacter pylori* antibiotic resistance surveillance needed and how can it be delivered? Aliment Pharmacol Ther. 2012; 35:1221-30.

[15] Oleastro M, Cabral J, Ramalho PM, *et al.* Primary antibiotic resistance of *Helicobacter pylori* strains isolated from Portuguese children: a prospective multicentre study over a 10 year period. J Antimicrob Chemother. 2011; 66: 2308-11.

[16] Kato S. *Helicobacter pylori* eradication therapy in children. Nippon Rinsho 2009; 67: 2311–16.

[17] Goh KL, Navaratnam P. High *Helicobacter pylori* resistance to metronidazole but zero or low resistance to clarithromycin, levofloxacin, and other antibiotics in Malaysia. Helicobacter. 2011; 16: 241-5.

[18] Sun QJ, Liang X, Zheng Q, *et al.* Resistance of *Helicobacter pylori* to antibiotics from 2000 to 2009 in Shanghai. World J Gastroenterol. 2010; 16: 5118-21.

[19] Bruce MG, Bruden DL, McMahon BJ, *et al.* Alaska sentinel surveillance for antimicrobial resistance in *Helicobacter pylori* isolates from Alaska native persons, 1999-2003. Helicobacter 2006; 11: 581–8.

[20] Tveit AH, Bruce MG, Bruden DL, *et al.* Alaska sentinel surveillance study of *Helicobacter pylori* isolates from Alaska Native persons from 2000 to 2008. J Clin Microbiol. 2011; 49: 3638-43

[21] Debets-Ossenkopp YJ, Herscheid AJ, Pot RG, Kuipers EJ, Kusters JG, Vandenbroucke-Grauls CM. Prevalence of *Helicobacter pylori* resistance to metronidazole, clarithromycin, amoxycillin, tetracycline and trovafloxacin in The Netherlands. J Antimicrob Chemother 1999; 43: 511–5.

[22] Pilotto A, Rassu M, Leandro G, Franceschi M, Di Mario F. Prevalence of *Helicobacter pylori* resistance to antibiotics in Northeast Italy: a multicentre study. GISU. Interdisciplinary Group for the Study of Ulcer. Dig Liver Dis 2000; 32: 763–8.

[23] Miendje Deyi VY, Bontems P, Vanderpas J, *et al.* Multicenter survey of routine determinations of resistance of *Helicobacter pylori* to antimicrobials over the last 20 years (1990 to 2009) in Belgium. J Clin Microbiol. 2011; 49: 2200-09.

[24] De Francesco V, Margiotta M, Zullo A, *et al.* Primary clarithromycin resistance in Italy assessed on *Helicobacter pylori* DNA sequences by TaqMan real-time polymerase chain reaction. Aliment Pharmacol Ther. 2006; 23: 429-35.

[25] Megraud F. *H. pylori* antibiotic resistance: prevalence, importance, and advances in testing. Gut 2004; 53: 1374-84.

[26] De Francesco V, Zullo A, Hassan C, Giorgio F, Rosania R, Ierardi E. Mechanisms of *Helicobacter pylori* antibiotic resistance: An updated appraisal. World J Gastrointest Pathophysiol. 2011; 2: 35-41.

[27] Cuadrado-Lavín A, Salcines-Caviedes JR, Carrascosa MF, *et al.* Antimicrobial susceptibility of *Helicobacter pylori* to six antibiotics currently used in Spain. J Antimicrob Chemother. 2012; 67: 170-3.

[28] Ndip RN, Malange Takang AE, Ojongokpoko JE, *et al. Helicobacter pylori* isolates recovered from gastric biopsies of patients with gastro-duodenal pathologies in Cameroon: current status of antibiogram. Trop Med Int Health 2008; 13: 848–854.

[29] Seck A, Mbengue M, Gassama-Sow A, Diouf L, Ka MM, Boye CS. Antibiotic susceptibility of *Helicobacter pylori* isolates in Dakar, Senegal. J Infect Dev Ctries 2009; 3: 137–140.

[30] Karczewska E, Wojtas-Bonior I, Sito E, Zwolińska-Wcisło M, Budak A Primary and secondary clarithromycin, metronidazole, amoxicillin and levofloxacin resistance to *Helicobacter pylori* in southern Poland. Pharmacol Rep. 2011; 63: 799-807.

[31] Hu CT, Wu CC, Lin CY, *et al.* Resistance rate to antibiotics of *Helicobacter pylori* isolates in eastern Taiwan. J Gastroenterol Hepatol 2007; 22: 720–23.

[32] Kim N, Kim JM, Kim CH, *et al.* Institutional difference of antibiotic resistance of *Helicobacter pylori* strains in Korea. J Clin Gastroenterol 2006; 40: 683–7.

[33] Horiki N, Omata F, Uemura M, *et al.* Annual change of primary resistance to clarithromycin among *Helicobacter pylori* isolates from 1996 through 2008 in Japan. Helicobacter 2009; 14: 86–90.

[34] Lee CC, Lee VW, Chan FK, Ling TK. Levofloxacin-resistant *Helicobacter pylori* in Hong Kong. Chemotherapy 2008; 54: 50–53.

[35] Chisholm SA, Teare EL, Davies K, Owen RJ. Surveillance of primary antibiotic resistance of *Helicobacter pylori* at centres in England and Wales over a six-year period (2000-2005). Euro Surveill 2007;12: E3–4.

[36] Nishizawa T, Suzuki H, Matsuzaki J, *et al. Helicobacter pylori* Resistance to Rifabutin in the Last 7 Years. Antimicrob Agents Chemother. 2011; 55: 5374-75.

[37] Wueppenhorst N, Stueger HP, Kist M, Glocker E. Identification and molecular characterization of triple- and quadruple-resistant *Helicobacter pylori* clinical isolates in Germany. J Antimicrob Chemother 2009; 63: 648–53.

[38] Versalovic J, Shortridge D, Kibler K, *et al.* Mutations in 23S rRNA are associated with clarithromycin resistance in *Helicobacter pylori.* Antimicrob Agents Chemother. 1996; 40: 477-80.

[39] van Doorn LJ, Debets-Ossenkopp YJ, Marais A, *et al.* Rapid detection, by PCR and reverse hybridization, of mutations in the *Helicobacter pylori* 23S rRNA gene, associated with macrolide resistance. Antimicrob Agents Chemother. 1999;43: 1779-82.

[40] García-Arata MI, Baquero F, de Rafael L, *et al.* Mutations in 23S rRNA in *Helicobacter pylori* conferring resistance to erythromycin do not always confer resistance to clarithromycin. Antimicrob Agents Chemother. 1999; 43: 374-6.

[41] Versalovic J, Osato MS, Spakovsky K, *et al.* Point mutations in the 23S rRNA gene of *Helicobacter pylori* associated with different levels of clarithromycin resistance. J Antimicrob Chemother. 1997; 40: 283-6.

[42] Stone GG, Shortridge D, Versalovic J, *et al.* A PCR-oligonucleotide ligation assay to determine the prevalence of 23S rRNA gene mutations in clarithromycin-resistant *Helicobacter pylori.* Antimicrob Agents Chemother 1997;41:712–14.

[43] De Francesco V, Margiotta M, Zullo A, *et al.* Clarithromycin-resistant genotypes and eradication of *Helicobacter pylori.* Ann Intern Med. 2006; 17; 144: 94-100.

[44] Paulsen IT. Multidrug efflux pumps and resistance: regulation and evolution. Curr Opin Microbiol. 2003;6:446-51.

[45] Zhang Z, Liu ZQ, Zheng PY, Tang FA, Yang PC. Influence of efflux pump inhibitors on the multidrug resistance of *Helicobacter pylori*. World J Gastroenterol. 2010 Mar 14;16:1279-84.

[46] Jenks PJ, Edwards DI. Metronidazole resistance in *Helicobacter pylori*. Int J Antimicrob Agents. 2002; 19: 1-7.

[47] Goodwin A, Kersulyte D, Sisson G, *et al*. Metronidazole resistance in *Helicobacter pylori* is due to null mutations in a gene (rdxA) that encodes an oxygen-insensitive NADPH nitroreductase. Mol Microbiol. 1998; 28: 383-93.

[48] Tankovic J, Lamarque D, Delchier JC, Soussy CJ, Labigne A, Jenks PJ. Frequent association between alteration of the rdxA gene and metronidazole resistance in French and North African isolates of *Helicobacter pylori*. Antimicrob Agents Chemother. 2000; 44:608-13.

[49] Yang YJ, Wu JJ, Sheu BS, Kao AW, Huang AH. The rdxA gene plays a more major role than frxA gene mutation in high-level metronidazole resistance of *Helicobacter pylori* in Taiwan. Helicobacter. 2004; 9:400-7.

[50] Matteo MJ, Pérez CV, Domingo MR, Olmos M, Sanchez C, Catalano M. DNA sequence analysis of rdxA and frxA from paired metronidazole-sensitive and -resistant *Helicobacter pylori* isolates obtained from patients with heteroresistance. Int J Antimicrob Agents. 2006; 27:152-8.

[51] van Amsterdam K, Bart A, van der Ende A. A *Helicobacter pylori* TolC efflux pump confers resistance to metronidazole. Antimicrob Agents Chemother. 2005; 49:1477-82.

[52] Choi SS, Chivers PT, Berg DE. Point mutations in *Helicobacter pylori's fur* regulatory gene that alter resistance to metronidazole, a prodrug activated by chemical reduction. PLoS One. 2011; 6: 1-10.

[53] Malfertheiner P, Megraud F, O'Morain CA, *et al*. Management of *Helicobacter pylori* infection--the Maastricht IV/ Florence Consensus Report. Gut. 2012; 61: 646-64.

[54] Dore MP, Osato MS, Realdi G, Mura I, Graham DY, Sepulveda AR. Amoxycillin tolerance in *Helicobacter pylori*. J Antimicrob Chemother. 1999; 43 :47-54.

[55] Rimbara E, Noguchi N, Kawai T, Sasatsu M. Correlation between substitutions in penicillin-binding protein 1 and amoxicillin resistance in *Helicobacter pylori*. Microbiol Immunol. 2007;51:939-44. PMID: 17951983.

[56] Gerrits MM, Godoy AP, Kuipers EJ, *et al*. Multiple mutations in or adjacent to the conserved penicillin-binding protein motifs of the penicillin-binding protein 1A confer amoxicillin resistance to *Helicobacter pylori*. Helicobacter. 2006;11:181-7.

[57] Rimbara E, Noguchi N, Kawai T, Sasatsu M. Mutations in penicillin-binding proteins 1, 2 and 3 are responsible for amoxicillin resistance in *Helicobacter pylori*. J Antimicrob Chemother. 2008; 61:995-8.

[58] Matteo MJ, Granados G, Olmos M, Wonaga A, Catalano M. *Helicobacter pylori* amoxicillin heteroresistance due to point mutations in PBP-1A in isogenic isolates. J Antimicrob Chemother. 2008; 61:474-7.

[59] Godoy AP, Reis FC, Ferraz LF, *et al*. Differentially expressed genes in response to amoxicillin in *Helicobacter pylori* analyzed by RNA arbitrarily primed PCR. FEMS Immunol Med Microbiol. 2007 ; 50:226-30.

[60] Kutschke A, de Jonge BL. Compound efflux in *Helicobacter pylori*. Antimicrob Agents Chemother. 2005;49:3009-10.

[61] Cattoir V, Nectoux J, Lascols C, *et al.* Update on fluoroquinolone resistance in *Helicobacter pylori*: new mutations leading to resistance and first description of a gyrA polymorphism associated with hypersusceptibility. Int J Antimicrob Agents. 2007;29:389-96.

[62] Glocker E, Kist M. Rapid detection of point mutations in the gyrA gene of *Helicobacter pylori* conferring resistance to ciprofloxacin by a fluorescence resonance energy transfer-based real-time PCR approach. J Clin Microbiol. 2004; 42:2241-6.

[63] Chopra I, Roberts M. Tetracycline antibiotics: mode of action, applications, molecular biology, and epidemiology of bacterial resistance. Microbiol Mol Biol Rev. 2001; 65: 232-60.

[64] Gerrits MM, Berning M, Van Vliet AH, Kuipers EJ, Kusters JG. Effects of 16S rRNA gene mutations on tetracycline resistance in *Helicobacter pylori*. Antimicrob Agents Chemother. 2003; 47: 2984-6.

[65] Wu JY, Kim JJ, Reddy R, Wang WM, Graham DY, Kwon DH. Tetracycline-resistant clinical *Helicobacter pylori* isolates with and without mutations in 16S rRNA-encoding genes. Antimicrob Agents Chemother. 2005; 49: 578-83.

[66] Trieber CA, Taylor DE. Mutations in the 16S rRNA genes of *Helicobacter pylori* mediate resistance to tetracycline. J Bacteriol. 2002; 184: 2131-40.

[67] Trieber CA, Burkhardt N, Nierhaus KH, Taylor DE. Ribosomal protection from tetracycline mediated by Tet(O): Tet(O) interaction with ribosomes is GTP-dependent. Biol Chem. 1998; 379: 847-55.

[68] Lawson AJ, Elviss NC, Owen RJ. Real-time PCR detection and frequency of 16S rDNA mutations associated with resistance and reduced susceptibility to tetracycline in *Helicobacter pylori* from England and Wales. J Antimicrob Chemother. 2005; 56: 282-6.

[69] Gisbert JP, Calvet X. Review article: rifabutin in the treatment of refractory *Helicobacter pylori* infection. Aliment Pharmacol Ther 2012; 35: 209-21.

[70] Moore JM, Salama NR. Mutational analysis of metronidazole resistance in *Helicobacter pylori*. Antimicrob Agents Chemother. 2005;49:1236–37.

[71] De Francesco V, Zullo A, Ierardi E, *et al.* Phenotypic and genotypic *Helicobacter pylori* clarithromycin resistance and therapeutic outcome: benefits and limits. J Antimicrob Chemother. 2010; 65: 327-32.

[72] Morris JM, Reasonover AL, Bruce MG, *et al.* Evaluation of seaFAST, a rapid fluorescent *in situ* hybridization test, for detection of *Helicobacter pylori* and resistance to clarithromycin in paraffin-embedded biopsy sections. J Clin Microbiol 2005;43:3494–96.

[73] Megraud F, Lehn N, Lind T, *et al.* Antimicrobial Susceptibility Testing of *Helicobacter pylori* in a Large Multicenter Trial: the MACH 2 Study. Antimicrob Agents Chemotherar 1999; 43: 2747-52.

[74] Lind T, Mégraud F, Unge P, *et al.* The MACH2 study: role of omeprazole in eradication of *Helicobacter pylori* with 1-week triple therapies. Gastroenterology. 1999;116: 248-53.

[75] Bardhan K, Bayerdörffer E, Veldhuyzen Van Zanten SJ, *et al.* The HOMER Study: the effect of increasing the dose of metronidazole when given with omeprazole and amoxicillin to cure *Helicobacter pylori* infection. Helicobacter. 2000; 5: 196-201.

[76] Bayerdoèrffer E,. Lonovics J, Dite P. *et al.* Efficacy of two different dosage regimens of omeprazole, amoxycillin and metronidazole for the cure of *Helicobacter pylori* infection. Aliment Pharmacol Ther 1999; 13: 1639-45.

[77] Perna, F, Zullo, A, Ricci, C, *et al*. Levofloxacin-based triple therapy for *Helicobacter pylori* re-treatment: Role of bacterial resistance. Dig Liver Dis 2007; 39: 1001-05.

Send Orders for Reprints to reprints@benthamscience.net
Helicobacter Pylori: A Worldwide Perspective 2014, **2014, 429-480** **429**

CHAPTER 19

Vulnerable Points of the *Helicobacter pylori* Story – Based on Animal and Human Observations (1975 – 2012)

Gyula Mózsik[*], Imre L. Szabo and Jozsef Czimmer

First Department of Medicine, Medical and Health Centre, University of Pécs, Hungary

Abstract: The pathological and therapeutical aspects of the *Helicobacter pylori* infection in patients with peptic ulcer disease, chronic atrophic gastritis and gastric cancer have been widely studied. However, various observations have indicated controversial results and highlighted a few questionable aspects of the broadly accepted role of *Helicobacter pylori* in generating certain gastroduodenal disorders. These are the following: 1. The sonicated *Helicobacter pylori* culture did not cause any direct cellular-damaging effect (at the level of the cell membrane, mitochondrion, DNA) in an application of 10^6-to 10^8 germ/mL given alone or in combination with indomethacin (10^{-8} to 10^{-4} M) on freshly isolated gastric mucosal cells. 2 Ethanol (EtOH) dose-dependently induced cellular damage (at the level of the cell membrane, mitochondrion and DNA), however, the sonicated *Helicobacter pylori* culture did not aggravate the damaging effect produced by EtOH. 3. The gastric acid secretory responses in patients with classical duodenal ulcer did not decrease depending on the patients' age and on the period since the onset of complaints, however, the gastric basal acid output (BAO) increased significantly in correlation with these parameters. Meanwhile the maximal acid output (MAO) did not change. 4. Authors never observed gastric cancer in duodenal ulcer patients without gastric surgery (in time period from 1962 to 2012), however, the gastric (stump) cancer developed after a partial gastrectomy in patients with duodenal ulcer. 5. The capsaicin-sensitive afferentation of the vagal nerve is involved in the development of gastric mucosal damage and prevention, which seems to be an independent pathway from the *Helicobacter pylori* infection or eradication treatment. Conclusions: the results of our experimental and clinical observations might offer some details underlying a reconsideration of the widely accepted etiological role of *Helicobacter pylori* in the development of gastric mucosal damage, gastroduodenal ulcers, chronic atrophic gastritis, gastric cancer and the treatment of *Helicobacter pylori* positive gastritis.

Keywords: *H. pylori*, Koch' postulates, *H. pylori* cultures, Isolated gastric mucosal cells, Damages of isolated cells, Trypan Blue exclusion test, Succinic dehydrogenase assay, Ethidium bromide-DNA flourescence assay, Testing of *H. pylori* on isolated gastric mucosal cells, Patients with duodenal ulcer, Gastric Basal and Maximal Acid

[*]**Address correspondence to Gyula Mózsik:** First Department of Medicine, Medical and Health Centre, University of Pécs, Pécs, Hungary; Tel: +36-72-536-494; Fax: +36-72-536-495; E-mail: gyula.mozsik@aok.pte.hu or gyula.mozsik@gmail.com

Buzás György Miklós (Ed.)

Outputs (BAO, MAO), Gastric acid secretory responses in patients with duodenal ulcer, BAO and MAO values *vs.* ages of patients with dodenal ulcer, BAO and MAO values *vs.* onset of complaints in DU patients, Unchanged gastric acid secretion in DU patients, Gastric surgery, Gastric stump cancer after gastric surgery, Gastric resection *vs.* appearance of gastric stump cancer, Capsaicin-sensitive afferentation, Capsaicin receptor (TRPV1), Calcitonin gen-related peptide (CGRP), Substance P (SP), Chronic gastritis, Chronic gastritis *vs.* capsaicin-sensitive afferentation, Eradication treatment, Eradication treatment *vs.* capsaicin-sensitive afferentation, Capsaicin-sensitive neural pathway in the mucosal protection, Capsaicin-sensitive afferention differs from eradication treatment, Vulnerable points of *Helicobacter pylori* story.

GENERAL INTRODUCTION

The *Helicobacter pylori* (*H. pylori*) infection is the subject of one of the most controversial medical opinions in everyday medical practice, including its role in the development of various gastrointestinal and extra-gastrointestinal disorders as well as the efficacy of the eradication treatment. The *H. pylori* bacterium was discovered in middle of the 1880s, while its pathological role in the development of different gastrointestinal diseases has been widely emphasised only from 1983, based on the observations of two Australian scientists, Warren and Marshall [1, 2]. They revealed the presence of this Gram-negative bacterium in the gastric mucosa of patients with chronic gastritis, which was first named *Campylobacter pylori* and later as *Helicobacter pylori*. Following their observations a great many observations were made internationally in patients with gastric ulcers, duodenal ulcers, gastritis, gastric cancer and different extragastric located disorders, such as MALT lymphoma, and allergic reactions. The number of the published papers in these fields has grown extremely fast (it is practically impossible to conduct a correct review of the published scientific data).

The involvement of *H. pylori* was suggested in the development of gastric and duodenal ulcers, leading later to chronic atrophic gastritis and gastric cancer. Consequently, everyone tried to find suitable treatment for *H. pylori*-induced disorders. Finally, “evidence-based” therapeutic recommendations were established consisting of antibiotic combinations, metronidazole and proton pump inhibitors (PPI). The efficacy of various therapeutic schemes that differed with small modifications has been widely studied by randomised, multicentre, multinational studies and their meta-analysis [3-6].

The nature of a new medical treatment has a unique curve of efficacy: in the first 5-10 years all new therapeutic approaches indicate very good results, during the following 10 years its real therapeutic value appears, and after about 15 years from the onset of new treatment, its real place in the medical treatment is finally established. This natural behaviour of treatments was also true for the *H. pylori* eradication treatment. The development of *H. pylori* resistance to antibiotics, mostly to metronidazole, appeared during recent decades; meanwhile the permanent application of proton pump inhibitors (PPI) caused serious side-effects in the regulation of bone structure as well as in hormonal regulation.

Research over the world can be divided into two groups based on their views of *H. pylori* importance: a larger group of researchers totally accept the role of *H. pylori* in all of afore- mentioned pathological circumstances, including the etiological role and eradication treatment of these *H. pylori*-induced diseases. A smaller group of researchers is spectical about *H. pylori* as being the exclusive factor in gastric and duodenal ulcers, gastric atrophic gastritis and gastric cancer development.

The aim of this chapter is to summarise the observations that are not in agreement with the main line of *H. pylori* infection and the need to eradicate it. On the other hand we are all aware that effective treatments have useful and harmful effects, and some can only be detected as late complications. This chapter briefly gives an overview of the following main problems:

1. Position of Koch's postulates in *H. pylori* infection,

2. Testing of *H. pylori* cultures on the isolated gastric mucosal cell alone, and in combination with other damaging agents (EtOH and IND),

3. Duodenal ulcers with *H. pylori* infection and gastric acid secretory responses depending on patients' ages and on the time from the onset of the disease,

4. Duodenal ulcer disease (with and without *H. pylori* infection) *vs.* gastric atrophic gastritis and gastric cancer after gastric partial resections,

5. Role of capsaicin-sensitive afferentation in chronic *H. pylori* positive and/or negative gastritis and after eradication treatment.

Application of Koch's Postulates for *H. pylori* Infection

General and Basic Definitions of Koch's Postulates in the Development of Various Infectious Diseases

Koch's postulates were established by Koch in 1891 [7]. They determine which organisms may be established directly as causes of diseases in general (aspecific technique as a means of disease prevention is only circumstantial evidence that microorganism cause disease). Koch's postulates are particularly used to demonstrate that a specific ***pathogen*** is the cause of a specific ***disease***. According to the Koch's postulates, the following criteria must hold for a given microorganism to be considered as the cause of a **disease [8, 9]:**

1. The **pathogen** must be present in all hosts diagnosed with the **disease,**

2. The **pathogen** must be isolatable from the diseased host,

3. The **pathogen** must be purifiable,

4. The purified **pathogen** must cause the specific **disease,**

5. The **pathogen** must be isolated from the host used in step 4,

6. The **pathogen** in step 5 must be shown to be the same pathogen purified in step 3.

Problems with Koch's Postulates:

a. There are a number of infectious diseases which agree with **Koch's postulates**, but does not fulfil all the criteria.

b. The most common exceptions:

   i. Have an inability to culture the **pathogen** outside of the normal host,

   ii. Lack of suitable, especially non-human hosts, that display the same symptoms.

Etiology of **Disease (Etiologic Agents):**

a. The **etiology of disease** is a description of the cause of that disease (*e.g.* as addressed by **Koch's postulates**).

b. **Etiologic Agent**:

   i. The agent responsible for the development of a microbial disease.

   ii. Pathogens are the etiologic agents of microbial diseases.

Infection (Colonisation):

a. Body Colonisation:

   i. Infection is typically considered in terms of colonisation of the body by microorganism causing a disease.

   ii. (Note, however, that the term colonisation actually has a specific meaning, *i.e.* microorganism growth on epithelial tissues, and most pathogens cause disease by invading tissues, rather than growing on their surfaces).

   iii. "Infection" refers to the multiplication of any parasitic organism within or upon the host's body.

b. There are actually numerous variations on this infection theme of bacteriemia, septicaemia, viremia and intracellular infection like symptomatic, asymptomatic, subclinical, unapparent, opportunistic, local, systemic, focal, primary, secondary, mixed, acute, chronic, sub-acute and latent.

Symptomatic Infection:

a. **Disease Symptoms:**

i. An infection by a microorganism which results in some sort of health impairment (disease) may be described as a symptomatic infection [8, 9]

ii. Typically an infection is only apparent symptomatically if it results in a noticeable disease

i. A symptomatic infection may lead to an asymptomatic infection or to a lack of **infection.**

Asymptomatic Infection

a. No disease, yet

iii. Colonisation of the body by a microorganism that does not cause symptoms must be described as an asymptomatic infection [8, 9].

iv. An asymptomatic infection may lead to a symptomatic infection or to a lack of **infection.**

v. If the asymptomatic infection does not change in status over time, the microorganisms involved are mostly part of the normal flora.

Subclinical (Inapparent) Infection:

a. Subclinical or inapperent infections are simply asymptomatic infections with different names.

Application of the Stress Theory to Approach Host Reactions Induced by Various Chemical, Bacterial, Viral and Physical Agents

Hans Selye published his original paper on stress theory in Nature in 1936 [10]. His theory has been widely used to approach various health problems and different diseases in animal experiments and in human observations.

Hans Selye's theory points out that the stimuli reaching a living organ **are non-specific**, but the reactions caused in the organisms **are specific**. So the stomach can respond to different chemicals and physical influences like drugs, bacteria and viruses with an increased or decreased function (*e.g.* gastric secretory responses, gastric emptying, alkali secretion, mucus secretion, *etc*).

During the last four decades we carried out many animal observations to examine the possible mechanisms of gastric mucosal damage and protection. Non-steroidal anti-inflammatory drugs (NSAIDs), various chemicals (HCl, NaOH, EtOH, concentrated NaCl solution and their combinations, as well as physical stress (cold water, immobilisation) were applied to produce gastric mucosal damage. Various biochemical parameters were analysed. Gastric mucosal changes, erosions, bleedings, ulcers and perforations in the stomach were obtained, and surprisingly in all cases biochemical changes were similar in all cases.

Main Classifications and Backgrounds of Gastritis

These observations were carried out in acute experimental circumstances. When the observations were extended for longer time, classical signs of inflammation (tumour, calor, dolor, pallor and function laesa) were noted. Stomach inflammation was seen in acute, subacute and chronic forms (depending on time).

Gastritis is an inflammation of the inner stomach lining, which is fairly common and can be induced by different causes. Many kinds of agents can lead to inflammation. Most commonly, this can be due to NSAIDs, such as aspirin, ibuprofen and naproxen, which are used in different treatments to reduce inflammation and pain caused by specific illnesses (*e.g.* rheumatoid arthritis and osteoarthritis). Sometimes inflammation can be due to abrasive compounds (alcohol, acids and others) or unbalanced diets, where the stomach is damaged by its own gastric acid; rarely, it can be caused by long-term physical and/or mental stress that resulting in the production of excessive amounts of stomach acid, or it can be due to the infection caused by *H. pylori*. If stomach inflammation is not treated, the illness can result gastric ulcers or in a worse scenario, gastric cancer.

The signs and symptoms of gastritis depend on the length of the disease. When it occurs suddenly, the inflammation is called acute gastritis. In the acute phase, the superficial inflammation of the stomach causes classic nausea, pain or discomfort in the upper abdomen. If it develops gradually it is called chronic gastritis; the symptoms are limited mainly to a sensation of dull pain in the upper abdomen or early satiety. However, in many cases, people with chronic gastritis cannot feel any of these symptoms. Another type of gastritis is the *reactive* or *chemical gastritis/gastropathy*, which is defined by foveolar elongation, tortuosity, and hypercellularity of the gastric surface epithelium together with oedema, vasodilatation, congestion of gastric mucosa propria, and paucity of inflammatory cells. This type of gastritis is kept as the result of duodenogastric bile reflux or use of NSAIDs [11-14].

Clinical classification differs on *non-specific chronic gastritis* (other than specific) forms since there is so much overlap in their development and pathological features. Other types of gastritis may be diagnosed:

a. *acute stress gastritis*, the most serious form of gastritis, that usually occurs in critically ill patients, such as those under intensive care, where stress erosions may develop suddenly as the result of severe trauma or stress to the stomach lining;

b. *atrophic gastritis* resulting from chronic gastritis leading to glandular atrophy, or a decrease in the size of the gastric lining. Gastric atrophy is the final state of chronic gastritis and may be a precursor to gastric cancer;

c. *superficial gastritis* is a term often used to describe the initial stages of chronic gastritis;

d. *uncommon, specific gastritis* includes granulomatous, eosinophilic and lymphocytic gastritis [14].

There is a specific position in the case of *H. pylori* infection. The classical points of the Koch's postulates cannot be applied to diseases caused *H. pylori* infection. One of the main points is missing in the case of *H. pylori* infection, since infection cannot be transferred to classical experimental animals (rats, mice). Professor Okabe from Japan was able to identify the Mongolian gerbil as the only animal species in which the *H. pylori* is able to produce similar pathological changes to those observed in patients.

Testing of *H. pylori* Cultures on the Isolated Gastric Mucosal Cell

Following the publication of Marshall's and Warren's letters in Lancet [1, 2], active research started throughout the world. Researchers tried to find an explanation how *H. pylori* could produce inflammation in the stomach and peptic ulcers, and the existence of the directly damaging effect of *H. pylori* was one of the possibilities. To answer the question, we analysed the direct cellular effect of sonicated *H. pylori* (at the level of membrane, mitochondrion and DNA) given alone and in different combinations on freshly isolated rat gastric mucosal cells. The aggravating effect of this sonicatum was also examined in the ethanol-induced cell injury model to evaluate the changes in cell resistance.

H. pylori Culture

Bacteria were obtained from biopsy samples. Urease test and histological positivity were both required to be definite in the tissue samples used. Bacterial suspensions (10^8 bacteria/ml in 20 mM Tris/HCl buffer, pH 7.0) were sonicated on ice (30 W) in six consecutive treatments lasting 30 seconds.

Preparation of Mixed Gastric Mucosal Cells (GMCs)

Gastric mucosal cells from 1-2 unfasted Sprague-Dawley strain rats were isolated using the method of Nagy *et al.* [15]. Briefly, segments of glandular stomach without blood vessels and surrounding connective tissue were sequentially incubated in a physiologic solution containing 0.5 mg/ml pronase E (Type XXV Sigma Chemical Co.) and 10^{-3} M EGTA. After several washes cells were resuspended and kept in a shaking water bath at 37 °C in a solution (0.157 M, pH 7.4) produced freshly with the following ingredients: 98.0 mM NaCl, 5.8 KCl, 2.5 mM NaH_2PO_4, 5.1mM Na pyruvate, 6.9 mM Na fumarate, 2.0 mM glutamine, 24.5 mM HEPES Na, 1.0 mM Trizma base, 11.1 mM D-glucose, 1.0 mM $CaCl_2$, 1.0 mM $MgCl_2$ and 2.0 mg/ml (w/v) bovine serum albumin. The mixed population of isolated rat GMCs contained at least three types of cells: parietal (20-25%), chief (40%) and epithelial (40-45%). 85-95% of the initial viability of the isolated cells was maintained for 6-7 hrs. The examinations were carried out in same media solution.

Toxicological Studies

H. pylori Culture

Cells were incubated with sonicated *H. pylori* (10^6-10^8 bacteria/mL) for 30 min in a shaking water bath at 37 °C. The equivalent volume of both diluted toxic agent and cell suspension were added. After 30 minutes, incubation cells were separated from the supernatant by centrifugation. The cell pellet was carefully resuspended and incubated for 10 minutes in a water bath, then it was centrifuged again (500 g, 10 min) to get the toxic agent-free supernatant. Cells were resuspended once more for further biochemical examinations.

Ethanol

Sonicated *H. pylori*-pretreated and washed cells were incubated with 15% ethanol (EtOH) for 5 minutes in a shaking water bath at 37 °C. Thereafter, the cells were treated as described above.

Indomethacin

Sonicated *H. pylori*-pretreated and washed cells were incubated with 10^{-8} – 10^{-6} M indomethacin (IND) (Chinoin, Hungary) for 5 min in a shaking water bath at 37 °C. Then cells were treated as described above.

Determination of Cell Viability with Trypan Blue Exclusion Test

Trypan Blue (TB) is excluded by viable cells, but taken up by damaged cells staining the cytoplasma blue [16]. A solution of 0.4 % TB (Sigma Chemical Co., St. Louis, USA) was mixed with the same volume of cell suspension, and 5 minutes later the rate of stained (dead) and unsustained (viable) cells was calculated as a %, by counting 100 cells in a hematocytometer.

Biochemical Assays

Lactate Dehydrogenase Assay

The lactate dehydrogenase (LDH) enzyme can be found in the cytoplasma of the cells. If it is presented in the supernatant, that indicates membrane damage of cells. Its activity was determined in samples of both toxic-agent free supernatant and the cell pellet destroyed by freezing. The colorimetric assay was based on the reduction of NAD^+ to NADH catalysed by LDH in the presence of lactate as substrate [17]. The colour product of the reduction of phenazine metosulphate (Sigma Chemical, St. Louis, USA) and tetrazonium salt isonicotinic acid hydrazide (Sigma Chemical, St. Louis, USA) was measured at 520 nm by a Hitachi 124 spectrophotometer. The results were expressed as mU/min/10^6 cells.

Succinic Dehydrogenase Assay

The succinic dehydrogenase (SDH) enzyme can be found in the mitochondria. The mitochondria integrity was tested in $2x10^6$ previously treated and redispersed cells [18]. The colour formazon product was quantified by a Hitachi 124 spectrophotometer at 500 nm and calculated as nmol/min/$2x10^6$ cells.

Ethidium Bromide-DNA Fluorescence Assay

The nuclear damage of cells was assessed by nuclear fluorescence with ethidium bromide-DNA binding [19]. 10^7 cells were mixed with EB solution (Sigma Chemical Co., St. Louis, USA), and the fluorescence intensity was measured by a Hitachi F-3000 spectrophotometer at 325-585 nm (excitation-emission). The results were expressed as arbitrary fluorescence units/10^7 cells.

Direct Cellular Effect of H. pylori, EtOH and IND

H. pylori

10^6 - 10^8 sonicated bacteria/ mL had no direct cellular toxicity on freshly isolated rats GMCs with a Trypan Blue exclusion test (Fig. **1**), LDH activity (Fig. **2**) or ethidium bromide-DNA fluorescence (Fig. **3**) [20, 21].

Combined Effect of *H. pylori* and EtOH

The preincubation of cells with sonicated *H. pylori* (10^6 - 10^8 bacteria/mL) did not aggravated the 15% EtOH-induced cell damage detected by TB (Fig. **1**) and biochemical assays (Figs. **2, 3**) [20-22]. The 5, 10, 15, 20 and 50 % concentration of ethanol dose-dependently decreased cell viability detected by TB (Fig. **4**) (ED_{50}=13.5%).

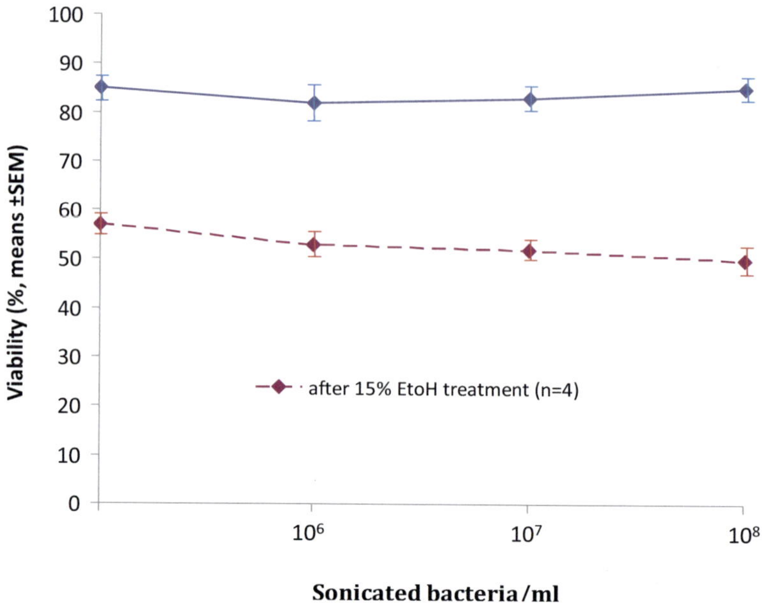

Figure 1: Effect of a 30 min incubation of sonicated 10^6-10^8 bacteria/mL *H. pylori* on the viability of freshly isolated rat gastric mucosal cells detected by Trypan blue exclusion test with or without 5 min 15% ethanol treatment (means ± SEM). From ref. [20], with permission.

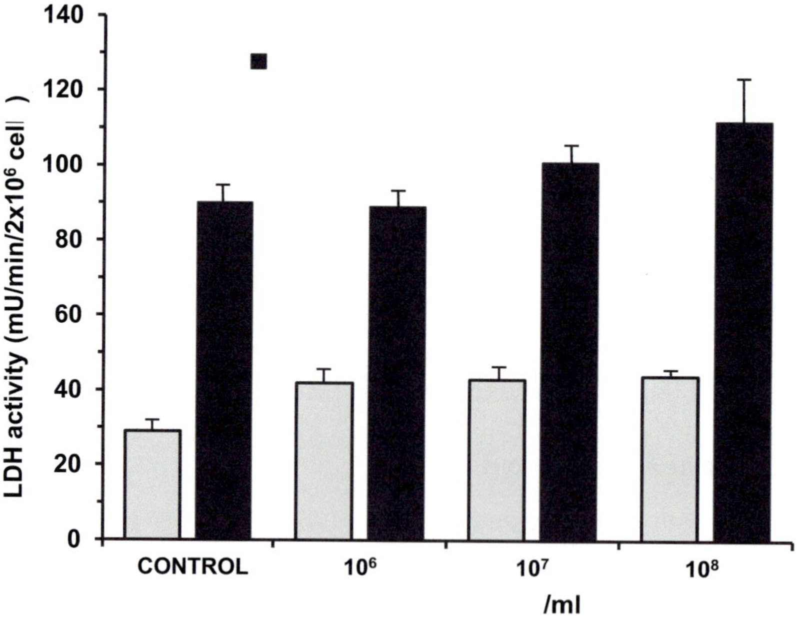

Figure 2: Changes in lactate dehydrogenase activity of freshly isolated rat gastric mucosal cells after 30 min incubation by sonicated 10^6-10^8 bacteria/mL *H. pylori* with or without 5 min 15% ethanol treatment (means ± SEM). From Ref [20], with permission.

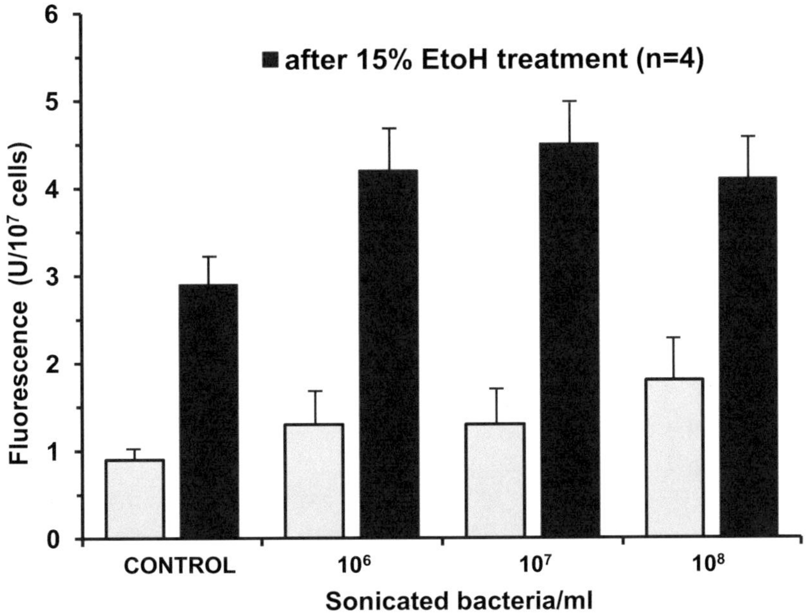

Figure 3: Changes in ethidium bromide-DNA fluorescence of freshly isolated rat gastric mucosal cells after 30 min incubation by sonicated 10^6 to 10^8 bacteria/mL *H. pylori* with or without 5 min 15% ethanol treatment (means ± SEM). From ref. [20], with permission.

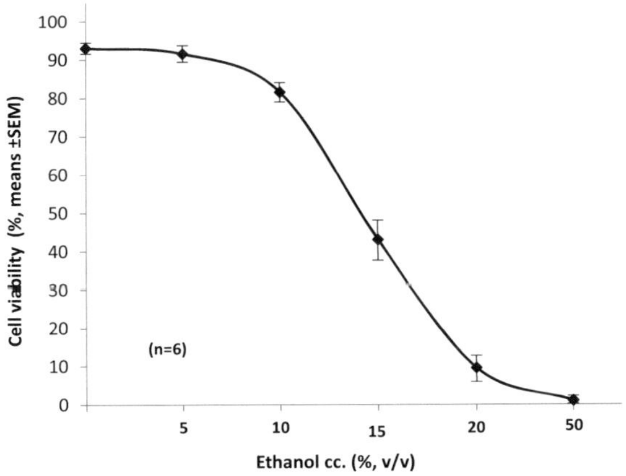

Figure 4: Changes in the viability of acutely (freshly) isolated rat gastric mucosal cells after 5 min incubation of 5 to 50 % (v/v) ethanol detected by Trypan Blue test. The EC_{50} = 13.5%) (means ± SDEM). From ref. [21], with permission.

Combined Effects of *H. pylori* and IND

After a 5 minute incubation of 10^{-8} – 10^{-3} M IND, only high doses (10^{-4}- 10^{-3} M) of IND significantly (P <0.01) decreased the number of viable cells (Fig. **5**).

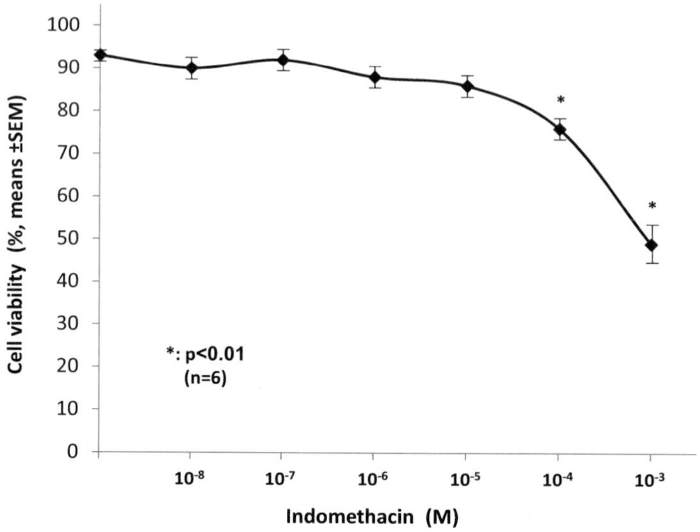

Figure 5: Changes in the viability of acutely (freshly) isolated rat gastric mucosal cells after 5 minute incubation of 10^{-8} to 10^{-3} M indomethacin (IND) detected by Trypan Blue exclusion test.* : $P < 0.01$ compared with untreated cells (means ± SEM). From ref. [22], with permission.

When the IND and *H. pylori* (10^7 sonicated bacteria/mL) were applied in combination, the number of viable cell did not change, compared to IND alone treatment (Fig. **6**), and no changes were obtained by biochemical assays either (Fig. **7**).

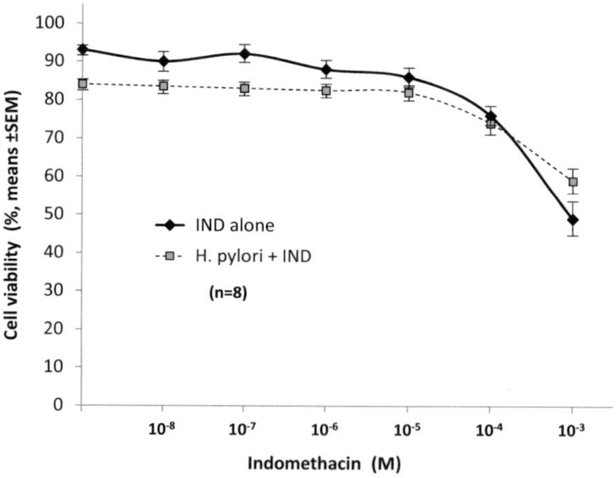

Figure 6: Effects of indomethacin (given in doses of 10^{-8} – to 10^{-3} M concentrations) with and without co-administration of sonicated *H. pylori* (given in a dose in 10^7 bacteria/mL together with all doses of indomethacin) on the viability of acutely (freshly) isolated gastric rat mucosal cells by Trypan Blue test. The incubation time was 30 minutes in all cases (means ± SEM).. From ref.[22], with permission.

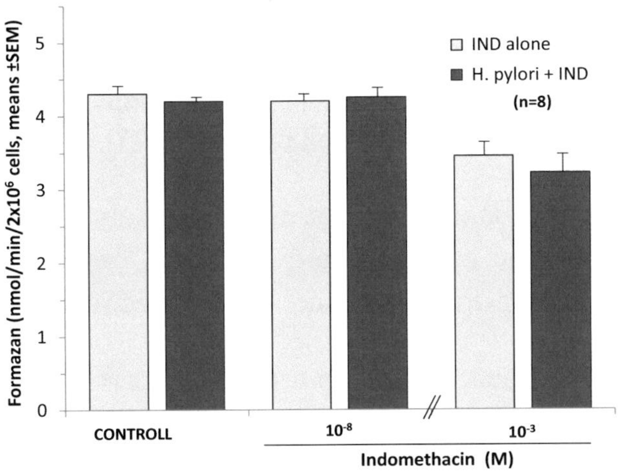

Figure 7: Effects of indomethacin (given in doses of 10^{-8} to 10^{-3} M concentrations) alone and in-co-administration with sonicated *H. pylori* (given in 10^7 bacteria /mL together with all doses of indomethacin) on the succinic dehydrogenase activity of acutely (freshly) isolated rat gastric mucosal cells. The incubation time was 30 min in all cases (means ± SEM). From ref. [22], with permission.

Combined Effect of EtOH and IND

Using these toxic agents, IND in all doses significantly aggravated the 15% EtOH-induced cell injury determined by Trypan Blue exclusion [20-22]

In these studies the direct effects of sonicated *H. pylori* were studied under different experimental circumstances (when it was given alone or in combination with EtOH and IND. This model was suitable for eliminating the additional effect of the immune system, which is naturally involved in a bacterial infection.

We found that sonicated *H. pylori* had no direct cellular toxicity.

These types of observations with freshly isolated gastric mucosal cells from rat stomach were widely used to study the direct actions of various aggressive and protective compounds under experimental circumstances.

For a correct understanding of the results obtained with *H. pylori* (given alone or in combination with EtOH or IND) we have to emphasise the following:

1. Rat (as an animal strain) may not represent the best model for studying the possible gastric mucosal mechanisms involved in *H. pylori* infection. The Mongolian gerbil might represent a better animal model to evaluate the mechanisms of *H. pylori*-induced pathology [23].

2. This *in vitro* model is an excellent model to study the direct cellular actions of different chemical and hormonal, natural compounds (EtOH, IND, pentagastrin, histamine, body protective compound, *etc*).

3. This experimental model is widely used in the research for preclinical selection of various drug candidates [15].

4. It is well known, that there is no absolute correlation between the direct cellular damaging and preventive effects obtained in freshly isolated gastric mucosal cells and *in vivo* observations [19].

Gastric Secretory Responses in Patients with Duodenal Ulcer (Dependinmg on Patient's Age and on the Time from the Onset of the Disease without Gastric Surgery)

It is well known that gastric H^+ secretion decreases as patients get older, without any gastrointestinal disease [24], which means a "senile decay" of different physiological functions in elderly age. Consequently, the number of persons with achlorhydria increases with age.

The following observations were made in the 1970s at a the time, when we had no clear knowledge of the possible role of *H. pylori*. We made systematic observations on the gastric secretory function of patients with duodenal ulcer [25].

In animal experiments, gastric parietal cell hyperplasia can be produced by the partial obstruction of the duodenum [26], which differs from that produced by chronically applied pentagastrin.

Our clinical observations indicated that the hyperacidity of patients with duodenal ulcers suffering from gastric retention syndrome was produced by disturbed gastric emptying. The pylorus can open when the milieu of gastric juice is at pH

4-5 (or higher). The gastric emptying is inhibited at a low pH (like 1-2), and consequently the gastric retention syndrome will appear in patients with duodenal ulcer. These observations clearly indicated that the gastric emptying is a pH dependent process. Gastric emptying is stimulated by a high (alkaline) pH of gastric juice [27]. These clinical investigations gave a rational explanation for the application of antacids in medical treatment. The delayed gastric emptying appears in practice as the main cause of dyspepsia.

We conducted a systematic study of gastric acid secretion in 120 patients with "classical duodenal ulcer" depending on the patient's age, and the time from the onset of the duodenal ulcer. We did not know the rate of *H. pylori* infection at that time, however, but now it is well known that almost all patients with duodenal ulcer are infected with *H. pylori.*

We studied the relationships between the different gastric secretory responses (volume, H^+ concentration, basal and maximal acid output, maximal acid output – basal acid output, basal acid output/maximal acid output x 100) in 120 patients with duodenal ulcer. These patients did not receive any ulcer inducer (salicylates, antirheumatic and antihypertensive agents, steroids) and did not suffer from renal, hepatic, endocrine, pulmonary and haematological diseases [25]. The gastric basal output (BAO) and maximal acid output (MAO) were measured in these patients. Gastric MAO was elicited by a subcutaneous injection of 6 µg/kg body weight pentagastrin (Acignost, VEB Berlin-Chemie, GDR). The results were expressed as means ± SEM. The correlation analysis between the two parameters followed Fischer's method [25, 28].

Age of Patients and Their Gastric Secretory Responses in Patients with Classical Duodenal Ulcer

Age of Patients *vs.* Gastric Basal Acid Secretory Response

A positive and mathematically significant correlations was found between the age of patients and H^+ concentration in gastric juice (mM/L) ($P< 0.001$; $r= 0.326$; $n= 120$) (Fig. **8**) and the age of patients *vs.* BAO (mM/h) ($P<0.05$; $r = 0.20$; $n= 120$) (Fig. **9**). No correlation was identified between the age of patients and the volume of gastric juice (mL/h) ($P>0.05$).

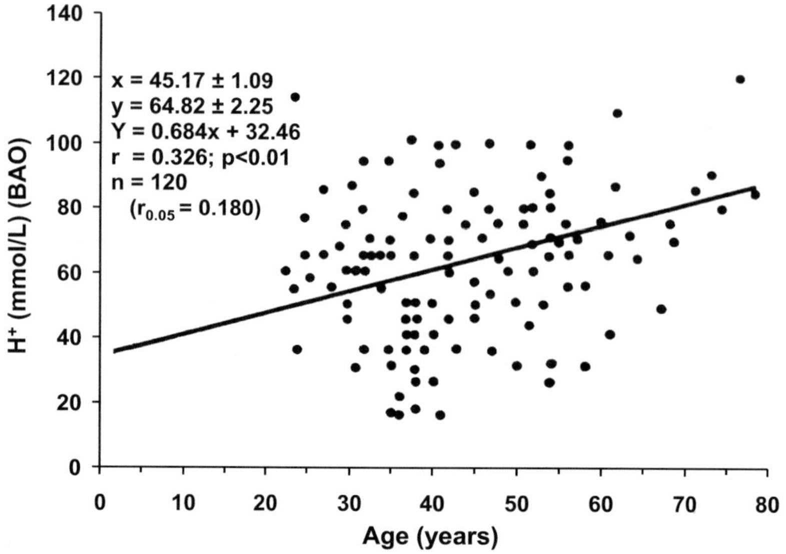

Figure 8: Correlation between age of patients *vs*. gastric H^+ concentration of gastric basal secretory responses in patients with classical duodenal ulcer. From ref. [25], with permission.

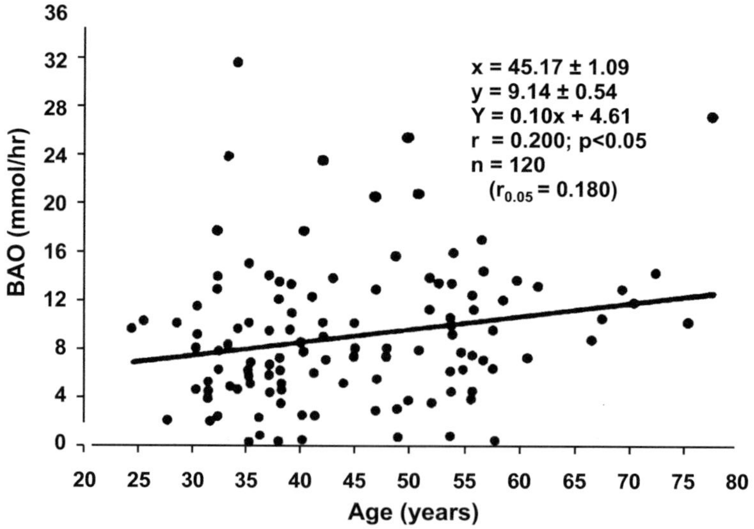

Figure 9: Correlation between the age of patients *vs*. the gastric basal acid output (BAO) in patients with classical duodenal ulcer. From ref [25], with permission.

Age of Patients *vs*. Gastric Maximal Acid Secretory Responses

The volume of gastric juice, H^+ concentration and MAO did not change (did not decreased!) significantly depending on the age of patients with duodenal ulcers (n=120).

Duration of Complaints and Gastric Acid Secretory Responses in Patients with Duodenal Ulcers

Duration of Complaints *vs.* Gastric Basal Acid Secretory Responses

A positive and statistically significant correlation was found between the volume (mL/h) *vs.* time from the onset of complaints (in years) ($P<0.05$; $r = 0.186$; $n=120$) (Fig. **10**) and between BAO values *vs.* time from the onset of complaints (in years) ($P<0.05$; $r = 0.237$; $n=120$) (Fig. **11**). No positive and significant correlation was found between the H^+ concentration *vs.* time from the onset of complaints (in years) in duodenal ulcer patients ($n=120$).

Duration of Complaints *vs.* Gastric Maximal Secretory Responses

No positive and statistically significant correlations was found between the time of onset of patients' complaints (in years) *vs.* volume of gastric juice, H^+ concentration and MAO values (P values were>0.05), however it is important to note that these values did not decrease.

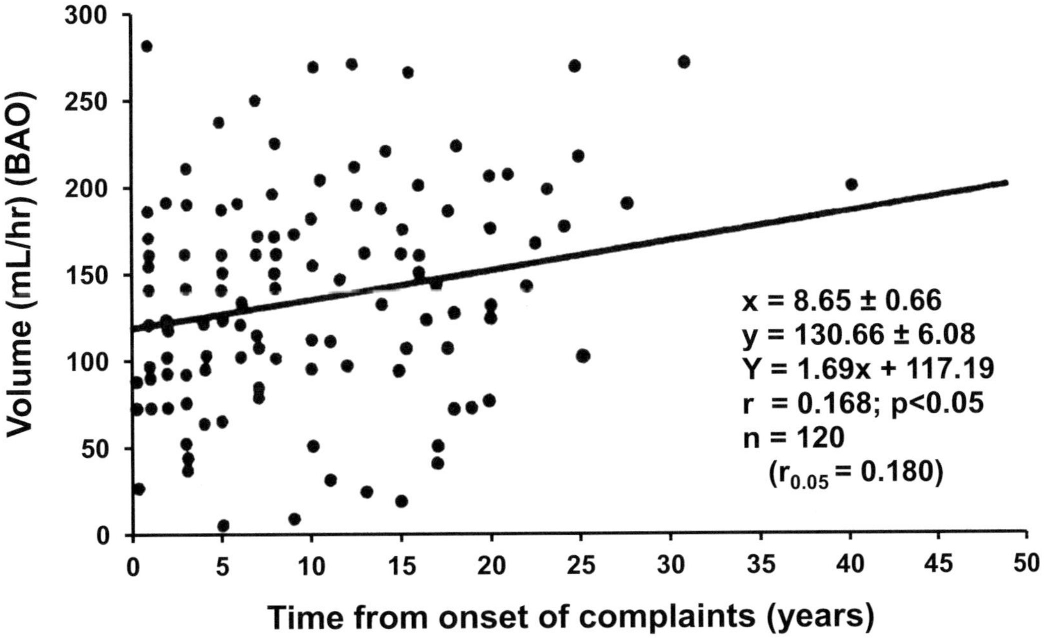

Figure 10: Correlation between the volumes of gastric basal secretory responses *vs.* the duration of time from the onset of complaints in patients with classical duodenal ulcer. From the ref. [25], with permission.

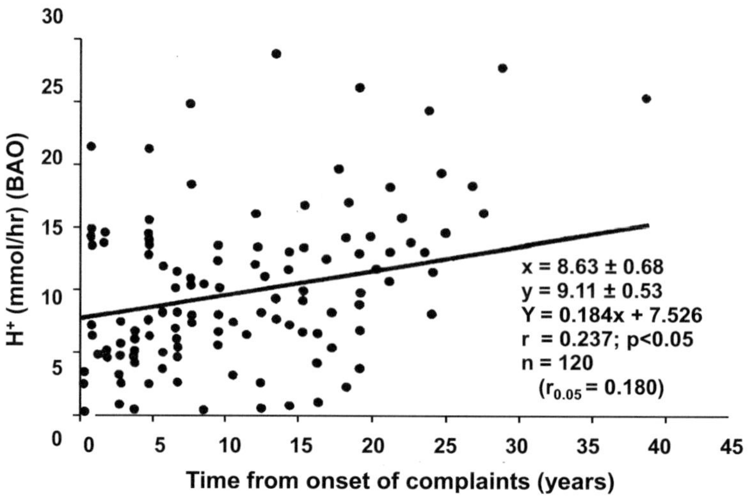

Figure 11: Correlation between the time from the onset of complaints *vs*. the gastric basal acid output (BAO) in patients with classical duodenal ulcers. From ref [25], with permission.

Interrelationships Between Age of Patients and Time of Onset of Patients' Complaints with Duodenal Ulcer

The complications of peptic ulcer diseases (activity of disease, vomitus of acidic taste of gastric juice, retention syndrome) *vs*. duration of patients' complaints showed a positive and mathematically significant correlation ($P<0.05$; $r=0.240$; $n=120$), however no bleedings, precancerous states or malignancy were found.

Interrelationships Between Gastric Basal and Maximal Secretory Responses in Patients with Duodenal Ulcer

Volume of Gastric Juice at the Time of Gastric Basal and Maximal Gastric Secretory Responses

A positive and mathematically significant correlation was found between the secreted volume of gastric juice in basal secretory responses *vs*. that of maximal acid secretory responses ($P<0.001$; $r=0.378$; $n=120$) (Fig. **12**).

H^+ Concentrations of Gastric Basal and Maximal Secretory Responses

A positive and mathematically significant correlation was found between the H^+ concentration (mEq/L) of gastric basal and maximal secretory responses ($P<0.001$; $r=0.480$; $n=120$) (Fig. **13**).

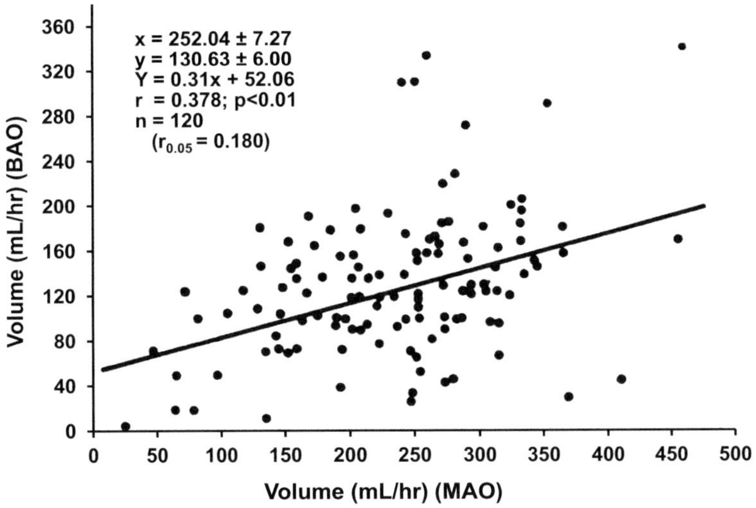

Figure 12: Correlation between the volumes of gastric maximal *vs*. basal secretory responses in patients with classical duodenal ulcers. From ref [25],with permission.

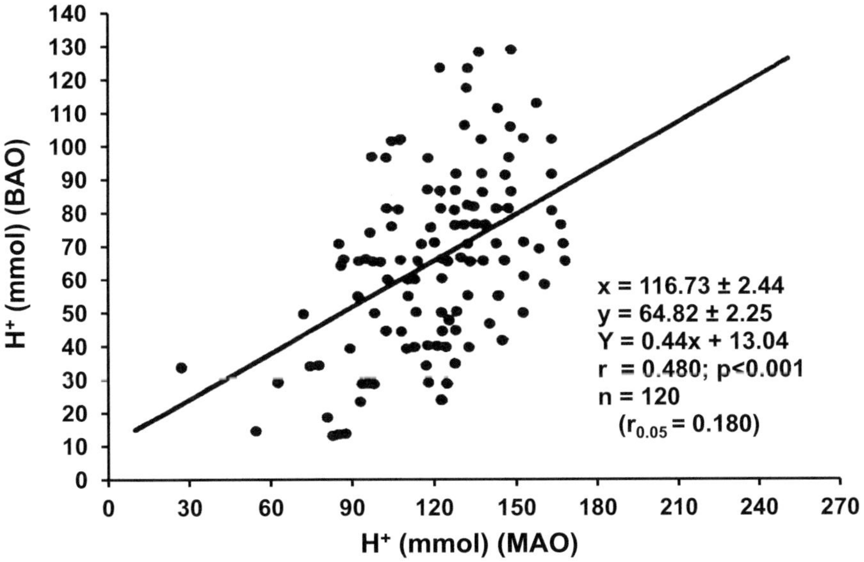

Figure 13: Correlation between H^+ concentration of the gastric maximal and basal secretory responses in patients with classical duodenal ulcers. From ref [25],with permission.

BAO and MAO Values in Patients with Duodenal Ulcer

A positive and mathematically significant correlation was found between them ($P<0.001$; $r=0.521$; $n=120$) (Fig. **14**).

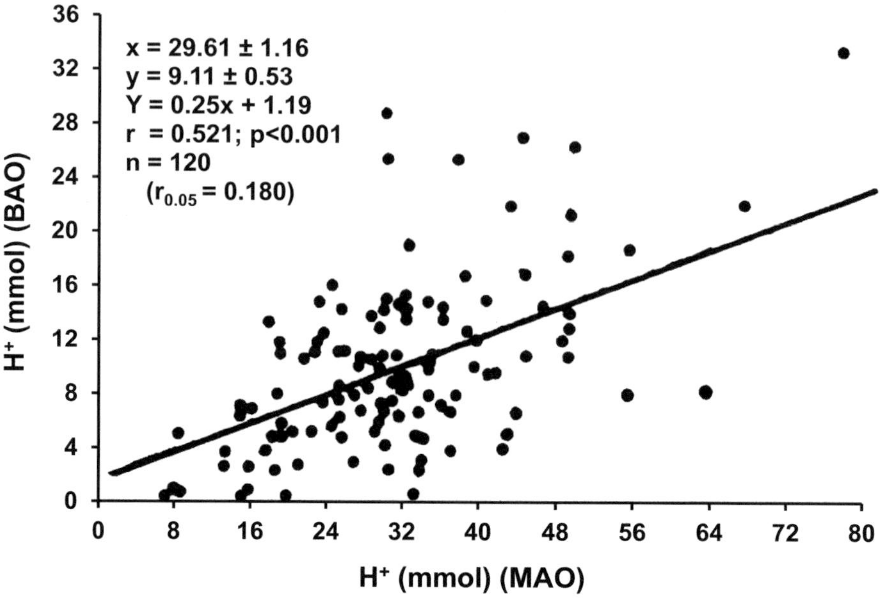

Figure 14: Correlation between gastric maximal (MAO) *vs*. basal acid output (BAO) in patients with classical duodenal ulcers. From ref [25],with permission.

Values of BAO / MAO x 100, MAO – BAO and Age of Patients

A negative and mathematically significant correlation was obtained between MAO-BAO and BAO/MAO x 100 ($P<0.001$; $r = -0.435$; $n=120$) (Fig. **15**).

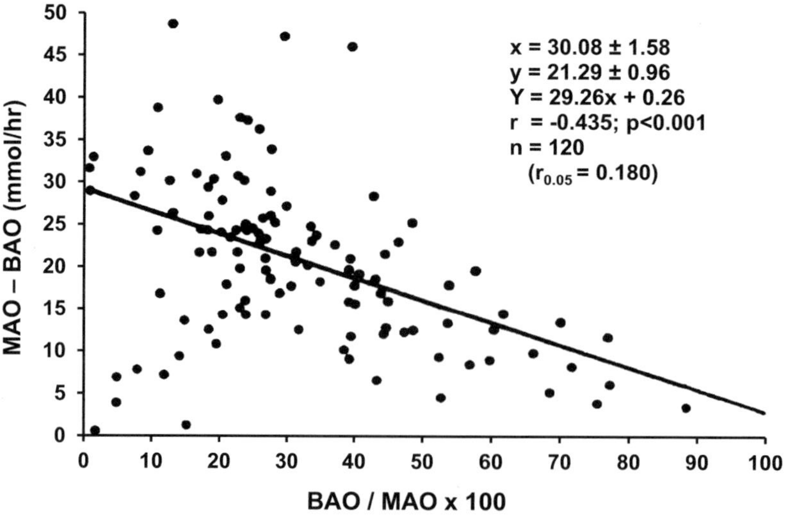

Figure 15: Correlation between the values of BAO/MAO x 100 *vs*. MAO-BAO in patients with classical duodenal ulcers. From ref [25],with permission.

Values of BAO/ MAO x 100 values *vs.* age of patients

A positive and mathematically significant correlation was found between these parameters (P<0.05; r=0.216; n=120) (Fig. **16**).

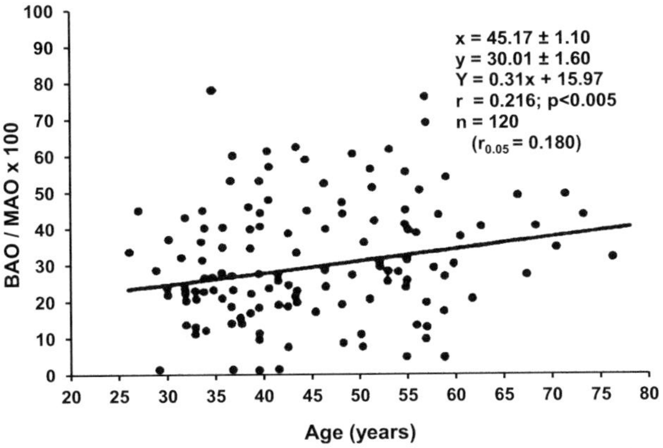

Figure 16: Correlation between the age of patients *vs.* the value of BAO / MAO x 100 in patients with classical duodenal ulcers. From ref [25],with permission.

Values of MAO – BAO *vs.* Age of Patients

No significant correlation was found.

Values of BAO/MAO x 100 *vs.* Age of Patients

A positive and mathematically significant correlation was observed (P<0.05; r=0.197) (Fig. **17**).

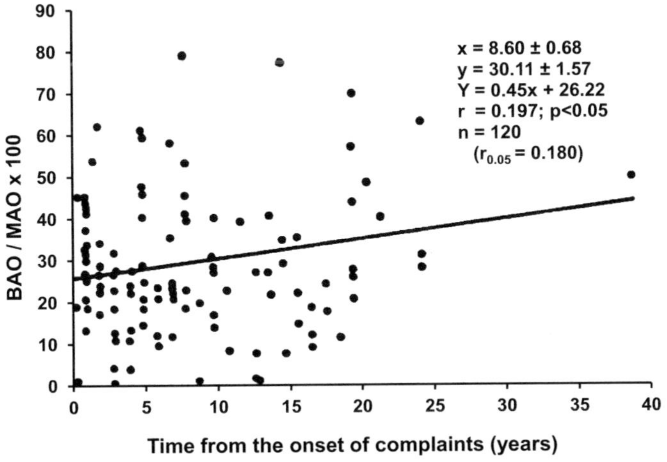

Figure 17: Correlation between the time from the onset of complaints of patients *vs.* values BAO / MAO x 100 in patients with classical duodenal ulcers. From ref [25],with permission.

MAO- BAO x 100 *vs.* Duration of Complaints

A positive and statistically significant correlation was found between these mentioned parameters (P<0.05; r=0.197) (Fig. **18**).

Other correlation analyses were carried out between the different parameters of gastric secretory (volume, H^+ concentration, output) and of gastric basal and maximal secretory responses in patients with duodenal ulcers, depending on the age of patients and on the time since the onset a complaints [25].

The results of the above observations clearly indicated:

a. The values of gastric BAO increased significantly in patients with duodenal ulcer depending on age;

b. The values of gastric BAO increased significantly in patients with duodenal ulcer depending on the onset of complaints,

c. No significant change was obtained in gastric MAO responses either depending on patient age, or depending on the time after the onset of patient complaints.

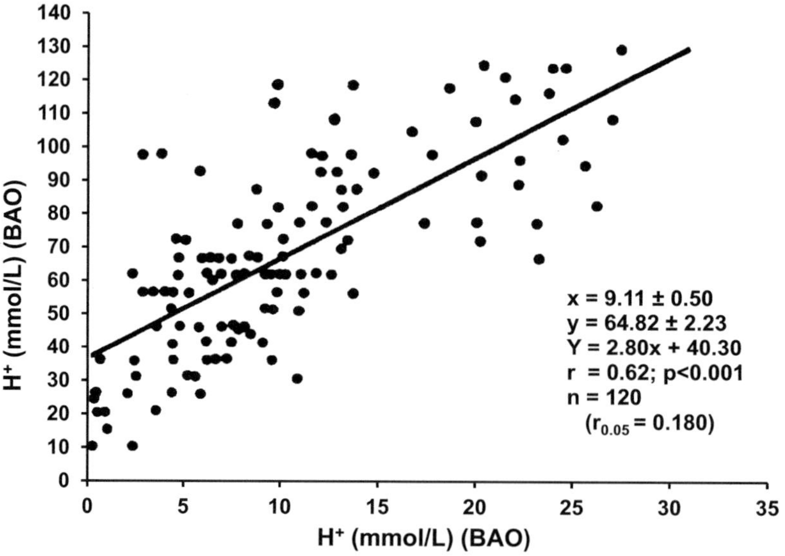

Figure 18: Correlation between gastric H+ output (BAO) *vs*. H^+ concentration of the gastric basal secretory responses in patients with classical duodenal ulcer. From ref. [25], with permission.

The analysis of these results excludes the presence of atrophic gastritis in patients with duodenal ulcers, since a gradually increased basal acid output and unchanged MAO value cannot be obtained in the case of atrophic gastritis. As mentioned earlier, we had no knowledge about the presence of *H. pylori* infection (especially on the immunological and toxicological behaviour of different strains *of H. pylori*), however, it is now well known that nearly all duodenal ulcer patients are infected in with *H. pylori.*

Development of Gastric Stump Cancer in Duodenal Ulcer Disease After Partial Gastrectomy

The criteria for the cancer development in the gastric stump after gastric surgery are well known in the literature:

a. Partial gastrectomy was carried out in patients with gastric and duodenal ulcer

b. No tumour-like pathological alterations found in the stomach at the time of gastric surgery,

c. Gastric resection was carried out in patients with other non-malignant diseases and 5 years or more after gastric resection.

The first paper on patients with gastric stump cancer was published by Prinz [29]. After his published paper many observations were made in the early decades of the 20th century. In the 1980s years we evaluated the ages of patients when cancer appeared in the stomach, without gastric surgery, and when gastric stump cancer appeared after gastric surgery. It was observed that the gastric cancer developed at an the average age of 61 years in about 3000 cases without gastric surgery. When gastric stump cancer appeared, the patients were in their 58th year (615 patients) on average, and originally suffered from gastric, duodenal ulcers or other non- malignant diseases.

According to literature, gastric surgery was carried out in about 60% of all patients due to gastric ulcer, in about 35-40 % of the cases due to duodenal ulcer and in about 5-6% due to gastric tumours (761 patients) [30].

The following types of gastric surgery were carried out in patients who later developed stump cancer: Billroth I resection was carried out in 6%, Billroth II resection in 67%, gastroenteric anatomosis in 27% and pyloroplasty in 0.4% of all the cases (720 patients) [30].

Jávor [31] reviewed the world literature examining the relationships between gastric cancer and the gastric HCl secretion. According to this review, three different correlations were put forward:

a. Gastric cancer develops and the gastric HCl secretion decreases as a result;

b. There is a common cause for both the decrease in gastric HCl secretion and the appearance of gastric cancer;

c. Gastric secretion decreases leading to the development of cancer.

Most of the data suubstantiated the reality of the third possibility. For example, HCl secretion plays a role in the location of gastric cancer. According to Strauss's observation, 50% of gastric cancer is located in the antrum-pylorus, which is only a small portion (about 20%) of the whole stomach; while 50% is located in the fundus and cardiac region, which is four fifths of the stomach.

About two-thirds of the stomach is removed by a partial gastrectomy (Billroth I and Billroth II resections); therefore, a relatively small gastric stump remains for cancer development. After gastric surgery, the frequency of the cancer locations is as follows: 16.4% in the cardiac region, 54.2% in the stump and 29.4% in the line of anastomosis [30]. By contrast, gastric cancer is located proportionally in the stomachs of patients with pernicious anaemia [31, 32].

The frequency of gastric cancer in patients with duodenal ulcers, without gastric surgery, is practically zero. Direct cancer development from duodenal ulcer is a real rarity (only 9 cases were described in literature before 1961) [33]. As an active internist since 1962 I have never identified gastric cancer in patients who originally suffered from duodenal ulcer.

The gastric secretory responses in duodenal ulcer increased significantly. We studied different parameters of gastric secretory responses in patients with duodenal ulcers in the years of 1973-1975 years (including 91 patients) and we found the following:

1. BAO (10.37 ± 0.59 mEq/h) *vs.* ages of patients (46.33 ± 1.22 years) (regression line: Y = 5.66 + 0.10. X; correlation coefficient: 0.208; P value < 0.05),

2. MAO (32.99 ± 1.17 mEq/ h) *vs.* ages of patients (46.33 ± 1.22 years) (regression line: Y = 34.03 + 0.02 ·X; regression coefficient: - 0.023; P value < 0.05),

3. BAO /MAO x 100 (32.67 ± 1.72 mEq/ h) *vs.* ages of patients (46.33 ± 1.22) (regression line: Y = 16.04 + 0.35 · X; correlation coefficient: 0.255; P values < 0.05),

4. BAO values (10.37 ± 0.59 mEq/h) *vs.* time after the first complaint (8.87 ± 0.81 years) (regression line: Y = 8.54 + 0.20 · X; correlation coefficient: 0.277; P < 0.01),

5. BAO /MAO x 100 (28.05 ± 1.72 mEq/h) and time after the first complaint (8.97 ± 1.22 years) (regression line: Y = 2.05 + 0.51 · X; correlation coefficient: 0.243; P value < 0.02),

6. MAO (32.99 ± 1.17 mEq/h) *vs.* BAO (10.37 ± 0.59 mEq/h) (regression line: 24.05 + 0.86 · X ; correlation coefficient: 0.438 ; P value < 0.001) [34].

These results agree with those detailed in the subchapter of section 3.

Twenty-five patients altogether were identified with cancer of the gastric stump who were admitted to the First Department of Surgery (between 1939 and 1973) and to the Department of Medicine at the University Medical School, Pécs (Hungary) between 1963 and 1973 [35]. The 25 patients is a relatively small group for a thorough analysis of the problem. Reviewing Hungarian literature, we found some other cases [36]. The two groups (our own cases and Szabolcs's patients), 45 in total. were used for a further analysis of the problem. These patients experienced partial gastric resection, due to a gastric ulcer according to the Billroth II resection model.

Between the time of gastric resection and the appearance of cancer in the gastric stump a nice correlation equation was found: $X = 40.25 \pm 1.54$; $Y = 59.80 \pm 1.07$; $Y = 46.70 + 0.32 \cdot X$; correlation coefficient: $r = 0.47$; $P<0.001$; n=45 [34].

The forty years was taken as a borderline age to indicate the gastric surgery (that was Billroth II type of gastric partial resection). To answer the correlation between the time elapsed after gastric resection and the ages of patients, a closed correlation was found: $X = 39.6 \pm 10.20$; $Y = 19.82 \pm 8.75$; $Y = 53.08 - 0.83 \cdot X$; correlation coefficient: 0.84; $P< 0.001$; n=46).

Twenty-eight cases of patients with gastric stump cancer, who underwent partial gastric resection (Billroth II type gastric resection), were collected throughout the 20 years period from 1956 to 1976 at the First Department of Medicine and First Department of Surgery, Medical School of Pécs (Hungary). These patients were all males and admitted with a typical clinical picture of malignant disease. Their ages ranged from 43 to 75 (mean ± SEM; 60.10 ± 1.57) years at the time of the stump cancer, and 26 to 61 (41.64 ± 2.16) years at the time of the partial gastrectomy due to duodenal ulcers.

The gastric stump cancer appeared at a significantly younger age, when the gastric resection had been carried out before the age of fourty years ($P<0.001$) (Table **1**).

A positive and statistically significant correlation was observed between the age of patients at the time the stump cancer appeared ($Y = 60.10 \pm 1.57$ years) and their at gastric resection ($X = 41.64 \pm 2.16$ years) (regression line: $Y = 45.04 + 0.36 \cdot X$; correlation coefficient = 0.497; $P<0.01$; n=28) (Fig. **19**).

A negative and statistically significant correlation was found to be present between the time of cancer development ($Y = 18.28 \pm 1.91$ years) and the age of patients at the time of gastric resection ($X = 41.64 \pm 2.16$ years) (regression line: $Y = 44.00 - 0.61 \cdot X$; correlation coefficient: - 0.699; $P<0.001$; n=28) (Fig. **20**).

Table 1: Development of gastric stump cancer in patients, who underwent partial Billroth II type gastrectomy because of duodenal ulcer. "n " indicates the number of patients, the results are expressed as means ± SEM.From the Ref. [95], with permission

Age of patients in years (means ± SEM) at the time of gastric resectio n (left column) and of the appearance of gastric stump cancer (right column)	
For all patients	
41.64 ± 2.16 (n = 28)	60.10 ± 1.57 (n = 28)
in patients for whom the gastric resection was carried out before the age of forty	
32.20 ± 1.45 (n = 16)	57.40 ± 2.10 (n = 16) **
in patients for whom the gastric resection has been carried out after age of forty	
52.80 ± 2.00 (n = 12)	63.70 ± 2.17 ** (n = 12)
** level of significance, P < 0.001	

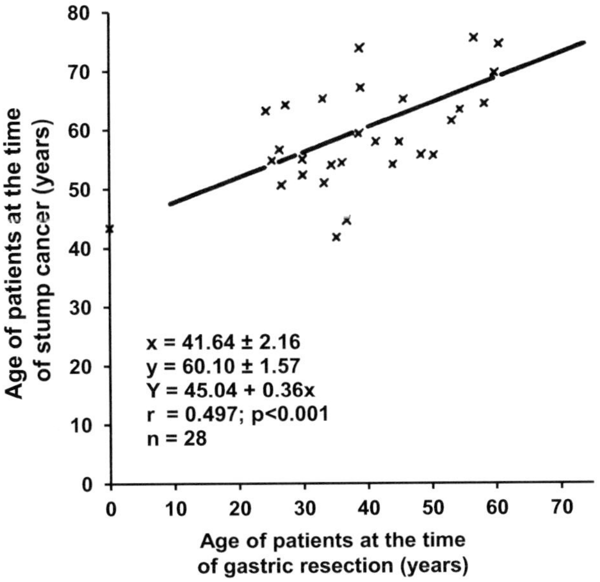

Figure 19: Correlation between the age of patients at the time of apperarance of gastric stump cancer *vs*. age of patients at the time of the gastric Billroth II gastric resection in patients, who suffered from classical duodenal ulcer. From ref. [95], with permission.

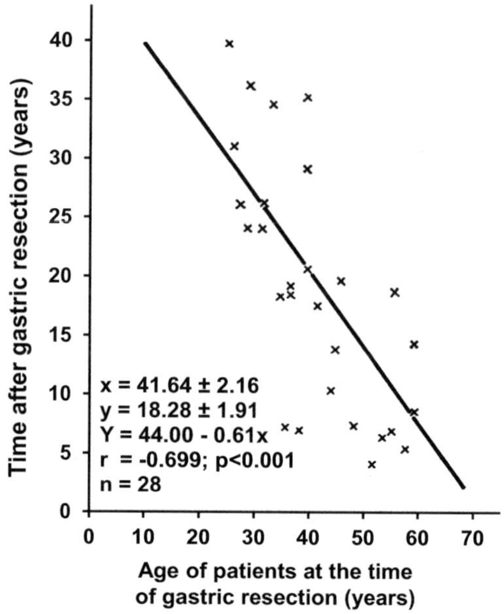

Figure 20: Correlation between the time elapsed (from the age of patients upon the gastric Billroth II gastric resection to the appearance of gastric stump cancer) *vs.* the age of patients of patients when the gastric partial resection was carried out in patients with classical duodenal ulcers. From ref. [95], with permission.

We found no differences when we compared the identical regressions lines between:

a. The age of patients when the gastric stump cancer appeared *vs.* their age at the the time of the gastric the resection, and

b. The elapsed time of cancer development and the age of patients upon gastric resection in those patients who originally suffered from gastric or duodenal ulcers before the partial Billroth II gastrectomy.

It is true that we had no knowledge of the presence of *H. pylori* infection, however, it was a very surprising to note that the gastric stump cancer developed in a relatively large number of patients (just after Billroth II type gastric resection) who originally had suffered from classical duodenal ulcers. Meanwhile, one of the authors (G. M.) never diagnosed gastric ulcer in duodenal ulcer patients without gastric surgery in his 50 years of his practice. Patients with duodenal ulcers are almost always infected with *H. pylori,* whereas the rate of gastric cancer development is very small [37] in contrast to gastric ulceration.

Furthermore, the gastric acid secretory responses did not decrease in patients with classical duodenal ulcers, as it was demonstrated in 210 patients with duodenal ulcers depending on the duration of the disease or the age of patients [25, 34]. The presence of a functional retention syndrome (produced by the high pH of gastric juice) has been suggested and permanently noted in duodenal ulcer patients (without gastric surgery) [37], which is able to increase the BAO value depending both on the age of patients and on the time since the onset of complaints. Similarly, when the pylorus was partially obstructed in animals then the gastric acid secretion was also increased [26, 38].

Many internists believed that the classical duodenal ulceration in patients without gastric surgery represents a line of defence against the development of gastric ulcers. We followed these patients from a clinical pharmacological perspective before 1983. They received intermittent treatment of with atropine plus permanent use of antacids (respecting the development of tolerance to atropine and pharmacological denervation phenomenon during chronic atropine treatment) [39]. These patients were in good health condition and gastric surgery never became necessary. We obtained similarly good results with the use of H_2A or PPI treatment. We never offered permanent antisecretory treatment for patients who suffered from peptic ulcer disease.

Relationship of Capsaicin-Sensitive Afferent Vagal Nerves and Chronic Gastritis

Introduction to Capsaicin-Sensitive Afferentation in the Human GI Tract

The principle role of the efferent vagal nerve has been emphasized in the development of gastrointestinal mucosal damage and prevention, as well as in medical treatment involving anticholinergic agents, histamine H_2 receptor inhibitors, antigastric agents and PPIs during the last century. From the initial observation of the capsaicin desensitisation phenomenon, a long-lasting chemoanalgesia and impairment of chemoregulation in the 1970s, a chain of new findings led to the discovery of the capsaicin receptor, a type of C-polymodal nociceptors [40, 41]. The effects of capsaicin depend on the applied doses and duration of exposure [41-46]. These different effects of capsaicin are:

1. excitation,
2. sensory-blocking effects,
3. long-term selective **neurotoxic impairment** and
4. irreversible cell destruction.

Neurogenic inflammation is mediated by the C-afferent fibres, which are supplied with the putative capsaicin receptor. These afferents are called capsaicin-sensitive chemoreceptive afferents. They opened up new avenues of local peptidergic regulation in peripheral tissues. In contrast to classical axon theory, it has been suggested that the capsaicin-sensitive sensory system has a dual sensory-afferent function, whereby the initiation of afferent signals and neuropeptide release are coupled at the same nerve endings. Capsaicin receptor, also named as transient receptor potential vanilloid-1 (TRPV1) [47] was detected in the postrema area and in the nucleus tractus solitary, where the afferent vagal nerve fibres end. Studies with the capsaicin receptor led to the discovery of the first temperature-gated ion channel exerting stimuli by noxious heat, protons, vanilloids and endogenous ligands such as anadamide, N-oleodopamine and lypoxygenase products. Another recent achievement was the discovery of a novel regulatory mechanisms mediated by somatostatin and glucagon. Somatostatin released from the TRPV1-expressing nerves endings reaches the circulation and elicits anti-inflammatory and analgetic functions [41, 48]; meanwhile the glucagon release *via* capsaicin indicates the interaction of capsaicin-sensitive afferentation with certain metabolic regulations [49].

The vagal nerve also contains also about 10% efferent and 90% of afferent fibres, and 9% of these afferent fibres are the capsaicin-sensitive afferent nerves [50, 51]. Thus, the amount of the efferent fibres and capsaicin-sensitive afferent fibres are roughly the same amount in the vagal nerve.

The possible role of the afferent vagal nerve has been studied during recent decades both in the development of gastrointestinal mucosal damage and production [39, 45, 52, 53]. Recently, the gastroprotective effect of capsaicin against chemical agents (EtOH, IND) has been proven in healthy human subjects [44-46, 54]. The beneficial effect of capsaicin has also been shown in patients with functional gastrointestinal disorders [55, 56].

The integrity of gastric mucosa relies on an equilibrium between aggressive and defensive factors, the development of gastric mucosal ulceration, and mostly likely chronic gastritis, are due to the distortion of this balance. One of the aggressive factors is *H. pylori* infection, which is a widely spread bacteria, one of the commonest pathogen bacillus in humans [57]. At least half of the world's population could be infected with this organism [58]. *H. pylori* – as a causative factor – increases the risk for the development of human gastrointestinal diseases such as acute gastritis, chronic gastritis, gastrointestinal ulcers, gastric mucosa-associated lymphoid tissue (MALT) lymphoma, gastric adenocarcinoma and duodenal ulcers, and it may be implicated in iron deficiency anaemia, ischemic cerebrovascular disease and atherosclerosis according to recent research [59-65].

On the other hand, the capsaicin-sensitive afferentation is a part of defensive mechanisms. During administration of small doses of capsaicin (from ng/kg to μg/kg body weight) neurotransmitters such as substance P (SP), calcitonin-gene related peptide (CGRP), somatostanin (SS) and glucagon are released from the capsaicin-sensitive afferent nerve endings [41, 53, 54, 66]. These mediators can increase the gastric mucosal blood flow [67], carbohydrate metabolism [68], can induce mast cells and immune cell activation in the GI mucosa [69]. Somatostatin can elicit systemic anti-inflammatory and analgetic functions. The immunodistribution of neuropeptides (SP, VIP, NPY, SOM, GAL, and TH) released from sensory neurons and their neuroimmune functions are known, but their role has not been examined in gastritis without *H. pylori* infection [70].

The presence of TRPV1 receptor and released neurotransmitters has been studied in the development of different human gastrointestinal disorders including gastritis, peptic ulcer, gastrointestinal polyps with and without dysplasia, tumour, and inflammatory bowel diseases by immunohistochemical methods [53, 54, 71].

Presentation of Capsaicin-Sensitive Afferentation in the H. pylori Positive and H. pylori Negative Chronic Gastritis in Patients

The symptoms of patient's suffering from chronic gastritis with or without *H. pylori* infection (21 *H. pylori* positive, 30 *H. pylori* negative) were nonspecific including epigastric discomfort, nausea, loss of appetite and vomiting. The patients underwent physical, laboratory, ultrasonographic, endoscopic and histological examinations. Twenty people with functional dyspepsia (all of whom underwent the afore-mentioned medical, laboratory, iconographic and histological examinations and all of these examinations indicated completely negative results) were taken as healthy controls. The age of the patients was 39 to 68 years; there were 22 males and 29 females with chronic gastritis, and 10 males and females in the functional dyspepsia group.

The *H. pylori* infection was detected by a [^{14}C] urea breath test, rapid urease test, Warthin-Starry silver staining and specific histological examinations. The gastric tissue samples from the stomach and antrum were examined by an independent histopathologist and classified as chronic gastritis according to the Sydney System [72].

The immuno-histological studies were carried out on formalin fixed, paraffin embedded tissue samples of gastric mucosa using the peroxidase-labelled polymer method (Lab Vision Co., Fremont, USA). SP was detected by the NC1/34HL rat monoclonal antibody, the TRPV1 receptor and CGRP were labelled using polyclonal rabbit antisera (all from Alcam Ltd., UK, Cambridge) [68] (Figs. **21-23**).

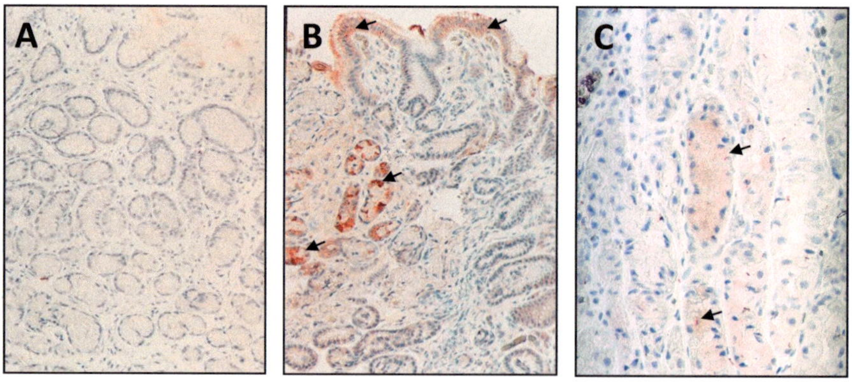

Figure 21: Immunohistochemical distribution of capsaicin receptor (transitoric receptor potential vanilloid) (TRPV1 in the gastric mucosa of a healthy patient (A) and of patients with *H. pylori* negative (B) and *H. pylori* positive (C) chronic gastritis. Arrows indicate the immuno-signs in the epithelial layer of the gastric mucosa (original magnification: 100x). From ref. [75], with permission.

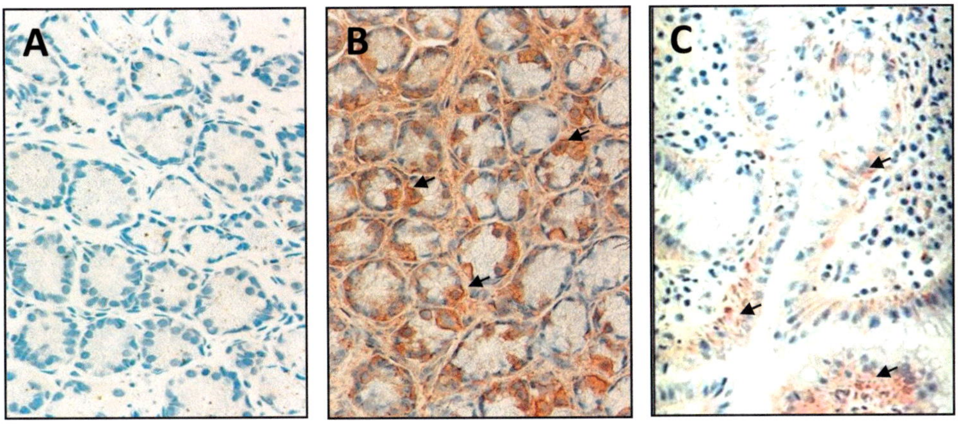

Figure 22: Immuno-histochemical distribution of calcitonin gene-related peptide (CGRP) in the gastric mucosa of healthy subject (A), of patient with *H. pylori* negative (B) and *H. pylori* positive (C) chronic gastritis. Arrows demonstrate the immuno-signs in the epithelial layer of the gastric mucosa (original magnification: 100x). From ref. [75], with permission.

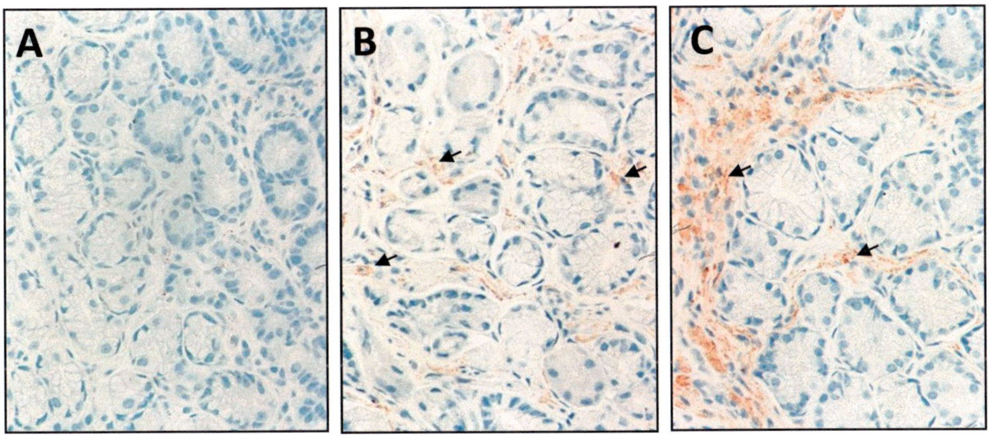

Figure 23: Immono-histochemical distribution of substance P (SP) in gastric mucosa of a healthy subject (A), of patients with *H. pylori* negative (B) and positive (C) chronic gastritis. Arrows show the immunosigns in the epithelial layer of the gastric mucosa (original magnification:100x). From ref. [75], with permission.

Presentation of Capsaicin-Sensitive Afferention in H. pylori Positive Chronic Gastritis Patients Before and After Eradication Treatment

Very recently the same clinical and immuno-histochemical examinations were carried out as those mentioned above (section 5.2.) in patients with *H. pylori* positive chronic gastritis before and after eradication treatment. These observations were carried out in 38 persons, including 20 healthy subjects and 18 patients with *H. pylori* positive gastritis. The age of persons with histologically intact gastric mucosa (controls) were between 41 and 67 years (mean=52.2 years). The age of patients (6 males, 12 females) was 39 to 68 years (mean = 56.4 years).

The period between the first and control gastroscopy was 6 weeks. The biopsies were taken from the corpus and antrum of patients with chronic gastritis, before and after eradication treatment, and from healthy persons. *H. pylori* positive patients underwent 7 days eradication treatment with combination of double dose PPI (pantoprazole 40 mg twice daily), amoxicillin (1000 mg twice daily) and clarithromycin (500 mg twice daily) according to current European guidelines [73]. After this one-week combination treatment, patients continued to take normal dose of PPI for another week.

The *H. pylori* infection was detected before and after treatment by [^{14} C] urea breath test, rapid urease test, Warthing-Starry silver staining and specific histological and immmunohistological examinations (see section 5.3. for further details).

The results of eradication treatment was successful in 89% of the cases, the gastric histology indicated normal picture in 22% of cases, while in 78 per cent patient the mucosa showed moderate gastritis [74].

Expression of TRPV1 Receptor, CGRP and SP in the Gastric Mucosa of Patients Before and After Eradication Treatment

The expression of TRPV1 and CGRP increased in the gastric mucosa of patients with chronic gastritis, however, that the increased expression of TRPV1 and CGRP did not depend on the presence of *H. pylori* infection was unexpected. The changes in the expression of SP were not significant between these groups of patients.

Another surprising result was obtained in patients with *H. pylori* positive chronic gastritis before and after successful eradication treatment. The extent in the expression of TRPV1, CGRP remained at a similar level after eradication. No significant changes were obtained in the expression of SP in the gastric mucosa of these patients (Fig. **24**) [75].

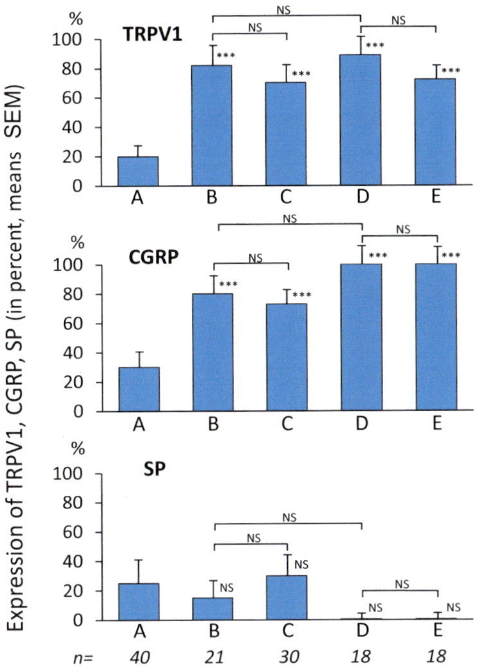

Figure 24: Changes in the expression of capsaicin receptor (TRPV1), calcitonin gene-related peptide (CGRP) and substabtance P (SP) in the human gastric mucosa of healthy volunteers (histologically intact) (A), *H. pylori* positive (B), *H. pylori* negative (C) and *H. pylori* positive before (D) and after eradication (pantoprazole 40, amoxicillin 1000 and clarithromycin 500 mg, all two times per day, for seven days) (n=number of patients).

General Discussion

It is practically impossible to get an overview on the possible role of *H. pylori* infection as an aspect of a bacteriological infection in the development of peptic ulcer disease, chronic atrophic gastritis, gastric cancer or *H. pylori*-associated diseases (Maltoma, lymphoma, allergic skin diseases, *etc.*) There is extensive literature on *H. pylori* including the experimental and clinical observations is extremely huge. However, all the literature emphasise the essential role of *H. pylori* infection in the development of these diseases (underlining ulcer disease, atrophic gastritis, gastric cancer) and the uniform application of eradication treatment on patients with peptic ulcer diseases and gastritis. It is also important to know what needs to be done with the *H. pylori* positive patients [76]. In addition to these mentioned dilemmas, the Nobel Committee gave Marshall and Warren a Nobel prize in 2005 for the research in this field.

We participated in the research of peptic ulcer diseases for several decades at the level of clinical practice, animal and clinical research (molecular biochemistry and pharmacology of gastric mucosa in animals and patients with peptic ulcer, innovative nutritional and pharmacological observations, cellular energetical biochemical observations, capsaicin-sensitive afferent fibres of the vagal nerve, clinical pharmacology, new drug production), organized 38 international congresses or symposia, published more than 350 papers, many monographs and edited books (G. M.). The first author was an founding member of the International Conferences on Ulcer Disease (in 1970 in Copenhagen, Denmark), one of the active leaders (from 1970 to 2009) of the Gastrointestinal Section of the International Union of Pharmacology (IUPHAR GI-Section, 1994 at Montreal, Canada), and also president of this section during the time period of 2002-2006. Consequently, we had good insight into international ulcer research involving animal experiments and human observations. Independently from the afore-mentioned possibilities, the details of this discussion are based on our original observations. Most part of our observations were carried out in the 1970-80s, when we had no knowledge of the existence of *H. pylori* and on its essential roles in the development of peptic ulcer, atrophic gastritis and gastric cancer.

Direct Toxic Actions of H. pylori, IND and EtOH on Isolated Rat Gastric Mucosal Cells

We used the freshly isolated rat gastric mucosal cells to test the direct actions of *H. pylori* on cells [15, 20-22, 77]. This method is widely used to test the different necrotising and beneficial effects of various biological and chemical compounds at the cell level [78].

The biochemical observations were able to demonstrate the damaging effects of noxious agents at the level of plasma membrane, mitochondrion and DNA (see chapter 2, for details). We used sonicated *H. pylori* culture obtained from *H. pylori* positive peptic ulcer patients. *H. pylori* was confirmed by a rapid urease test, special positive histological staining, a UBT test and by cultures obtained from biopsy samples in these patients. The applied number of germs of *H. pylori* ranged from 10^6 to 10^8/ mL. We used EtOH and IND as control-damaging agents in these systems. Furthermore, since IND inhibits the prostaglandin (PG) synthesis in the cells, this offered an approach to examine the possible role of decreased PG synthesis in the development of direct cell injuries induced by various agents.

These experiments produced surprising results; *H. pylori* did not cause any damaging effects at the levels of plasma membrane, mitochondria and DNA (testing alone or in combination with IND). Similar results were obtained with IND in this experimental model. On the other hand, EtOH produced cellular damage at the level of plasma membrane, mitochondria and DNA. Interestingly the EtOH-induced cellular damaging effect at the level of plasma membrane, mitochondria and DNA was enhanced by the co-administration of IND.

These results lead us to conclude the followings:

1. *H. pylori* has no direct cell damaging effect in this freshly isolated gastric mucosal cells (similar results were obtained with IND); however, EtOH could produce direct damage at the level of plasma membrane, mitochondria and DNA.

2. The co-administration of *H. pylori* with IND was not able to produce any direct cellular damaging effect at the level of plasma membrane, mitochondria or DNA in this experimental circumstance. These results allow us to conclude:

   a. the two main emphasised etiological agents cannot produce any direct cellular damage at the level of plasma membrane, mitochondria or DNA.

   b. the freshly isolated preparation of rat gastric mucosal cells contains parietal and non-secreting cells; however, the agents did not produce any damaging effect on these different types of gastric mucosal cells.

   c. although many *in vivo* research data suggest (or clearly accept) that parietal cells are the major susceptible cell type of the gastric mucosa for direct cellular damage during mucosal injury, we did not observe this in our experiments; this statement also did not seem to be true for other types of gastric cells either.

d. Very surprisingly, gastric mucosal damage caused by *H. pylori* cannot be enhanced by the co-administration of IND (clinical observation literature, on this standpoint is extremely contradictory).

e. *H. pylori* cannot enhance the damaging effect of IND on the isolated gastric mucosal cells (these questions are the most focussed issues in gastroenterology).

3. The decrease of gastric acid secretion in *H. pylori* infected patients will probably result clinically enhanced direct damaging effects on parietal cells.

4. If we accept that *H. pylori* produces a significant decrease in gastric acid secretion in an indirect way (namely by producing chronic inflammation in the gastric mucosa), then we are not able to find any explanation for the suggested standpoints.

Gastric Secretory Responses, Chronic Atrophic Gastritis, Gastric Cancer in Patients with Duodenal Ulcer (With and Without H. pylori Infection)

There are many crucial problems in this field, namely the decrease of gastric acid secretion, development of chronic atrophic gastritis resulting in a precancerous state, and gastric cancer patients with classical duodenal ulcer and *H. pylori* infection.

To analyse these problems we need to mention the different scientific arguments to avoid misunderstanding the standpoints, and the background of changed medical practice during the last decades:

1. The clear definition of "ulcer disease" relies on the histological presentation of mucosal damage reaching the muscularis mucosae. Many other types of mucosal damage, like erosions produced by anti-inflammatory compounds, do not represent the classical ulcer disease.

On the other hand, in the 1990s and 2000s, mostly Scandinavian researchers introduced the terminology of "non-ulcer dyspepsia" (NUD) when the clinical picture indicated the typical framework of this disease; but there were no abnormalities found in the endoscopy and gastric histology. Consequently, the use of peptic ulcer terminology, especially duodenal ulcers, is a little confusing in international literature.

2. When Marshall and Warren received the Nobel prize for their *H. pylori* research, almost every researchers put aside their previously obtained and published results in this field.

3. At present there is no clinically used method for the direct measurement of gastric acid secretory responses in patients with peptic ulcer diseases in everyday medical practice, while the measurements of gastric basal and maximal secretory responses were incorporated into the everyday medical practice in earlier decades (1970-80s).

4. Research into gastrointestinal pharmacology produced different types of antisecretory drugs (like anticholinergic, antigastrinic, H_2RA and PPI), that have been introduced into clinical practice. These represent different periods in the medical treatment of patients with peptic ulcer disease during recent decades.

5. The discovery of "gastric cytoprotection" in animal experiments [79, 80] and patients [81] opened up a new pathway to understand the role of etiological factors in peptic ulcer and related treatment. These observations emphasised the potential roles of gastric mucosal defensive mechanisms (1979).

After the 1983, many researchers were eager to study the role of *H. pylori* infection in this disease. The gastrointestinal endoscopists wanted to demonstrate the presence of *H. pylori* in the gastric mucosa, while other different methods were introduced into clinical practice (like UBT, rapid urease test, *etc.*). As new methods were developed for testing the presence of *H. pylori* in the gastric mucosa, different medical therapeutic approaches were introduced into clinical practice for eradication. Consequently, a clear line can be observed in the medical treatment of ulcer patients before and after the era of *H. pylori* (1983).

It is now well known that the presence of *H. pylori* in the gastric mucosa was first observed in the late 1800s, but nobody paid any attention to this observation. Probably, it is due to its difficult cultivation. We also have to mention that clinical pharmacology was established in the 1960s and was soon used in analysing the efficacy of various ulcer treatments (we were one of the pioneers in developing clinical pharmacology). We need to mention that the healing rate induced by various studied drugs differed at 2 weeks after the onset of treatment, but no significant difference in healing was observed at 4 weeks [82-84]. As pharmacological and pharmaceutical research and products of these activities appeared in clinical practice, the need for multicentre randomised, prospective examinations soon arose. Following this era, the after the publication of Marshall and Warren [1, 2], most of clinicians accepted the introduction of eradication treatment for patients with peptic ulcer. Unfortunately, clinicians forgot the internationally accepted results previously obtained.

Our goal is to point out the importance of the changes in gastric acid secretory responses in duodenal ulcers with and without *H. pylori* infection. The BAO increased with the age of patients with duodenal ulcers; meanwhile the MAO remained the same in the elderly as well as in young patients. We are sure that gastric acid secretory responses in patient with duodenal ulcer do not decrease either with the age of patients or based on the time from the onset of complaints. As the secretory responses of these patients' stomachs do not decrease, then there is no real proof for the presence of chronic atrophic gastritis [31, 32, 85]. In other words, the existence of gastric hypersecretory responses in patients with duodenal ulcers exclude the possibility for developing of chronic gastritis (with and without *H. pylori* infection) in these patients. If we accept that the *H. pylori* infection is present in almost every in duodenal ulcer, then afore-mentioned results contradict to those suggested by Marshall, Warren and by other researchers following them [86-90].

The impaired function (*e.g.* decrease in gastric secretion) should be apparent in the existing inflammation. The intact gastric secretory responses were obtained in about 200 patients with duodenal ulcers, thus the duodenal ulcer does not represent a precancerous state (because there is no de- differention in the gastric mucosa). We never diagnosed gastric cancer in patients with duodenal ulcer and with no surgery. The number of parietal cells remained unchanged in these patients. Surprisingly the values of gastric acid outputs increased as the patient got older and with the time from the onset of complaints. In our explanation the presence of functional retention syndrome with impaired gastric emptying is due to the lower pH [25].

The explanation for the fact that no gastric cancer develops in patients with duodenal ulcers is the gastric hypersecretory state that might defend against the development of gastric cancer. Looking through our observation and its possible explanation, there is a vulnerable point regarding the emphasis of *H. pylori's* action in carcinogenesis obtained by the data from duodenal ulcer patient.

Duodenal ulcer patients who underwent gastric surgery point out significantly changed clinical problems. The unity of gastric function interrupted after the surgical intervention consists of the decrease in gastric secretion, the development of different types of refluxes, the disappearance of pyloric function and developing stump gastritis. This state of duodenal patients induced by gastric surgery really represents a precancerous state. We were able to collect 28 gastric stump cancer patients for observations, who originally suffered from duodenal ulcer and underwent gastric surgery [91-95]. It was surprising to note, that the correlations between the ages of patients at the development of gastric stump cancer *vs.* the ages of patients at the time of surgery and the time elapsed (in years) between the gastric surgery *vs.* the ages of patients at the surgical intervention were the same in those patients who underwent gastric surgery owing to previous duodenal ulcers as in patients with gastric cancer [91, 92]. In other words, the dedifferention time was longer in patients who underwent gastric surgery before their ages of 40 years, than in those who underwent gastric surgery after then 40 years. It was also important to note that stump cancer appeared around the age of 60, independently of time or indications of gastric surgery.

These observations, at least in the case of stump cancer, support the development of atrophic chronic gastritis before the development of cancer.

Potential Role of Capsaicin-Sensitive Afferent Vagal Nerve in the Development of Chronic Gastritis

After doing many animal experiments from the 1980s, we started human observations from 1997 [96, 97]. These were carried out in healthy human persons [45, 46] and in patients with different gastrointestinal disorders [54, 98, 99]. Different doses of capsaicin were applied to evaluate the possible roles of capsaicin-sensitive afferent vagal fibres. From the experimental observations we learned that the actions of capsaicin are dose-dependent [42, 98, 99]. We produced gastric mucosal damage in healthy human beings by applying IND (orally given) and EtOH (applied topically to gastric mucosa). The extent of gastric mucosal damage was approached by the measurements of blood loss and direct measurements of gastric transmucosal potential difference (GTPD). The IND increased the extent of gastric microbleedings and the EtOH decreased of GTPD values [98]. Various types of gastric mucosal damage could be prevented with the oral application of small doses (200 to 800μg/person) of capsaicin [42]. The results of these observations focused our attention on the mucosal protecting effect of capsaicin (acting *via* the stimulation of capsaicin-sensitive afferent fibres of the vagal nerve) in healthy human subjects.

We carried out specific enzyme histochemical examinations, using specific antisera to detect the expression of TRPV1, CGRP and SP. In the previous human observations, we carried out specific immuno-histochemical examinations in the biopsy samples from the upper (stomach, duodenum) and distal (colon) parts of the gastrointestinal tract in patients with different gastrointestinal disorders [75]. The results of these observations indicated that the capsaicin-sensitive afferentation is involved in these different gastrointestinal disorders in a different manner. As a next step we performed immuno-histochemical examinations in the gastric mucosa of patients with *H. pylori* negative and positive chronic gastritis [74]. The healthy subjects taken as controls had complaints of functional dyspepsia (however the gastric biopsy indicated an intact histological picture qualified by an independent pathologist).

These observations indicated that the expression of TRPV1 and CGRP increased significantly in chronic gastritis, and no significant change was obtained in SP levels. However, these immunohistochemical results did not differ in patients with *H. pylori* positive and negative chronic gastritis.

The last step of our observations indicated that capsaicin-sensitive afferention did not differ before and 6 weeks after successful eradication treatment in patients with chronic *H. pylori* positive gastritis (meanwhile the control biopsy was normal in 22% of the cases, and indicated a moderated histological picture of gastritis in 78%) [74]. Our explanation for the unchanged immunohistochemical distribution of TRPV1, CGRP and SP of gastric *H. pylori* positive chronic gastritis before *vs*. after eradication treatment:

1. A six-week time period might not be enough for the complete healing of chronic gastritis.

2. A six-week period (after eradication treatment) is probably not enough for a complete histological recovery of chronic *H. pylori* positive infection in patients in term of histology and immunohistology.

3. *H. pylori* as an etiological factor might represent only one of factor causing chronic gastritis (in terms of histology);

4. The immunohistological distribution of TRPV1, CGRP and SP are independent from gastritis produced by different physical, chemical, bacteriological or immunological agents. However, the increased expression of TRPV1, CGRP is involved in the gastric mucosal damage and the normalisation of these changes can be obtained by ways other than the classical eradication treatment [74].

After a careful analysis of these results, it can be stated that the capsaicin-sensitive afferentation represents an essential pathway in the healing of chronic gastritis (probably with and without *H. pylori* infection or eradication). These results suggest an independent mechanism in the healing of chronic gastritis which differs from the eradication treatment. In other words, besides the *H. pylori* infection there is a new problem, namely the capsaicin-sensitive afferention is involved in either or both of the development (with and without *H. pylori* positivity) and in the healing of chronic gastritis in patients.

The *H. pylori* infection can be taken as one (but probably the most important) exogenous factor; however, the capsaicin-sensitive afferent fibres of the vagal nerve represents an endogenous factor in the damage and protection of gastric mucosa. We have gathered lot of information on the *H. pylori* infection; however, we have very little information on the capsaicin-sensitive afferent fibres of the vagal nerve. The details of these mechanisms are still unknown, especially the possible correlation between them. It seems clear, that *H. pylori* infection has no privileged role in the development of chronic gastritis. The result of our studies on gastric mucosal damage and the prevention in both animal experiments and in healthy human subjects and patients with different gastrointestinal disorders, including the chronic gastritis [42, 43-47, 100, 101] agree with Kozlowski *et al.* [102], who concluded that: 1. chronic superficial gastritis coexists with significantly higher proliferative activity of gastric mucosal glandular epithelium, particularly in relation to the prepyloric area, and 2. changes of proliferative activity of the gastric mucosal glandular epithelium are independent of age, histotopography and of *H. pylori* colonisation.

ACKNOWLEDGEMENT

None Declared.

CONFLICT OF INTEREST

The author(s) confirm that this chapter content has no conflict of interest.

REFERENCES

[1] Warren JR, Marshall BJ. Unidentified curved bacilli on gastric epitelium in active chronic gastritis. Lancet 1983; 1: 1273-75.

[2] Marshall BJ, Warren RJ. Unidentified curved bacilli in the stomach of patients with peptic ulceration. Lancet 1983; 1:1311-15.

[3] National Cancer Institue: *Helicobacter pylori* and Cancer. www.cancer.gov/cancertopics/factsheet/Risk/p-pylori-cancer 2012.04.01.

[4] Wong BCY, Ching CK, Lam SK, Li ZL, Chen BW, Li YN, Liu JB, Wang BE, Yuan SZ, Xu CP, Hou XH, Zhang AT, Zheng ZT. Differential north to south gastric cancer – duodenal ulcer gradient in China. J Gastroenterol Hepatol 1998, 13: 1050-57.

[5] Molloy RM, Sonneberg A. Relationship between gastric cancer and previous peptic ulcer disease. Gut 1997; 40: 247-52.

[6] Mabe K, Takahashi M, Oizumi H, Tsukuma H, Shibata A, Fukase K, Matsuda T, Takeda H, Kawata S. Does *Helicobacter pylori* eradication therapy for peptic ulcer prevent gastric cancer. World J Gastroenterol 2009; 14: 4290-97.

[7] Koch R. Über bakteriologische Forschung. In: Verhandlungen X. Int. Med. Congr. Verlag von August Hirscwald 1891: 35-7.

[8] Black JG. Microbiology.Principles and Applications. 3rd Edition,.Prentice Hall.Upper Saddle River, New Yersey. 1996. pp. 392-412.

[9] Tortola GJ, Funke BR, Case CL. Microbiology. 4th Edition. The Benjamin/Cumming Publishing Co., Inc. Redwood City, CA. 1995. pp. 369-73.

[10] Selye H. Syndrome produced by diverse noxious agents. Nature 1936; 138: 32-45.

[11] Voutilainen M, Juhola M, Färkkilä M, Sipponen P. Foveolar hyperplasia at the gastric cardia: prevalence and associations. J Clin Pathol 2002; 55: 352-4.

[12] Voutilainen M, Mäntynen T, Färkkilä M, Juhola M, Sipponen P. Impact of non-steroidal anti-inflammatory drug and aspirin use on the prevalence of dyspepsia and uncomplicated peptic ulcer disease. Scand J Gastroenterol 2001; 36: 817-21.

[13] Enomoto S, Watanabe M, Mukoubayashi C, *et al.* Gastric cancer risk - diagnosis and prevention in subjects with *Helicobacter pylori*-related chronic gastritis. In: Tonoto P, Ed. Gastritis and Gastric Cancer – New Insights in Gastroprotection, Diagnosis and Treatments. 2011 inTech, Rijeka, Croatia 2011, pp. 179-96.

[14] Sipponen P, Price AB. The Sydney System for classification of gastritis 20 years ago. J Gastroenterol Hepatol 2011; 26 Suppl 1: 31-4.

[15] Nagy L, Szabo S, Morales RE, Plebani M, Jenkins JM. Identification of subcellular targets and sensitive tests on ethanol-induced damage in isolated gastric mucosal cells. Gastroenterology 1994; 107: 907-14.

[16] Bauer H, Kasperek S, Pfaff E. Criteria of viabilty of liver isolated cells. Z Physiol Chem 1975; 356: 827-38.

[17] Bergmeyer HU, Bern TE. Colorimetric assay with L(+)lactase, NAD, phenazole methosulphate and INT. In: Bergmeyer HU, Ed. Methods in Enzymatic Analysis. New York, Academic Press 1972, pp. 579-82.

[18] Mosmann T. Rapid colorimetric assay for cellular growth and survival. Application to proliferation and cytotoxicity assays. J Immunol Methods 1983; 65: 55-63.

[19] Dey CS, Majumder GC. A simple quantitative method of estimation of cell-intactness based on ethidium bromide fluorescence. Biochem Int 1988; 17: 367-74.

[20] Bodis B, Karádi O, Voros S, Mozsik Gy. Has sonicated *Helicobacter pylori* any direct cellular effect? In: Bajtai A, Papp J, Racz I, Simon L, Eds. *Helicobacter pylori*. Budapest, Hungarian Society of Gastroenterology. Medicom. 1995; pp 137-42.

[21] Bódis B, Karadi O, Abdel-Salam OME, Voros S, Nagy L., Mozsik Gy. Direct cellular effect of *Helicobacter pylori* alone with co-treatment of ethanol and indomethacin in mixed isolated rats gastric mucosal cells. Dig Dis Sci 1996; 41: 430.

[22] Bodis B, Nemeth P, Mozsik Gy. Organoprotection and Cytoprotection in the Stomach. Akadémiai Kiadó, Budapest 1998.

[23] Takahashi S, Keto Y, Fujita H, Muramatsu H, Nishino T, Okabe S. Pathological changes in the formation of *Helicobacter pylori*-induced gastric lesions in Mongolian gerbils. Dig Dis Sci 1998; 43: 754-65.

[24] Krentz K. Gastric secretion in relation to gastric cancer and precancerous state. In: Semb L, Myren J, Eds. The Physiology of Gastric Secretion. Universitetsforlaget, Oslo, 1968. pp 595-604.

[25] Mozsik Gy, Venter E, Schmelczer M, Kutas J. A critical analysis of the the gastric secretory response of patients with duodenal ulcer in dependence their age and duration of complaints. Acta Medica Acad Sci Hung 1981; 38: 117-28

[26] Crena G, Rumsey P, Hogg RDE, Marscall MV. Experimental hyperplasia of the gastric mucosa. In: Semb L., Myren J., Eds. The Physiology of Gastric Secterion. Universitesforlaget, Oslo, 1968. pp 62-85.

[27] Javor T. The roles of gastric secretion, gastric emptying and blood flow supply in the development of peptic ulcer. Sc.D. Thesis, Debrecen, 1968.

[28] Fischer SR. Statistical Methods for Research Workers. Oliver and Boyed Ltd., Edinburg, UK 1958.

[29] Prinz H. Über Krebsbildung im Anastomosenring und deren Bedeutung für die Lehre von der Krebsentstehungen in Magen. Lagerbecks Arch klin Chir 1938; 191: 140-148.

[30] Peters H, Schubert HJ, Reihherschheid M. Das Carcinom im Restmagen nach Resekion wegen gutartiger Befunde. Arch klin Chir 1974; 336: 219-33.

[31] Javor T. Correlation between the acidity of the gastric juice and gastric cancer. Acta Med Acad Sci Hung 1965; 21: 159-68.

[32] Mozsik Gy. The interrelationship between the gastric secretion and gastric carcinoma. Magyar Belorvosi Archivum (Hung Med Arch) Suppl 1970, 45-52.

[33] Hardt A. Über ein primäres Ulkus-Carcinom des Duodenum. Chirurg 1961; 32: 322-330.

[34] Mozsik Gy, Javor T, Bero T, Kutas J, Palotai Z, Polyak L. Late complication of gastric surgery. In: Luohija A, Valtonen V, Eds. Internal Medicine:1976 Topics.13th International Congress of Internal Medicine., Helsinki 1976. Karger, Basel 1977, pp 200-208.

[35] Kutas J, Poka L, Laky D. Klinische Probleme des Magenstumpfkarcinoms. Bruns' Beitr. Klin Chir 1969; 217: 597-603.

[36] Szabolcs Z. Gastric Cancer. Akadémiai Kiadó, Budapest, 1966.

[37] Hansson LE, Nyrén O, Hsing AW, Bergström R, Joseffsonn S, Cwow WH, Fraumeni FF, Adam HO. The risk of stomach cancer in patients with gastric or duodenal ulcer diseseas. N Engl J Med 1996; 335: 242-49.

[38] Pober Z. An explanation of gastric hypersecretion in the pylorus-ligated rat. Arch Physiol Biochem. 1999; 107: 376-82.

[39] Mozsik G, Hunyady B, Garamszegi M, Nemeth A, Pakodi F, Vincze A. Dynamism of cytoprotective and antisecretory drugs in patients with unhealed gastric and duodenal ulcers. J Gastroenterol Hepatol 1994; 9 Suppl 1: S88-92.

[40] Szolcsanyi J. Capsaicin and neurogen inflammation history and early findins. In: Chahl LA, Szolcsanyi J, Lembeck F, Eds. Antidromic Vasodilation and Neurogenic Inflammation. Akadémiai Kiadó, Budapest 1984; pp. 27-56.

[41] Szolcsanyi J. Forty years in capsaicin research for sensory pharmacology and physiology. Neuropeptides 2004; 38: 377-84.

[42] Mozsik Gy, Vincze A, Szolcsanyi J. Four response of capsaicin-sensitive primary neurones to capsaicin and its analoque. Gastric secretion, gastric mucosal damage and protection. J Gastroenterol Hepatol 2001; 16: 193-97.

[43] Abdel Salam OME, Debreceni A, Mozsik Gy. Capsaicin-sensitive afferent sensory nerves in modulating gastric mucosal defense againts noxious agents. J Physiol Paris 1999; 93: 443-54.

[44] Mozsik Gy, Abdel-Salam OME, Szolcsanyi J. Capsaicin-Sensitive Afferent Nerves in Gastric Mucosal Damage and Protection. Akadémiai Kiadó, Budapest. 1997.

[45] Mozsik Gy, Belagyi J, Szolcsanyi J, Par G, Par A, Rumi Gy, Racz I. Capsaicin-sensitive afferent nerves and gastric mucosal protection in human healthy subjects. A critical overview. In: Takeuchi K, Mozsik Gy, Eds. Mediators in Gastrointestinal Protection and Repair. Reseach Singpost, Kerala 2004; pp. 43-62.

[46] Mozsik Gy, Szolcsanyi J, Racz I. Gastroprotection induced by capsaicin in healthy human subjects. World J Gastroenterol 2005; 11: 5180-84.

[47] Caterina MJ, Chumacher MA, Tominaga M, Rosen TA, Levine JD, Julius D. The capsaicin receptor: a heat-activated ion channel in the pain pathway. Nature 1997; 389: 816-24.

[48] Helyes Zs, Szabo A, Nemeth J, Jakab B, Pinter E, Banvolgyi A, Kereskai L, Szolcsanyi J. Anti-antifalammatory and analgetic effects of somatostatin released from capsaicin-sensitive sensory nerves terminals in a Freund's adjuvant-induced chronic arthritis model in the rats. Arthritis Rheumatism 2005; 50: 1677-85.

[49] Dömötör A, Szolcsanyi J, Mozsik Gy. Capsaicin and glucose absorption and utilization in healthy human subjects. Eur J Pharmacol 2006; 534: 280-83.

[50] Gabella G, Pease H. Number of axons in the abdominal vagus of the rat. Brain Research 1973; 52: 411-7.

[51] Grivalja CV, Novin D. The role of hypothalamus and dorsal vagal complex in the gastrointestinal gunction and pathophysiology. Ann N York Acad Sci 1990; 597: 207- 21.

[52] Mózsik Gy, Szolcsányi J, Dömötör A. Capsaicin research as a new tool to approach of the human gastrointestinal physiology, pathology and pharmacology. Inflammopharmacology 2007; 15: 232-45.

[53] Holzer P. Capsaicin cellular targets, mechanisms of action and selectivity for thin sensory neurons. Pharmacol Rev 1999; 43: 143-201.

[54] Dömötör A, Peidl Zs, Vincze Á, Hunyady B, Szolcsanyi J, Kereskai L, Szekeres Gy, Mozsik Gy. Immunohistochemical distribution of vanilloid receptor receptor, calcitonin gene-related peptide and substance P in the gastrointestinal mucosa of patients with different gastrointestinal disorders. Inflammopharmacology 2005; 13: 161-77.

[55] Bartolotti M, Coccia G, Grossi G, Miglioni M. The treatment of functional dyspepsia with red pepper. Aliment Pharmacol Ther 2002; 16: 1075-85.

[56] Bhat YM, Bielefeldt K. Capsaicin receptor (TRPV1) and non-erosive reflux disease. Eur J Gastroenterol Hepatol 2006; 18: 63-70.

[57] Hocker M, Hohenberger P. *Helicobacter pylori* virulence factors – one part of a big picture. Lancet 2003; 362: 1231-3.

[58] Logan RPH, Walker MN. Epidemiology and diagnosis of *Helicobacter pylori* infection. Brit Med J 2001; 323: 902.

[59] Parsonnet J. The incidence of *Helicobacter pylori* infection. Pharmacol Ther 1995; 2: 45-51.

[60] Peng H, Ranaldi R, Diss TC, Isaacson PG, Bearzi I, Pant L. High frequency of CagA+ *Helicobacter pylori* infection in high-grade gastric MALT B-cell lymphomas. J Pathol 1998; 185: 409-12.

[61] Pakodi F, Abdel-Salam OME, Debreceni A, Mozsik Gy. *Helicobacter pylori.* One bacterium and a broad sprectum of human disease! An overview. J Physiol Paris 2003; 94: 139-62.

[62] Mitani K, Tatsuta M, Iishi H, Yano H, Uedo N, Iseki K, Narahara H. *Helicobacter pylori* infection as a risk factor for gastric ulceration. Hepatogastroenterology 2004; 51: 309-12.

[63] Janulaite-Gunther D, Kucinskiene R, Kupcinskas L, Pavilonis A, Lbanauskas L, Cizeuskas A, Schmith U, Wadstrom T, Andersen LP. Humoral immune response to *Helicobater pylori* in children with gastrointestinal symptoms. FEMS Immunology Medical Microbiology 2005; 44: 205-12.

[64] Salih BA, Abasiyanik MF, Saribasak H, Juten O, Sander E. A follow-up study on the effect of *Helicobacter pylori* eradication on the severity of gastric histology. Dig Dis Sci 2005; 50: 1517-22.

[65] Zhang C, Yamada N, Wu YL, Wen M, Matsuhisa T, Matsukura N. Comparison of *Helicobacter pylori* infection and gastric mucosal features of gastric ulcer patients with chronic gastritis patients. World J Gastroenterol 2005; 11: 976-81.

[66] Holzer P. Neural emergency system in the stomach. Gastroenterology 1998; 114: 823-83.

[67] Holzer P, Livingston EH, Saria A, Guth P. Sensory neurones mediate protective vasodilatation in the rat gastric mucosa. Am J Physiol 1991; 260: 363-70.

[68] Dömötör A, Kereskai L, Szekeres G, Hunyady B, Szolcsanyi J, Mozsik Gy. Participation of capsaicin-sensitive afferent nerves in the gastric mucosa of patients with *Helicobacter pylori*-positve or negative chronic gastritis. Dig Dis Sci 2006; 52: 411-7.

[69] Stead RH. Innervation of mucosal immune cells in the gastrointestinal tract. 1992; 4: 91-9.

[70] Sipos G, Altdorfer K, Pongor É, Chen LP, Fehér E. Neuroimmune-link in the mucosa of chronic gastritis with Helicobater pylori infection. Dig Dis Sci 2006; 51: 1810-17.

[71] Zhang C, Yamada N, Wu YL, Wen M, Matsuhisa T, Matsukura N. *Helicobacter pylori* infection, glandular atrophy and intestinal metaplasia in superficial gastritis, erosion, erosive gastritis, gastric ulcer and early gastric cancer. World J Gastroenterol 2005; 11: 791-96.

[72] Price AB, Misiewicz JJ. Sydney classification for gastritis. Lancet. 1991; 337: 174.

[73] Malfertheiner P, Megraud F, O'Morain C, Bazzoli F, El-Omar E. Graham D, Hunt R, Rokkas T, Vakiel N, Kuipers EJ. Current concepts in the management of *Helicobacter pylori* infection. The Maastricht III. Consensus Report. Gut 2007; 56: 772-81.

[74] Lakner L, Dömötör A, Tóth Cs, Szabo IL, Mecker A, Hajos R, Kereskai L, Szekeres Gy, Döbrönte Z, Mozsik Gy. Capsaicin-sensitive afferentation represents an indifferent defensive pathway from eradication in patients with *H. pylori* gastritis. World J Gastrointest Pharmacol Ther 2011; 2: 36-41

[75] Mozsik Gy, Szabo IL, Dömötör A. Approach to role of capsaicin-sensitive afferent nerves in the development and healing in patients with chronic gastritis. In: Tonino P (ed). Gastritis and New Gastric Cancer – New Insights in Gastroprotection, Diagnosis and Treatment. 2011 Publisher by inTech. Rijeka, Croatia 2011. pp. 25-46.

[76] Gold BD, Colletti RB, Abbott M, Czinn SJ, Elitsur Y, Hassall E, Macarthur C, Snyder J, Sherman PM; North American Society for Pediatric Gastroenterology and Nutrition. *Helicobacter pylori* infection in children: recommendations for diagnosis and treatment. J Pediatr Gastroenterol Nutr 2000; 31: 490-7.

[77] Bodis B, Karadi O, Nagy L, Dohocki Cs, Kolega M, Mozsik Gy. Direct cellular effects of some mediators, hormones and growth factor-like agents on denervated (isolated) rat gastric mucosal cells. J Physiol Paris. 1997; 91: 183-87.

[78] Bodis B, Abdel-Salam OME, Karadi O, Mozsik Gy. Protective effect of prostacyclin against indomethacin on isolated gastric mucosal cells. Z Gastroenterol 1995; 33: 282.

[79] Robert A. Cytoprotection by prostaglandins. Gastroenterology 1979; 77: 761-7.

[80] Mozsik G. Gastric cytoprotection 30 years after its discovery by André Robert: a personal perspective. Inflammopharmacology 2010;18: 209-21.

[81] Mozsik G, Szabo IL, Czimmer J. Approaches to gastrointestinal cytoprotection: from isolated cells, *via* animal experiments to healthy human subjects and patients with different gastrointestinal disorders. Curr Pharm Des. 2011; 17:1556-72.

[82] Mozsik G, Jávor T, Doby S, Petrassi K, Szabó A. Development of pharmacological denervation phenomena in patients treated with atropine. Eur J Phramacol 1967; 1; 391-5.

[83] Mozsik G, Javor T. Development of drug cross- tolerance in patients treated chronically with atropine. Eur J Pharmacol 1969; 6: 169-74.

[84] Mozsik G, Berstad A, Myren J, Setekeiv. Absorption and uninary exresion of oxyphencyclimide HCl in patients before and after prolonged oxyphencyclimide treatment. Med Exp 1969; 19: 10-16.

[85] McColl KEL, El-omar E, Gillen D. Interactions between *H. pylori* infection, gastric acid secretion and antisecretory therapy. Brit Med Bull 1998; 54: 121-38.

[86] Graham DY,Yamaoka Y. *H. pylori* and cagA : relationships with gastric cancer, duodenal ulcer, and reflux esophagitis and its complications. Helicobacter 1998; 3: 145-51.

[87] Goodwin CS. *Helicobacter pylori* gastritis, peptic ulcer, and gastric cancer: clinical and molecular aspects. Clin Infect Dis 1996; 25: 1017-9.

[88] Wu CY, Kuo KN, Wu MS, Chen YJ, Wang CB, Lin JT. Early *Helicobacter pylori* eradication decreases risk of gastric cancer in patients with peptic ulcer disease. Gastroenterology 2009 137: 1641-8.

[89] Zhang Z, Zheng Q, Chen X, Xiao S, Liu W, Lu H. The *Helicobacter pylori* duodenal ulcer promoting gene, dupA in China. BCM Gastroenterology 2008; 8: 49-57.

[90] Fuccio L, Zagari RM, Minardi ME, Bazzoli F. Sytemic review: *Helicobacter pylori* eradication for the prevention of gastric cancer. Aliment Pharmacol Ther 2007; 25: 133-41.

[91] Mozsik Gy, Kutas J, Kulcsar I. Conditions after gastric surgery from the point of view of gastric carcinogenesis. In: Figus IA, Simon L, Eds. Gastric Precanceroses. Akadémiai Kiadó, Budapest, 1977. pp. 123-29.

[92] Mozsik Gy. The problems of "followup" of gastric precanceroses. In: Figus IA, Simon L, Eds. Gastric Precanceroses. Akadémiai Kiadó, 1977. pp. 231-32.

[93] Figus IA, Simon L, Eds. Gastric Precanceroses. Akadémiai Kiadó, Budapest.1977.
[94] Figus IA, Simon L, Mozsik Gy. Operated stomach as a possible precancerous state. In: Varró V, Bálint GA, Eds. Current Views in Gastroenterology. Vol. I. Hungarian Society of Gastroenterology, Budapest.1976. pp. 563-68.
[95] Mozsik G, Kutas J. Some regularities in the development of gastric stump cancer in patients partially gastrectomized for duodenal ulcer. Acta Med Acad Sci Hung. 1980; 37:67-72.
[96] Mozsik G, Debreceni A, Abdel-Salam OM, Szabo I, Figler M, Ludany A, Juricskay I, Szolcsanyi J. Small doses of capsaicin given intragastrically inhibit gastric basal acid secretion in healthy human subjects. J Physiol Paris 1999; 93: 433-6.
[97] Debreceni A, Abdel-Salam OM, Figler M, Juricskay I, Szolcsanyi J, Mozsik G. Capsaicin increases gastric emptying rate in healthy human subjects measured by ^{13}C-labeled octanoic acid breath test. J Physiol Paris 1999; 93: 455-60.
[98] Czimmer J, Szabo IL, Szolcsányi J, Mózsik G. Capsaicin-sensitive afferentation represent a new mucosal defensive neural pathway system in the gastric muxcosa in patients with chronic gastritis. In Mózsik G, ed., Current Topics in Gastritis – 2012, in Tech, Rijeka, 2013, 61-75.
[99] Mozsik G, Past T, Abdel Salam OM, Kuzma M, Perjesi P. Interdisciplinary review for correlation between the plant origin capsaicinoids, non-steroidal antiinflammatory drugs, gastrointestinal mucosal damage and prevention in animals and human beings. Inflammopharmacology. 2009; 17: 113-50.
[100] Mozsik Gy, Dömötör A, Past T, Vas V, Perjesi P, Kuzma M, Blazsik Gy, Szolcsanyi J. Capsaicinoids: from the Plant Cultivation to the Production of Human Medical Therapy. Akadémiai Kiadó, Budapest. 2009.
[101] Mozsik Gy, Past T, Dömötör A, Kuzma M, Perjesi P. Production of orally applicable new drug or drug combinations from natural origin capsaicinoids for human medical therapy. Curr Phar Des 2011; 16: 1197-208.
[102] Kozlowski W, Jochymski C, Markiewiocz T. Chronic gastritis. In: Tonino P, Ed. Gastritis and Gastric Cancer – New Insights in Gastroportection, Diagnosis and Treatment. Publisher by inTech, Rijeka, Croatia. 2011, pp 75-92.

Send Orders for Reprints to reprints@benthamscience.net
Helicobacter Pylori: A Worldwide Perspective 2014, **2014, 481-499** **481**

CHAPTER 20

Development and Current State of *Helicobacter pylori Research* in Hungary

György M. Buzás*

Division of Gastroenterology, Ferencváros Health Center Non-Profit Ltd., Budapest, Hungary

Abstract: The discovery of *H. pylori* led to a paradigm shift in the Hungarian medical community about the pathogenesis and treatment of peptic ulcer disease. *H. pylori* is the most prevalent infection also in our country. Epidemiologic studies revealed an overall prevalence of 52-63% of the infection in healthy blood donors with an age-dependent increase and no geographic differences. Endoscopic studies found a 83-92% prevalence in duodenal and 63-92% in gastric ulcer patients. All known diagnostic methods are available in Hungary: serology and endoscopic biopsy + histology are mainly used in practice, urea breath tests are reserved for eradication control. The test-and treat, search-and-treat and scope-and treat strategies are not, however, used systematically and their cost-benefit ratio has not been determined. Antimicrobial resistance testing encounters the same difficulties as in Western countries, while fluorescence *in situ* hybridisation and polymerase chain reaction-based methods are used in research centres. The first consensus meeting of the *Helicobacter pylori* Working Group of the Hungarian Society of Gastroentrerology was held in 2000 and the results updated in 2002, following the Maastricht I provisions. A meta-analysis of the Hungarian studies showed that between 1992-2002, the proton pump inhibitor- based triple therapies achieved an overall eradication rate of 82.9% (71.3-93.7%) on an intention-to-treat basis, and are the most extensively used regimens. The efficiency of second- and third-line therapies is, unfortunately, unacceptably low. Several groups of researchers participated in randomised controlled trials which were later incorporated in international guidelines. Resistance to chlarithromycin was low in the 1990's, then increased to 18% between 2005-2009 in Budapest, came it at 10% in towns around the country and remained low in rural areas. Basic research on *H. pylori* has been developed in university centres from Budapest, Pécs and Szeged and published in major journals of gastroenterology.

Keywords: *Helicobacter pylori,* epidemiology, eradication therapy, chlarithromycin resistance, extraintestinal manifestations.

INTRODUCTION AND SHORT HISTORY

Helicobacter pylori is the most prevalent infection in Hungary. The possibility of

***Address correspondence to György M. Buzás:** Division of Gastroenterology Ferencváros Health Center Non-Profit Ltd., Budapest, Hungary; Tel: +36 1 455-4571; Fax: +36-72-536-495; E-mail: drbgym@gmail.com an infectious origin of peptic ulcer disease occurred as early as 1896, when in a 5-volume textbook of internal medicine the author of the chapter on ulcer disease, citing contemporary publications, mentioned that some infections could lead to gastric ulcers [1]. However, the subject was forgotten and in the first half of the 20th century the forerunners of Hungarian gastroenterology did not mention the infectious etiology of this disease. One of the founders of modern Hungarian gastroenterology, *Géza Hetényi* (1894-1959) stated in his monograph in 1954 that the infectious theory of ulcer disease could be relevant only in the case of acute gastric mucosal lesions [2]. Knowledge about the newly discovered *Campylobacter pyloridis* entered medical thinking after some delay: although the seminal publication of *Marshall* and *Warren* [3] was referred in local medical journals, the first Hungarian paper on *Campylobacter pyloridis* was published in 1987 dealing with the histological diagnosis of the infection [4] and was followed by review articles written by leading gastroenterologists [5,6]. The first therapeutic attempt to eradicate the infection was published in 1988: the authors used either penicillin, metronidazole, cimetidine or an antacid [7]. In a bibliometric analysis of the Hungarian weekly medical journal, *Orvosi Hetilap* (published continuously since 1857), 42 original Hungarian papers on *Helicobacter pylori* were found between 1989 and 2008 [8]. Using the search terms "*Helicobacter pylori*" and "*Campylobacter pylori"* and "*Hungary"* 107 titles of national and international studies were identified according to PUBMED [9]. The first position statement concerning the diagnosis and treatment of the infection occurred in 1994. The *Helicobacter pylori Working Group* of the Hungarian Society of Gastroenterology was founded in 1996 by *István Rácz* (Petz Aladár Teaching Hospital, Győr) and organised successful sessions on the topic each year at the Annual Meetings of the Society. The 1998 meeting of the European *Helicobacter pylori* Study Group was held in Budapest and with its over 3000 participants was the second largest workshop of this organisation according to *Francis Mégraud* [10]. The first monograph about the bacterium was published in 1998 [11] and in 2000 the first Consensus Meeting was held, which largely adopted the provisions of the Maastricht I consensus [12,13] and was revised in 2002 [14]. *Helicobacter pylori* gradually became a fashionable research topic for specialists, doctoral and post-doctoral fellows and was included in PhD programs. Some of the leading gastroenterologists participated in international studies

(GU-MACH, DU-MACH, *etc.*) (see below). A meta-analysis of the Hungarian eradication trials was published in 2004 showing an overall eradication rate of 80% [15], but an increase in antimicrobial resistance rates also occurred in Hungary.

The purpose of this review chapter is to analyse the development and current state of *Helicobacter pylori*-related research and practices in Hungary, with its local peculiarities.

EPIDEMIOLOGY

The prevalence of *H. pylori* infection in the Hungarian population was studied by serology in healthy adults from different regions of the country and by endoscopy/histology in several groups of patients with dyspeptic complaints. The first relevant study was published in 1995 by *Klára Tamás*sy *et al.* in which the presence of anti-*H. pylori* IgG was tested in sera collected from a military hospital blood bank; an overall rate of seropositivity of 63.3% was found along with an age-related increase in prevalence (20-24 years: 44%, 25-29 years: 40%, 30-34 years: 52%, 35-39 years: 64%, 40-44 years: 75%, 45-49 years: 73%, 50-54 years: 77%, 55-59 years: 83%). Gender, living in urban/rural areas, type of work and level of education did not influence the prevalence of infection [16]. In a further seroepidemiologic study on 996 blood donors, seropositivity was identified in 52.3% of the cases with the same trend increasing by age [17]. The same group compared the seroprevalence of the infection in 400-400 healthy volunteers from the eastern and western parts of the country. Although the industrial and socio-economic conditions are more developed in the western part as compared to the eastern region, the overall prevalence was 60.3% in the western and 57.0% in eastern Hungary. In positive cases, the cag A seropositivity rate was 63.1% in the west and 66.6% in the east [18].

In another serologic study performed in an eastern county with 756 adults, the overall rate of anti-IgG antibodies was 58.6%, and higher in rural than in urban areas. From these *H. pylori* positives, 67.5% of the cases were anti-CagA positives too [19].

Data from the 1990s acquired by *Mégraud et al.* showed that the prevalence of the infection is lower in Hungary than in most Eastern European countries (Albania: 96.1%, Romania 90.7%, Poland 89.5%, Bulgaria 82.6%, Czech Republic 70.4%) [19]. In a newer study, young male recruits (19-23 years) in the Hungarian Army were seropositive in 23% of the cases [20].

With Hungarian recruits, the seroprevalence of *H. pylori* was found in 23% of the cases in 2004 [21].

Several groups were examined endoscopically and the prevalence of the infection in patients with dyspeptic symptoms and in healthy persons was as follows: with duodenal ulcers, *H. pylori* was present in 83-92%, with gastric ulcers in 63-92%, with chronic gastritis in 40-75%, and with healthy controls in 17-40% of the cases [22-25].

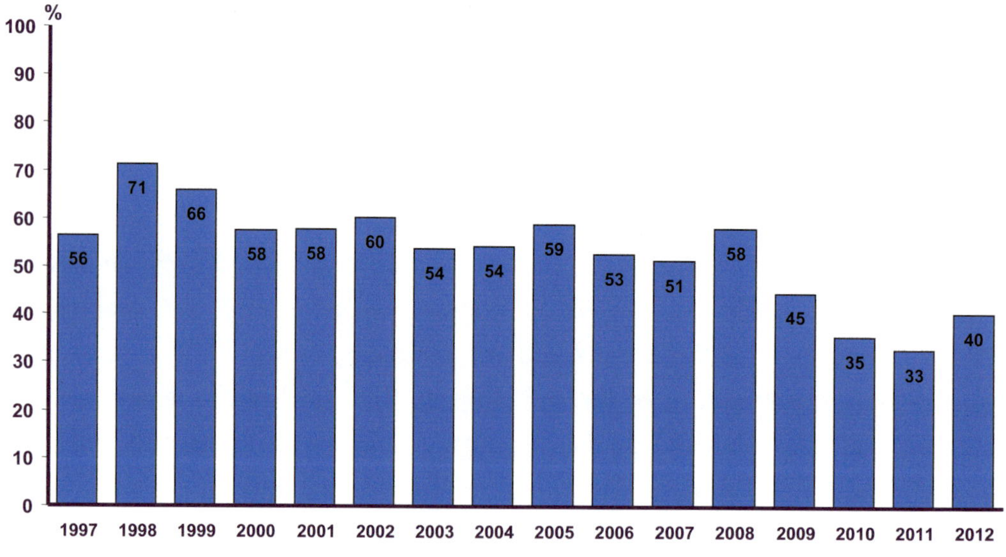

Figure 1: Prevalence of *Helicobacter pylori* infection in dyspeptic patients in Ferencváros, Budapest, according to the year of examination (1997-2012). By permission of Akadémiai Kiadó, Budapest.

Fortunately, in line with developed countries, the prevalence of infection in Hungary is decreasing. In a university centre with large endoscopic workload, the prevalence of *H. pylori* decreased from 40 % in 1995 to 19 % in 2011 [26]. In our retrospective study, in 4647 dyspeptic patients examined endoscopically, the overall prevalence was 55%, which decreased from 71.3% in 1997 to 32,7% in 2011. The mean prevalence on infection was 62.5% in the birth cohorts of 10 years, born between 1920 and 1960 and decreased significantly from the late 1960's and 1970', s process which is continuous until the 1990's (Fig. **1** and Table **1**) [27]. This proves that the birth-cohort effect is also operating in Hungarian population, emphasizing the role of environmental factors.

Table 1: The prevalence of *H. pylori* according to age decades and 10-year birth cohorts

Age (Years)	**<19**	**20-29**	**30-39**	**40-49**	**50-59**	**60-69**	**70-79**	**>80**
Prevalence %	21.8	34.9	46.5	63.7	63.2	59.2	61.8	57.6
Birth cohorts	1920-29	1930-39	1940-49	1950-59	1960-69	1970-79	1980-89	1990-94
Prevalence %	63.6	62.8	63.0	62.1	57.4.	39.0	26.7	12.2

DIAGNOSIS

A diagnosis of *Helicobacter pylori* infection is made by invasive and non-invasive tests: they are listed along with their year of introduction and actual price in Table **2**.

Table 2: Diagnostic methods of *Helicobacter pylori* infection available in Hungary

Method	**Availability**	**Cost ($)[1]**
Serology	1987	5
Upper digestive endoscopy	available[2]	25
Histology: (haematoxilin-eosin or Giemsa stain)	available	26/bioptic sample
Rapid urease tests: - commercial - house-made	1985	2-3 Few cents/probe
$^{13/14}$urea breath test	1997	35
Antimicrobial resistance testing E test FISH PCR	 available 2002 2001	 12-15 100 120
Stool monoclonal antigen	2005	5

[1)] $ = 226 Hungarian forint; [2)] methods available before *H. pylori*-era.

Diagnosing using histological methods was introduced because in the 1980s, endoscopy was the first-choice examination method for dyspeptic patients; haematoxilin-eosin and modified Giemsa stains were initially used, while

Warthin-Starry silver impregnation became familiar to pathologists later on [28]. Rapid urease tests were rapidly available either as original packs or as in-house prepared solutions: their accuracy has been tested by different authors [29,30].

Serologic methods were used extensively after the epidemiologic studies and many different kits for laboratory and in-office tests became available with variable levels of sensitivity and specificity. Although they were mainly proposed by experts for epidemiologic studies, they continue to be used extensively for diagnostic purposes by family physicians [30].

The first ^{13}C-urea breath tests were performed in 1997 and now there are sufficient mass- or infrared isotope-selective spectrometric devices to cover examinations all over the country. Breath tests are mainly used as controls after eradication treatment, and less so as a primary diagnostic tool in children, with pregnancies, extra-gastric manifestations of the infection without dyspeptic symptoms and in patients who are not willing/suitable to undergo endoscopies. The ^{13}C-urea breath test was found to be the most sensitive for detecting *H pylori* in comparison with histologies and rapid urease tests [31]. Moreover, the serial determination of UBT after successive treatments showed a tendency to increase over time in failed cases. Higher pre-treatment UBT values were associated with lower eradication rates (< 60%) [32]. This might be a local peculiarity, while the predictive value of UBT has not been confirmed by others [33].

Stool antigen determination has recently become available and its use is restricted to the county epidemiological centres.

Antimicrobial sensibility determination is available only in some centres, however, it encounters the well-known methodological difficulties related to transport and culture media, so it is seldom applied.

Polymerase chain reactions (PCR) and fluorescent *in-situ* hybridisation (FISH) were introduced in Hungary in the early 2000s: because of their limited availability and high cost they are mainly used in academic centres and research settings [34,35].

INDICATIONS OF ERADICATION THERAPY

The provisions of the Maastricht I consensus were accepted in the 2000 and 2002 consensus of the Hungarian *Helicobacter pylori Working Group*; thereafter, the Maastricht II and IV guidelines for diagnosis and treatment of the infection were adopted and spread among family physicians and gastroenterologists, although a new consensus meeting was not held. There are no particularly Hungarian indications of eradication that are distinct from the common European guidelines. The recommended first-line regimens consist of any proton pump inhibitors (PPI) in a standard dose + amoxicillin 1000 mg and either clarithromycin 500 mg bi.d. or metronidazole 4-500 mg b.i.d./t.i.d. for 7-14 days. As a second-line regimen, the bismuth-based quadruple therapy (bismuth subsalicylate 100 mg q.i.d., tetracycline 500 mg q.i.d., metronidazole 500 mg t.i.d., PPI b.i.d.) is proposed. Ranitidin bismuth citrate and colloidal bismuth subcitrate were only temporarily available; instead, unpalatable galenic bismuth formulas were used in many places. Third-line regimens or rescue treatments are not exactly defined and antimicrobial sensibility determination is seldom performed. Levofloxacin is increasingly used either in second- or third-line regimens, but other rescue drugs as furazolidone or rifabutin are not on the market. Although the "test-and treat", "scope and treat" and "search-and treat" strategies are well known to practitioners, their cost-benefit ratio under the ever-changing healthcare reimbursement system has not been examined.

Meta-Analysis of Hungarian Eradication Trials

As in most countries, the advent of eradication therapy for the infection resulted in a large variety of empiric regimens with unacceptably low and surprisingly high rates of success. After the Maastricht I consensus, however, most practitioners and gastroenterologists adhered to the standard triple regimens (see above). A meta-analysis performed in 2004 summarised the results of 42 Hungarian studies using 72 treatment arms and 31 different regimens in 3939 patients: the main results are presented in Table **3**.

PPI-based triple therapies were given extensively and achieved a pooled eradication rate on an intention-to-treat (ITT) basis of 82.9% (95% confidence limit 72.1-93.7) [15]. The results obtained in Hungary overlap with those obtained by a meta-analysis of European congress abstracts from the same period [36]. According to *Graham et al.* physicians should prescribe regimens that have a > 80% eradication rate on an ITT basis and >90%, or even better > 95% on a per-protocol (PP) basis [37]: the overall results obtained in Hungary seldom satisfy these criteria.

Table 3: Meta-analysis of Hungarian (1992-2002)[1] and European eradication trials[2] (1997-2004)

Type of Treatment	Regimen Used	Hungarian Patients No. of Cases	Pooled Eradication Rates (Mean±95% CI) %	European Patients No. of Cases	Pooled Eradication Rates (Mean±95%CI), %
First-line therapies	PPI+2AB	2265	82.9 (71.1-93.7%)	20.998	80.4 (78.9-81.8)
	RBC+2AB	289	83.6 (74.1-92.4)	2643	79.9 (75.7-84.0)
	H_2B+2AB	344	86.8 (72.7-99.8)	928	68.0 (59.0-78.1)
	Quadruple	198	82.8 (76.5-87.9)	1456	81.1 (76.6-85.6)
Second-line therapies	PPI+2AB	132	65.8 (50.7-81.1)	645	75.5 (69.9-82.0)
	RBC+2AB	125	59.8 (51.6-67.5)	1086	71.0 (62.3-79.3)
	Quadruple	416	73.8 (62.3-81.4)	417	75.5 (69.9-82.0)
Antibiotic-based analysis	PPI+C+A	3010	81.7 (72.5-92.7)	10.710	79.6 (77-8-81.4)
	PPI+C+N	1190	82.8 (72.6-92.7)	6823	84.2 (81.7-86.4)
	PPI+A+C	1659	69.4 (60.1-78.7)	2547	72.5 (66.6-78.5)

Notes: [1]Based on Hungarian full papers and congress abstracts, [2]Based on abstracts published at European Helicobacter Study Group meetings, United European Gastroenterology Week and Digestive Disease Week; CI= confidence interval, PPI: proton pump inhibitors, AB: antibiotics, RBC: ranitidin bistmuth citrate, H2B: histamine H_2 receptor blockers; quadruple regimen: PPI +colloidal bismuth subcitrate/bismuth subsalicylate + tetracyclin + metronidazole; C=clarithromycin, A=amoxicillin, N=nitroimidazole.

Ranitidin bismuth citrate-based triple therapies achieved comparable results with the standard triple therapies. Surprisingly, H_2-blocker-based triple regimens given for 10-14 days obtained better results than PPI-based triple combinations, however, the studies were open and date from the pre-Maastricht years.

Studies from the same period showed that PPI or RBC-based double combinations obtained a success rate of (78.1 %CI: 62.3-93.9) and 80.3 % (CI: 76.0-84.6).

Second-line standard triple therapies were efficient only in 65.8% (CI: 50-7-81.1) of the cases. There is a single prospective study on the third-line therapy, in which 2 quadruple regimens (pantoprazole, amoxicillin, tetracyclin and either nitrofurantoin or bismuth subsalicylate were given, obtaining eradication in 61.9 and 55.0% on an ITT and 65.01 and 70.6%, respectively, on a PP basis [38]. In a retrospective study of 1027 patients, assessed by urea breath test, a disappointingly low rate of eradication after second (36%) and third line therapies (20%) was found [39].

Antibiotic-based analysis showed that either PPI + clarithromycin+amoxicillin or clarithromycin + nitrodimidazole combinations achieved >80% eradication rates in Hungary, while amoxicillin-nitroimidazole combinations were less efficient (69.4%). Use of tinidazole achieved by 10% higher eradication rates than metronidazole, being thus the preferable nitroimidazole for eradication [15].

Several controlled studies from different geographical regions suggest that the efficiency of standard triple therapies decreased in the past decadc: while this is true for North America, some European and Eastern-Asia countries, in other countries such as Spain, the effectiveness of standard triple therapy has not been decreased between 1997 and 2008, being of 80% (CI:72-82%) on an ITT and 83% (CI: 81-86%) in PP basis [40]. In our retrospective study, we showed that between 2000 and 2010 the eradication rates obtained with standard triple regimens in 512 duodenal ulcer and functional dyspepsia patients undergo rather seasonal variations than a continuous decrease: the eradication rates peaked in winter and in summer and were lowest in the spring and autumn (Figs. **2** and **3**).The reasons of these circannual fluctuations are unknown [41].

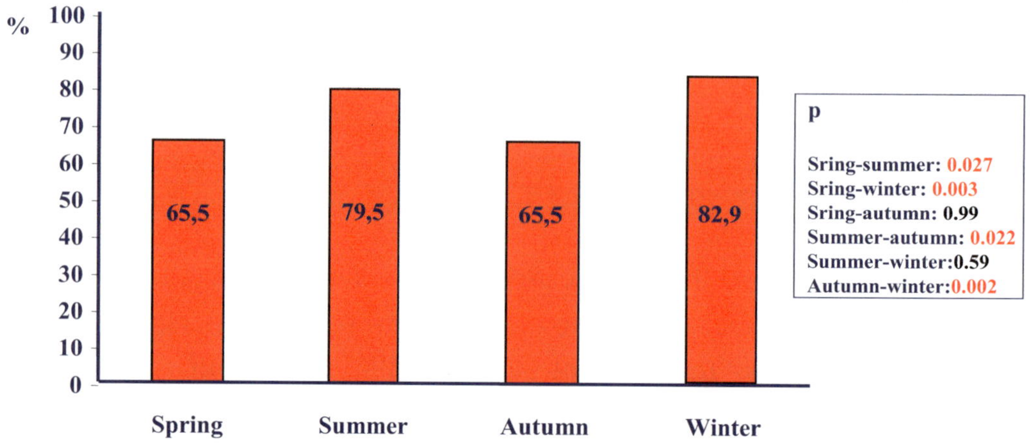

Figure 2: Seasonal variations of the eradication rates obtained with standard triple regimens in duodenal ulcer and functional dyspepsia patients between 2000-2010 (by permission of the Akadémiai Kiadó, Budapest)

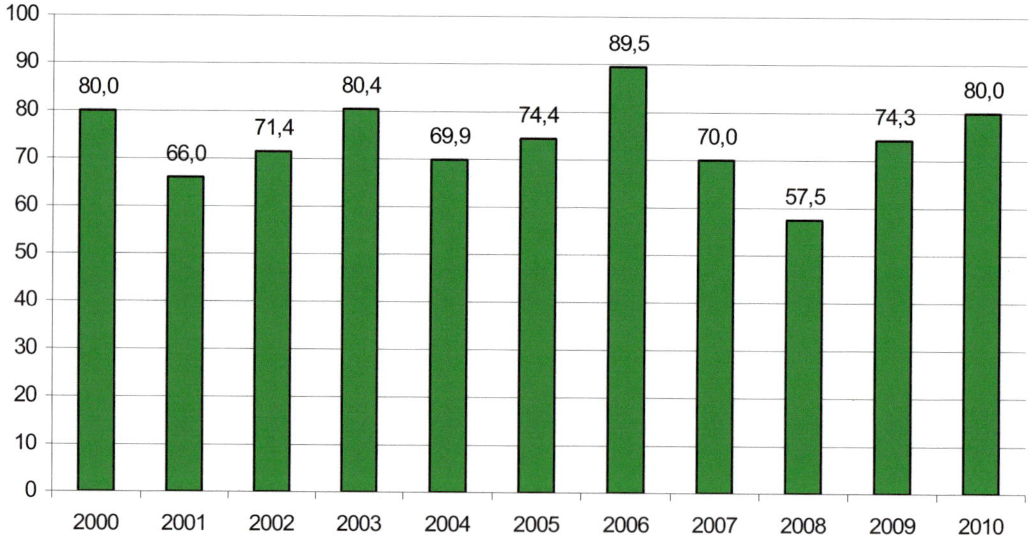

Figure 3: Overall eradication rates of *H. pylori* with standard triple regimens between 2000-2010 (by permission of the Akadémiai Kiadó, Budapest)

International Studies

Leaders of the Hungarian *H. pylori* research participated in international multicentre and randomised controlled trials, thus contributing to the evidence-based data which was subsequently cited on a regular basis and incorporated into consensus statements. The main results are summarised in Table **4** [42-48].

Table 4: Randomised controlled trials performed with Hungarian participation for *H. pylori* eradication

Ref.No.	Year	Hungarian Author and Institute	No. of Cases	Eradication Regimen + Duration and Follo-Wup	Results	Comments
42	1998	Tulassay I, 2nd Medical Clinic, Budapest	143/142 cases with past/present ulcer	OAC *vs* O+placebo ± for 7 days+ NSAIDs	Probability of being ulcer free at 6 months: 0.56 (0.44-0.62) *vs* 0.53 (0.44-0.62)	*H. pylori* eradication in long-term NSAID-users with ulcer led to impaired gastric ulcer healing
43	1999	Ujszászy, L., County Hospital Miskolc (GU-MACH study)	160 gastric ulcer cases	OAC *vs* OMC for 7 days	ITT: OAC: 79% (65-90%), OMC: 86% (73-94%); PP: OAC: 93% (68-93%), OMC: 93% (80-98%)	1-week OAC and OMC regimens are effective and safe for eradication of *H. pylori* in gastric ulcer patients
42	1999	Lonovics, J., Ist Medical Clinic, Szeged; Domján, L., County Hospital Kecskemét, Pap, Á., Szent Imre Hospital, Budapest	255 duodenal ulcer patients	OAM b.i.d. *vs* OAM t.i.d. for 7 days + O for 3 weeks endoscopic follow-up	ITT: OAM b.i.d.: 77% (69-85%), OAM t.i.d.: 76% (67-83%); PP: OAM b.i.d.: 81% (73-89%), OAM t.i.d.: 83% (75-91%). Ulcer healing: OAM b.i.d.: 95%, OAM t.i.d.: 97%	OAM given b.i.d. or t.i.d. achieve rates of > 80% in *H. pylori* eradication and healing of duodenal ulcer in 95-97% of the cases. The daily doses (b.i.d. *vs* t.i.d.) do not seem critical with OAM regimen.
45	1999	Rácz, I., Petz Aladár Teaching Hospital, Győr	278 functional dyspepsia patients	OAC *vs* placebo for 7 days + symptoms follow-up for 1 year	OAC: 85% (77-97%), Placebo: 4% (2-7%)	Successful eradication does not relieved dyspeptic symptoms 12 months after treatment
46	2001	Tulassay, Z	222/224 duodenal ulcer patients	EAC+ placebo *vs* OAC + O for 7 days + 3 weeks	ITT: EAC: 86% (81-90%), OAC: 88% (83-92%); PP: EAC: 89% (84-93%), OAC: 90%	EAC and OAC triple regimens is efficient in eradication and duodenal ulcer healing

Table 3: contd...

					(85-93%). Ulcer healing: EAC: 91% (8795%), OAC: 92% (88-95%)	
47		Tulassay Z, 2nd Medical Clinic, Budapest, Nagy,P., County Hospital, Miskolc	401 *H. pylori* positive gastric ulcer patients	EAC for 7 days +placebo for 3 weeks EAC+E for 3 weeks E+placebo antimicrobials 7 days + E for 3 weeks	ITT:EAC+E: 82% (74-90%) EAC + placebo E: 77% (65-79%) E + placebo antimicrobials +E: 9,5% (6,6-12,4%)	E-based triple therapy is effective for eradication of *H. pylori*, healing and prevention of gastric ulcer relapses.
48	2010	Tulassay Z	401 gastric ulcer patients	EAC for 7 days + placebo for 3 weeks vs EAC for 7 days+ E for 3 weeks, endoscopic and histologic follow-up	ITT: EAC + placedo: 80% (71-91%), EAC +E: 82% (73-92%)	Endoscopic/histologic abnormalities are common in gastric ulcer partients and persist after successful eradication, requiring follow-up to detect gastric malignancy

Notes: O=omeprazol, A=amoxicillin, C=claerithromycion, M=metzronidazole,. E=esomeprazole, ITT: inmtentiuon-totreat,. PP: per protocol.

Chlarithromycin Resistance

Antimicrobial resistance is the main, but not the only culprit for the lower eradication rates obtained in some, but not all studies from the past decade. Meta-analyses showed that macrolide resistance reduced there success rate of standard triple regimens by 20-55%, and nitroimidazole resistance by 25-50% [49,50]. Low compliance rate, the CYP2C19, cagA and dupA status could all influence the success of eradication. Early determinations of macrolid resistance in Hungary performed in the 1990's by E-test revealed values of 3,9 % [11,51]. With the advent of FISH, a study done in a central district of Budapest between 2005 and 2009 included 454 patients and found a mean primary clarithromycin resistance in 18% of the cases, showing yearly fluctuations, without tendency to increase (Table **5**).

Table 5: Prevalence of primary clarithromycin resistance between 2005 and 2009 in Ferencváros, Budapest, Hungary

Year	No. of Cases	C-Sensitive (%)	C-Resistant (Total) (%)	Complete Resistance (%)	Partial Resistance (%)
2005	28	78.5	**21.4**	33.3	66.6
2006	241	82.8	**16.1**	43.6	60.0
2007	46	78.3	**21.7**	60.0	40.0
2008	57	77.2	**22.8**	46.1	53.8
2009	81	82.7	**17.3**	28.5	71.4
Total	**454**	**81.9**	**18.1**	**42.7**	**57.3**

Secondary resistance was observed in 55% of the cases. Resistance was complete in 42.7% and partial (incomplete) in 57.3% of the cases. It is not known whether or not complete or incomplete resistance influences the outcome of eradication in the same way. In an another study from 2010, however, the clarithromycin resistance rate as determined by FISH was 10.9% in county cities and only 1.9% in rural media [52]. It seems that clarithromycin resistance in Hungary followed the general increasing tendency seen in Western countries only in the 1990's, reaching a plateau in the 2000's. There is a gradient between the urban and rural areas, probably reflecting the access to medical facilities and differences in use of macrolides.

Extraintestinal Manifestations

The provisions of the Maastricht consensuses regarding eradication in extraintestinal manifestations of *H. pylori* infection are followed, while treatment is offered to patients having unexplained iron deficiency anaemia and idiopathic thrombocytopenic purpura. The Hungarian contributions are worth mentioning. In cases with hereditary angioedema, it was shown that successful eradication led to a decrease in the intensity and frequency of abdominal symptoms and oedema [53,54]. In another multicentre study, an increased prevalence of anti-*H. pylori* IgA and IgG was found in Henoch-Schönlein purpura patients and the authors concluded that the infection may be associated with the development and progression of this autoimmune disease [55].

Basic Research

Beside implementing the diagnostic methods and eradication regimens in practice, as recommended by the national and Maastricht consensus meetings, several research teams were organized in academic centres which performed basic research either alone or with international co-operation. A research group lead by *Zsolt Tulassay* at the 2nd Medical Clinic of the Semmelweis University, Budapest has been involved in genetic and immunologic research, introducing the PCR-based methods from 2001 [34]. By determining cagA ands vacA genotypes and epidermal growth factor receptor (EGFR) expression, they showed that in cagA positive patients, the proliferation of mucosal cells and EGFR expression is augmented as compared to cagA-negative cases. Furthermore, it was shown that in the absence of intestinal metaplasia, *H. pylori* increases apoptotic activity ands p53 expression in the gastric mucosa [56]. The synthesis of secretory leukocyte protease inhibitor is downregulated in the antral mucosa by *H. pylori,* thus decreasing the antimicrobial and anti-inflammatory capacity of the mucosa [57].

The research group from Szeged university, showed that genetic polymorphism of interleukin 8 (IL-8) influences the occurrence of duodenal ulcer: the IL-8 A/T heterozygote mutant form seems to promote, the normal allelic genotype (TT) offer a relative protection from duodenal ulcer [58]. NOD1 and interleukin 8 (IL-8), but not that of toll-like receptor 4 (TLR4) is also associated with increased risk of chronic gastritis and duodenal ulcer [59]. Polymorphism of the IL-8 gene in patients with chronic gastritis, gastric atrophy and intestinal metaplasia was related to occurrence of premalignant histologic changes and macroscopic gastric erosions [60]. Finally, it was shown that mutations of the p53 gene reduce the risk of intestinal metaplasia in *H. pylori* positive patients as compared to normal controls: the genetic background of this is reflected by the expression of p53 protein, involved in gastric carcinogenesis [61].

The Szeged group demonstrated that *H. pylori* induced the release of alpha-defensin from mucosal granulocytes which may be of importance in the local host response to the infection [62].

A group lead by *Gyula Mózsik* from the 1st Medical Clinic, University Pécs, investigated the role of capsaicin-sensitive afferent nerves in chronic gastritis and found, that immunostaining for capsaicin receptor, substance P and calcitonin gene-related peptide is modified in chronic gastritis, changes which are not reversed at 6 weeks after successful eradication. The authors concluded that *H. pylori* infection might not represent a central pathogenetic factor in the development of chronic gastritis [63].

All these studies suggest that the more and more sophisticated genetic and immunologic methods could reveal new aspects of the pathogenesis of chronic gastritis, peptic ulcer and gastric cancer: some of these methods might be of diagnostic importance in the future [64].

ACKNOWLEDGEMENTS

The secretarial assistance of Mrs. Jolán Józan (Semmelweis University, Department of Physiology, Budapest) and correction of the English manuscript of the preface and other chapters by Mr. Douglas Arnott (EDMF Language Services Ltd., Budapest, Hungary) is highly acknowledged.

CONFLICT OF INTEREST

The author(s) confirm that this chapter content has no conflict of interest.

REFERENCES

[1] Hirschler Á. 1896. Peptikus gyomorfekély, in: A belgyógyászat kézikönyve (Peptic gastric ulcer, in: Handbook of Internal Medicine), Bókay A., Kétli, K., Korányi, F. Magyar Orvosi Könyvkiadó Társulat, Budapest, vol 3, pp 271-273. (Hungarian)

[2] Hetényi G. A fekélybetegség aktuális kérdései (Actual questions of ulcer disease), Academic Publishing House, Budapest,1954, pp 31-2.(Hungarian)

[3] Marshall BJ, Warren JR Unidentified curved bacilli in the stomach of patients with gastritis and peptic ulceration. Lancet 1984; 1:1311-15.

[4] Csiszár K, Gyepes P, Bujalka R. Detection of *Campylobacter pyloridis* from gastric biopsies) Orv. Hetil 1987; 28: 1419-21. (Hungarian)

[5] Simon L A fekélybetegség gyógyszeres kezelése: az utolsó öt év eredményei. (Medical treatment of ulcer disease: results of the past 5 years). Gyógyszereink 1990; 40: 65-782. (Hungarian)

[6] Varró V. Fekélybetegség. Tények és gondolatok. (Ulcer disease. Facts and thoughts). Lege Artis Medicinae 1996;6: 527-532. (Hungarian)

[7] Erdei A, Győri I, Kazsuba A.: Antibakteriális kezelés *Campylobacter pylori* pozitiv gastroduodenalis kórképekben.(Antibacterial treatment in *Campylobacter pylori* positive gastroduodenal diseases) Magyar Belorv. Arch. 1988; 41: 167-73. (Hungarian)

[8] Buzás GM 2009. The role of *Orvosi Hetilap* in the development of contemporary Hungarian gastroenterology. Part 4: 1989-2008.Orv Hetil, 2009; 150: 703-709. (Hungarian)

[9] http://www.pubmed.com., accessed on June 8, 2013.

[10] Mégraud F. Evolution of *Helicobacter pylori* research as observed through the workshops of the European Helicobacter Study Group. *Helicobacter* 1997;12: Suppl.2: 1-5.

[11] Buzás GM. 1998. *Helicobacter pylori*. Medicina Publishing House, Budapest, pp. 9-17, and 35-52. (Hungarian)

[12] Rácz I, Bajtai A, Lonovics J, Simon L. Consensus Meeting of the *Helicobacter pylori Working Group* of the Hungarian Society of Gastroenterology. Medicom, Budapest, 2000.

[13] European *Helicobacter pylori* Study Group. Current European concepts in the management of *Helicobacter pylori* infection. The Maastricht Consensus Report. Gut 1997; 41: 8-13.

[14] Rácz I, Bajtai A, Lonovics J, Simon L. Tulassay Z. Current problems of the *Helicobacter pylori* infection. Eur J Gastroenterol Hepatol (Hungarian edition) 2002; 7: 215-220.

[15] Buzás GM Eradication of *Helicobacter pylori* infection in Hungary, 1993-2002). Orv Hetil 2003; 144: 1077-83. (Hungarian)

[16] Tamássy K, Simon L Mégraud F. Epidemiology of *Helicobacter pylori* infection in Hungary (comparative seroepidemiologic study). Orv Hetil 1995;136: 1387-91.

[17] Lakner L, Jáger R, Toldy E, Sarang K, Varga L, Kovács GL, Döbrönte Z. Seroepidemiology of *Helicobacter pylori* infection in Western Hungary. Z. Gastroenterol. 1999; 128: A136

[18] Lakner L, Iszlai É, Toldy E, Jáger R, Döbrönte Z. Comparing *Helicobacter pylori* sero-prevalence in West- and East Hungary. Z. Gastroenterol. 2002; 40: A126

[19] Iszlai E, Kiss E, Toldy E, Ágoston S, Sipos B, Vén L, Rácz F, Szerafin L. Seroprevalence of *Helicobacter pylori* infection and anti-cagA positivity in the county of Szabolcs-Szatmár Bereg. Orv Hetil 2003; 144: 1713-1718. (Hungarian)

[20] Mégraud F, Bouchard L, Drugmand D.. Seroprevalence of *H. pylori* infection in six countries in Eastern Europe using a common methodology. Gut 1995; 37: Supplement 1, A283.

[21] Fűrész J, Lakatos S, Németh K, Fritz PO, Simon L, Kacserka K.. The prevalence and incidence of *Helicobacter pylori* infections among young recruits during service in the Hugarian Army. Helicobacter 2004; 9: 77-80.

[22] Döbrönte Z, Lakatos F, Brittig F, Löcsei Z, Bokor N, Stöckert A, Varga L. Has *Campylobacter pylori* infection any clinical relevance? Methodologic, epidemiologic and clinical study. Orv Hetil 1989; 130: 2563-68.

[23] Simon, L., Tornóczky, Z., Tóth, B, Jámbor M, Sugár, Z. The significance of Campylobacter *pylori* in gastroenterologic and diabetic practice. Orv Hetil 130: 1325-29. (Hungarian)

[24] Herszényi L, Zalatnai A, Schaff Zs, Lengyel G, Tóth J, Dank M., Fehér J, Szalay L.: Chronic gastritis and the presence of *Helicobacter pylori* in patients with non-ulcerative dyspepsia. Orv Hetil 1991; 132: 1915-19. (Hungarian)

[25] Joós Á, Németh A, Zsolnay G, Kővári E, Papp, J. *Helicobacter pylori* in benign gastroduodenal diseases. Orv Hetil 1995;136: 709-13.

[26] Varga, M., Bittera, B., Láng, J. *et al.* Significant decrease in prevalence of *Helicobacter pylori* and peptic ulcer disease over a 17-year period. Z Gastroenterol 2012, 50, 386, A84 (abstract)

[27] Buzás, G.M., Lotz, G, Schneider F., Józan J.: A *Helicobacter pylori* –fertőzés epidemiológiája Ferencvárosban.. Orv Hetil 2013, 154, 899-906 (Hungarian)

[28] Cserni, L., Serényi, P., Domján, L, Lehoczki N. Detection of *Helicobacter pylori* in biopsy specimens. Methodological studies. Orv Hetil 1995; 136: 2225-30. (Hungarian)

[29] Buzás GyM, Győrffy H, Illyés Gy, Széles I. 2000. Performance of Controloc rapid urease test in the pre-treatment diagnosis of *Helicobacter pylori* infection. Gut 2000; 3: Suppl.1, A126.

[30] Juhász M, Prónai L, Zágoni T, Németh A, Herszényi L, Schandl, Tulassay Z.. Comparison of various methods in the detection of *Helicobacter pylori* infection. Orv Hetil 2000; 141: 911-14.

[31] Sütő G, Vincze Á, Pákodi F, Hunyadi B, Karádi O, Garamszegi M, László T, Mózsik Gy. ^{13}C-urea breath test is superior in sensitivty to detect *Helicobacter pylori* infection than either antral histology or rapid urease test. J. Physiol. Paris 2000; 94: 153-6.

[32] Buzás GM, Széles I. Interpretation of the 13C-urea breath test in the choice of second- and third-line eradication of *Helicobacter pylori* infection. J Gastroenterol 2008; 43: 108-14.

[33] De Francesco, VB., Zullo, A., Perna, F., Giorgio, F., Hassan, C., Vanella, L., Cristofari, F., Panelèla, C., Vaira, D,l Ierardi, E. *Helicobacter pylori* antibiotic resistance and 13C urea breath test values. J Med Microbiol 2010; 59: 588-91.

[34] Ruzsovics A, Molnár B, Unger Z, Tulassay Z, Prónai L. Determination of *Helicobacter pylori* cagAS, vacA genotypes with real-time PCR melting curve analysis. J Physiol Paris 2001;95: 369-377.

[35] Buzás GM, Lotz G, Kiss A.. The epidemiology of clarithromycin resistance of *Helicobacter pylori* infection in Hungary. Orv Hetil 2007; 148: 1461-67. (Hungarian)

[36] Buzás GM, Józan J. First-line eradication of *H. pylori* infection in Europe: a meta-analysis based on congress abstracts, 1997-21004. World J Gastroenterol. 2006;12: 5311-19

[37] Rimbara E, Fischbach LA, Graham DY Optimal therapy for *Helicobacter pylori* infections. *Nat Rev Gastroenterol Hepatol* 2011; 8: 79-88.

[38] Buzás GM, Győrffy H, Széles I, Szentmihályi A. Second-line and third-line trial for *Helicobacter pylori* infection in patients with duodenal ulcers: a prospective, crossover, controlled study. Curr. Therap Res 2004; 65: 13-25.

[39] Prónai L, Tulassay Z. Failure of *Helicobacter* eradication: suggestions for further therapy. Orv Hetil 2003; 144: 1299-1302. (Hungarian)

[40] Gisbert JP, Calvet X. Review article: the effectiveness of standard triple therapy for *Helicobacter pylori* has not been changed over the last decade, but t is not good enough. Aliment Pharmacol Ther 2011; 34: 1255-1568.

[41] Buzás GM, Józan J, Visnay B, Nagy J, Szilágyi É. Seasonal variation of *H. pylori* eradication rates with standard triple therapies: a 10-year retrospective study. Helicobacter 2010: 15: 340, P2.07 (abstract)

[42] Hawkey CJ, Tulassay Z, Szcepanski L, van Rensburg CJ, Filipowicz-Sosnowska A, Lanas A, Watson CM, Peacock RA, and Gillon KR Randomized controlled trial of *Helicobacter pylori* eradication in patients on non.steroidal anti-inflammatory drugs: HELP-NSAID study. *Lancet*, 1998;1: 352-58.

[43] Malfertheiner P, Bayerdörffer E, Diete U, Gil L, Lind T, Misiuna P, O'Morain C, Sipponen P, Spiller RC, Stasiewicz J, Treichel H, Újszászy L, Unge P, Zanten SJV, Zeijlon L. The GU-MACH study: the effect of 1-week omeprazole triple therapy on *Helicobacter pylori* infection in patients with gastric ulcers., Aliment Pharmacol Ther 1999; 13: 703-13.

[44] Bayerdörffer E, Lonovics J, Dité P, Diete U, Domján L, Kisfalvi I, Mégraud F, Pap Á, Sipponen P, Burman CF, Zeijlon L. Efficacy of two different dosage regimens of omeprazole, amoxycillin and metronidazole for cure of *Helicobacter pylori* infection., Aliment Pharmacol Ther.1999; 13: 1639-45.

[45] Talley NJ, Janssen J, Lauritsen K, Rácz I, Boling-Sternerwald E. Eradication of *Helicobacter pylori* in functional dyspepsia: randomised double blind placebo controlled trial with 12 months follow up. The Optimal Regimen Cures *Helicobacter* Induced Dyspepsia (ORCHID) Study Group. Brit Med J 1999; 318: 833-838.

[46] Tulassay Z, Kryszewski A, Dite P, Kleczkowski D, Rudzinski J, Bartuzi Z, Hasselgren, G, Larkö A, Wrangstadh, H. One week treatmnent with esomepraszole-based triple therapy eradicates *Helicobacter pylori* and heals patients with duodenal ulcer disease. Eur J Gastroenterol Hepatol 2001; 13: 1457-65.

[47] Tulassay Z, Stolte M, Slöjund M. Effect of esomperazole triple therapy on eradication rates of *Helicobacter pylori*, gastric ulcer healing and prevention of relapse in gastric ulcer patients. Eur J Gastroenterol Hepatol 2008; 20: 526-36

[48] Tulassay Z, Stolte M, Engstrand L, Butruk E, Malfertheiner P, Dité P, Tchernev K, Wong BC, Gottlow M, Eklund S, Wrangstadh M, Herszényi L, Nagy P, and The Helix Study Investigators. Twelve-month endoscopic and histological analysis following proton-pump inhibitor-based triple therapy in *Helicobacter pylori*-positive patients with gastric ulcers. Scand J Gastroenterol. 2010; 45: 1048-58.

[49] Fischbach L. and Evans EL. Meta-analysis: the effect of antibiotic resistance status on the efficacy of triple and quadruple first-line therapies for *Helicobacter pylori.* Aliment Pharmacol Ther 2007; 26: 343-57.

[50] De Francesco V, Giorgio F, Hassan C, Manes G, Vanella L, Panella C, Ierardi E, and Zullo A. Worldwide *H. pylori* antibiotic resisatance: a systematic review. J Gastrointestin Liver Dis 2010; 19: 409-14.

[51] Buzás G.M. *Helicobacter pylori* – 2010. Orv Hetil 2010 151: 2003-10. (Hungarian)

[52] Tiszai A. Sükösd F, Lénárt Z, Bálint L, Kiss Z, Rosztoczy A, Garamszegi M, Váry A, Fricz P, Rácz I, Wittmann T. Primary resistance of *Helicobacter pylori* to chlarithromycin in different regions of Hungary. Z Gastroenterol 2010; 58: 619 (abstract)

[53] Farkas H, Füst G, Fekete B, Karádi I Varga L. Eradication of *Helicobacter pylori* and improvement of hereditary angioneurotic oedema. Lancet 2001; 358: 1695-96.

[54] Visy B, Füst G, Bygumn A, Bork K, Longhzuirst H, Bucher C, Boillet L, Cicardi M, Farkas H. *Helicobacter pylori* infection as a triggering factor of attacks in patients with hereditary angioedema, Helicobacter 2007; 12: 251-57.

[55] Novák J, Szekanecz Z, Sebes, J, Takáts A, Demeter P, Bene L, Sipka S, and Csiki Z. Elevated levels of anti-*Helicobacter pylori* antibodies in Henoch-Schönlein purpura. Autoimmunity 2003; 36: 307-11.

[56] Unger Z, Molnár B, Prónai L, Szaleczky E, Zágoni T, and Tulassay Z. 2003. Mutant p53 expression and apoptotic activity of *Helicobacter pylori* positive and negative gastritis in correlation with the presence of intestinal metaplasia. Eur J Gastroenterol Hepatol 2003; 15: 389-93.

[57] Hritz I. Kuester D, Vieth M, Herszényi L, Stolte M, Roessner A, Tulassay Z, Wex T and Malfertheiner P. Secretory leukocyte protease inhibitor expression in various types of gastritis: a specific role of *Helicobacter pylori* infection. Eur J Gastroenterol Hepatol 2006; 18: 277-82.

[58] Gyulai Zs, Klausz G, Tiszai A, Lénárt Zs, Kása IT, Lonovics J, and Mándi Y. Genetic polymorphism of interleukin-8 (IL-8) is associated with *Helicobacter pylori*-induced duodenal ulcer. Eur Cytokine Netw 2004; 15: 353-58.

[59] Hofner P, Gyulai Z, Kiss ZF, Tiszai A, Tiszlavicz L, Tóth G, Szőke D, Molnár B, Lonovics J, Tulassay Z, Mándi Y. Genetic polymorphisms of NOD1 and IL-8, but not polymorphisms of TLR4 genes are associated with *Helicobacter pylori*-induced duodenal ulcer and gastritis. Helicobacter 2007; 12: 124-31.

[60] Szőke D, Molnár B, Solymossi N, Klausz G, Gyulai Z, Tóth M, Mándi Y, Tulassay Z.. T252A polymorphism of IL-8 relating to the development of histological gastritis and G-308A polymorphism of TNF-alpha realting to the development of macroscopic erosion. Eur J Gastroenterol Hepatol 2008; 20: 191-95.

[61] Szőke D, Molnár B, Solymosi N, Sipos F, Galamb O, Győrffy A, Tulassay Z. The RR genotype of codon 72 of p53 gene reduces the development of intestinal mucosa. Dig Liver Dis 2009; 41: 179-84.

[62] Kocsis AK, Ocsovszky I, Tiszlavicz L, Tiszlavicz Z, Mándi Y. *Helicobacter pylori* induces the release of alpha-defensin by human granulocytes. Inflamm Res 2009; 58: 241-47.

[63] Lakner L, Dömötör A, Tóth C, Szabó IL, Meczker A, Hajós R, Kereskai L, Szekeres G, Döbrönte Z.and Mózsik Gy. Capsaicin-sensitive afferentation represents an indifferernt defensive pathway from eradication in patients with *H. pylori* gastritis. World J Gastrointest Pharmacol Ther 2011; 2: 36-41.

[64] Molnár B, Galamb O, Sipos F, Leiszter K, Tulassay Z. Molecular pathogenesis of *Helicobacter pylori* infection: the role of bacterial virulence factors. Dig Dis 2010; 128: 604-8.

Author Index

Subject Index

A

B

C

D

E

F

G

H

I

K

L

M

N

Q

R

S

T

U

V

Z

Made in the USA
Las Vegas, NV
04 November 2026

57436058R00314